Quick Find Guide

Foundations of Periodontics for the Dental Hygienist

FOURTH EDITION

Jill S. Gehrig, RDH, MA

Dean Emeritus, Division of Allied Health & Public Service Education
Asheville-Buncombe Technical Community College
Asheville, North Carolina

Donald E. Willmann, DDS, MS

Professor Emeritus, Department of Periodontics
University of Texas Health Science Center at San Antonio
San Antonio, Texas

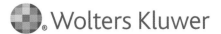. Wolters Kluwer

Philadelphia • Baltimore • New York • London
Buenos Aires • Hong Kong • Sydney • Tokyo

Senior Acquisitions Editor: Jonathan Joyce
Product Development Editor: John Larkin
Production Project Manager: David Saltzberg
Design Coordinator: Steve Druding
Marketing Manager: Leah Thompson
Manufacturing Coordinator: Margie Orzech
Prepress Vendor: Aptara, Inc.

4th Edition

Library of Congress Cataloging-in-Publication Data
Gehrig, Jill S. (Jill Shiffer), author.
  Foundations of periodontics for the dental hygienist/Jill S. Gehrig,
Donald E. Willmann. – Fourth edition.
       p. ; cm.
  Includes bibliographical references and index.
  ISBN 978-1-4511-9415-9
  I. Willmann, Donald E., author. II. Title.
  [DNLM: 1. Periodontics. 2. Dental Hygienists. 3. Periodontal
Diseases–therapy. WU 240]
  RK361
  617.6'32–dc23
                                    2015006097

Liability Statement

This textbook endeavors to present an evidence-based discussion of periodontology based on information from recent research. Periodontology, however, is a rapidly changing science. The authors, editors, and publisher have made every effort to confirm the accuracy of the information presented and to describe generally accepted practices at the time of publication. However, as new information becomes available, changes in treatment may become necessary. The reader is encouraged to keep up with dental and medical research through the many peer-reviewed journals available to verify information found here and to determine the best treatment for each individual patient. The authors, contributors, editors, and publisher are not responsible for errors or omissions or for any consequences from application of the information in this book and make no warranty, express or implied, with respect to the contents of this publication.

Contributors

Ralph M. Arnold, DDS
Associate Professor, Retired
Department of Periodontics
University of Texas Health Science
    Center at San Antonio
San Antonio, Texas

Ann M. Bruhn, BSDH, MS
Assistant Professor and Continuing
    Education Coordinator
School of Dental Hygiene
Old Dominion University
Norfolk, Virginia

Elizabeth Carr, RDH, MDH
Assistant Professor of Dental Hygiene
University of Mississippi Medical
    Center
Jackson, Mississippi

Delwyn Catley, PhD
Professor of Psychology and Dentistry
Director of Health Behavior
    Change Laboratory
Department of Psychology
University of Missouri – Kansas City
Kansas City, Missouri

Charles Cobb, DDS, MS, PhD
Professor Emeritus
Department of Periodontics
School of Dentistry
University of Missouri – Kansas City
Kansas City, Missouri

Teresa Butler Duncan, RDH, MDH
Assistant Professor
Department of Dental Hygiene
School of Health Related Professions
University of Mississippi Medical
    Center
Jackson, Mississippi

Pinar Emecen-Huja, DDS, MS
Assistant Professor
Department of Periodontics
University of Kentucky College
    of Dentistry
Lexington, Kentucky

Richard Foster, DMD
Department Chair, Dental Science
Guilford Technical Community
    College
Jamestown, North Carolina

Carol A. Jahn, RDH, MS
Senior Professional Relations
    Manager
Water Pik, Inc.
Fort Collins, Colorado

Archie A. Jones, DDS, MBA
Professor
Department of Periodontics
University of Texas Health Science
    Center at San Antonio
San Antonio, Texas

Margaret Lemaster, BSDH, MS
Assistant Professor
School of Dental Hygiene
Old Dominion University
Norfolk, Virginia

Sharon Logue, RDH, MPH
Virginia Department of Health
Richmond, Virginia
Dental Health Program

Robin Blatt Matloff, RDH, BSDH, JD
Professor
Mount Ida College
Dental Hygiene Program
Newton, Massachusetts

Deborah P. Milliken, BS, DMD
Professor and Chair, Dental
    Education
South Florida Community College
Avon Park, Florida

Craig S. Miller, DMD, MS
Professor of Oral Medicine
Division of Oral Diagnosis, Oral
    Medicine and Oral Radiology
Department of Oral Health
    Practice
College of Dentistry
Lexington, Kentucky

William S. Moore, DDS, MS
Assistant Professor and Radiology
    Clinic Director
Department of Comprehensive
    Dentistry
School of Dentistry
University of Texas Health Science
    Center at San Antonio
San Antonio, Texas

John Preece, DDS, MS
Professor, Retired
Division of Oral & Maxillofacial
    Radiology
Department of Dental Diagnostic
    Science
University of Texas Health Science
    Center at San Antonio
San Antonio, Texas

**Christoph A. Ramseier, MAS
Dr. Med. Dent.**
Assistant Professor
Department of Periodontology
University of Berne, School of
    Dental Medicine
Bern, Switzerland

Keerthana Satheesh, DDS, MS
Associate Professor and Director of
    Advanced Education
Department of Periodontics
School of Dentistry
University of Missouri – Kansas City
Kansas City, Missouri

Carol Southard, RN, MSN
Tobacco Treatment Specialist
Osher Center for Integrative
    Medicine
Northwestern Medical Group
Northwestern Medicine
Chicago, Illinois

Rebecca Sroda, RDH, MS
Dean, Health Sciences
South Florida State College
Avon Park, Florida

**Dianne Glasscoe Watterson,
RDH, MBA**
Chief Executive Officer
Professional Dental Management, Inc.
Frederick, Maryland

Karen Williams, RDH, MS, PhD
Professor and Chair
Department of Biomedical and
    Health Informatics
School of Medicine
University of Missouri – Kansas City
Kansas City, Missouri

Reviewers

Genevieve Benoit, RDH, MEd
Professor
Dental Hygiene
LSUHSC School of Dentistry
New Orleans, Louisiana

Bonnie Blank, MA
Instructor – Dental Hygiene
Camosun College
Victoria, British Columbia, Canada

Megan Brightbilk, RDH, MEd
Instructor, Dental Hygiene
Harrisburg Area Community
   College
Harrisburg, Pennsylvania

Lynnann B. Bryan, BSDH, MEd
Associate Clinical Professor
Marquette University School of
   Dentistry
Milwaukee, Wisconsin

April Catlett, MDH
Program Chair
Dental Hygiene
Central Georgia Technical College
Macon, Georgia

Christine Chore
Vancouver College of Dental Hygiene
Vancouver, British Columbia, Canada

Tammy Clossen, RDH, PhD
Associate Professor, Dental Hygiene
Pennsylvania College of Technology
Williamsport, Pennsylvania

Lori DeFore, RDH, BS, BTh
Dental Hygiene Instructor
Southeastern Technical College
Vidalia, Georgia

Diane Estes, BS, MEd
Instructor/Clinical Coordinator
Dental Hygiene
Athens Technical College
Athens, Georgia

Lisa Fleck, RDH, MS
Chairperson, Advisor
College of Allied Health &
   Nursing – Dental Hygiene
Minnesota State University –
   Mankato
Mankato, Minnesota

Linda Hecker, CDA, RDH, BS, MA
Director of Dental Hygiene
Burlington County College
Pemberton, New Jersey

Rosemary Herman, RDH, MEd
First Year Dental Hygiene
   Coordinator
Montgomery County Community
   College
Blue Bell, Pennsylvania

Jennifer K.L. Hew, RDH, MSHCM, FADPO
Assistant Professor
LSUHSC School of Dentistry
New Orleans, Louisiana

Sandra Horne, MHSA, RDH
Associate Professor of Dental
   Hygiene
University of Mississippi Medical
   Center
Jackson, Mississippi

Lisa Hunter, CDA, MA
Dental Assisting Program Director
Ozarks Technical Community
   College
Springfield, Missouri

Debra James, MSDS
Dental Programs Director
Fortis College – Phoenix
Phoenix, Arizona

Lori Kaczor, RDH, MS
Associate Professor
Dental Hygiene
Erie Community College
Williamsville, New York

Connie Kracher, PhD, MSD
Director of Dental Assisting Program
Department of Dental Education
Indiana University – Purdue
   University Fort Wayne
Fort Wayne, Indiana

Nancy Mann, RDH, MSEd
Clinical Professor
Indiana University – Purdue
   University Fort Wayne
Fort Wayne, Indiana

Joy Osborn, RDH, BS, MA
Associate Professor
School of Dentistry
University of Minnesota
Minneapolis, Minnesota

Mary Ann Schneiderman, RDH, MS
Clinical Assistant Professor and
   Senior Clinic Coordinator
University of Maryland School of
   Dentistry
Baltimore, Maryland

Stacie Scrivner, RDH, MEd
Ahead of Dental Hygiene
    Department
Missouri Southern State University
Joplin, Missouri

Phyllis Spragge, RDH, MA
Dental Hygiene Director
Foothill College
Los Altos Hill, California

Maribeth Stitt, BSDH, RDH, MEd
Professor and Director of Dental
    Hygiene Program
Lone Star College – Kingwood
Kingwood, Texas

Melanie Taverna, MS, RDH
Assistant Professor/Clinical Faculty
University of Texas Health Care
    Center at San Antonio
San Antonio, Texas

Maria Tigner, DDS
Professor of Dental Programs
Health, Safety and Community
    Service
Algonquin College
Ottawa, Ontario, Canada

Kristy Unterbrink, BSDH, MEd
Allied Health and Nursing
Lorain County Community College
Elyria, Ohio

Laura Webb, RDH, MS, CDA
LJW Education Services
Fallon, Nevada

Preface for Course Instructors

Foundations of Periodontics for the Dental Hygienist, 4th edition, is written with two primary goals in mind. First and foremost, this textbook focuses on the dental hygienist's role in periodontics. Our second goal was to develop a book with an instructional design that facilitates the teaching and learning of the complex subject of periodontics—as it relates to dental hygiene practice—without omitting salient concepts or "watering down" the material. Written primarily for dental hygiene students, *Foundations of Periodontics for the Dental Hygienist* also would be a valuable resource on current concepts in periodontics for the practicing dental hygienist or general dentist.

ONLINE INSTRUCTOR AND STUDENT RESOURCES

Follow the steps in Box 1 to access the online instructor resources.

Box 1. Accessing Online Instructor Resources

1. Open an internet browser and select: **http://thepoint.lww.com**

2. Existing users: Click on **"Return User"** to log on.

3. New users: Select **"New User."** Complete all required field on the online access request form.
   - Educators: Instructor access codes come directly from your sales representative. Access codes in the product packaging are intended only for access to student resources. If you need additional help entering a code, please contact your sales representative.
   - Students: Access codes are located inside the front or back cover of the book.
4. Locate **Foundations of Periodontics for the Dental Hygienist.** Select either "Student Resources" or "Instructor Resources."

TEXTBOOK FEATURES

The fourth edition of *Foundations of Periodontics for the Dental Hygienist* has many features designed to facilitate learning and teaching.

1. **Module Overview and Outline.** Each module begins with a concise overview of the module content. The module outline makes it easier to locate material within the module. The outline provides the reader with an organizational framework with which to approach new material.

2. **Learning Objectives and Key Terms.** Learning objectives assist students in recognizing and studying important concepts in each chapter. Key terms are listed at the beginning of each chapter. One of the most challenging tasks for any student is learning a whole new dental vocabulary and gaining the confidence to use new terms with accuracy and ease. The key terms list assists students in this task by identifying important terminology and facilitating the study and review of terminology in each chapter. Terms are highlighted in bold type and clearly defined within the chapter.

3. **Instructional Design**
   - Each chapter is subdivided into sections to help the reader recognize major content areas.
   - Chapters are written in an expanded outline format that makes it easy for students to identify, learn, and review key concepts.
   - Material is presented in a manner that recognizes that students have different learning styles. Hundreds of illustrations and clinical photographs visually reinforce chapter content.
   - Chapter content is supplemented in a visual format with boxes, tables, and flow charts.

4. **Focus on Patients.** The "*Focus on Patients*" items allow the reader to apply chapter content in the context of clinical practice. The cases provide opportunities for students to integrate knowledge into their clinical work. Three types of scenarios help students to apply content to the real world setting.
   - Clinical Patient Care scenarios
   - Evidence in Action scenarios
   - Ethical Dilemma scenarios

5. **Patient Case Studies**

   Chapter 36 presents five fictitious patient cases. Patient assessment data pertinent to the periodontium challenges the student to interpret and use the information in periodontal care planning for the patient.

   Chapter 38 provides radiographs for several cases. These cases give students the opportunity to develop skills in radiographic analysis as it pertains to the hard tissues of the periodontium in health and disease.

6. **Glossary. An online audio glossary** provides quick access to common periodontal terminology and pronunciation.

7. **Online Resources**
   - Chapter 37: Patient Cases Radiographic Analysis
   - Instructor Resources
   - Student Resources

NEW CONTENT SEQUENCING FOR THE FOURTH EDITION

The book is divided into nine major content areas:

Part 1: The Periodontium in Health

Part 2: Diseases Affecting the Periodontium

Part 3: Risk Factors for Periodontal Diseases

Part 4: Assessment and Planning for Patients with Periodontal Disease

Part 5: Implementation of Therapy for Patients with Periodontal Disease

Part 6: Health Maintenance in Treated Periodontal Patients

Part 7: Other Aspects of the Management of Patients with Periodontal Diseases

Part 8: Comprehensive Patient Cases

Part 9: Online Resources

Foundations of Periodontics for the Dental Hygienist, 4th edition, strives to present the complex subject of periodontics in a reader-friendly manner. The authors greatly appreciate the comments and suggestions from educators and students about previous editions of this book. It is our sincere hope that this textbook will help students and practitioners alike to acquire knowledge that will serve as a foundation for the prevention and management of periodontal diseases.

Jill S. Gehrig, RDH, MA
Donald E. Willmann, DDS, MS

Acknowledgments

It is a great pleasure to acknowledge the following individuals whose assistance was indispensable to this third edition:

- **Charles D. Whitehead and Holly R. Fischer,** MFA the highly skilled medical illustrators, who created all the wonderful illustrations for the book.

- **Kevin Dietz,** a colleague and friend for his vision and guidance for all four editions of this book.

- And with great thanks to our wonderful team at Wolters Kluwer without whose expertise and support this book would not have been possible: **Jonathan Joyce, John Larkin,** and **Jennifer Clements.**

Jill S. Gehrig, RDH, MA
Donald E. Willmann, DDS, MS

Contents

PART 3: RISK FACTORS FOR PERIODONTAL DISEASES

11 Etiologic Factors: Risk for Periodontitis   174

Jill Gehrig and Donald Willmann; Ethical Dilemma by Robin Matloff

12 Oral Biofilms and Periodontal Infections   189

Jill Gehrig and Donald Willmann

13 Basic Concepts of Immunity and Inflammation   210

Jill Gehrig and Donald Willmann

14 Host Immune Response to Plaque Biofilm   229

Jill Gehrig and Donald Willmann; Ethical Dilemma by Robin Matloff

15 Systemic Conditions that Amplify Susceptibility to Periodontal Disease   246

Jill Gehrig and Donald Willmann; Ethical Dilemma by Robin Matloff

16 Local Factors Contributing to Periodontal Disease   274

Donald Willmann and Jill Gehrig

17   Nutrition, Inflammation, and Periodontal Disease   290

Rebecca Sroda and Jill Gehrig; Ethical Dilemma by Robin Matloff

18   Tobacco, Smoking, and Periodontal Disease   304

Keerthana Satheesh, Charles Cobb, Carol Southard

PART 4: ASSESSMENT AND PLANNING FOR PATIENTS WITH PERIODONTAL DISEASE

19   Clinical Periodontal Assessment   319

Donald Willmann and Jill Gehrig; Ethical Dilemma by Robin Matloff

20   Radiographic Analysis of the Periodontium   339

William Moore; Ethical Dilemma by Robin Matloff

21   Best Practices for Periodontal Care   352

Carol Jahn: Ethical Dilemma by Robin Matloff

28 Periodontal Emergencies   511

Donald Willmann and Jill Gehrig; Ethical Dilemma by Robin Matloff

PART 6: HEALTH MAINTENANCE IN TREATED PERIODONTAL PATIENTS

29 Using Motivational Interviewing to Enhance Patient Behavior Change   531

*Delwyn Catley, Karen Williams, Christoph Ramseier;
Ethical Dilemma by Robin Matloff*

30 Maintenance for the Periodontal Patient   551

Donald Willmann and Teresa Butler Duncan

31 Periodontal Maintenance of Dental Implants   576

Archie Jones

PART 7: OTHER ASPECTS OF THE MANAGEMENT OF PATIENTS WITH PERIODONTAL DISEASES

PART 8: COMPREHENSIVE PATIENT CASES

PART 9: ONLINE RESOURCES

The Point: Online Instructor & Student Resources (http://thePoint.lww.com)

Sharon Logue, Margaret Lemaster, Rebecca Sroda, Donald Willmann, and Jill Gehrig

CHAPTER 1

Periodontium: The Tooth-Supporting Structures

Clinical Application.
The dental hygienist is involved in a continuous process of interacting with patients, making clinical decisions, performing clinical procedures, evaluating new techniques, and adapting to evolving technologies. Nearly every action taken by a hygienist throughout a successful career requires a detailed knowledge of the anatomy of the tooth-supporting structures—the periodontium. Chapters 1 and 2 outline current knowledge of the anatomy of the periodontium. Chapter 1 deals with what is known about the fundamental structure of the complex system of tissues that support the teeth and can serve as a basis for organizing thoughts about additional anatomical information as it becomes available through additional research. Chapter 2 deals with the microscopic anatomy of these same structures.

Learning Objectives

- Identify the tissues of the periodontium on an unlabeled drawing depicting the periodontium in cross section.
- Describe the function that each tissue serves in the periodontium, including the gingiva, periodontal ligament, cementum, and alveolar bone.
- In a clinical setting or on a color photograph, identify the following anatomical areas of the gingiva: free gingiva, gingival sulcus, interdental gingiva, and attached gingiva.
- In a clinical setting or on a color photograph, identify the following boundaries of the gingiva: gingival margin, free gingival groove, and mucogingival junction.
- In a clinical setting, identify the free gingiva on an anterior tooth by inserting a periodontal probe to the base of the sulcus.

- In a clinical setting, contrast the coral pink tissue of the attached gingiva with the darker, shiny tissue of the alveolar mucosa.
- In the clinical setting, use compressed air to detect the presence or absence of stippling of the attached gingiva.
- Identify the alveolar process (alveolar bone) on a human skull.
- Describe the position and contours of the alveolar crest of the bone in health.
- Describe the nerve and blood supply to the periodontium.
- Explain the role of the lymphatic system in the health of the periodontium.

Key Terms

Periodontium	Attached gingiva	Cortical bone
Gingiva	Stippling	Alveolar crest
Periodontal ligament	Interdental gingiva	Cancellous bone
Cementum	Papillae	Periosteum
Alveolar bone	Gingival col	Innervation
Gingival margin	Gingival sulcus	Trigeminal nerve
Alveolar mucosa	Gingival crevicular fluid	Anastomose
Free gingival groove	Alveolar process	Lymphatic system
Mucogingival junction	Alveolar bone proper	Lymph nodes
Free gingiva	Alveolus	

Section 1
Tissues of the Periodontium

The **periodontium** (peri = around and odontos = tooth) is the functional system of tissues that surrounds the teeth and attaches them to the jawbone (Figs. 1-1 and 1-2). An excellent overview of the periodontium is located on the Madison Area Technical College website at http://learningobjects.madisoncollege.edu/window_holder.asp?f=16654_Periodontium_ Gingiva.swf. The periodontium is also called the "**supporting tissues of the teeth**" and "the **attachment apparatus**." The tissues of the periodontium include the following:

1. **Gingiva**—the tissue that covers the cervical portions of the teeth and the alveolar processes of the jaws.
2. **Periodontal ligament (PDL)**—the fibers that surround the root of the tooth. These fibers attach to the bone of the socket on one side and to the cementum of the root on the other side.
3. **Cementum**—the thin layer of mineralized tissue that covers the root of the tooth.
4. **Alveolar bone**—the bone that surrounds the roots of the teeth. It forms the bony sockets that support and protect the roots of the teeth.

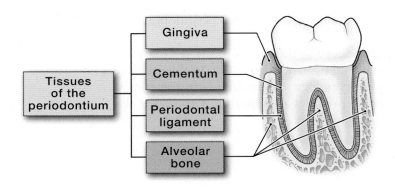

Figure 1-1. Tissues Comprising the Periodontium. A graphic representation of the periodontium in cross section.

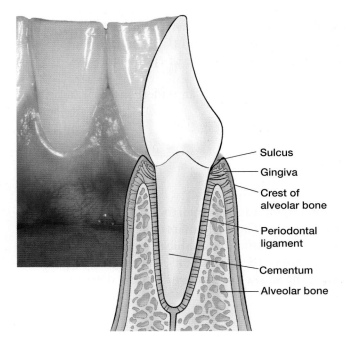

Figure 1-2. Healthy Periodontium. Clinical photograph and drawing depicting the structures of the periodontium.

TABLE 1-1. THE PERIODONTIUM	
Structure	**Brief Description of Its Function**
Gingiva	• Provides a tissue seal around the cervical portion (neck) of the tooth • Covers the alveolar processes of the jaws • Holds the tissue against the tooth during mastication
Periodontal ligament	• Suspends and maintains the tooth in its socket
Cementum	• Anchors the ends of the periodontal ligament fibers to the tooth, so that the tooth stays in its socket • Protects the dentin of the root
Alveolar bone	• Surrounds and supports the roots of the tooth

Each of the tissues of the periodontium plays a vital role in maintaining the health and function of the periodontium (Table 1-1). Knowledge of the periodontal tissues in health is a necessary foundation for understanding the concepts of (1) normal function of the periodontium, (2) disease prevention, and (3) the periodontal disease process.

Dental hygiene students usually are introduced to the tissues of the periodontium during the first semester or quarter of the dental hygiene curriculum. In the preclinical stages of the curriculum, mastering dental terminology and anatomy can sometimes be overwhelming and confusing. This chapter provides an opportunity to review this complex system of tissues known as the periodontium.

THE GINGIVA

1. Overview of the Gingiva
   A. **Description.** The gingiva is the part of the mucosa that surrounds the cervical portions of the teeth and covers the alveolar processes of the jaws (Fig. 1-3).
      1. The gingiva ends coronal to the cementoenamel junction (CEJ) of each tooth and attaches to the tooth by means of a specialized type of epithelial tissue (junctional epithelium).
      2. It is composed of a thin outer layer of epithelium and an underlying core of connective tissue.
      3. The gingiva is divided into four anatomical areas (Fig. 1-4).
         a. Free gingiva
         b. Gingival sulcus
         c. Interdental gingiva
         d. Attached gingiva
   B. **Function.** The gingiva protects the underlying tooth-supporting structures of the periodontium from the oral environment. The oral environment is exposed to a wide range of temperatures in food and drink, mechanical forces, and a large number of oral bacteria. To accomplish these functions, the gingiva has several defense mechanisms, including the saliva and immune system defense mechanisms.

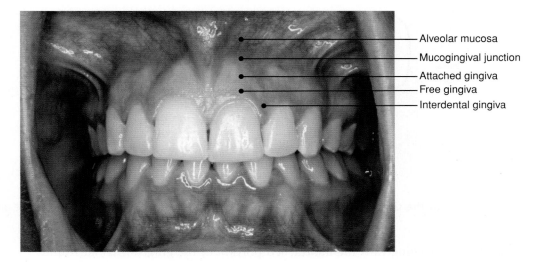

Alveolar mucosa
Mucogingival junction
Attached gingiva
Free gingiva
Interdental gingiva

Figure 1-3. The Gingival Tissues. Photograph of healthy gingival tissues showing the free, attached, and interdental gingiva.

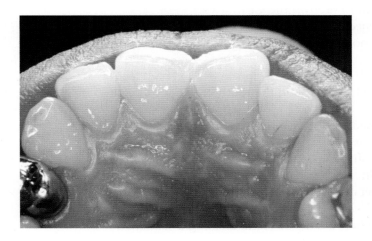

Figure 1-4. Gingival Tissue of the Palate. On the palate, the lingual gingiva is directly continuous with the keratinized masticatory mucosa.

C. Boundaries of the Gingiva
1. The coronal boundary, or upper edge, of the gingiva is the **gingival margin** (Fig. 1-5).
2. The apical boundary, or lower edge, of the gingiva is the alveolar mucosa. The **alveolar mucosa** can be distinguished easily from the gingiva by its dark red color and smooth, shiny surface.

D. Demarcations of the Gingiva
1. The **free gingival groove** is a shallow linear depression that separates the free and attached gingiva (this line may be visible clinically but is not obvious in many instances).
2. The **mucogingival junction** is the clinically visible boundary where the pink attached gingiva meets the red, shiny alveolar mucosa. (Clinically visible means that this landmark can be seen in the oral cavity.)

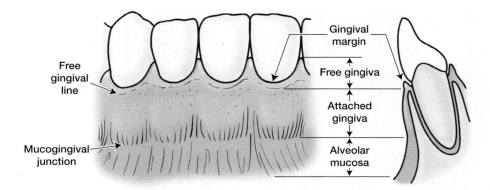

Free
gingival
line

Mucogingival
junction

Gingival
margin

Free gingiva

Attached
gingiva

Alveolar
mucosa

Figure 1-5. Boundaries of the Gingiva. Illustration showing the boundaries and anatomical areas of the gingiva.

2. **Free Gingiva.** The **free gingiva** is the unattached portion of the gingiva that surrounds the tooth in the region of the CEJ. The free gingiva is also known as the unattached gingiva or the marginal gingiva.
   A. **Location of the Free Gingiva**
      1. The free gingiva is located coronal to (above) the CEJ.
      2. It surrounds the tooth in a turtleneck or cuff-like manner.
      3. The free gingiva attaches to the tooth by means of a specialized epithelium—the junctional epithelium.
   B. **Characteristics of the Free Gingiva**
      1. The tissue of the free gingiva fits closely around the tooth but is not directly attached to it.
      2. This tissue, because it is unattached, may be gently stretched away from the tooth surface with a periodontal probe.
      3. The free gingiva also forms the soft tissue wall of the gingival sulcus.
   C. **Contour of the Free Gingival Margin**
      1. The tissue of the free gingiva meets the tooth in a thin rounded edge called the **gingival margin**.
      2. The gingival margin follows the contours of the teeth, creating a scalloped (wavy) outline around them.
3. **Attached Gingiva.** The **attached gingiva** is the part of the gingiva that is tightly connected to the cementum on the cervical-third of the root and to the periosteum (connective tissue cover) of the alveolar bone.
   A. **Location of the Attached Gingiva.** The attached gingiva lies between the free gingiva and the alveolar mucosa (Fig. 1-6).
   B. **Width of the Attached Gingiva**
      1. The attached gingiva is widest in the incisor and molar regions, ranging from 3.3 to 3.9 mm on the mandible and 3.5 to 4.5 mm on the maxilla (Fig. 1-7).
      2. The attached gingiva is narrowest in premolar regions (1.8 mm on mandible and 1.9 mm on maxilla).
      3. The width of the attached gingiva is not measured on the palate since clinically it is not possible to determine where the attached gingiva ends and the palatal mucosa begins (Fig. 1-4).
      4. It was once believed that a minimum 2-mm width of attached gingiva is necessary to maintain the health of the periodontium; this concept is not accepted today (1).

C. Color of the Attached Gingiva
  1. In health, the attached gingiva is pale or coral pink.
  2. The attached gingiva may be pigmented (Fig. 1-8).
     a. Pigmentation occurs more frequently in dark-skinned individuals (2).
     b. The pigmented areas of the attached gingiva may range from light brown to black.

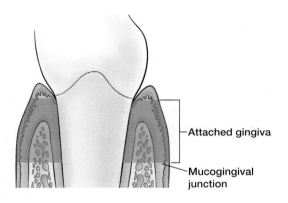

Figure 1-6. Location of the Attached Gingiva. The attached gingiva extends from the free gingival groove to the mucogingival junction.

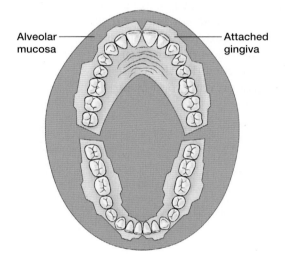

Figure 1-7. Mean Width of the Attached Gingiva. The attached gingiva is widest in the incisor and molar regions and narrowest in premolar regions.

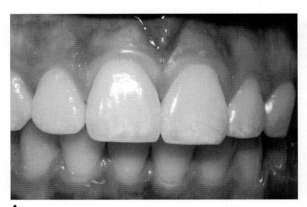

A

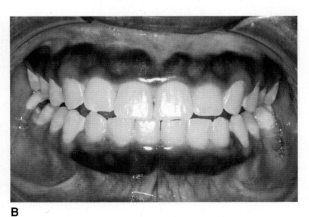

B

Figure 1-8. Color Variations of Normal Gingiva. The color of the normal gingiva varies among different persons. **A:** The color is a lighter, coral pink in individuals with fair complexions. **B:** In individuals with dark skin and hair, the gingiva may be pigmented. (Courtesy of Elizabeth Carr, University of Mississippi Medical Center, Jackson, MS)

D. **Texture of the Attached Gingiva.** In health, the surface of the attached gingiva may have a dimpled appearance similar to the skin of an orange peel. This dimpled appearance is known as **stippling** (Fig. 1-9). Healthy tissue may or may not exhibit a stippled appearance as the presence of stippling varies greatly from individual to individual. Stippling is present in 40% of adults.

E. **Function of the Attached Gingiva**
   1. The attached gingiva allows the gingival tissue to withstand the mechanical forces created during activities such as mastication, speaking, and toothbrushing.
   2. The attached gingiva prevents the free gingiva from being pulled away from the tooth when tension is applied to the alveolar mucosa.

4. **Interdental Gingiva.** The **interdental gingiva** is the portion of the gingiva that fills the interdental embrasure between two adjacent teeth apical to the contact area (Fig. 1-10).
   A. **Parts of Interdental Gingiva**
      1. The interdental gingiva consists of two interdental **papillae**—one facial papilla and one lingual papilla (papilla = singular noun; papillae = plural noun).
         a. The lateral borders and tip of an interdental papilla are formed by the free gingiva from the adjacent teeth.
         b. The center portion of the interdental papilla is formed by the attached gingiva.
      2. The **gingival col** is a valley-like depression in the portion of the interdental gingiva that lies directly apical to the contact area of two adjacent (touching) teeth and connects the facial and lingual papillae. ***The col is not present if the adjacent teeth are not in contact*** (i.e., there is a space between two adjacent teeth), there is no adjacent tooth (i.e., the lingual surface of the posterior most tooth in the arch), or if the interdental gingiva has receded (Fig. 1-11).
   B. **Function of Interdental Gingiva.** The interdental gingiva prevents food from becoming packed between the teeth during mastication.

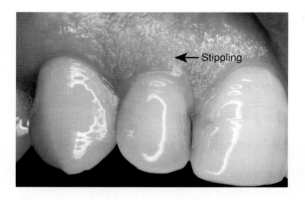

Figure 1-9. Gingival Stippling. In health, the surface of the attached gingiva may have a dimpled appearance known as gingival stippling.

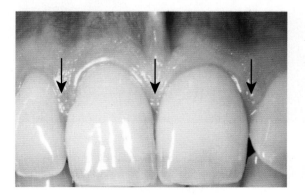

Figure 1-10. The Interdental Gingiva. The interdental tissue fills the area between two adjacent teeth.

5. **Gingival Sulcus.** The **gingival sulcus** is the *space* between the free gingiva and the tooth surface (Fig. 1-12).
   A. **Description.** The sulcus is a V-shaped, shallow space around the tooth (3).
      1. The depth of a clinically normal gingival sulcus is from 1 to 3 mm, as measured using a periodontal probe.
      2. **Base of Sulcus.** The base of the sulcus is formed by the junctional epithelium (a specialized type of epithelium that attaches to the tooth surface).
   B. **Gingival Crevicular Fluid.** The **gingival crevicular fluid**, also called the gingival sulcular fluid, is a fluid that seeps from the underlying connective tissue into the sulcular space.
      1. Little or no fluid is found in the healthy gingival sulcus but the fluid flow increases in the presence of dental plaque biofilm and the resulting gingival inflammation (4).
      2. Fluid flow increases in response to toothbrushing, mastication, or other stimulation of the gingivae. The flow is greatly increased when the gingivae are inflamed.
      3. If a filter strip is inserted into the sulcus, it aborbs the fluid in the sulcus. Using the filter strip the amount of gingival crevicular fluid can be measured and used as an index of gingival inflammation.

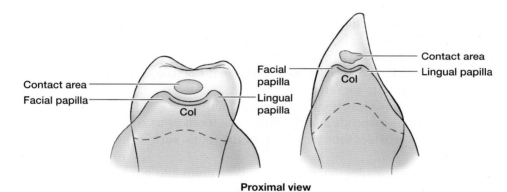

Proximal view

Figure 1-11. Interdental Col. Apical to the contact area between two teeth, the interdental gingiva has a concave (depressed) form. The concavity, the "col" is located between the facial and lingual papillae and extends beneath the contact area of two adjacent teeth.

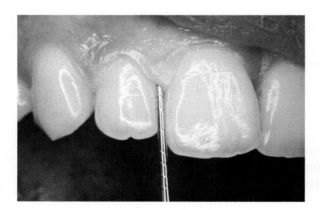

Figure 1-12. Gingival Sulcus. This photograph shows a periodontal probe inserted into the gingival sulcus, the space between the free gingiva and the tooth.

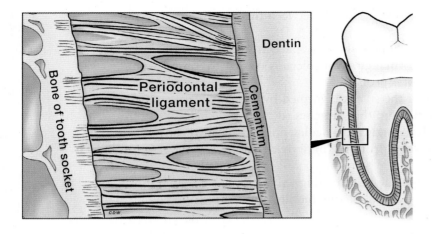

Figure 1-13. Periodontal Ligament.

- **On tooth side**, the ends of the periodontal ligament fibers are anchored in the cementum of the root.
- **On the bone side**, the ends of the periodontal ligament fibers are anchored in the alveolar bone of the tooth socket.

PERIODONTAL LIGAMENT

1. Description
   A. The PDL is a layer of soft connective tissue that covers the root of the tooth and attaches it to the bone of the tooth socket (Fig. 1-13).
      1. The PDL is composed mainly of dense fibrous connective tissue (3).
      2. The fibers of the PDL attach on one side to the root cementum and on the other side to the alveolar bone of the tooth socket (5).
   B. The PDL not only connects the tooth to the alveolar process, but also supports the tooth in the socket and absorbs mechanical loads placed on the tooth, thus protecting the tooth in its socket.
2. Functions. The PDL has five functions in the periodontium:
   A. Supportive function—suspends and maintains the tooth in its socket.
   B. Sensory function—provides sensory feeling to the tooth, such as pressure and pain sensations.
   C. Nutritive function—provides nutrients to the cementum and bone.
   D. Formative function—builds and maintains cementum and the alveolar bone of the tooth socket. The tissues of the PDL contain specialized cells such as fibroblasts, cementoblasts, and osteoblasts.
   E. Resorptive function—can remodel the alveolar bone in response to pressure, such as that applied during orthodontic treatment (braces).

ROOT CEMENTUM

1. Description. Cementum is a thin layer of hard, mineralized connective tissue that covers the surface of the tooth root (Fig. 1-14).
2. Characteristics of Cementum
   A. Cementum overlies and is attached to the dentin of the root. It is light yellow in color and softer than dentin or enamel.
   B. Cementum is a bone-like tissue that is more resistant to resorption than bone (6).
      1. Resistance to resorption (loss of substance) is an important characteristic of cementum that makes it possible for the teeth to be moved during orthodontic treatment (7).

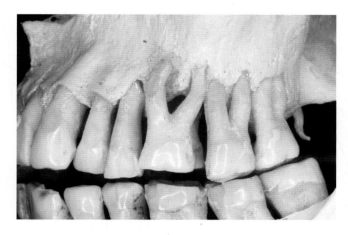

Figure 1-14. Cementum. Cementum is mineralized connective tissue that covers the root of the tooth; it is light yellow in color.

2. The high resistance of cementum to resorption allows the pressure applied during orthodontics to cause resorption of the alveolar bone, for tooth movement, without resulting in root resorption.
   C. Cementum is formed slowly throughout life. There are two main types of cementum: cellular and acellular.
   D. Cementum does not have its own blood or nutrient supply; it receives its nutrients from the PDL.
3. **Functions of Cementum in the Periodontium.** Cementum performs several important roles in the periodontium, and, therefore, conservation of cementum should be a goal of periodontal instrumentation.
   A. The primary function of cementum is to give attachment to the collagen fibers of the PDL. Cementum anchors the ends of the PDL fibers to the tooth; without cementum, the tooth would fall out of its socket.
   B. The outer layer of cementum protects the underlying dentin and seals the ends of the open dentinal tubules.
   C. Cementum formation compensates for tooth wear at the occlusal or incisal surface due to attrition. Cementum is formed at the apical area of the root to compensate for occlusal attrition.

ALVEOLAR BONE

1. Description
   A. The **alveolar process** or **alveolar bone** is the bone of the upper or lower jaw that surrounds and supports the roots of the teeth (Fig. 1-15).
   B. Bone is mineralized connective tissue and consists by weight of about 60% inorganic material, 25% organic material and about 15% water.
   C. The existence of the alveolar bone is dependent on the presence of teeth; when teeth are extracted, in time, the alveolar bone resorbs. If teeth do not erupt, the alveolar bone does not develop.
2. **Function of the Alveolar Bone in the Periodontium.** The alveolar bone forms the bony sockets that provide support and protection for the roots of the teeth.

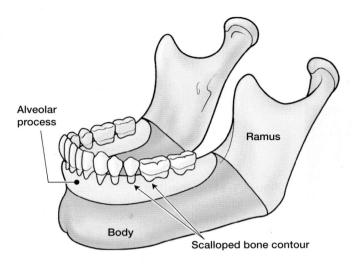

Figure 1-15. Alveolar Process. The alveolar process is the bone that surrounds and supports the roots of the teeth.

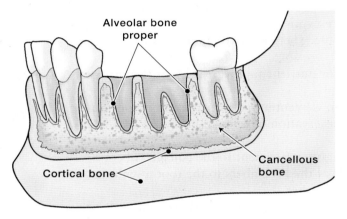

Figure 1-16. Layers of the Alveolar Process. A lateral section of the mandible reveals the three bony layers: the alveolar bone proper, cancellous bone, and cortical bone.

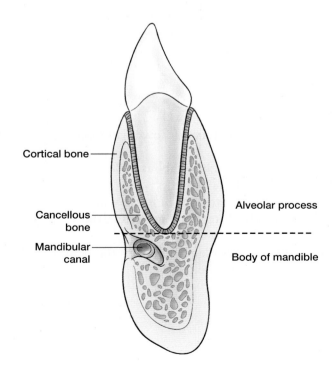

Figure 1-17. Cross Section of the Mandible. The dotted line indicates the boundary of the alveolar process with the body of the mandible.

3. **Layers that compose the Alveolar Process.** When viewed in cross section, the alveolar process is composed of three layers of hard tissue and covered by a thin layer of connective tissue (Figs. 1-16 and 1-17).
   A. The **alveolar bone proper** (or **cribriform plate**) is the thin layer of bone that lines the socket to surround the root of the tooth.
      1. The **alveolus** is the bony socket, a cavity in the alveolar bone that houses the root of a tooth (alveolus = singular; alveoli = plural) (Fig. 1-18).
      2. The alveolar bone proper has numerous holes that allow blood vessels from the cancellous bone to connect with the vessels of the PDL space.
      3. The ends of the PDL fibers are embedded in the alveolar bone proper.
   B. The **cortical bone** is a layer of compact bone that forms the hard, outside wall of the mandible and maxilla on the facial and lingual aspects. This cortical bone surrounds the alveolar bone proper and gives support to the socket.
      1. The buccal cortical bone is thin in the incisor, canine, and premolar regions; cortical bone is thicker in molar regions.
      2. Since the cortical plate is only on the facial and lingual sides of the jaw, it will not show up in a radiograph; only the cancellous bone and the alveolar bone proper can be seen on a radiograph.
      3. The **alveolar crest** is the coronal most portion of the alveolar process.
         a. In health, the alveolar crest is located 1 to 2 mm apical to (below) the CEJs of the teeth (Fig. 1-19).
         b. When viewed from the facial or lingual aspect, the alveolar crest meets the teeth in a scalloped (wavy) line that follows the countours of the CEJs.
   C. The **cancellous bone** (or **spongy bone**) is the lattice-like bone that fills the interior portion of the alveolar process (between the cortical bone and the alveolar bone proper). The cancellous bone is oriented around the tooth to form support for the alveolar bone proper.
   D. The **periosteum** is a layer of connective soft tissue covering the outer surface of bone; it consists of an outer layer of collagenous tissue and an inner layer of fine elastic fibers.

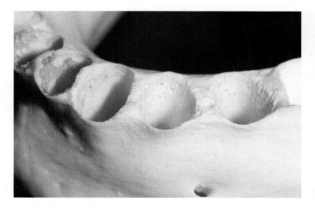

Figure 1-18. Alveoli of the Mandible. The alveoli are the sockets in the alveolar bone that house the roots of the teeth. (Courtesy of Dr. Don Rolfs, Periodontal Foundations, Wenatchee, WA)

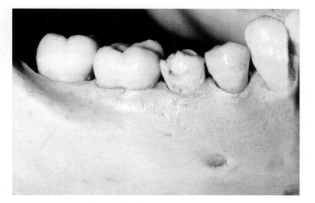

Figure 1-19. Bony Contours. The alveolar crest meets the teeth in a scalloped line that follows the contours of the cementoenamel junctions. (Courtesy of Dr. Don Rolfs, Periodontal Foundations, Wenatchee, WA)

Section 2
Nerve Supply, Blood Supply, and Lymphatic System

NERVE SUPPLY TO THE PERIODONTIUM

1. **Description.** The innervation of the periodontium—nerve supply to the periodontium—occurs via the branches of the **trigeminal nerve** (Fig. 1-20). Innervation to the maxilla (Fig. 1-21) is by the second branch of the trigeminal nerve (the maxillary nerve) and the mandible by the third branch (the mandibular nerve).
   A. The trigeminal nerves have sensory, motor, and intermediate roots that attach directly to the brain.
   B. The trigeminal nerve is responsible for the sensory sensibility of most of the skin on the front part of the face and head, the teeth, oral cavity, maxillary sinus, and nasal cavity.
   C. The motor function of the trigeminal nerve is essential for the act of chewing.
2. **Functions of the Nerve Supply to the Periodontium**
   A. Nerve receptors in the gingiva, alveolar bone, and PDL register pain, touch, and pressure.
   B. Nerves in the PDL provide information about movement and tooth position. These nerves provide the sensations of light touch or pressure against the teeth and play an important role in the regulation of chewing forces and movements. When biting down on something hard, it is the nerves of the PDL that are stimulated, allowing the individual to experience a sense of pressure with the teeth against the hard object.
3. **Innervation of the Periodontium**
   A. **Innervation of the Gingiva**
      1. Innervation of the gingiva of the maxillary arch is from the superior alveolar nerves (anterior, middle, and posterior branches), infraorbital nerve, and the greater palatine and nasopalatine nerves.
      2. Innervation of the gingiva of the mandibular arch is from the mental nerve, buccal nerve, and the sublingual branch of the lingual nerve (Fig. 1-22).
   B. **Innervation of the Teeth and PDL**
      1. Innervation of the teeth and PDL of the maxillary arch is from the superior alveolar nerves (anterior, middle, and posterior branches).
      2. Innervation of the teeth and PDL of the mandibular arch is from the inferior alveolar nerve.

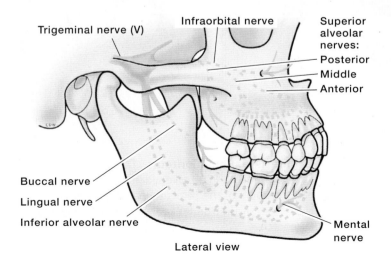

Figure 1-20. Nerve Supply to the Periodontium (Lateral View). The nerve supply to the periodontium is derived from the branches of the trigeminal nerve.

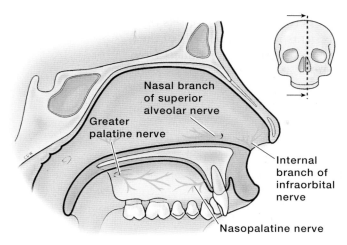

Figure 1-21. Nerve Innervation to the Palate.

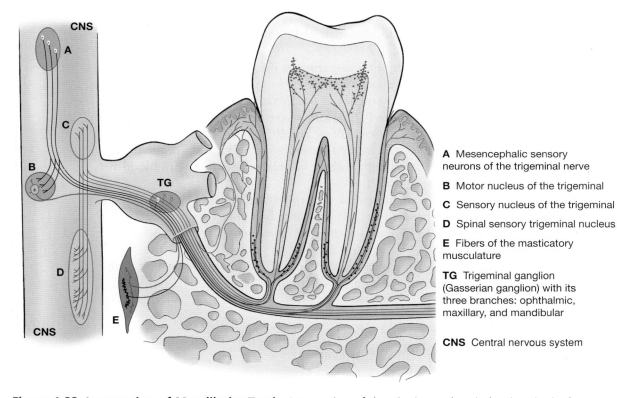

A Mesencephalic sensory neurons of the trigeminal nerve

B Motor nucleus of the trigeminal

C Sensory nucleus of the trigeminal

D Spinal sensory trigeminal nucleus

E Fibers of the masticatory musculature

TG Trigeminal ganglion (Gasserian ganglion) with its three branches: ophthalmic, maxillary, and mandibular

CNS Central nervous system

Figure 1-22. Innervation of Mandibular Teeth. Innervation of the gingiva and periodontium is via the mandibular nerve.

BLOOD SUPPLY TO THE PERIODONTIUM

1. **Description.** The vessels of the periodontium **anastomose** (join together) to create a complex *system of blood vessels* that supply blood to the periodontal tissues.
   A. This network of blood vessels acts as a unit, supplying blood to the soft and hard tissues of the maxilla and mandible.
   B. It is the proliferation of this rich blood supply to the gingiva that accounts for the dramatic color changes that are seen in gingivitis.

2. **Function.** The major function of the complex network of blood vessels of the periodontium is to transport oxygen and nutrients to the tissue cells of the periodontium and to remove carbon dioxide and other waste products from the cells for elimination.

3. **Vascular Supply to the Periodontium** (Fig. 1-23)
   A. Maxillary gingiva, PDL, and alveolar bone
      1. Anterior and posterior-superior alveolar arteries
      2. Infraorbital artery
      3. Greater palatine artery
   B. Mandibular gingiva, PDL, and alveolar bone
      1. Inferior alveolar artery
      2. Branches of the inferior alveolar artery: the buccal, facial, mental, and sublingual arteries

4. **Vascular Supply to the Teeth and Periodontal Tissues**
   A. The major arteries
      1. Superior alveolar arteries—maxillary periodontal tissues
      2. Inferior alveolar artery—mandibular periodontal tissues
   B. Branch arteries (Figs. 1-24 and 1-25)
      1. The dental artery: a branch of the superior or inferior alveolar artery
      2. Intraseptal artery: enters the tooth socket
      3. Rami perforantes: terminal branches of the intraseptal artery; they penetrate the tooth socket and enter the PDL space where they anastomose (join) with the blood vessels from the alveolar bone and PDL
      4. Supraperiosteal blood vessels: located in the free gingiva and are the main supply of blood to the free gingiva; these vessels anastomose with blood vessels from the alveolar bone and PDL
      5. Subepithelial plexus: branches of the supraperiosteal blood vessels located in the connective tissue beneath the free and attached gingiva
      6. PDL vessels: supply the PDL and form a complex network of vessels that surrounds the root
      7. Dentogingival plexus: a fine-meshed network of blood vessels located in the connective tissue beneath the gingival sulcus

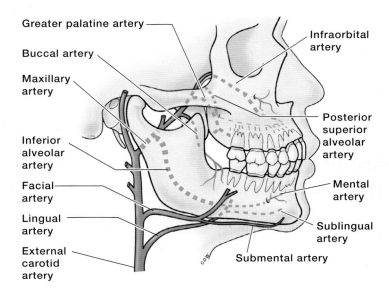

Figure 1-23. Vascular Supply to the Periodontium. A complex network of blood vessels supplies blood to the periodontium.

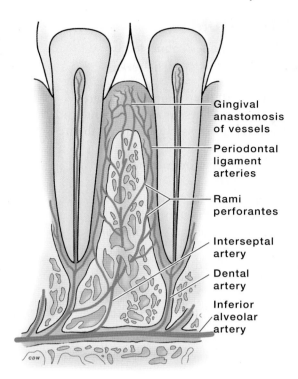

Gingival anastomosis of vessels

Periodontal ligament arteries

Rami perforantes

Interseptal artery

Dental artery

Inferior alveolar artery

Figure 1-24. Branch Arteries. The branch arteries supply blood to the teeth and periodontium.

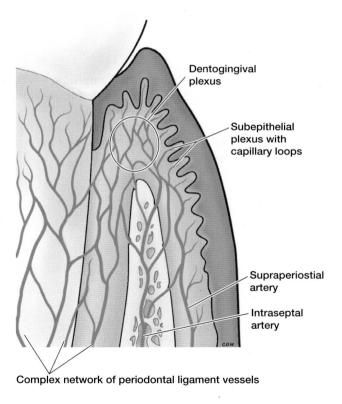

Dentogingival plexus

Subepithelial plexus with capillary loops

Supraperiostial artery

Intraseptal artery

Complex network of periodontal ligament vessels

Figure 1-25. Network of Vessels. A fine network of vessels supplies blood to gingiva, gingival connective tissue, and periodontal ligament.

LYMPHATIC SYSTEM AND THE PERIODONTIUM

1. **Description.** The **lymphatic system** is a network of lymph nodes connected by lymphatic vessels that plays an important role in the body's defense against infection.
2. **Function.** Lymph nodes (pronounced: limf nodes) are small bean shaped structures located on either side of the head, neck, armpits, and groin. These nodes filter out and trap bacteria, fungi, viruses, and other unwanted substances to safely eliminate them from the body.
3. **Lymph Drainage of the Periodontium.** The lymph from the periodontal tissues is drained to the lymph nodes of the head and neck (Fig. 1-26).
   A. Submandibular lymph nodes—drain most of the periodontal tissues
   B. Deep cervical lymph nodes—drain the palatal gingiva of the maxilla
   C. Submental lymph nodes—drain the gingiva in the region of the mandibular incisors
   D. Jugulodigastric lymph nodes—drain the gingiva in the third molar region

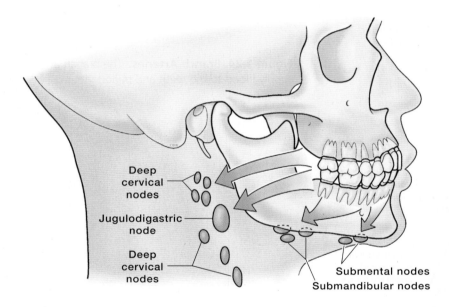

Figure 1-26. Lymphatic System of the Periodontium. The lymph from the periodontium is drained to the lymph nodes of the head and neck.

Chapter Summary Statement

The gingiva, PDL, cementum, and alveolar bone make up a system of tissues that surround the teeth and attach them to the alveolar bone. Each tissue of the periodontium plays a vital role in the functioning and retention of the teeth.

- The gingiva provides a tissue seal around the cervical portion of the teeth and covers the alveolar process.
- The PDL supports the tooth in its socket, provides nutrients and sensory feeling to the tooth, and maintains cementum and the alveolar bone of the tooth socket.
- The cementum anchors the PDL to the tooth and seals the ends of the open dentinal tubules. Cementum formation compensates for tooth wear due to occlusal attrition.
- The alveolar bone forms the bony sockets that provide support and protection for the roots of the teeth.

Section 3
Focus on Patients

Clinical Patient Care

CASE 1

A patient involved in an automobile accident receives a penetrating wound involving the oral cavity. The wound enters the alveolar mucosa near the apex of a lower premolar tooth and extends from the surface mucosa all the way through the tissues to the premolar tooth root. List periodontal tissues most likely injured by this penetrating wound.

CASE 2

A patient who has lost a maxillary lateral incisor tooth is scheduled to have a dental implant placed. The dental implant placement will require the clinician to prepare a hole with a drill in the bone formerly occupied by the lateral incisor tooth. Name the types of bone that will most probably be penetrated by the drill.

CASE 3

A dentist injects a local anesthetic before working on a maxillary molar tooth. The injection results in complete loss of sensation in the molar tooth and in most of the gingiva surrounding the molar tooth. Name the nerves that most likely have been affected by the injection of the local anesthetic.

References

1. Lang NP, Loe H. The relationship between the width of keratinized gingiva and gingival health. *J Periodontol.* 1972;43(10):623–627.
2. Ainamo J, Loe H. Anatomical characteristics of gingiva. A clinical and microscopic study of the free and attached gingiva. *J Periodontol.* 1966;37(1):5–13.
3. Cho MI, Garant PR. Development and general structure of the periodontium. *Periodontol 2000.* 2000;24:9–27.
4. Cimasoni G. Crevicular fluid updated. *Monogr Oral Sci.* 1983;12:III-VII, 1–152.
5. Saygin NE, Giannobile WV, Somerman MJ. Molecular and cell biology of cementum. *Periodontol 2000.* 2000;24:73–98.
6. Diekwisch TG. The developmental biology of cementum. *Int J Dev Biol.* 2001;45(5–6):695–706.
7. Sodek J, McKee MD. Molecular and cellular biology of alveolar bone. *Periodontol 2000.* 2000;24:99–126.

 STUDENT ANCILLARY RESOURCES

A wide variety of resources to enhance your learning and understanding of this chapter are available on thePoint®.

- Visit thePoint to access:
  - Audio Glossary
  - Animations
  - Suggested Readings
  - Answers to Review Questions
  - Case Studies

CHAPTER

2

Microscopic Anatomy of the Periodontium

Clinical Application. The dental hygienist is involved in a continuous process of interacting with patients, making clinical decisions, performing clinical procedures, evaluating new techniques, and adapting to evolving technologies. Nearly every action taken by a hygienist throughout a successful career requires a detailed knowledge of the anatomy of the tooth-supporting structures—the periodontium. Chapter 1 dealt with what is known about the fundamental structure of the complex system of tissues that support the teeth. Chapter 2 deals with the microscopic anatomy of these same structures. The information presented in these two chapters can serve as a basis for organizing thoughts about additional anatomical information as it becomes available through additional research.

Learning Objectives

- Describe the histology of the tissues and the function that each serves in the human body.
- List and define the layers that comprise the stratified squamous epithelium of the skin.
- Define keratin and describe its function in the epithelium.
- Describe the composition and function of the connective tissue.
- Describe the epithelium–connective tissue interface found in most tissues of the body, such as the interface between the epithelium and connective tissues of the skin.

- Define the term *cell junction* and describe its function in the epithelial tissues.
- Compare and contrast the terms *desmosome* and *hemidesmosome.*
- Identify the three anatomical areas of the gingival epithelium on an unlabeled drawing depicting the microscopic anatomy of the gingival epithelium.
- Describe the location and function of the following regions of the gingival epithelium: oral epithelium, sulcular epithelium, and junctional epithelium.
- State the level of keratinization present in each of the three anatomical areas of the gingival epithelium (keratinized, nonkeratinized, or parakeratinized).
- State which of the anatomical areas of the gingival epithelium have an uneven, wavy epithelium–connective tissue interface **in health** and which have a smooth junction in **health**.
- Identify the enamel, gingival connective tissue, junctional epithelium, internal basal lamina, external basal lamina, epithelial cells, desmosomes, and hemidesmosomes on an unlabeled drawing depicting the microscopic anatomy of the junctional epithelium and surrounding tissues.
- Define and describe the function of the supragingival fiber bundles and the periodontal ligament in the periodontium.
- Identify the principal fiber groups of the periodontal ligament on an unlabeled drawing.
- Define the terms *cementum* and *Sharpey fibers* and describe their function in the periodontium.
- State the three relationships that the cementum may have in relation to the enamel at the cementoenamel junction.
- Define the term alveolar bone and describe its function in the periodontium.

Key Terms

Histology
Tissue
Cells
Extracellular matrix
Epithelial tissue
Stratified squamous
 epithelium
Basal lamina
Keratinization
Keratinized epithelial cells
Nonkeratinized epithelial cells
Connective tissue
Epithelial–connective tissue
 interface

Basement membrane
Epithelial ridges
Connective tissue papillae
Cell junctions
Desmosome
Hemidesmosome
Gingival epithelium
Oral epithelium (OE)
Sulcular epithelium (SE)
Junctional epithelium (JE)
Keratinized
Parakeratinized
Keratin
Gingival crevicular fluid

Internal basal lamina
External basal lamina
Collagen fibers
Supragingival fiber bundles
Dentogingival unit
Periosteum
Periodontal ligament (PDL)
Fiber bundles of the PDL
Sharpey fibers
Cementum
OMG (overlap, meet, gap)
Alveolar process

Section 1
Histology of the Body's Tissues

Histology is a branch of anatomy concerned with the study of microscopic structures of tissues. Knowledge of the microscopic characteristics of tissues is a prerequisite for understanding the microscopic anatomy of the periodontium. Section 1 reviews the microscopic anatomy of the epithelial and connective tissues of the body.

MICROSCOPIC ANATOMY OF A TISSUE

A **tissue** is a group of interconnected cells that perform a similar function within an organism. For example, muscle cells group together to form muscle tissue that functions to move parts of the body. The tissues and organs of the body are composed of several different types of cells and extracellular elements outside of the cells.

1. Cells
   A. **Cells** are the smallest structural unit of living matter capable of functioning independently.
   B. Cells group together to form a tissue.
   C. The four basic types of tissues are epithelial, connective, nerve, and muscle tissues.
2. **Extracellular Matrix.** Tissues are not made up solely of cells. A gel-like substance containing interwoven protein fibers surrounds most cells.
   A. The **extracellular matrix** is a mesh-like material that surrounds the cells (Fig. 2-1). It is like scaffolding for the cells. This material helps hold cells together and provides a framework within which cells can migrate and interact with one another.
   B. The extracellular matrix consists of ground substance and fibers.
      1. The ground substance is a gel-like material that fills the space between the cells.
      2. The fibers consist of collagen, elastin, and reticular fibers. Collagens are the major proteins of the extracellular matrix.
   C. Amount of Extracellular Matrix
      1. In epithelial tissue, the extracellular matrix is scanty, consisting mainly of a thin mat called the basal lamina, which underlies the epithelium.
      2. In connective tissue, the extracellular matrix is more plentiful than the cells that it surrounds.

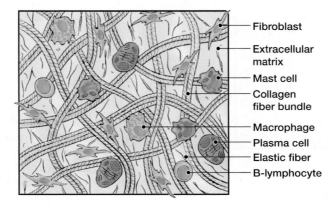

Fibroblast
Extracellular matrix
Mast cell
Collagen fiber bundle
Macrophage
Plasma cell
Elastic fiber
B-lymphocyte

Figure 2-1. Extracellular Matrix. The extracellular matrix surrounds the cells of a tissue and comprises fibers and a gel-like substance.

MICROSCOPIC ANATOMY OF EPITHELIAL TISSUE

1. **Description.** The epithelial tissue is the tissue that makes up the outer surface of the body (skin) and lines the body cavities such as the mouth, stomach, and intestines (mucosa). The skin and mucosa of the oral cavity are made up of **stratified squamous epithelium**—a type of epithelium that comprises flat cells arranged in several layers.
2. **Composition of Epithelial Tissue**
   A. **Plentiful Cells.** Most of the volume of epithelial tissue consists of many closely packed epithelial cells (Fig. 2-2). Epithelial cells are bound together into sheets.
   B. **Sparse Extracellular Matrix**
      1. The extracellular matrix is a minor component of the epithelial tissue consisting mainly the basal lamina.
      2. The **basal lamina** is a thin mat of extracellular matrix secreted by the epithelial cells. This basal lamina mat supports the epithelium (somewhat like the scaffolding of a building).
3. **Keratinization.** Keratinization—the process by which epithelial cells on the surface of the skin become stronger and waterproof.
   A. **Keratinized Epithelial Cells**
      1. **Keratinized epithelial cells** have no nuclei and form a tough, resistant layer on the surface of the skin.
      2. The most heavily keratinized epithelium of the body is found on the palms of the hands and soles of the feet.
   B. **Nonkeratinized Epithelial Cells**
      1. **Nonkeratinized epithelial cells** have nuclei and act as a cushion against mechanical stress and wear. Nonkeratinized epithelial cells are softer and more flexible.
      2. Nonkeratinized epithelium is found in areas such as the mucosal lining of the cheeks—permitting the mobility needed to speak, chew, and make facial expressions.
4. **Blood Supply.** Epithelial tissues do not contain blood vessels; nourishment is received from blood vessels contained in the underlying connective tissue (Fig. 2-2).

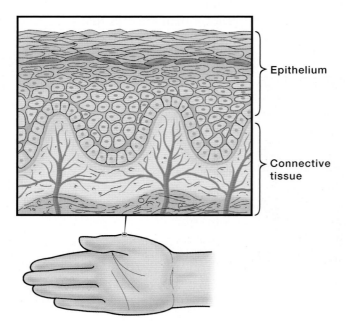

Epithelium

Connective tissue

Figure 2-2. Stratified Squamous Epithelium and Connective Tissue of the Skin. The epithelium of the skin consists of many closely packed epithelial cells and a thin basal lamina. The epithelium of the skin rests on a supporting bed of connective tissue. The epithelium does not contain blood vessels; nourishment is received from blood vessels in the underlying connective tissue.

MICROSCOPIC ANATOMY OF CONNECTIVE TISSUE

1. Description. Connective tissue fills the spaces between the tissues and organs in the body. It supports and binds other tissues. Connective tissue consists of cells separated by abundant extracellular substance.
2. **Composition of Connective Tissue**
   A. **Sparse Cells.** Connective tissue cells are sparsely distributed in the extracellular matrix.
      1. Fibroblasts ("fiber-builders")—cells that form the extracellular matrix (fibers and ground substance) and secrete it into the intercellular spaces
      2. Macrophages and neutrophils—phagocytes ("cell-eaters") that devour dying cells and microorganisms that invade the body
      3. Lymphocytes—cells that play a major role in the immune response
   B. **Plentiful Extracellular Matrix.** The extracellular matrix—a rich gel-like substance containing a network of strong fibers—is the major component of connective tissue. The network of fibers matrix, rather than the cells, gives connective tissue the strength to withstand mechanical forces.
3. Dental Connective Tissue. All dental tissues of the tooth—cementum, dentin, alveolar bone, and the pulp—are specialized forms of connective tissue *except enamel*. Enamel is an epithelial tissue.

EPITHELIAL–CONNECTIVE TISSUE INTERFACE

1. Description. The epithelial–connective tissue interface is the boundary where the epithelial and connective tissues meet.
2. **The Basement Membrane and Basal Lamina**
   A. As discussed previously, the basal lamina is a thin layer secreted by the epithelial cells on which the epithelium sits. The term *basal lamina* often is confused with the term *basement membrane* and is sometimes used inconsistently in the literature.
   B. The basal lamina is not visible under the light microscope but can be distinguished under the higher magnification of an electron microscope. The basal lamina assists the attachment of the epithelial cells to adjacent structures, such as the tooth surface.
   C. The term basement membrane specifies a thin layer of tissue visible with a light microscope beneath the epithelium. The basement membrane is formed by the combination of a basal lamina and a reticular lamina.
3. **Characteristics of the Epithelial–Connective Tissue Boundary**
   A. **Wavy Boundary.** In most places in the body, the epithelium meets the connective in a wavy, uneven manner (Fig. 2-3).
      1. Epithelial ridges—deep extensions of epithelium that reach down into the connective tissue. The epithelial ridges are also known as rete pegs.
      2. Connective tissue papillae—finger-like extensions of connective tissue that extend up into the epithelium.
   B. **Smooth Boundary**
      1. Some specialized epithelial tissues in the body meet the connective tissue in a smooth interface that has no epithelial ridges or connective tissue papillae.
      2. Some anatomical areas of the gingiva have an epithelial–connective tissue interface that is smooth.

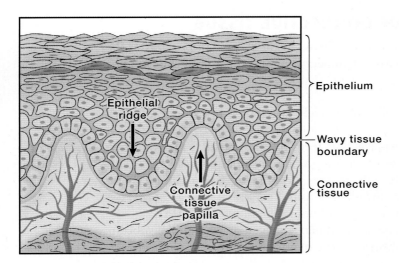

Figure 2-3. Wavy Epithelial–Connective Tissue Interface. In most cases, the epithelium meets the connective tissue at an uneven, wavy border. Epithelial ridges extend down into the connective tissue. Connective tissue papillae extend upward into the epithelium.

4. **Function of the Wavy Tissue Boundary**
   A. **Enhances Adhesion.** The wavy tissue interface enhances the adhesion of the epithelium to the connective tissue by increasing the surface area of the junction between the two tissues. This strong adhesion of the epithelium allows the skin to resist mechanical forces.
   B. **Provides Nourishment.** The wavy junction between the epithelium and connective tissue also increases the area from which the epithelium can receive nourishment from the underlying connective tissue. The epithelium does not have its own blood supply; blood vessels are carried close to the epithelium in the connective tissue papillae.

EPITHELIAL CELL JUNCTIONS

Neighboring epithelial cells attach to one another by specialized cell junctions that give the tissue strength to withstand mechanical forces and to form a protective barrier.

1. **Definition.** Cell junctions are cellular structures that mechanically attach a cell and its cytoskeleton to its neighboring cells or to the basal lamina.
2. **Purpose.** Cell junctions bind cells together, so that they can function as a strong structural unit. Tissues such as the epithelium of the skin that must withstand severe mechanical stresses have the most abundant number of cell junctions.
3. **Forms of Epithelial Cell Junctions**
   A. **Desmosome**—a specialized cell junction that connects two neighboring epithelial cells and their cytoskeletons together. You might think of desmosomes as being like the snaps used to close a denim jacket. Instead of fastening the front of a jacket together, desmosomes fasten epithelial cells together (Fig. 2-4A,B).
      1. A cell-to-cell connection
      2. An important form of cell junction found in the gingival epithelium
   B. **Hemidesmosome**—a specialized cell junction that connects the epithelial cells to the basal lamina (Fig. 2-4B).
      1. A cell-to-basal lamina connection
      2. An important form of cell junction found in the gingival epithelium

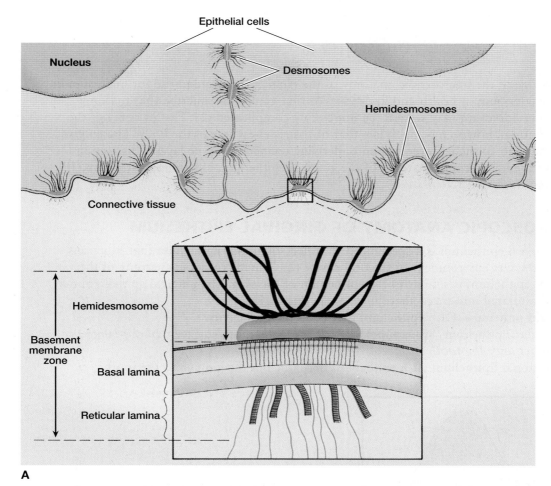

Figure 2-4. A: The Epithelium–Connective Tissue Interface. The epithelium–connective tissue interface is the site of the basement membrane zone, a complex structure mostly synthesized by the epithelial cells. **Inset:** A representation of an electron micrograph showing the hemidesmosomal attachment to the basal lamina. (Adapted with permission from Rubin R, Strayer DS. *Rubin's Pathology: Clinicopathologic Foundations of Medicine.* 5th ed. Philadelphia, PA: Lippincott Williams & Wilkins; 2008.)

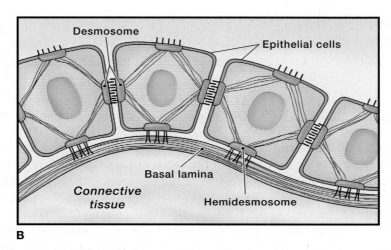

Figure 2-4. B: Epithelial Cell Junctions. Epithelial cells attach to each other with specialized cell junctions called desmosomes. Hemidesmosomes attach the epithelial cells to the basal lamina.

Section 2
Histology of the Gingiva

Knowledge of the microscopic anatomy of the gingiva is a prerequisite for understanding the periodontium in health and in disease. At first glance, the microscopic anatomy of the periodontium may seem to be impossibly complicated (1). The anatomy of the periodontium, however, is much like that of tissues elsewhere in the body. **The gingiva consists of an epithelial layer and an underlying connective tissue layer.** This section reviews the microscopic anatomy of the gingival epithelium, junctional epithelium (JE), and gingival connective tissues.

MICROSCOPIC ANATOMY OF GINGIVAL EPITHELIUM

The gingival epithelium is a specialized stratified squamous epithelium that functions well in the wet environment of the oral cavity (2). The microscopic anatomy of the gingival epithelium is similar to the epithelium of the skin. The gingival epithelium may be differentiated into three anatomical areas (Fig. 2-5):
1. Oral Epithelium (OE): epithelium that faces the oral cavity
2. Sulcular Epithelium (SE): epithelium that faces the tooth surface *without being in contact with the tooth surface*
3. Junctional Epithelium (JE): epithelium that attaches the gingiva to the tooth

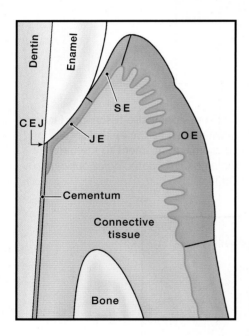

Figure 2-5. Three Areas of the Gingival Epithelium. The gingival epithelium has three distinct areas:

- **JE**—junctional epithelium at the base of the sulcus
- **SE**—sulcular epithelium that lines the sulcus
- **OE**—oral epithelium covering the free and attached gingiva

1. Oral epithelium (OE). The oral epithelium covers the outer surface of the free gingiva and attached gingiva; it extends from the crest of the gingival margin to the mucogingival junction. The OE is the only part of the periodontium that is visible to the unaided eye.
   A. Cellular Structure of the Oral Epithelium
      1. The OE may be keratinized or parakeratinized (partially keratinized). Keratin is a tough, fibrous structural protein that occurs in the outer layer of the skin and the OE (Fig. 2-6).

2. The OE is stratified squamous epithelium that can be divided into the following cell layers (Fig. 2-6):
   a. Basal cell layer: cube-shaped cells
   b. Prickle cell layer: spine-like cells with large intercellular spaces. The cells of both the basal and prickle cell layers attach to each other with desmosomes
   c. Granular cell layer: flattened cells and increased intracellular keratin
   d. Keratinized cell layer: flattened cells with extensive intracellular keratin

   B. **Interface with Gingival Connective Tissue.** *In health, OE joins with the connective tissue in a **wavy interface with epithelial ridges** (Figs. 2-7 and 2-8).*

2. **Sulcular Epithelium.** Sulcular epithelium (SE) is the epithelial lining of the gingival sulcus. It extends from the crest of the gingival margin to the coronal edge of the JE.

   A. **Cellular Structure of the Sulcular Epithelium**
   1. The SE is a thin, nonkeratinized epithelium (3).
   2. The SE has three cellular layers (Fig. 2-6):
      a. Basal cell layer
      b. Prickle cell layer
      c. Superficial cell layer: flattened cells without keratin
   3. The SE is permeable allowing fluid to flow from the gingival connective tissue into the sulcus. This fluid is known as the **gingival crevicular fluid**. The flow of gingival crevicular fluid is slight in health and increases in disease.

   B. **Interface with Gingival Connective Tissue.** In health, the SE joins the connective tissue at a *smooth interface* with no epithelial ridges (no wavy junction).

3. **Junctional Epithelium.** Junctional epithelium (JE) is the specialized epithelium that forms the base of the sulcus and joins the gingiva to the tooth surface. ***The gingiva surrounds the cervix of the tooth and attaches to the tooth by means of the JE. The base of the sulcus is made up of the coronal-most cells of the JE.*** In health, the JE attaches to the tooth at a level that is slightly coronal to the cementoenamel junction (CEJ).

   A. **Cellular Structure of the Junctional Epithelium**
   1. Keratinization of JE
      a. The JE is a thin, nonkeratinized epithelium.
      b. Nonkeratinized epithelial cells of both the sulcular and junctional areas of the gingival epithelium make them a less effective protective covering. Thus, the sulcular and junctional areas provide the easiest point of entry for bacteria or bacterial products to invade the connective tissue of the gingiva.
   2. The JE has only two cell layers (Figs. 2-6 and 2-7):
      a. Basal cell layer
      b. Prickle cell layer
   3. Length and Width of the JE
      a. The JE ranges from 0.71 to 1.35 mm in length (4).
      b. The JE is about 15 to 30 cells thick at the coronal zone—the zone that attaches highest on the crown of the tooth.
      c. The JE tapers to 4 to 5 cells thick at the apical zone.

   B. **JE Interface with Gingival Connective Tissue.** In health, the JE has a *smooth tissue interface* with the connective tissue (no wavy junctions).

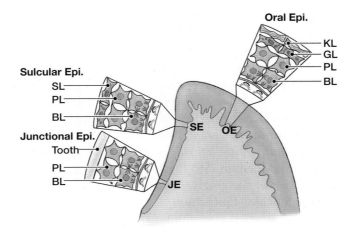

Figure 2-6. Cell Layers of the Gingival Epithelium. The cell layers of the oral, sulcular, and junctional epithelium. Illustration key: KL, keratinized cell layer; GL, granular cell layer; SL, superficial cell layer; PL, prickle cell layer; BL, basal cell layer.

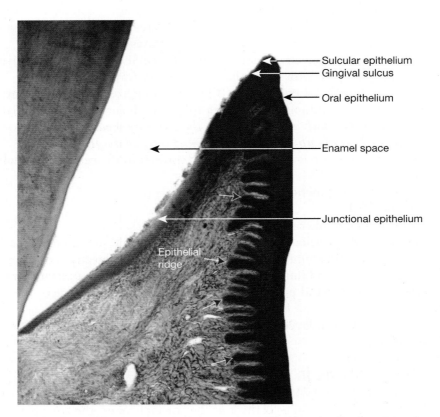

Figure 2-7. Human Gingiva. This photograph shows a decalcified longitudinal section of an incisor tooth as seen through an ordinary light microscope. All of the calcium hydroxyapatite crystals have been extracted from the tooth and from its bony alveolus. Since enamel is composed almost completely of calcium hydroxyapatite crystals, only the space where enamel used to be—the enamel space—is represented in this photograph. The sulcular epithelium of the free gingiva borders a space known as the gingival sulcus. Observe the well-developed epithelial ridges (identified by label and *arrows*) of the oral epithelium. (Adapted with permission from Gartner LP, Hiatt JL. *Color Atlas and Text of Histology*. Philadelphia, PA: Lippincott Williams & Wilkins; 2013.)

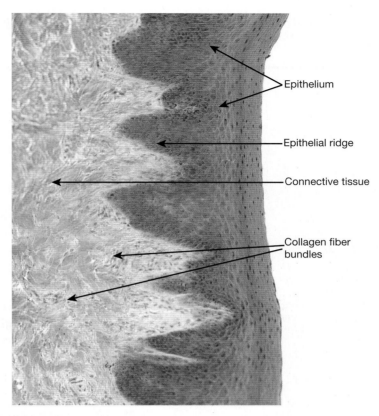

Epithelium

Epithelial ridge

Connective tissue

Collagen fiber bundles

Figure 2-8. Epithelial Ridges. This photograph shows the epithelial–connective junction as seen through an ordinary light microscope. The tall epithelial ridges of the epithelium (in *dark red*) extend down into the underlying connective tissue. Collagen fiber bundles are visible in the connective tissue. (Adapted with permission from Gartner LP, Hiatt JL. *Color Atlas and Text of Histology*. Philadelphia, PA: Lippincott Williams & Wilkins; 2013.)

WHY THE TEETH NEED A JUNCTIONAL EPITHELIUM?

1. **The Teeth Create a Break in the Epithelial Protective Covering**
   A. **Protective Epithelial Sheet Covers the Body**
      1. A continuous sheet of epithelium protects the body by covering its outer surfaces and lining the body's cavities, including the oral cavity.
      2. The teeth penetrate this protective covering by erupting through the epithelium, thus creating an opening through which microorganisms can enter the body.
   B. **The Teeth Puncture the Protective Epithelial Sheet**
      1. The body attempts to seal the opening created when a tooth penetrates the epithelium by attaching the epithelium to the tooth.
      2. The word "junction" means "connection"; thus, the epithelium that is connected to the tooth is termed the "junctional epithelium."
2. **Functions of Junctional Epithelium**
   A. **Epithelial Attachment.** The JE provides an attachment between the gingiva and the tooth surface, thus providing a seal at the base of the gingival sulcus or periodontal pocket (Fig. 2-9).
   B. **Barrier.** The JE provides a protective barrier between the plaque biofilm and the connective tissue of the periodontium.

C. **Host Defense.** The epithelial cells play a role in defending the periodontium from bacterial infection by signaling the immune response (5).

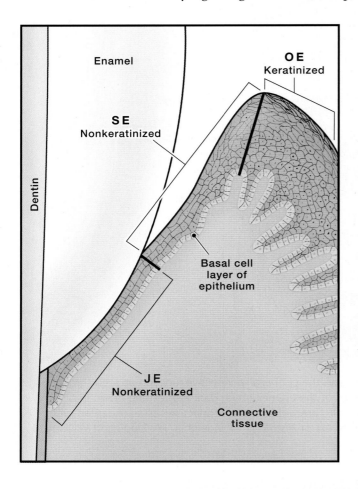

Figure 2-9. Microscopic Anatomy of the Three Areas of the Gingival Epithelium. Interface with Connective Tissue.

- **OE** (oral epithelium)—these epithelial cells form the outer layer of the free and attached gingiva.

- **SE** (sulcular epithelium)—these epithelial cells extend from the edge of the JE coronally to the crest of the gingival margin.

- **JE** (junctional epithelium)—these epithelial cells join the gingiva to the tooth surface at the base of the sulcus.

ATTACHMENT OF THE CELLS OF THE JUNCTIONAL EPITHELIUM

1. **Microscopic Anatomy of Junctional Epithelium**
   A. **Components of the Junctional Epithelium (JE).** The JE consists of the following:
      1. Plentiful Cells
         a. Layers of closely packed epithelial cells
         b. Desmosomes and hemidesmosomes—specialized cell junctions
      2. A Sparse Extracellular Matrix
         a. Internal basal lamina—a thin basal lamina between the JE and the tooth surface.
         b. External basal lamina—a thin basal lamina between the JE and the gingival connective tissue.
2. **Attachment of Junctional Epithelium to the Tooth Surface**
   A. **Attachment to the Tooth Surface**
      1. The JE cells next to the tooth surface form *hemidesmosomes* that enable these cells to attach to the *internal basal lamina* and the surface of the tooth (6–9).
      2. The internal basal lamina is a thin sheet of extracellular matrix adjacent to the tooth surface.

3. The epithelial cells physically attach to the tooth surface by four to eight hemidesmosomes per micron at the coronal zone and two hemidesmosomes per micron in the apical zone of the JE (10,11). The apical zone is the area of the JE with the least adhesiveness.
4. The attachment of the hemidesmosomes and internal basal lamina to the tooth surface is not static; rather, the cells of the JE appear to be capable of moving along the tooth surface.

B. **Attachment to the Underlying Gingival Connective Tissue**
1. The epithelial cells of the JE attach to the underlying *gingival connective tissue* via **hemidesmosomes** and the **external basal lamina** (Fig. 2-10) (8,12,13).
2. In health, the JE has a *smooth tissue interface* with the connective tissue (no wavy junctions).

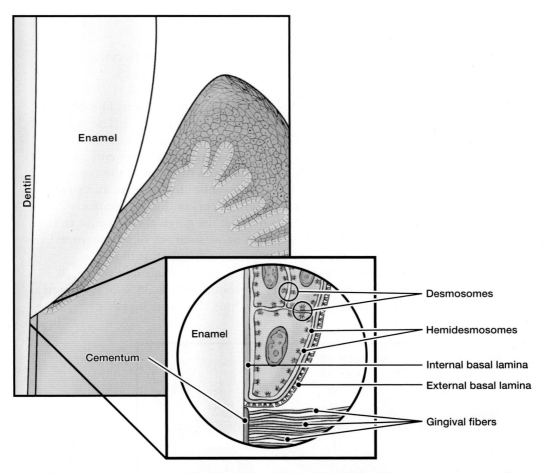

Figure 2-10. Microscopic Anatomy of the Junctional Epithelium (JE). Microscopic structures of the junctional epithelium include the epithelial cells, desmosomes, external and internal basal laminae, and hemidesmosomes.

MICROSCOPIC ANATOMY OF GINGIVAL CONNECTIVE TISSUE

1. **Function of Gingival Connective Tissue.** The gingival connective tissue of the free and attached gingiva provides solidity to the gingiva and attaches the gingiva to the cementum of the root and the alveolar bone (14–16). The gingival connective tissue is also known as the lamina propria.

2. **Components of the Gingival Connective Tissue**
   A. **Cells**
      1. In contrast to the gingival epithelium (which has an abundance of cells and sparse extracellular matrix), the gingival connective tissue has an abundance of extracellular matrix and few cells (Fig. 2-11).
      2. Cells comprise about 5% of the gingival connective tissue.
      3. The different types of cells present in the gingival connective tissue are the following
         a. Fibroblasts
         b. Mast cells
         c. Immune cells, such as macrophages, neutrophils, and lymphocytes
      4. The fibers of the connective tissue are produced by the fibroblasts.
   B. **Extracellular Matrix**
      1. The major components of the connective tissue are protein fibers, fibroblasts, vessels, and nerves that are embedded in the extracellular matrix. The matrix of the connective tissue is produced mainly by the fibroblasts.
      2. The matrix is the medium in which the connective tissue cells are embedded and it is essential for the maintenance of the normal function of the connective tissue. The transportation of water, nutrients, metabolites, oxygen, and so on to and from the individual connective tissue cells occurs within the matrix.
      3. Protein fibers account for about 55% to 65% of the gingival connective tissue. Most of these are **collagen fibers** that form a dense network of strong, rope-like cables that secure and hold the gingival connective tissues together.
      4. The collagen fibers enable the gingiva to form a rigid cuff around the tooth.
      5. Gel-like material between the cells makes up about 30% to 35% of the gingival connective tissue. This gel-like material helps hold the tissue together.

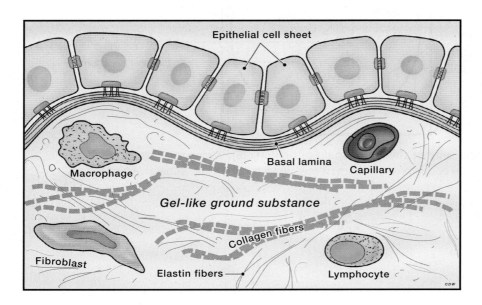

Figure 2-11. Microscopic Anatomy of Gingival Connective Tissue. The gingival connective tissue comprises a gel-like substance, protein fibers, and cells.

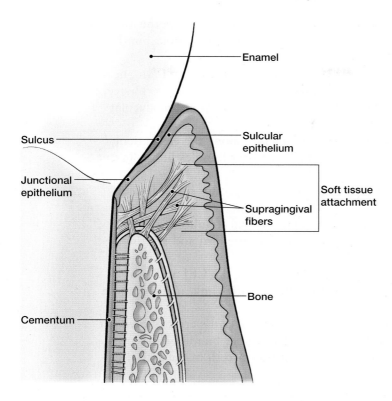

Figure 2-12. Supragingival Fibers of Gingival Connective Tissue. The gingival fibers are rope-like collagen fiber bundles in the gingival connective tissue. These fibers form a soft tissue attachment coronal to the alveolar bone.

3. **The Supragingival Fiber Bundles of the Gingival Connective Tissue.** The supragingival fiber bundles (gingival fibers) are a network of rope-like collagen fiber bundles in the gingival connective tissue (Fig. 2-12). These fibers are located coronal to (above) the crest of the alveolar bone.

   A. **Characteristics of the Fiber Bundles**
      1. The fiber bundles are embedded in the gel-like extracellular matrix of the gingival connective tissue.
      2. The subgingival fiber bundles strengthen the attachment of the JE to the tooth by bracing the gingival margin against the tooth surface.
      3. Together the JE and the gingival fibers are referred to as the **dentogingival unit**. The dentogingival unit acts to provide structural support to the gingival tissue.

   B. **Functions of the Gingival Fiber Bundles**
      1. Brace the free gingiva firmly against the tooth and reinforce the attachment of the JE to the tooth.
      2. Provide the free gingiva with the rigidity needed to withstand the frictional forces that result during mastication.
      3. Unite the free gingiva with the cementum of the root and alveolar bone.
      4. Connect adjacent teeth to one another to control tooth positioning within the dental arch.

   C. **Classification of Gingival Fiber Groups.** The supragingival fiber bundles are classified based on their orientation, sites of insertion, and the structures that they connect (Figs. 2-13 and 2-14).
      1. **Alveologingival fibers**—extend from the periosteum of the alveolar crest into the gingival connective tissue. These fiber bundles attach the gingiva to the bone. (The **periosteum** is a dense membrane composed of fibrous connective tissue that closely wraps the outer surface of the alveolar bone.)

2. **Circular fibers**—encircle the tooth in a ring-like manner coronal to the alveolar crest and are not attached to the cementum of the tooth. These fiber bundles connect adjacent teeth to one another.

3. **Dentogingival fibers**—embedded in the cementum near the CEJ and fan out into the gingival connective tissue. These fibers act to attach the gingiva to the teeth.

4. **Periostogingival fibers**—extend laterally from the periosteum of the alveolar bone. These fibers attach the gingiva to the bone.

5. **Intergingival fibers**—extend in a mesiodistal direction along the entire dental arch and around the last molars in the arch. These fiber bundles link adjacent teeth into a dental arch unit.

6. **Intercircular fibers**—encircle several teeth. These fiber groups link adjacent teeth into a dental arch unit.

7. **Interpapillary fibers**—are located in the papillae coronal to (above) the transseptal fiber bundles. These fiber groups connect the oral and vestibular interdental papillae of posterior teeth.

8. **Transgingival fibers**—extend from the cementum near the CEJ and run horizontally between adjacent teeth. These fiber bundles link adjacent teeth into a dental arch unit.

9. **Transseptal**—pass from the cementum of one tooth, over the crest of alveolar bone, to the cementum of the adjacent tooth. These fiber bundles connect adjacent teeth to one another and secure alignment of teeth in the arch.

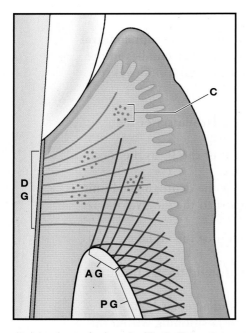

Figure 2-13. Supragingival Fiber Groups.

- C—circular
- AG—alveologingival
- DG—dentogingival
- PG—periostogingival

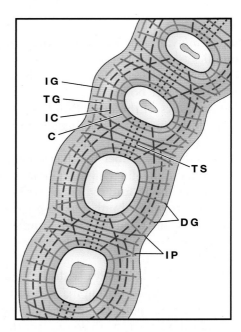

Figure 2-14. Supragingival Fiber Groups of the Mandibular Arch (Occlusal View, Looking Down on the Mandibular Arch).

- C—circular
- IG—intergingival
- IC—intercircular
- IP—interpapillary
- DG—dentogingival
- TG—transgingival
- TS—transseptal

4. **The Periodontal Ligament Fibers of the Gingival Connective Tissue**
   A. **Definition.** The **periodontal ligament (PDL)** is a thin sheet of fibrous connective tissue that surrounds the roots of the teeth and joins the root cementum with the socket wall. The thickness of the PDL ranges from 0.05 to 0.25 mm depending on the age of the patient and the function of the tooth (17,18).

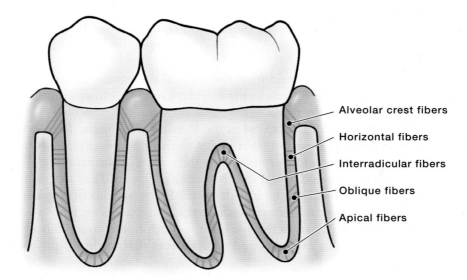

Alveolar crest fibers

Horizontal fibers

Interradicular fibers

Oblique fibers

Apical fibers

Figure 2-15. Principal Fiber Groups of the Periodontal Ligament. The fibers of the PDL are classified as the alveolar crest, horizontal, interradicular, oblique, and apical.

   B. **Components of the Periodontal Ligament.** The PDL consists of connective tissue fibers, cells, and extracellular matrix.
      1. **Cells.** The cells of the PDL are mainly fibroblasts with some cementoblasts and osteoblasts.
      2. **Extracellular Matrix.**
         a. The extracellular matrix of the PDL is similar to the extracellular matrix of other connective tissue. This rich gel-like substance contains specialized connective fibers.
      3. **Fiber Bundles.** The **fiber bundles of the PDL** are a specialized connective tissue that surrounds the root of the tooth and connects it with the alveolar bone. These fibers are the largest component of the PDL.
         a. The rope-like collagen fiber bundles of the PDL stretch across the space between the cementum and the alveolar bone of the tooth socket (Fig. 2-15).
         b. The collagen fiber bundles are anchored on one side in the cementum covering the tooth root; on the other side, they are embedded in the bone of the tooth socket.
      4. **Blood Vessels and Nerve Supply.** The PDL has a rich supply of nerves and blood vessels.
   C. **Functions of the Periodontal Ligament**
      1. Supportive function—the major function of the PDL is to anchor the tooth to its bony socket and to separate the tooth from the socket wall, so that the root does not collide with the bone during mastication.
      2. Sensory function—the PDL is supplied with nerve fibers that transmit tactile pressure (such as a tap with dental instrument against tooth) and pain sensations.

3. Nutritive function—the PDL is supplied with blood vessels that provide nutrients to the cementum and bone.

4. Formative function—the PDL contains cementoblasts ("cementum builders") that produce cementum throughout the life of the tooth while the osteoblasts ("bone builders") maintain the bone of the tooth socket.

5. Resorptive function—in response to severe pressure, cells of the PDL (osteoclasts) can produce rapid bone resorption and, sometimes, resorption of cementum.

D. **Principal Fiber Groups of the PDL.** The tooth is joined to the bone by bundles of collagen fibers that can be divided into the five groups based on their location and orientation (Fig. 2-15).

1. **Alveolar crest fiber group**—extend from the cervical cementum, running downward in a diagonal direction, to the alveolar crest. This fiber group resists horizontal movements of the tooth.

2. **Horizontal fiber group**—located apical to the alveolar crest fibers. They extend from the cementum to the bone at right angles to the long axis to the root. This fiber group resists horizontal pressure against the crown of the tooth.

3. **Oblique fiber group**—located apical to the horizontal group. They extend from the cementum to the bone, running in a diagonal direction. This fiber group resists vertical pressures that threaten to drive the root into its socket.

4. **Apical fiber group**—extend from the apex of the tooth to the bone. This fiber group secures the tooth in its socket and resists forces that might lift the tooth out of the socket.

5. **Interradicular fiber group** (present only in multirooted teeth)—extend from the cementum in the furcation area of the tooth to the interradicular septum of the alveolar bone. These fiber groups help to stabilize the tooth in its socket.

E. **Sharpey Fibers of the Periodontal Ligament**

1. The ends of the PDL fibers that are embedded in the cementum and alveolar bone are known as **Sharpey fibers** (Figs. 2-16 and 2-17).

2. The attachment of the fiber bundles occurs when the cementum and bone are forming. As cementum forms, the tissue hardens around the ends of the periodontal fibers (Sharpey fibers) surrounding them with cementum. The same process occurs during bone formation. As the bony wall of the tooth socket hardens, it surrounds the ends of the periodontal fibers with bone. The ends of the fiber bundles become trapped in the bone that forms around them.

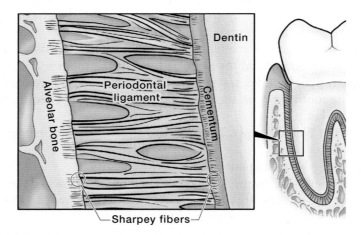

Figure 2-16. Sharpey Fibers. The ends of the periodontal ligament fibers that are embedded in the alveolar bone and the cementum are known as Sharpey Fibers.

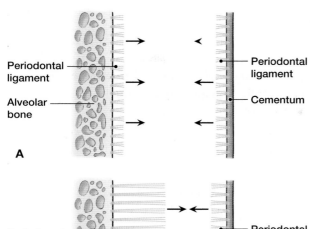

Periodontal ligament

Alveolar bone

A

Periodontal ligament

Cementum

Figure 2-17. Development of the Periodontal Ligament Fibers.

A: Fine collagen fibers arise from the root cementum. Similarly, collagen fibers arise from the alveolar bone proper.

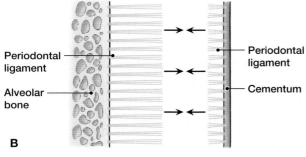

Periodontal ligament

Alveolar bone

B

Periodontal ligament

Cementum

B: The fibers grow into the midportion of periodontal ligament space.

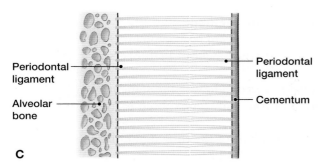

Periodontal ligament

Alveolar bone

C

Periodontal ligament

Cementum

C: The fibers from the root cementum fuse with fibers from the alveolar bone proper.

Section 3
Histology of the Root Cementum and Alveolar Bone

Section 3 reviews the microscopic anatomy of the cementum and alveolar bone. Knowledge of the microscopic anatomy of these structures is a prerequisite to understanding the function of these structures in health and the alterations in disease.

MICROSCOPIC ANATOMY OF CEMENTUM

1. **Definition.** Cementum is a mineralized layer of connective tissue that covers the root of the tooth. Anatomically, cementum is part of the tooth; however, it is also a part of the periodontium.
   A. **Functions of Cementum**
      1. Seals and covers the open dentinal tubules and acts to protect the underlying dentin (Fig. 2-18).
      2. Attaches the periodontal fibers to the tooth.
      3. Compensates for attrition of teeth at their occlusal or incisal surfaces. Over time, teeth experience wear at their occlusal or incisal surfaces. Cementum is formed at the apical areas of the roots to compensate for loss of tooth tissues due to attrition.
   B. **Conservation of Cementum During Periodontal Instrumentation**
      1. Conservation of cementum is ideal since loss of cementum is accompanied by exposure of the dentinal tubules and by a loss of attachment of PDL fibers to the root surface.
      2. Until recently, intentional aggressive removal of cementum was the standard of care for treatment during instrumentation of root surfaces exposed by the apical migration of the JE.
         a. Intentional removal cementum on the coronal half of the root should be avoided as the cementum is important to the health of the periodontium.
         b. Over the course of many years, overzealous instrumentation can result in removal of all cementum and exposure of the underlying dentin.

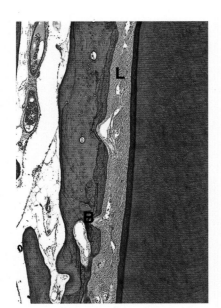

Figure 2-18. Cementum and Tooth-Supporting Structures.

- A thin layer of cementum (appearing as a **blue band**) covers the dentin of the root.
- The periodontal ligament (**L**) holds the tooth in the bony socket of the alveolar bone (**B**).

(Used with permission from Mills SE. *Histology for Pathologists*. 3rd ed. Philadelphia, PA: Lippincott Williams & Wilkins; 2006:423, Figure 15-39.)

2. **Components of Mature Cementum.** Cementum contains collagen fibers embedded in an organic matrix (19).
   A. **Collagen Fibers.** The organic matrix of cementum is composed of a framework of densely packed collagen fibers held together by the gel-like extracellular ground substance. These fibers are oriented more or less parallel to the long axis of the tooth.
   B. **Mineralized Portion.** The mineralized portion of cementum is made up of hydroxyapatite crystals (calcium and phosphate).
   C. **Vessels and Innervation.** Cementum contains no blood vessels or nerves. (Hypersensitivity of the root surface occurs when the cementum is removed exposing the dentin. It is the dentin that is sensitive to brushing or the touch of a dental instrument.)
3. **Types of Cementum**
   A. **Acellular Cementum.** Acellular cementum is primarily responsible for attaching the tooth to the alveolar bone (Fig. 2-19).
      1. Contains no living cells within its mineralized tissue
      2. First to be formed and covers approximately the cervical-third or half of the root
      3. No new acellular cementum is produced during the life of the tooth
      4. Thickness ranges from 30 to 60 microns
      5. Sharpey fibers make up most of the structure of acellular cementum
   B. **Cellular Cementum**
      1. Contains cementoblasts and fibroblasts within its mineralized tissue (Fig. 2-19)
      2. Formed after the tooth has erupted and is less calcified than acellular cementum
      3. Deposited in intervals throughout the life of the tooth (thickness increases with age)
      4. Thickness ranges from 150 to 200 microns
      5. Sharpey fibers make up a smaller portion of cellular cementum

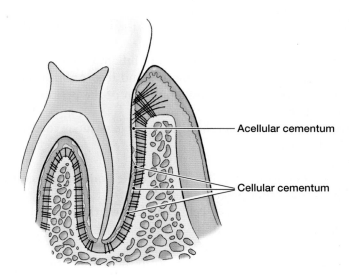

Figure 2-19. Types of Cementum. Acellular cementum covers approximately the cervical third or half of the root. New acellular cementum normally is not produced during the life of the tooth. Cellular cementum covers the apical half of the root. It is deposited throughout the life of the tooth and increases in thickness with age.

4. **Relationship of Cementum to Enamel at the CEJ.** The cementum covering the root may have any one of three relationships with the enamel of the tooth crown. In order of frequency, the cementum may overlap the enamel, meet the enamel, or there is a gap between the cementum and enamel. This order of frequency is known as the OMG (overlap, meet, gap) (Fig. 2-20).
   A. **Overlap**—in 60% of all cases, the cementum overlaps the enamel for a short distance.
   B. **Meet**—in 30% of all cases, the cementum meets the enamel.
   C. **Gap**—in 10% of all cases, there is a small gap between the cementum and enamel (exposing the dentin in this area). The patient may experience discomfort (dentinal sensitivity) during instrumentation. The use of local anesthesia may be helpful during instrumentation, and desensitization of sensitive areas should be performed following instrumentation.

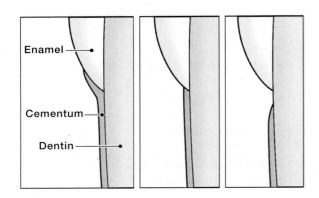

Figure 2-20. Relationship of Cementum to Enamel at the Cementoenamel Junction. In order of frequency, the cementum may (1) overlap the enamel, (2) meet the enamel, or (3) not meet, leaving a gap between the cementum and enamel.

MICROSCOPIC ANATOMY OF ALVEOLAR BONE

1. **Definition.** The alveolar process or alveolar bone is the part of the maxilla and mandible that form and support the sockets of the teeth (Fig. 2-21).
2. **Function of Alveolar Bone in the Periodontium**
   A. **Protects Roots of Teeth.** The alveolar bone forms the bony sockets that provide support and protection for the roots of the teeth.
   B. **Remodels in Response to Mechanical Forces and Inflammation.** Alveolar bone constantly undergoes periods of bone formation and resorption (loss) in response to mechanical forces on the tooth and inflammation of the periodontium.
3. **Characteristics of Alveolar Bone**
   A. **Components.** Alveolar bone is mineralized connective tissue made by cells called osteoblasts ("bone builders") (20).
      1. Major Cell Types
         a. Osteoblasts—bone-forming cells—produce the bone matrix consisting of collagen fibers and other protein fibers.
         b. Osteoclasts—bone consumers—cells that remove the mineral materials and organic matrix of alveolar bone.
      2. Extracellular Matrix
         a. Collagen fibers and gel-like substance form the major component of the alveolar bone.
         b. The bone matrix is rigid because it undergoes mineralization by the deposition of minerals such as calcium and phosphate, which are subsequently transformed into hydroxyapatite (Fig. 2-22).
   B. **Vessels and Innervation.** The alveolar bone has blood vessels and nerve innervation.

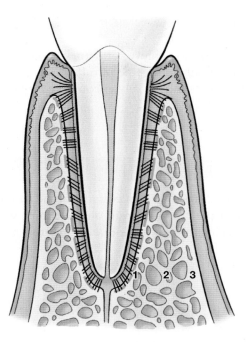

Figure 2-21. Anatomy of Alveolar Bone.
(**1**) Alveolar bone proper, (**2**) trabecular bone, and (**3**) compact bone.

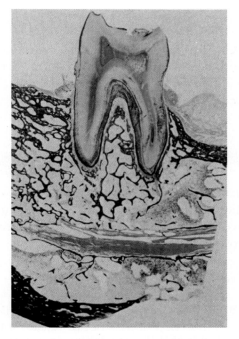

Figure 2-22. Histology of Alveolar Bone. A histologic section through a mandibular first molar and its alveolar process. (Used with permission from Melfi RC. *Permar's Oral Embryology and Microscopic Anatomy*. 10th ed. Philadelphia, PA: Lippincott Williams & Wilkins; 2000:215, Figure 9-20.)

Chapter Summary Statement

Knowledge of the microscopic anatomy of the periodontium is fundamental in understanding the (1) function of the periodontium in health and (2) changes that occur during the periodontal disease process. The JE plays an important role in the health of the periodontium by attaching the gingival epithelium to the tooth via hemidesmosomes and an internal basal lamina. In health, the PDL, cementum, and alveolar bone act as a functional unit to support and maintain the teeth in the oral cavity.

Section 4
Focus on Patients

Clinical Patient Care

CASE 1

A clinician penetrates the oral mucosa with a needle before injecting a local anesthetic. The needle tip stops in the loose connective tissue underlying the surface structures. Name the layers of epithelium that have been penetrated by the needle.

CASE 2

A clinician finds it necessary to use a unique type of injection to achieve total anesthesia of a tooth being treated. The injection involves sliding a small-diameter needle into the PDL space to a point halfway down the tooth root. Name the PDL fibers most likely encountered by the needle tip during insertion.

CASE 3

Recession of the gingival margin exposes a portion of tooth root on a maxillary canine tooth. Microscopic examination of the cementum in the area of the crown margin on the canine will reveal what possible relationships between the level of cementum and the level of the tooth crown?

References

1. Cho MI, Garant PR. Development and general structure of the periodontium. *Periodontol 2000.* 2000;24:9–27.
2. Bartold PM, Walsh LJ, Narayanan AS. Molecular and cell biology of the gingiva. *Periodontol 2000.* 2000;24:28–55.
3. Weinmann JP, Meyer J. Types of keratinization in the human gingiva. *J Invest Dermatol.* 1959;32(2, Part 1):87–94.
4. Listgarten MA. Electron microscopic study of the gingivo-dental junction of man. *Am J Anat.* 1966;119(1):147–177.
5. Dale BA. Periodontal epithelium: a newly recognized role in health and disease. *Periodontol 2000.* 2002;30:70–78.
6. Schroeder HE. Ultrastructure of the junctional epithelium of the human gingiva. *Helv Odontol Acta.* 1969;13(2):65–83.
7. Listgarten MA. The ultrastructure of human gingival epithelium. *Am J Anat.* 1964;114:49–69.
8. Schroeder HE, Listgarten MA. The gingival tissues: the architecture of periodontal protection. *Periodontol 2000.* 1997; 13:91–120.
9. Thilander H, Bloom GD. Cell contacts in oral epithelia. *J Periodontal Res.* 1968;3(2):96–110.
10. Sabag N, Saglie R, Mery C. Ultrastructure of the normal human epithelial attachment to the cementum root surface. *J Periodontol.* 1981;52(2):94–95.
11. Pollanen MT, Salonen JI, Uitto VJ. Structure and function of the tooth-epithelial interface in health and disease. *Periodontol 2000.* 2003;31:12–31.
12. Schroeder HE, Listgarten MA. The junctional epithelium: from strength to defense. *J Dent Res.* 2003;82(3):158–161.
13. Schroeder HE, Theilade J. Electron microscopy of normal human gingival epithelium. *J Periodontal Res.* 1966;1(2):95–119.
14. Bartold PM. Connective tissues of the periodontium. Research and clinical implications. *Aust Dent J.* 1991;36(4):255–268.
15. Bartold PM. Connective tissues of the periodontium–preface. *Periodontol 2000.* 2000;24:7–8.
16. Wang Y, Wang Q, D Arora P, et al. Cell adhesion proteins: roles in periodontal physiology and discovery by proteomics. *Periodontol 2000.* 2013;63(1):48–58.
17. Ho SP, Marshall SJ, Ryder MI, et al. The tooth attachment mechanism defined by structure, chemical composition and mechanical properties of collagen fibers in the periodontium. *Biomaterials.* 2007;28(35):5238–5245.
18. Beertsen W, McCulloch CA, Sodek J. The periodontal ligament: a unique, multifunctional connective tissue. *Periodontol 2000.* 1997;13:20–40.
19. Saygin NE, Giannobile WV, Somerman MJ. Molecular and cell biology of cementum. *Periodontol 2000.* 2000;24:73–98.
20. Sodek J, McKee MD. Molecular and cellular biology of alveolar bone. *Periodontol 2000.* 2000;24:99–126.

 STUDENT ANCILLARY RESOURCES

A wide variety of resources to enhance your learning and understanding of this chapter are available on thePoint°.

- Visit thePoint to access:
  - Audio Glossary
  - Animations
  - Suggested Readings
  - Answers to Review Questions
  - Case Studies

CHAPTER 3

Overview of Diseases of the Periodontium

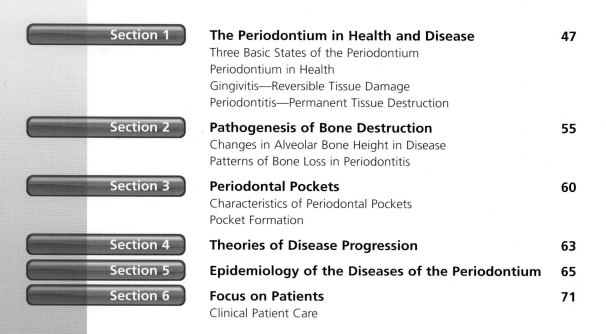

Clinical Application.   Each of the various types of diseases that affect the periodontium will be discussed in detail in subsequent chapters of this book. To understand these upcoming detailed discussions, clinicians need to be aware of a few important ideas that relate to most of these disease conditions, and these topics are discussed in Chapter 3. This overview gives the student an understanding of the fundamental changes seen in the diseased periodontium and discusses concepts related to the epidemiology, occurrence, and progression of periodontal diseases.

Learning Objectives

- Define the term *disease progression*.

- Define the term *periodontal disease* and contrast it with the term *periodontitis*.

- Describe and contrast the (1) position of the junctional epithelium, (2) characteristics of the epithelial–connective tissue junction, and (3) position of the crest of the alveolar bone in health, gingivitis, and periodontitis.

- Explain why there is a band of intact transseptal fibers even in the presence of severe bone loss.

- Describe the progressive destruction of alveolar bone loss that occurs in periodontitis.

- Describe the pathway of inflammation that occurs in horizontal bone loss and contrast it with the pathway of inflammation that occurs in vertical bone loss.

- Contrast the characteristics of gingival and periodontal pockets.

- For patients in the clinical setting, identify visible clinical signs of health and periodontal disease for your clinic instructor.

- For a patient with periodontal disease, measure the probing depth of the sulci or pockets on the facial aspect of one sextant of the mouth. Using the information gathered visually and with the periodontal probe, explain whether this patient's disease is gingivitis or periodontitis.

- Given a drawing of a periodontal pocket, determine whether the pocket illustrated is a suprabony or infrabony pocket.

- Describe variables associated with periodontal disease that an epidemiologist might include in a research study.

- Define prevalence and incidence as measurements of disease within a population.

- Describe how clinical dental hygiene practice can be affected by epidemiological research.

Key Terms

Disease progression
Gingivitis
Acute gingivitis
Chronic gingivitis
Reversible (tissue damage)
Periodontitis
Apical migration of the
    junctional epithelium
Inflammation
Alveolar bone loss

Horizontal bone loss
Vertical bone loss
Osseous defect
Infrabony defect
Osseous crater
Furcation involvement
Attachment loss
Disease site
Inactive disease site
Active disease site

Gingival pocket
Periodontal pocket
Suprabony pocket
Infrabony pocket
Intermittent disease
    progression theory
Epidemiology
Incidence
Prevalence

Section 1
The Periodontium in Health and Disease

THREE BASIC STATES OF THE PERIODONTIUM

Disease progression (pathogenesis) is the sequence of events that occur during the development of a disease or abnormal condition. The periodontium exists in three basic states: health, gingivitis, and periodontitis (Fig. 3-1). It is important to recognize the differences among health, gingivitis, and periodontitis (Figs. 3-2 to 3-4). This section provides an overview of these three basic states at the clinical and microscopic levels.

The term *periodontal disease* should not be confused with the term *periodontitis*. Gingivitis and periodontitis are the two basic categories of periodontal disease (1–4).

- Gingivitis is a bacterial infection that is confined to the gingiva. The tissue damage that occurs in gingivitis results in reversible destruction to the tissues of the periodontium (Fig. 3-3).
- Periodontitis is a bacterial infection of all parts of the periodontium including the gingiva, periodontal ligament, bone, and cementum. The tissue damage that occurs in periodontitis results in irreversible destruction to the tissues of the periodontium (Fig. 3-4).

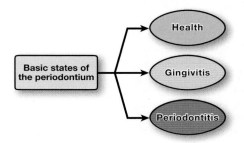

Figure 3-1. Three Basic States of the Periodontium. In the absence of disease, the periodontium is healthy. The two basic categories of periodontal disease are gingivitis and periodontitis.

TABLE 3-1. HISTOLOGIC CHANGES IN GINGIVITIS AND PERIODONTITIS

State	Junctional Epithelium	Connective Tissue Attachment	Periodontal Ligament Fibers	Alveolar Bone
Health	JE coronal to CEJ Tight intercellular junctions	Intact; supragingival fiber bundles provide support to gingiva and JE	Intact: attach root to the bone of the tooth socket	Intact; supports and protects root of tooth
Gingivitis	JE at CEJ Widened intercellular junctions; epithelial extensions into connective tissue	Connective tissue damage	Intact	Intact
Periodontitis	JE apical to CEJ Widened intercellular junctions; epithelial extensions into connective tissue	Destruction of supragingival fiber bundles	Destruction of periodontal ligament fibers; exposure of cementum to pocket environment	Destruction of bone Eventual tooth loss

JE, junctional epithelium; CEJ, cementoenamel junction.

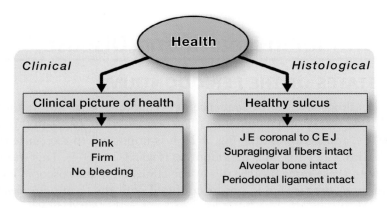

Figure 3-2. Characteristics of Healthy Periodontium. The clinical and histologic characteristics of the tissues of the periodontium in health.

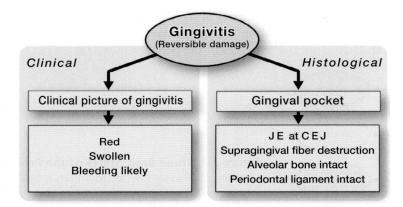

Figure 3-3. Characteristics of Gingivitis. The clinical and histologic characteristics of gingivitis. Some reversible tissue damage occurs in gingivitis.

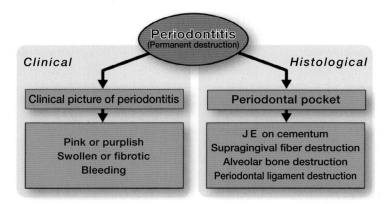

Figure 3-4. Characteristics of Periodontitis. The clinical and histologic characteristics of periodontitis. Permanent tissue damage occurs in periodontitis.

PERIODONTIUM IN HEALTH

1. Clinical Picture of Healthy Gingiva
   A. **Color:** Pink, may be pigmented, and is resilient in consistency.
   B. **Gingival Margin**
      1. Scalloped outline.
      2. Located coronal to (above) the cementoenamel junction (CEJ).
   C. **Interdental Papillae:** Firm and occupy the embrasure spaces apical to the contact areas.
   D. **Absence of Bleeding:** No bleeding upon probing.
   E. **Sulcus:** Probing depths range from 1 to 3 mm.
2. The Microscopic Picture of Healthy Gingiva (Fig. 3-5)
   A. **Junctional Epithelium:** The JE is firmly attached by hemidesmosomes to the enamel slightly coronal to (above) the CEJ.
   B. **Epithelial–Connective Tissue Junction:** In health, the junctional epithelium has no epithelial ridges.
   C. **Gingival Fibers:** Intact supragingival fiber bundles support the junctional epithelium.
   D. **Alveolar Bone:** The crest of the alveolar bone is intact and located 2 to 3 mm apical to (below) the base of the junctional epithelium.
   E. **Periodontal Ligament Fibers:** Intact periodontal ligament fiber bundles stretch between the bony walls of the tooth socket to the cementum of the root.
   F. **Cementum:** Cementum is normal.

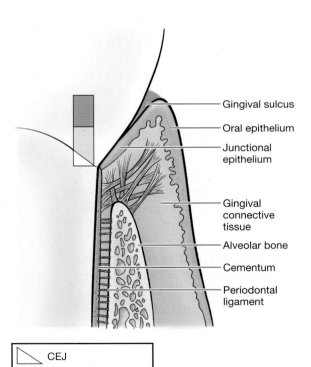

Gingival sulcus
Oral epithelium
Junctional epithelium
Gingival connective tissue
Alveolar bone
Cementum
Periodontal ligament

CEJ
Probing depth
Junctional epithelium

Figure 3-5. The Healthy Periodontium.

- **Plaque Biofilm:** light accumulation
- **Junctional epithelium:** slightly coronal to the CEJ, no epithelial ridge formation
- **Supragingival fibers:** intact
- **Periodontal ligament fibers:** intact
- **Alveolar bone:** intact

Illustration Key: The *white wedge* indicates the location of the CEJ; the depth of the sulcus is shown by the *blue vertical rectangle;* the length of junctional epithelium is indicated by the *pink vertical rectangle.*

GINGIVITIS—REVERSIBLE TISSUE DAMAGE

1. **Characteristics of Gingivitis.** Gingivitis is *a type of periodontal disease* characterized by changes in the color, contour, and consistency of the gingival tissues (Fig. 3-6).
   A. **Onset of Gingivitis.** Gingivitis is observed clinically from 4 to 14 days after plaque biofilm accumulates in the gingival sulcus (5).
      1. **Acute gingivitis** is a gingivitis that lasts for a short period of time. Acute gingivitis often is characterized by fluid in the gingival connective tissues that results in swollen gingiva.
      2. **Chronic gingivitis** is a gingivitis that lasts for months or years.
         a. When gingivitis is chronic, the body may attempt to repair the tissue damage by forming new collagen fibers in the gingival connective tissue.
         b. Excess collagen fibers lead to gingival tissues that are enlarged and fibrotic (leathery) in consistency.
         c. The excess collagen fibers conceal the redness caused by the increased blood flow, making the tissue appear less red.
   B. **Tissue Enlargement.** Gingival enlargement may be caused by swelling (acute gingivitis) or fibrosis (chronic gingivitis).
      1. Tissue enlargement causes the gingival margin to cover more of the crown of the tooth and results in deeper probing depths.
      2. This enlargement of the gingival tissue is said to produce a false or gingival pocket.
      3. A gingival pocket has a sulcus depth over 3 mm. This increased probing depth is caused solely by enlarged gingival tissue. Microscopically, the junctional epithelium remains in its normal position coronal to CEJ on the tooth in a gingival pocket.
   C. **Reversible Tissue Damage.** *The tissue damage in gingivitis is reversible*—that is, with good patient self-care the body can repair the damage.
   D. **Duration of Gingivitis.** In many cases, gingivitis may persist for years without ever progressing to the next stage, periodontitis. In some cases, a combination of risk factors may result in gingivitis progressing to periodontitis.
2. **Clinical Picture of Gingivitis**
   A. **Color:** In gingivitis, the gingival tissue usually is red or reddish blue in color (Table 3-1).
      1. The blood flow increases in the gingival connective tissue and the gingival blood vessels become engorged with blood, causing the gingiva to appear red.
      2. If the gingivitis persists, the gingival blood vessels may become congested. This slow-moving blood flow causes the gingiva to have a bluish color.
   B. **Gingival Margin**
      1. The gingival margin is swollen and loses its knife-edge adaptation to the tooth.
      2. Gingival tissue may cover more of the crown of the tooth due to tissue swelling or fibrosis.
   C. **Interdental Papillae.** The interdental papillae often are bulbous and swollen.
   D. **Bleeding.** There is bleeding upon gentle probing.
   E. **Sulcus.** Probing depths may be greater than 3 mm due to swelling of the tissues. It is important to note that *there is NO apical migration of the junctional epithelium* in gingivitis.
3. **The Microscopic Picture of Gingivitis**
   A. **Junctional Epithelium:** The hemidesmosomes still attach to the enamel coronal to the CEJ (Fig. 3-6 and Table 3-2).
   B. **Epithelial–Connective Tissue Junction**
      1. The junctional epithelium extends epithelial ridges down into the connective tissue.

2. *Such extension of the epithelial ridges only can occur because destruction of the gingival fibers creates space for the growing epithelium.*

C. **Gingival Fibers.** Damage has occurred to the supragingival fiber bundles. This damage is reversible if the bacterial infection is brought under control.

D. **Alveolar Bone.** The bacterial infection has not progressed into the alveolar bone. There is no destruction of alveolar bone.

E. **Periodontal Ligament Fibers.** The bacterial infection has not progressed into the periodontal ligament fibers.

F. **Cementum.** The cementum covering the root of the tooth is normal.

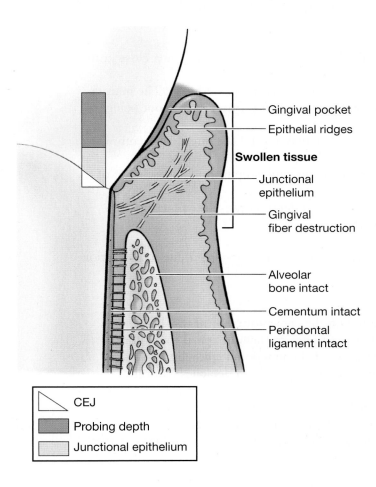

CEJ

Probing depth

Junctional epithelium

Figure 3-6. Gingivitis.

- **Plaque Biofilm:** increased numbers of bacteria
- **Junctional epithelium:** slightly coronal to the CEJ; the coronal portion of the JE detaches from the tooth; probing depth increases; epithelial ridges extend down into gingival connective tissue
- **Supragingival fibers:** some fiber destruction
- **Periodontal ligament fibers:** intact
- **Alveolar bone:** intact

Illustration Key: Note in this illustration that the JE, as indicated by the *pink rectangle,* is still coronal to the CEJ (*white wedge*). The *blue rectangle* has increased in depth due to the swelling of the gingival margin, so that the gingival tissue covers more of the crown of the tooth.

PERIODONTITIS—PERMANENT TISSUE DESTRUCTION

1. **Characteristics of Periodontitis**
   A. **Extent of Tissue Destruction**
      1. Periodontitis is *a type of periodontal disease* that is characterized by the (1) apical migration of the junctional epithelium, (2) loss of connective tissue attachment, and (3) loss of alveolar bone (6).
      2. The tissue damage of periodontitis is permanent.
   B. **Process of Tissue Destruction**
      1. The tissue destruction of periodontitis is not a continuous process. Rather, the disease process occurs in an intermittent manner with extended periods of disease inactivity followed by short periods of destruction (3).

2. Tissue destruction progresses at different rates throughout the mouth. Destruction does not occur in all parts of the mouth at the same time, but instead, destruction usually occurs in only a few specific sites (tooth surfaces) at a time.

2. **Clinical Picture of Periodontitis**
   A. **Color:** The gingival tissue shows visible alternations in color, contour, and consistency.
      1. Edematous tissue (spongy tissue)—bluish red or purplish red with a smooth, shiny appearance.
      2. Fibrotic tissue (firm, nodular tissue)—light pink with a leathery consistency. Beginning clinicians often mistakenly interpret this light pink color as a sign of tissue health.
   B. **Gingival Margin**
      1. The gingival margin may be swollen or fibrotic and does not have a close knife-edged adaptation to the tooth.
      2. The position of the gingival margin varies greatly in periodontitis. The margin may be apical to the CEJ (recession) resulting in a portion of the root being visible in the mouth.
   C. **Interdental Papillae.** The interdental papillae may not fill the interdental embrasure spaces.
   D. **Bleeding.** There often is bleeding upon probing, and suppuration (a discharge of pus) may be visible.
   E. **Pocket.** Probing depths are 4 mm or greater in depth because the junctional epithelium is attached to the root surface.
      1. Pus may be evident upon probing.
      2. Pain is usually absent; however, probing may cause some pain due to ulceration of the pocket epithelium.

3. **The Microscopic Picture of Periodontitis**
   A. **Junctional Epithelium**
      1. The junctional epithelium is located on the cementum, apical to—below—its normal location. Movement of the junctional epithelium apical to its normal location is termed the **apical migration of the junctional epithelium.**
      2. The coronal-most portion of the junctional epithelium detaches from the tooth surface. As the bacterial infection progresses, the apical portion of the junctional epithelium moves further in an apical direction along the root surface creating a periodontal pocket (Fig. 3-7 and Table 3-2).
      3. The extracellular matrix of the gingiva and the attached collagen fibers at the apical edge of the junctional epithelium are destroyed.
   B. **Epithelial–Connective Tissue Junction**
      1. The *junctional* epithelium proliferates and extends epithelial ridges into the connective tissue.
      2. The *sulcular* epithelium of the pocket wall thickens and extends epithelial ridges deep into the connective tissue. Small ulcerations of the pocket epithelium expose the underlying inflamed connective tissue.
   C. **Gingival Connective Tissue**
      1. Changes in the gingival connective tissue are severe. Collagen destruction in the area of inflammation is almost complete.
      2. There is widespread destruction of the supragingival fiber bundles, reducing them to fiber fragments. The destruction of the periodontal ligament fiber bundles makes it easier for the junctional epithelium to migrate apically along the root surface.

3. The transseptal fiber bundles, however, are regenerated continuously across the crest of bone. A band of intact transseptal fibers separates the site of inflammation from the remaining alveolar bone even in cases of extensive bone loss (Fig. 3-8).

4. Epithelium grows over the root surface in areas where the fiber bundles have been destroyed. *The loss of fiber attachment is permanent because the epithelium growing over the root surface prevents the reinsertion of the periodontal ligament fibers in the cementum.*

D. **Alveolar Bone.** There is permanent destruction of the alveolar bone that supports the teeth. Tooth mobility may be present.

E. **Periodontal Ligament Fibers.** There is permanent destruction of some or all of the periodontal ligament fiber bundles.

F. **Cementum.** Cementum within the periodontal pocket is exposed to dental plaque biofilm.

G. **Pulp.** Histologic studies of the dental pulp of patients with severe periodontitis show inflamed, edematous pulps, pulpal necrosis, vascular congestion, and dentin demineralization (7,8).

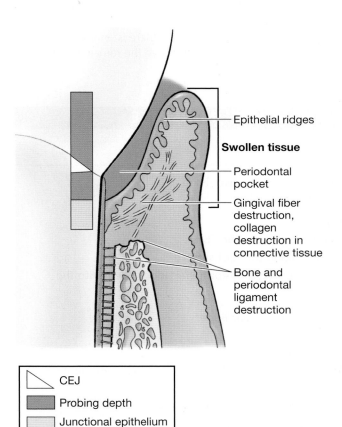

Epithelial ridges

Swollen tissue

Periodontal pocket

Gingival fiber destruction, collagen destruction in connective tissue

Bone and periodontal ligament destruction

CEJ

Probing depth

Junctional epithelium

Figure 3-7. Periodontitis.

- **Plaque Biofilm:** vast numbers of bacteria
- **Junctional epithelium:** apical to the CEJ with attachment on cementum; a remnant of the JE persists at the base of the periodontal pocket: epithelial ridges extend down into gingival connective tissue
- **Supragingival fibers:** fiber destruction
- **Periodontal ligament fibers:** fiber destruction
- **Alveolar bone:** portions of alveolar bone destroyed

Illustration Key: Note the *blue rectangle* shows that the pocket in this illustration is increased by (1) the swollen gingiva margin and (2) the location of the JE apical to (below) the CEJ. The level of the CEJ is indicated by the *white wedge*.

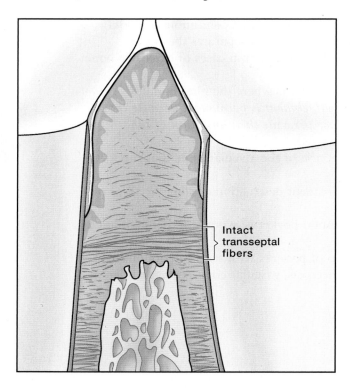

Figure 3-8. Band of Intact Transseptal Fibers. Even in the presence of severe horizontal bone loss, there is an intact band of transseptal fibers above the remaining alveolar bone.

TABLE 3-2. HISTOLOGIC CHANGES IN DISEASE

Disease State	Histology
Gingivitis	Epithelial ridges extend down into connective tissue Destruction of supragingival fiber bundles
Periodontitis	*Changes in Epithelial Tissues:* • Junctional epithelium located apical to the CEJ • Junctional epithelium grows along the root surface • Sulcular epithelium thickens and extends epithelial ridges down into the connective tissue *Changes in Connective Tissues and Alveolar Bone:* • Collagen destruction • Destruction of supragingival fiber bundles • Destruction of periodontal ligament fibers; transseptal fibers regenerate and remain intact • Junctional epithelium grows over the root surface in areas where the periodontal ligament fibers are destroyed • Root cementum is exposed to the plaque biofilm • Destruction of alveolar bone

Section 2
Pathogenesis of Bone Destruction

Inflammation is the body's reaction to injury or invasion by disease-producing organisms. The inflammatory process that occurs in periodontitis results in permanent destruction to the tissues of the periodontium, including the destruction of gingival connective tissue, periodontal ligament, and alveolar bone. **Alveolar bone loss** is the resorption of alveolar bone as a result of periodontitis. This section discusses the patterns of bone destruction that occur in periodontitis. *The pattern of bone destruction that occurs depends on the pathway of inflammation as it spreads from the gingiva into the alveolar bone.* It is important to understand the changes that occur in the alveolar bone because it is the reduction in bone height that eventually results in tooth loss.

CHANGES IN ALVEOLAR BONE HEIGHT IN DISEASE

1. Reduction in Bone Height
   A. **Bone Height in Health and Gingivitis.** In health and gingivitis, the crest of the alveolar bone is located approximately 2 mm apical to (below) the CEJs of the teeth (Fig. 3-9).
   B. **Bone Height in Periodontitis.** In periodontitis, the bone destruction may be severe (Fig. 3-10). As periodontal disease progresses (worsens) tooth loss may occur from lack of alveolar bone support (Fig. 3-11).

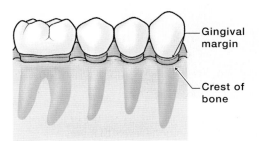

Figure 3-9. Level of Alveolar Crest in Health and Gingivitis. In health, crest of the alveolar bone is located approximately 2 mm apical to the cementoenamel junction.

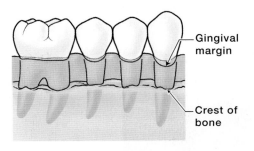

Figure 3-10. Level of Alveolar Crest in Disease. In periodontitis, the crest of the alveolar bone is located more than 2 mm apical to the cementoenamel junction.

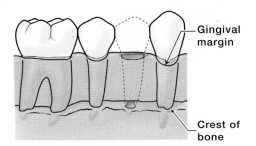

Figure 3-11. Level of Alveolar Crest as Disease Progresses. There is a progressive alveolar bone loss in periodontitis. Bone destruction may eventually lead to tooth mobility or loss due to insufficient bone support for the teeth.

PATTERNS OF BONE LOSS IN PERIODONTITIS

1. **Patterns of Bone Loss.** The two types of bone loss are (1) horizontal and (2) vertical bone loss.
   A. **Horizontal Bone Loss**
      1. Horizontal bone loss is the most common pattern of bone loss (Fig. 3-12).
      2. This type of bone loss results in a fairly even, overall reduction in the height of the alveolar bone.
      3. The alveolar bone is reduced in height, but the margin of the alveolar crest remains more or less perpendicular to the long axis of the tooth.
   B. **Vertical Bone Loss**
      1. Vertical bone loss is a less common pattern of bone loss (Fig. 3-13). Vertical bone loss is also known as angular bone loss.
      2. This type of bone loss results in an uneven reduction in the height of the alveolar bone.
      3. In vertical bone loss, the resorption progresses *more rapidly* in the bone next to the root surface. This uneven pattern of bone loss leaves a trench-like area of missing bone alongside the root.

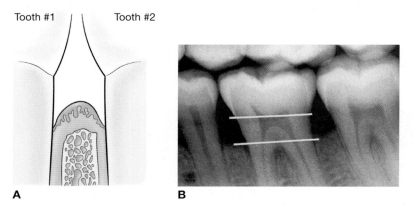

Figure 3-12. Horizontal Pattern of Bone Loss. **A:** Horizontal bone loss results in bone levels that are approximately at the same height on adjacent tooth roots. **B:** On a radiograph, if an imaginary line drawn between the CEJs of adjacent teeth is approximately parallel, then the bone loss is described as horizontal bone loss.

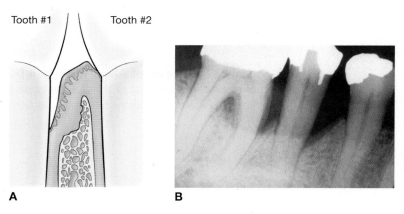

Figure 3-13. Vertical Pattern of Bone Loss. **A:** Vertical bone loss results in an uneven reduction in bone height on adjacent tooth roots, resulting in a trench-like area of missing bone alongside the root of one tooth. **B:** On a radiograph, if an imaginary line drawn between the CEJs of adjacent teeth is not parallel, then the bone loss is described as vertical bone loss.

2. Pathways of Inflammation into the Alveolar Bone
   A. Pathway of Inflammation in Horizontal Bone Loss
      1. In horizontal bone loss, inflammation spreads into the tissues in this order: (1) within the gingival connective tissue along the connective tissue sheaths surrounding the blood vessels, (2) into the alveolar bone, and (3) finally, into the periodontal ligament space (Fig. 3-14A).
      2. Inflammation usually spreads in this manner because it is the *path of least resistance*. The periodontal ligament fiber bundles act as an effective barrier to the spread of inflammation. Thus, the inflammation spreads into the alveolar bone and then into the periodontal ligament space.
   B. Pathway of Inflammation in Vertical Bone Loss
      1. In vertical bone loss, inflammation spreads into the tissues in this order (1) within the gingival connective tissue, (2) directly into the periodontal ligament space, and (3) finally, into the alveolar bone (Fig. 3-14B).
      2. Inflammation spreads in this manner whenever the crestal periodontal ligament fiber bundles are weakened and no longer present an effective barrier. Prior events such as occlusal trauma can be responsible for the weakened condition of the fiber bundles.

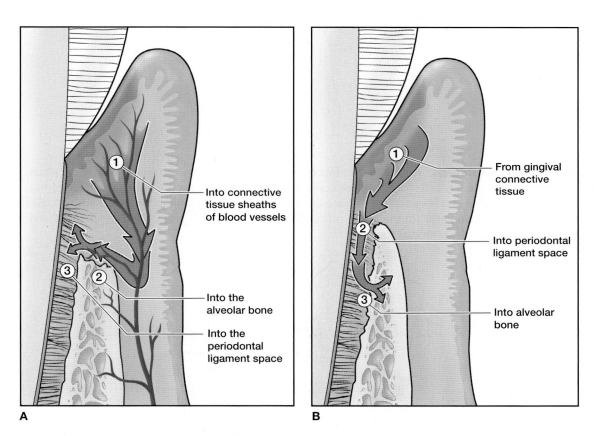

A   **B**

Figure 3-14. Pathway of Inflammation into Alveolar Bone. A: In horizontal bone loss, inflammation spreads through the tissues in this order: 1—Into the gingival connective tissue; 2—Into the alveolar bone; 3—Finally, into the periodontal ligament; **B:** In vertical bone loss, inflammation spreads through the tissues in this order: 1—Into the gingival connective tissue; 2—Into the periodontal ligament; 3—Finally, into the alveolar bone.

3. **Bone Defects in Periodontal Disease.** Periodontitis results in different types of defects in the alveolar bone. These bony defects are called **osseous defects**.
   A. **Infrabony Defects.**
      1. **Infrabony defects** result when bone resorption occurs in an uneven, oblique direction. In infrabony defects, the bone resorption primarily affects one tooth.
      2. Classification of Infrabony Defects. Infrabony defects are classified on the basis of the number of osseous walls. Infrabony defects may have one, two, or three walls (Fig. 3-15).
   B. **Osseous Craters.** An **osseous crater** is a bowl-shaped defect in the interdental alveolar bone with bone loss nearly equal on the roots of two adjacent teeth (Fig. 3-16A,B).
      1. Whereas infrabony defects primarily affect one tooth, in craters the defect affects two adjacent root surfaces to a similar extent.
      2. The presence of an osseous crater causes dental plaque biofilm to collect and makes it difficult to clean the interdental area.

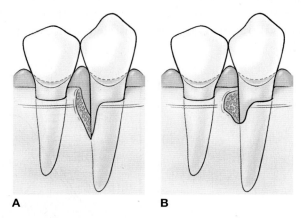

A **B**

Figure 3-15. Osseous Defects. A: One-wall infrabony defect, looking from the canine tooth root distally toward the premolar, there is only "one" wall of bone remaining, and that is on the mesial surface of the premolar. The facial plate and lingual plate of bone are missing. **B:** Two-wall infrabony defect with facial plate of bone missing. The "two walls" of the bone surrounding this defect are the remaining lingual plate and bone on the mesial surface of the premolar tooth root.

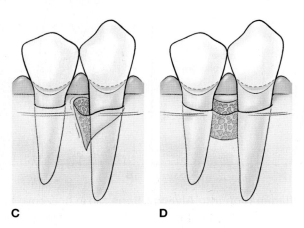

C **D**

Figure 3-15. C: Three-wall infrabony defect, the "three walls" of remaining bone that surround this defect are the lingual plate, facial plate, and the bone on the mesial surface of the adjacent premolar root. **D:** Interproximal osseous crater with the lingual plate and facial plate of bone remaining. The bone between these plates is missing resulting in bone being lost on the mesial surface of the premolar and the distal surface of the adjacent canine. The term crater refers to the dip in the contour of the interproximal bone between the facial and lingual plates.

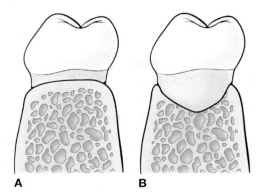

Figure 3-16. Contour of Interdental Bone. A: Normal contour of the alveolar bone on the proximal (mesial or distal) surface of a posterior tooth. Note that the bone contour from the facial to lingual is a relatively flat interproximal contour. **B:** Osseous crater on the proximal surface of a posterior tooth. Note that the contour of the bone from the facial to the lingual dips apically and forms what is described as a "crater" between the facial and lingual bone margins.

C. Bone Loss in Furcation Areas
   1. **Furcation involvement** occurs on a multirooted tooth when periodontal infection invades the area between and around the roots, resulting in a loss of alveolar bone between the roots of the teeth.
   2. Bone loss in the furcation area may be hidden by the gingival tissue or may be clinically visible in the mouth (Fig. 3-17).

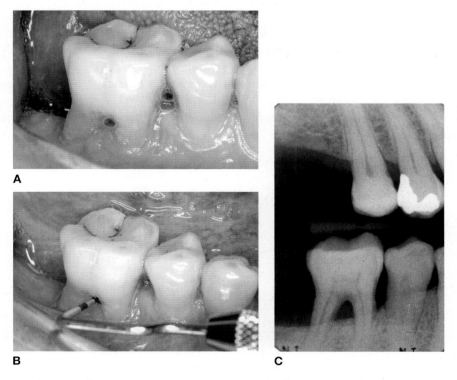

Figure 3-17. Furcation Involvement. A: Due to recession, the furcation involvement on this molar is clinically evident. **B:** A periodontal probe easily can be inserted between the two roots of this mandibular molar. **C:** A radiograph shows the extensive bone loss around this molar. (Images courtesy of Dr. Richard J. Foster, Guilford Technical Community College, Jamestown, N.C.)

Section 3
Periodontal Pockets

CHARACTERISTICS OF PERIODONTAL POCKETS

1. Attachment Loss in Periodontal Pockets
   A. **Attachment loss** is the destruction of the fibers and bone that support the teeth.
   B. Tissue destruction does not spread only in an apical (vertical) direction but also in a lateral (side-to-side) direction.
   C. *A pocket on different root surfaces of the same tooth can have different depths.* The loss of attachment may vary from surface to surface of the tooth, with the base of the pocket exhibiting very irregular patterns of tissue destruction (Fig. 3-18).
2. Disease Sites. A **disease site** is an area of tissue destruction. A disease site may involve only a single surface of a tooth, for example, the distal surface of a tooth. The disease site may involve several surfaces of the tooth or all four surfaces (mesial, distal, facial, and lingual).
   A. **Inactive disease site**—a disease site that is stable, with the attachment level of the junctional epithelium remaining the same over time.
   B. **Active disease site**—a disease site that shows continued apical migration of the junctional epithelium over time.
   C. **Assessment of Disease Activity.** The disease activity of each site in the mouth should be assessed using a periodontal probe and recorded in the patient chart at regular intervals (scheduled check-up appointments).
   D. **Periodontal Pockets.** *A periodontal pocket is an area of tissue destruction left by the disease process.* The pocket is much like a demolished home that is left after a hurricane.
      1. The presence of a periodontal pocket does not indicate necessarily that there is active disease at that site. Likewise, a demolished house does not necessarily indicate that a hurricane still is pounding the shoreline. A demolished house may indicate that the hurricane is still active or that a hurricane passed through a day, a week, or a year ago.
      2. *The majority of pockets in most adult patients with periodontitis are inactive disease sites.*

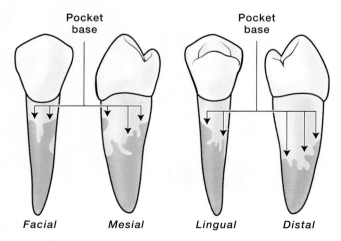

Pocket base   Pocket base

Facial   *Mesial*   *Lingual*   *Distal*

Figure 3-18. Irregular Pattern of Attachment Loss. The amount of attachment loss can vary greatly on different surfaces of the same tooth. The base of a pocket may exhibit very irregular patterns of destruction.

POCKET FORMATION

1. **Gingival Sulcus.** In health, the sulcus is 0.5 to 3 mm in depth. The junctional epithelium is coronal to the CEJ and *attaches along its entire length to the tooth* (Fig. 3-19).
2. **Gingival Pockets.** A gingival pocket is a deepening of the gingival sulcus as a result of swelling or enlargement of the gingival tissue (Fig. 3-20A,B).
   A. **Why are gingival pockets "false" pockets?**
      1. Gingival pockets sometimes are referred to "pseudopockets," meaning "false pockets," because there is *no apical migration of the junctional epithelium.*
      2. *In gingivitis, however, the coronal portion of the junctional epithelium detaches from the tooth resulting in a slight increase in probing depth.*
   B. **What causes the increased probing depth of a gingival pocket?** The increased probing depth seen in a gingival pocket is due to (1) detachment of the coronal portion of the JE from the tooth and/or (2) increased tissue size due to swelling of the tissue.

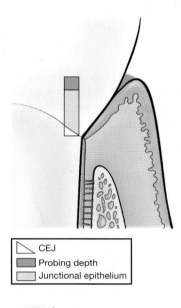

Figure 3-19. Gingival Sulcus. In health, the gingival sulcus has a shallow probing depth ranging from 0.5 to 2 mm (indicated by the *blue rectangle*). *The junctional epithelium (JE) attaches along its entire length to the enamel of the tooth* (as represented by the pink rectangle).

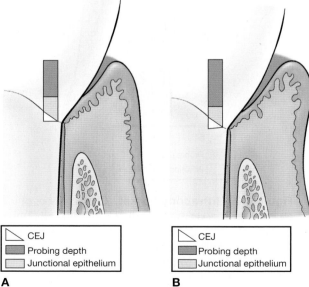

Figure 3-20. Gingival Pockets. A: There is no apical migration of the JE; however the coronal portion of the JE detaches from the tooth resulting in increased probing depth. **B:** In some cases the gingival tissue swells, resulting in a pseudo-pocket.

3. Periodontal Pockets
    A. A **periodontal pocket** is a pathologic deepening of the gingival sulcus.
        1. Pocket formation occurs as the result of the (1) apical migration of the junctional epithelium, (2) destruction of the periodontal ligament fibers, and (3) destruction of alveolar bone.
        2. Apical migration is the movement of the cells of the junctional epithelium from their normal position—coronal to the CEJ—to a position apical to the CEJ. In health, the junctional epithelial cells attach to the enamel of the tooth crown. In periodontitis, the junctional epithelial cells attach to the cementum of the tooth root.
    B. Two Types of Periodontal Pockets. The type of periodontal pocket is determined based on *the relationship of the junctional epithelium to the crest of the alveolar bone.*
        1. Suprabony Pocket
            a. **Suprabony pockets** occur when there is horizontal bone loss (Fig. 3-21).
            b. The junctional epithelium, forming the base of the pocket, is located *coronal* to (above) the crest of the alveolar bone.
        2. Infrabony Pocket
            a. **Infrabony pockets** occur when there is vertical bone loss (Fig. 3-22).
            b. The junctional epithelium, forming the base of the pocket, is located *apical* to (below) the crest of the alveolar bone. The base of the pocket is located within the cratered out area of the bone alongside of the root surface.

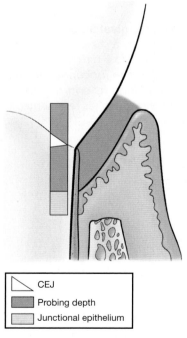

CEJ
Probing depth
Junctional epithelium

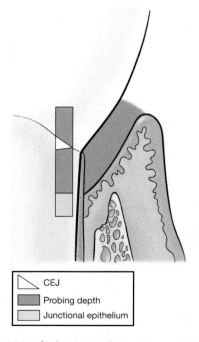

CEJ
Probing depth
Junctional epithelium

Figure 3-21. Suprabony Pocket. Characteristics of a suprabony pocket are (1) horizontal bone loss and (2) a pocket base located coronal to (above) the crest of the alveolar bone. Note the position of the JE (indicated by the *pink rectangle*) in relation to the level of the alveolar bone).

Figure 3-22. Infrabony Pocket. Characteristics of an infrabony pocket are (1) vertical bone loss and (2) a pocket base located below the crest of the alveolar bone within a trench-like area of the bone. Note the position of the JE (indicated by the *pink rectangle*) indicated below the uppermost level of the alveolar bone.

Section 4
Theories of Disease Progression

For years, clinical researchers have been trying to find an answer to the question, "How does untreated periodontal disease progress?" In this context, disease progression means that the disease gets worse. Data from ongoing studies suggest that the pattern of disease progression may vary from (1) one individual to another, (2) one site to another in a person's mouth, and (3) one type of periodontal disease to another.

1. **Historical Perspective on Disease Progression**
   A. **Continuous Progression Theory (Historical View of Disease Progression: Prior to 1980).** The continuous disease progression theory states that periodontal disease progresses throughout the entire mouth in a slow and constant rate over the adult life of the patient (Fig. 3-23).
      1. This theory suggests that:
         a. All cases of untreated gingivitis lead to periodontitis.
         b. All cases of periodontitis progress at a slow and steady rate of tissue destruction.
      2. Research studies conducted in the early 1980s indicated that periodontal disease does not progress at a constant rate nor affect all areas of the mouth simultaneously. The continuous progression theory does not accurately reflect the complex nature of periodontal disease.

2. **Current Theory of Disease Progression**
   A. **Intermittent Progression Theory (Current View).** Intermittent disease progression theory states that periodontal disease is characterized by periods of disease activity and inactivity (remission) (Fig. 3-24).
      1. Tissue destruction is sporadic, with short periods of tissue destruction alternating with periods of disease inactivity (no tissue destruction). The period of inactivity with no disease progression may last for months or for a much longer period of time.
      2. Tissue destruction progresses at different rates throughout the mouth. Destruction does not occur in all parts of the mouth at the same time. Instead, tissue destruction occurs in only a few specific sites (tooth surfaces) at a time.
      3. In the majority of cases, untreated gingivitis does not progress to periodontitis.
      4. Different forms of periodontitis progress at widely different rates.
      5. Susceptibility to periodontitis varies greatly from individual to individual and appears to be determined by the host response to periodontal pathogens.

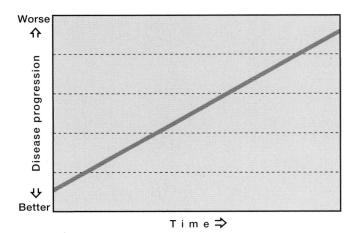

Figure 3-23. The Continuous Disease Model of Disease Progression (Prior to 1980). In the past, clinicians believed that periodontal disease progresses (worsens) throughout the entire mouth in a slow and constant rate over the life of the patient. It was believed that all cases of untreated gingivitis led to periodontitis.

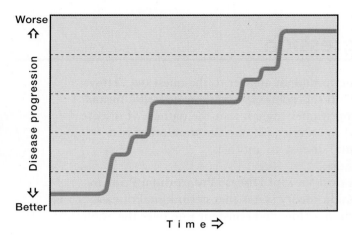

Figure 3-24. Intermittent Disease Progression Theory. Current research suggests that periodontal disease is characterized by periods of disease activity and inactivity. Furthermore, destruction does not occur in all parts of the mouth at the same time.

Section 5
Epidemiology of the Diseases of the Periodontium

Many generations of researchers have asked the question, "What causes periodontal disease?" while clinicians have asked, "What is the best care for my patients with periodontal disease?" This section discusses the study of disease in the population (epidemiology) and reviews historical and current perspectives on the causes and progression of periodontal disease.

1. What is Epidemiology?
    A. **Epidemiology** is the study of the health and disease within the total population (rather than an individual) and the behavioral, environmental, and genetic risk factors that influence health and disease. An epidemiologist assesses how much disease, investigates possible causes and applies results to treatment recommendations.
        1. Epidemiological research has three objectives: (1) to determine the amount and distribution of a disease in the total population and in subgroups, (2) to investigate the causes of a disease, and (3) to apply this knowledge to the control and prevention of disease.
        2. Through research of population groups, epidemiologists strive to identify the risk factors associated with disease such as race/ethnicity, heredity, gender, physical environment, systemic factors, socioeconomic status, and personal behavior.
        3. An understanding of the risk factors associated with a certain disease can lead to theories of the cause of that disease and then to treatment standards for patient care.
    B. Epidemiology of Periodontal Disease
        1. A large percentage of the adult population has periodontal disease. Epidemiologists study periodontal disease to determine its occurrence in the population and to identify risk factors for periodontal disease. Some of the questions epidemiologists ask when researching periodontal disease are illustrated in Figure 3-25.
        2. Epidemiological research also provides current information to the clinical dental hygienist about methods and behaviors that are successful in the treatment and prevention of periodontal disease. Current research also may define the level of risk a patient may have for periodontal disease.

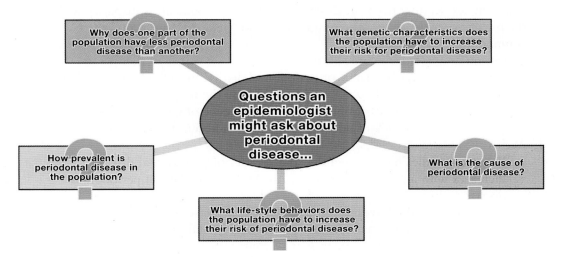

Figure 3-25. Researching Periodontal Disease. This diagram illustrates the types of questions asked by epidemiologists when studying periodontal disease.

3. Studies can be designed to look at the disparities or inequities of disease patterns. For instance a study may explore why more periodontal disease is found in a specific segment of the population than in another group of people. Oral diseases occur disproportionately more among individuals with low socioeconomic status and with poor general health (9).

2. Prevalence and Incidence of Disease
   A. Incidence and Prevalence
      1. **Incidence** is the number of *new disease cases* in a population that occur over a given period of time.

         For example, a 2011 clinical study evaluated 250 white adult males with the Gingival Index (GI) to assess gingivitis. The results of this study indicated that 125 of the men had gingivitis. In 2012 a follow-up study evaluated the same population and the results were that 150 of the men exhibited clinical signs of gingivitis. Therefore, the *incidence* of new cases of gingivitis in this study population was 25 cases.

      2. **Prevalence** refers to the number of all cases (both old and new) of a disease that can be identified within a specified population at a given point in time.

         For example, given the above example, the *prevalence* of gingivitis within the total 2011 study population was 50% (125/250). On the date of examination using the GI, the clinician does not know the length of time the men have had gingivitis, and cannot classify them as new cases of disease (or incidence).

   B. **Variables Associated with the Prevalence of Disease.** Research findings show that variables associated with the prevalence of periodontal disease include a person's gender, race, socioeconomic status, and age.
      1. Gender
         a. Males have a greater prevalence and severity of periodontal disease than females. (10) 2009–2010 National Health and Nutrition Examination Survey (NHANES) reports periodontal disease in about 56% men versus 38% women (11).
         b. There has been some speculation that females have a tendency to practice better and more frequent self-care than males. These differences in self-care behaviors may lead to the greater prevalence of disease in males.
      2. Race/ethnicity. Black and Hispanic males living in the United States have poorer periodontal health and a greater incidence of periodontal disease than White males. Results from the 2009–2010 NHANES indicate a disparity with the highest prevalence of periodontal disease in Mexican Americans when compared to other races.
      3. Education and Socioeconomic Status
         a. There is a greater incidence of periodontal disease in individuals with less than a high school education and living below the federal poverty level.
         b. Underdeveloped countries have a higher incidence of chronic periodontitis, possibly due to a lack of adequate information about disease prevention.
      4. Age
         a. Research studies have shown that the severity of periodontal disease increases with age; however, the exact role that age plays in periodontal disease is difficult to assess.
            1) As an individual lives longer, the chances increase that he will be exposed to additional risk factors for periodontal disease. Systemic illness, medications, and stress may contribute to disease risk in this population. With less edentulism, the elderly population has a greater

risk of developing periodontal disease. Results from the 2009–2010 NHANES indicate that 64% of adults over 65 years of age were found to have moderate to severe periodontitis.

2) The higher incidence of periodontal disease in the elderly, therefore, may not be due to age, but rather other risk factors to which an individual has been exposed during his or her long life.

b. Diminished dexterity is sometimes a problem in elderly individuals and can impact the individual's ability to perform self-care. Limited dexterity may also shorten the length of time that self-care is performed on a daily basis.

5. Behavior

a. Tobacco use has been identified as a behavioral risk factor for the development of periodontal disease. Both smoking tobacco and the use of smokeless tobacco products negatively impacts the periodontium (12,13). The 2009–2010 NHANES found over 64% of current smokers examined had periodontal disease.

b. With tobacco use as a risk factor, dental offices may consider stronger efforts toward including tobacco cessation programs with patient education.

6. Access to Dental Care. Individuals who desire care or need care may not have access to dental care. Barriers to obtaining dental care include transportation, geographic distances to a dental office, financial expense of dental care, and time available to seek care.

C. **Measuring the Disease Prevalence**

1. The prevalence of periodontal disease in the U.S. adult population is determined by performing clinical examinations on cross sections of groups using indices. Indices measure the amount and severity of disease. Indices used to measure both gingivitis and periodontitis vary across epidemiological studies, as does the extent of disease present when a study begins. Refer to Table 3-3 for a list of indices commonly used to assess periodontal disease.

2. Prevalence is affected by: new cases of disease (incidence), cures or deaths within a population, and the longer lives of subjects.

3. Historically gingival indices have used criteria to measure variables of inflammation such as color changes, presence of edema, and bleeding upon probing. Clinical indices for measuring periodontitis include variable of probing depth, clinical attachment level (CAL), and interpretation of radiographic bone levels (BL). Many studies use sample groups numbering in the thousands. Several groups are then compared and statistically analyzed. Epidemiologists will have different approaches to research and will include different variables in studies. The selected population can be studied over time.

D. **Difficulties in Measurement of Periodontal Disease**

1. It is far easier to evaluate a population for prevalence and incidence of dental caries than for periodontal disease because caries lends itself for more objective measurement. The development and process of caries is well known and involves only tooth structure. The Centers for Disease Control and Prevention (CDC) has provided guidance and standardized methods for public health surveillance of dental caries for many years.

2. Periodontal disease, on the other hand, involves both hard and soft tissues and has multiple variables that must be considered. Determining the presence of gingivitis with or without the presence of periodontitis further complicates the assessment of disease. Assessment can include:

a. Soft tissue color changes (redness)

b. Tissue swelling (edema)

    c. Loss of periodontal ligament fibers that support the teeth

    d. Loss of alveolar bone/furcation involvement

    e. Bleeding upon probing/spontaneous bleeding

    f. Probing depths

3. The multiple variables used to define periodontal disease make the numbers for prevalence and incidence of periodontal disease less specific, more of a range, and more subject to change. NHANES most recently used the definition/classification of periodontal disease, as determined by the collaboration of CDC and the American Academy of Periodontology (AAP) to assess the population.

4. Historically national periodontal health surveys (NHANES) have used partial mouth examination protocols that may not accurately represent disease as periodontal disease is not evenly distributed in the entire mouth. For example, attachment loss can vary on tooth surfaces being examined. The 2009–2010 NHANES did use a full-mouth examination and is being described as the most comprehensive survey of periodontal health in the United States (14).

TABLE 3-3. COMMONLY USED PERIODONTAL INDICES

Index	Measurement
Community and Periodontal Index of Treatment Needs (CPITN) (Federation Dentaire Internationale: Ainamo et al.)	Assesses probing depths and bleeding; developed to attain more uniform worldwide epidemiologic data; maybe used for measuring group periodontal needs
Eastman Interdental Bleeding Index (EIBI) (Abrams, Caton, and Polson) (Caton and Polson)	Assesses presence of inflammation and bleeding in the interdental area upon toothpick insertion
Gingival Bleeding Index (GBI) (Carter and Barnes)	Assesses presence of gingival inflammation by bleeding from interproximal sulcus within 10 s of flossing
Gingival Index (GI) (Loe and Silness)	Assesses severity of gingivitis based on color, consistency, and bleeding on probing
Modified Gingival Index (MGI)	Similar to GI but assesses severity of gingivitis without probing; redefined scoring for inflammation
Periodontal Index (PI) (Russell)	Assesses the severity of gingival inflammation without probing
Periodontal Disease Index (PDI) (Ramfjord)	Assesses the severity of gingival inflammation, pocket depth, and the level of gingival attachment
Periodontal Screening and Recording (PSR) (American Academy of Periodontology and the American Dental Association)	Assesses periodontal health in a rapid manner including probing depths, bleeding, and presence of hard deposits

E. **What the Research Shows.** Research on periodontal disease indicates it is one of the most widespread diseases in adult Americans, with most individuals who have periodontal disease being unaware of its presence. The findings are based on data collected as part of CDC's 2009–2010 NHANES, designed to assess the health and nutritional status of adults and children in the United States. The 2009–2010 NHANES included for the first time a full-mouth periodontal examination to assess for mild, moderate, or severe periodontitis, making it the most comprehensive survey of periodontal health ever conducted in the United States. Researchers measured periodontitis because it is the most destructive form of periodontal disease. Gingivitis, the earliest stage of periodontal disease, was not assessed.

1. Prevalence or Periodontitis
   a. A study titled *Prevalence of Periodontitis in Adults in the United States: 2009 and 2010* estimates that 47.2%, or 64.7 million American adults, have mild, moderate, or severe periodontitis. In adults 65 and older, prevalence rates increase to 70.1% (14). The findings also indicate disparities among certain segments of the U.S. population. Periodontal disease is higher in men than women (56.4% vs. 38.4%) and is highest in Mexican Americans (66.7%) compared to other races. Other segments with high prevalence rates include current smokers (64.2%); those living below the federal poverty level (65.4%); and those with less than a high school education (66.9%).
   b. According to data from 2009–2012 NHANES over 47% of the population had periodontitis:
      1) 8.7% had mild periodontitis
      2) 30.0% had moderate periodontitis
      3) 8.5% had severe periodontitis
   c. According to data from 2009–2012 NHANES, adults over 65 years of age, 64% had moderate/severe periodontitis.
2. Prevalence of Chronic Periodontitis
   a. The presence of periodontal disease is measured clinically in several ways. NHANES 2009–2010 used attachment loss and probing depths to assess periodontal disease. Loss of attachment is the term used to describe the destruction of periodontal ligament fibers and alveolar bone that support the teeth. Figure 5-3 shows that attachment loss of 4 mm or more affects approximately half of adults aged 50 to 59 (11).
   b. By age 60 to 69 less than half of all adults in the United States have retained 21 teeth or more (11).

F. **Public Health Surveillance of Periodontal Disease.** The most recent NHANES data suggests that the amount of periodontal disease may have been underestimated in the general population (14). Both AAP and CDC describe periodontal disease as a public health concern and are working toward improved disease surveillance. CDC's Division of Oral Health and the Association of State and Territorial Dental Directors collaborate to monitor the burden of oral disease and track state data sources.

Chapter Summary Statement

Periodontal pathogenesis is the sequence of events that occurs during the development of periodontal disease. The two types of periodontal disease are gingivitis and periodontitis.

- Gingivitis is a *reversible condition* that is characterized by changes in the color, contour, and consistency of the gingiva. There is no apical migration of the junctional epithelium or bone loss in gingivitis.
- Periodontitis results in some extent of *permanent tissue destruction* characterized by pocket formation, destruction of the periodontal ligament fibers, and resorption of alveolar bone. The pattern of alveolar bone loss and periodontal ligament destruction depends on the pathway that the inflammatory process takes as it spreads from the gingiva into the alveolar bone. It is the destruction of periodontal ligament fibers and resorption of alveolar bone that leads to tooth mobility and the possibility of tooth loss.

Epidemiological research of periodontal disease has three objectives: (1) to determine the amount and distribution of periodontal disease in a population, (2) to investigate the causes of periodontal disease, and (3) to apply this knowledge to the control of periodontal disease.

Advances in research have led to many changes in the understanding, prevention, and treatment of periodontal disease. In the future, ideas about causes and treatment will continue to be refined and changed as researchers delve further into the mysteries of periodontal disease.

Section 6
Focus on Patients

Clinical Patient Care

CASE 1

Your patient has 6 to 7 mm attachment loss on all surfaces of the maxillary first molar. Which of the tissues of the periodontium have experienced tissue destruction surrounding this tooth?

CASE 2

Your dental team provides appropriate therapy for a patient with periodontitis. When you began treatment, your initial findings were redness and edema (swelling) of the gingiva, bleeding on probing, periodontal pockets, and attachment loss. Successful control of the periodontal disease in the patient should *not* be expected to result in elimination of which of these initial clinical findings?

CASE 3

You find a newspaper article that estimates that in your home state 73% of state residents have some form of periodontal disease. You would like to use this statistic in a homework assignment. When you include this information in your homework assignment should you describe this statistic as incidence or prevalence of periodontitis?

CASE 4

Your dental team has a new patient who has gingivitis. The patient has poor daily self-care, generalized calculus deposits, poorly controlled diabetes mellitus, a history of smoking cigarettes, and inadequate dietary intake of calcium. In your patient counseling how would you characterize the likelihood that the patient will develop periodontitis in the future and what might you tell the patient about this?

References

1. Armitage GC. Development of a classification system for periodontal diseases and conditions. *Ann Periodontol.* 1999;4(1):1–6.
2. Armitage GC. Periodontal diagnoses and classification of periodontal diseases. *Periodontol 2000.* 2004;34:9–21.
3. Armitage GC. Learned and unlearned concepts in periodontal diagnostics: a 50-year perspective. *Periodontol 2000.* 2013;62(1):20–36.
4. Armitage GC. Classifying periodontal diseases–a long-standing dilemma. *Periodontol 2000.* 2002;30:9–23.
5. The pathogenesis of periodontal diseases. *J Periodontol.* 1999;70(4):457–470.
6. Armitage GC, Cullinan MP. Comparison of the clinical features of chronic and aggressive periodontitis. *Periodontol 2000.* 2010;53:12–27.
7. Caraivan O, Manolea H, Corlan Puscu D, et al. Microscopic aspects of pulpal changes in patients with chronic marginal periodontitis. *Rom J Morphol Embryol.* 2012;53(3 suppl):725–729.
8. Fatemi K, Disfani R, Zare R, et al. Influence of moderate to severe chronic periodontitis on dental pulp. *J Indian Soc Periodontol.* 2012;16(4):558–561.
9. United States. Public Health Service, Office of the Surgeon General, National Institute of Dental and Craniofacial Research (U.S.). *Oral Health in America: A Report of the Surgeon General.* Rockville, MD: Department of Health and Human Services, U.S. Public Health Service; 2000.
10. Shiau HJ, Reynolds MA. Sex differences in destructive periodontal disease: a systematic review. *J Periodontol.* 2010;81(10):1379–1389.
11. www.cdc.gov/nchs/nhanes/nhanes2009-2010/current_nhanes_09_10.htm. Accessed on January 19, 2015
12. Kibayashi M, Tanaka M, Nishida N, et al. Longitudinal study of the association between smoking as a periodontitis risk and salivary biomarkers related to periodontitis. *J Periodontol.* 2007;78(5):859–867.
13. Laxman VK, Annaji S. Tobacco use and its effects on the periodontium and periodontal therapy. *J Contemp Dent Pract.* 2008;9(7):97–107.
14. Eke PI, Dye BA, Wei L, et al; CDC Periodontal Disease Surveillance workgroup: James Beck GDRP. Prevalence of periodontitis in adults in the United States: 2009 and 2010. *J Dent Res.* 2012;91(10):914–920.

 STUDENT ANCILLARY RESOURCES

A wide variety of resources to enhance your learning and understanding of this chapter are available on **thePoint®**.

- Visit thePoint to access:
  - Audio Glossary
  - Animations
  - Suggested Readings
  - Answers to Review Questions
  - Case Studies

CHAPTER

4

Classification of Periodontal Diseases and Conditions

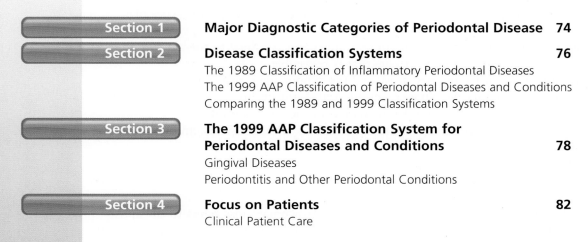
Clinical Application. A periodontal disease classification system assists the dental hygienist in communicating clinical findings accurately to other dental healthcare providers, patients, and dental insurance providers and provides a starting point for formulating an individualized treatment plan.

Learning Objectives

* Name the two major categories of periodontal disease.
* Define and contrast the terms gingival disease, periodontal disease, and periodontitis.
* Explain the historical background of the periodontal classification systems.
* Explain the importance of a classification system for periodontal disease.
* List, describe, and differentiate the various periodontal diseases according to the current classification system established by the American Academy of Periodontology.

Key Terms

Gingivitis
Periodontitis

Periodontal disease
Classification system

American Academy of
Periodontology

The reader should be aware that at the time of publication of this edition, the American Academy of Periodontology task force is reviewing the *1999 Classification of Periodontal Diseases and Conditions*. The work of the task force will take some time, but if an updated classification is made available, it will be posted on the LWW instructor/student website, The Point (http://thepoint.lww.com).

Section 1
Major Diagnostic Categories of Periodontal Disease

"Periodontal disease" is a broad term used to refer to a bacterial infection of the periodontium, just as "heart disease" is a general term. There are many different diseases of the heart, such as coronary artery disease, congestive heart failure, valvular disease, rheumatic heart disease, and infectious endocarditis. As with heart disease, there are many specific periodontal diseases that affect the gingival tissues, periodontal connective tissues, and/or the supporting alveolar bone.

   The two major diagnostic categories of periodontal disease are (1) gingivitis and (2) periodontitis (Fig. 4-1). Within each of these major categories specific types of diseases are identified.

1. **Gingivitis** is inflammation of the periodontium that is confined to the gingiva. It results in damage to the gingival tissue that is reversible.
2. **Periodontitis** is an inflammatory disease of the supporting structures of the periodontium including the gingiva, periodontal ligament, bone, and cementum. It results in irreversible destruction to the tissues of the periodontium.
3. It is important to recognize the differences among health, gingivitis, and periodontitis (Fig. 4-2).
   A. In health, no clinical signs of inflammation are present.
   B. In gingivitis, there are clinical signs of inflammation such as bleeding, redness, and swelling.
      1. There is no attachment loss in gingivitis. Attachment loss refers to the apical migration of the junctional epithelium and the destruction of connective tissue, periodontal ligament fibers, and alveolar bone.
      2. The tissue destruction in gingivitis can be reversed with professional treatment and good self-care by the patient.
   C. Periodontitis is characterized by inflammation, apical migration of the junctional epithelium, and attachment loss. In periodontitis there is irreversible tissue destruction including destruction of connective tissue, periodontal ligament fibers, and alveolar bone.

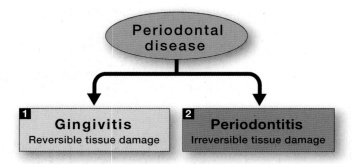

Figure 4-1. Periodontal Disease. There are two major categories of periodontal disease: (1) gingivitis and (2) periodontitis.

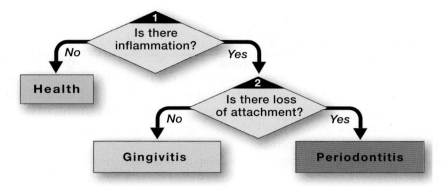

Figure 4-2. Decision Tree. Is it health, gingivitis, or periodontitis?

4. Terminology: Periodontal Disease Versus Periodontitis
   A. Many beginning clinicians confuse the meaning of the terms "*periodontal disease*" and "*periodontitis*." Often these terms are used interchangeably as if they mean the same thing. They do not.
   B. **Periodontal disease** refers to inflammation of the periodontium.
      1. Periodontal disease that is limited to an inflammation of the gingival tissues is called gingivitis.
      2. Periodontal disease that involves all the structures of the periodontium is called periodontitis.
   C. **Correct Terminology.** It is important to understand that the terms "*periodontal disease*" and "*periodontitis*" are not identical in their meaning and not interchangeable in their use.
      1. When a dental hygienist says to the dentist, "My patient has periodontal disease," the hygienist is conveying the general information that the patient has an inflammation of the periodontium that could be gingivitis or periodontitis.
      2. When the hygienist says, "My patient has periodontitis," the hygienist is conveying the specific information that the patient has a bacterial infection that involves all tissues of the periodontium including the periodontal ligament, cementum, and alveolar bone.

Section 2
Disease Classification Systems

A classification system is a grouping of similar entities on the basis of certain differing characteristics. An everyday example of a classification system is grouping vehicles into categories such as passenger cars, crossover vehicles, sport utility vehicles, and trucks. Classification systems provide a tool to study the etiology, pathogenesis, and treatment of periodontal diseases in an orderly manner.

Clinicians and researchers have struggled to develop a classification of the various forms of periodontal disease. Over the years, classification systems have changed in response to new scientific knowledge about the etiology and pathogenesis of periodontal diseases and conditions. In recent years, there have been several attempts to classify periodontal diseases. *A disease classification system, however, should not be regarded as a permanent structure. Rather it must evolve with the development of new knowledge. It is expected that systems of classification will change over time.* There has never been a perfect disease classification of periodontal diseases; as more is learned about the nature of periodontal diseases further revisions in the current classification system will be necessary.

A periodontal classification system provides information necessary in (1) communicating clinical findings accurately to other dental healthcare providers and to dental insurance providers, (2) presenting information to the patient about his or her disease, (3) formulating a diagnosis and individualized treatment plan, and (4) predicting treatment outcomes (prognosis).

THE 1989 CLASSIFICATION OF INFLAMMATORY PERIODONTAL DISEASES

The 1989 classification system (Table 4-1) included five types of periodontitis (Table 4-1) (1). The 1989 classification system emphasized the age of onset of disease and rates of disease progression. The main problems with the 1989 classification system were (1) unclear and overlapping disease categories, (2) inappropriate emphasis on age of onset of disease and rates of progression, and (3) absence of a gingival disease classification (2).

TABLE 4-1. 1989 CLASSIFICATION OF INFLAMMATORY PERIODONTAL DISEASES

Adult Periodontitis (AP)

Early Onset Periodontitis (EOP)
A. Prepubertal periodontitis (PPP)
B. Juvenile periodontitis (JP)
C. Rapidly progressive periodontitis (RPP)

Periodontitis Associated with Systemic Disease

Necrotizing Ulcerative Periodontitis (NUG)

Refractory Periodontitis (RP)

THE 1999 AAP CLASSIFICATION OF PERIODONTAL DISEASES AND CONDITIONS

The American Academy of Periodontology (AAP) initiated the currently accepted classification system by organizing the *International Workshop for a Classification of Periodontal Diseases and Conditions* in 1999 (3). The AAP Classification of Periodontal Diseases and Conditions attempts to correct some of the deficiencies of the 1989 classification system. The 1999 AAP classification system was established to identify types of periodontal disease by taking into consideration factors such as clinical manifestations, pathogenic microbial flora and the host response to these bacteria, rate of disease progression, and systemic influences. The 1999 classification includes eight main categories (Table 4-2). At the time of publication of this textbook, the 1999 AAP Classification of Periodontal Diseases and Conditions represents the most recent, internationally accepted classification system.

TABLE 4-2. MAIN CATEGORIES: AAP CLASSIFICATION OF PERIODONTAL DISEASES AND CONDITIONS, 1999
Gingival Diseases
Plaque-induced gingival diseases
Non–plaque-induced gingival lesions
Chronic Periodontitis
Localized
Generalized
Aggressive Periodontitis
Localized
Generalized
Periodontitis as a Manifestation of Systemic Disease
Necrotizing Periodontal Diseases
Abscesses of the Periodontium
Periodontitis Associated with Endodontic Lesions
Developmental or Acquired Deformities and Conditions

COMPARING THE 1989 AND 1999 CLASSIFICATION SYSTEMS

Much of the periodontal literature found in periodontal journals and textbooks is based on the earlier 1989 classification. For this reason, readers need to be somewhat familiar with both the 1989 and 1999 classification systems (Table 4-3).

TABLE 4-3. CHANGES FROM 1989 TO 1999 CLASSIFICATION	
New Terminology	• *Chronic periodontitis* replaces the term *adult periodontitis* since epidemiological evidence suggests that chronic periodontitis is also seen in some adolescents. • *Aggressive periodontitis* replaces the term *early onset periodontitis* because it is difficult to determine the age of onset of periodontitis in many cases. • *Necrotizing periodontal disease* replaces *necrotizing ulcerative periodontitis*.
Additions	• Gingival disorders • Periodontitis as a manifestation of systemic disease • Periodontal abscess • Periodontitis in conjunction with endodontic lesions • Developmental or genetic conditions
Deletion	• The category of *refractory periodontitis* is eliminated. In the 1999 classification, the designation *refractory* can be applied to *all types* of periodontal disease that do not respond to treatment.

Section 3
The 1999 AAP Classification System for Periodontal Diseases and Conditions

GINGIVAL DISEASES

The 1999 AAP Classification of Periodontal Diseases and Conditions (Table 4-4A,B) subdivides the major diagnostic category of gingivitis into specific types of diseases: (1) dental plaque-induced gingival diseases and (2) non–plaque-induced gingival lesions. Each gingivitis disease type has two or more subcategories (Fig. 4-3).

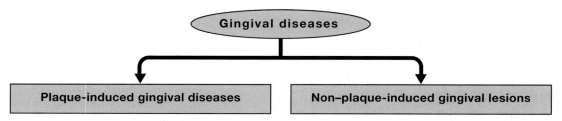

Figure 4-3. Two Major Diagnostic Categories of Gingival Diseases. The 1999 AAP Classification of Periodontal Diseases and Conditions subdivides into two major categories. Each of the two major categories has several subcategories.

TABLE 4-4A. AAP CLASSIFICATION OF GINGIVAL DISEASES	
Gingival Diseases	**I. Gingival Diseases**
• **Plaque-Induced Gingival Diseases**	**A. Dental plaque-induced gingival diseases**[a]
○ Caused solely by plaque	1. Gingivitis associated with dental plaque biofilm only
	a. Without other local contributing factors
	b. With local contributing factors
○ Modified by systemic factors	2. Gingival diseases modified by systemic factors
	a. Associated with the endocrine system
	1) Puberty-associated gingivitis
	2) Menstrual cycle-associated gingivitis
	3) Pregnancy-associated
	a) Gingivitis
	b) Pyogenic granuloma
	4) Diabetes mellitus-associated gingivitis
	b. Associated with blood dyscrasias
	1) Leukemia-associated gingivitis
	2) Other
○ Modified by medications	3. Gingival diseases modified by medications
	a. Drug-influenced gingival diseases
	1) Drug-influenced gingival enlargements
	2) Drug-influenced gingivitis
	a) Oral contraceptive-associated gingivitis
	b) Other
○ Modified by malnutrition	4. Gingival diseases modified by malnutrition
	a. Ascorbic acid deficiency gingivitis
	b. Other

TABLE 4-4A. AAP CLASSIFICATION OF GINGIVAL DISEASES (*Continued*)

- **Non–Plaque-Induced Gingival Lesions**
  - Bacterial infections

  - Viral infections

  - Fungal infections

  - Genetic origin

  - Systemically related

  - Trauma

  - Reactions to foreign bodies
  - Other

B. Non–plaque-induced gingival lesions

1. Gingival diseases of specific bacterial origin
   a. *Neisseria gonorrhoeae*-associated lesions
   b. *Treponema pallidum*-associated lesions
   c. Streptococcal species-associated lesions
   d. Other
2. Gingival diseases of viral origin
   a. Herpes virus infections
      1) Primary herpetic gingivostomatitis
      2) Recurrent oral herpes
      3) Varicella zoster infections
   b. Other
3. Gingival diseases of fungal origin
   a. *Candida* species infections
      1) Generalized gingival candidiasis
   b. Linear gingival erythema
   c. Histoplasmosis
   d. Other
4. Gingival lesions of genetic origin
   a. Hereditary gingival fibromatosis
   b. Other
5. Gingival manifestations of systemic conditions
   - Mucocutaneous disorders
     - Lichen planus
     - Pemphigoid
     - Pemphigus vulgaris
     - Erythema multiforme
     - Lupus erythematosus
     - Drug induced
     - Other
   - Allergic reactions
     - Dental restorative materials
       - Mercury
       - Nickel
       - Acrylic
       - Other
     - Reactions attributable to
       - Toothpastes/dentifrices
       - Mouthrinses/mouthwashes
       - Chewing gum additives
       - Foods and additives
     - Other
6. Traumatic lesions (factitious, iatrogenic, accidental)
   a. Chemical injury
   b. Physical injury
   c. Thermal injury
7. Foreign body reactions
8. Not otherwise specified (NOS)

[a]Can occur on a periodontium with no attachment loss or on a periodontium with attachment loss that is not progressing. Data from Armitage GC. Development of a classification system for periodontal disease and conditions. (Used with permission from *Ann Periodontol.* 1999;(4):1–6.)

PERIODONTITIS AND OTHER PERIODONTAL CONDITIONS

The 1999 AAP Classification of Periodontal Diseases and Conditions subdivides the major diagnostic category of periodontitis into specific types of diseases: (1) chronic periodontitis, (2) aggressive periodontitis, and (3) less common types of periodontitis. Each periodontitis disease type has two or more subcategories (Fig. 4-4).

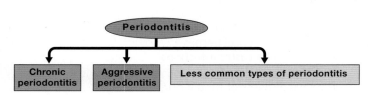

Figure 4-4. Three Major Categories of Periodontitis. The 1999 AAP Classification of Periodontal Diseases and Conditions subdivides periodontitis into three major categories of periodontitis. Each of the three major categories has two or more subcategories.

TABLE 4-4B. AAP CLASSIFICATION OF PERIODONTITIS AND OTHER PERIODONTAL CONDITIONS	
Chronic Periodontitis (CP)	II. Chronic Periodontitis[a] A. Localized B. Generalized
Aggressive Periodontitis (AP)	III. Aggressive Periodontitis[a] A. Localized B. Generalized
Periodontitis as Manifestation of Systemic Disease • Blood disorders • Genetic factors	IV. Periodontitis as a Manifestation of Systemic Disease A. Associated with hematological disorders 　1. Acquired neutropenia 　2. Leukemias 　3. Other B. Associated with genetic disorders 　1. Familial and cyclic neutropenia 　2. Down syndrome 　3. Leukocyte adhesion deficiency syndromes 　4. Papillon–Lefèvre syndrome 　5. Chédiak–Higashi syndrome 　6. Histiocytosis syndromes 　7. Glycogen storage disease 　8. Infantile genetic agranulocytosis 　9. Cohen syndrome 　10. Ehlers–Danlos syndrome (Types IV and VIII) 　11. Hypophosphatasia 　12. Other C. Not otherwise specified (NOS)
Necrotizing Periodontal Diseases	V. Necrotizing Periodontal Diseases A. Necrotizing ulcerative gingivitis (NUG) B. Necrotizing ulcerative periodontitis (NUP)
Abscesses of the Periodontium	VI. Abscesses of the Periodontium A. Gingival abscess B. Periodontal abscess C. Pericoronal abscess
Periodontitis Associated with Endodontic Lesions	VII. Periodontitis Associated with Endodontic Lesions A. Combined periodontic–endodontic lesions

TABLE 4-4B. AAP CLASSIFICATION OF PERIODONTITIS AND OTHER PERIODONTAL CONDITIONS (*Continued*)	
Deformities and Conditions	**VIII. Developmental or Acquired Deformities and Conditions**

• Tooth-related	A. Localized tooth-related factors that modify or predispose to plaque-induced gingival diseases or periodontitis
	   1. Tooth anatomic factors
	   2. Dental restorations/appliances
	   3. Root fractures
	   4. Cervical root resorption and cemental tears

• Mucogingival conditions	B. Mucogingival deformities and conditions around teeth
	   1. Gingival/soft tissue recession
	     a. Facial or lingual surfaces
	     b. Interproximal (papillary)
	   2. Lack of keratinized gingiva
	   3. Decreased vestibular depth
	   4. Aberrant frenum/muscle position
	   5. Gingival excess
	     a. Pseudopocket
	     b. Inconsistent gingival margin
	     c. Excessive gingival display
	     d. Gingival enlargement
	   6. Abnormal color

• Mucogingival deformities	C. Mucogingival deformities and conditions on edentulous ridges
	   1. Vertical and/or horizontal ridge deficiency
	   2. Lack of gingiva/keratinized tissue
	   3. Gingival/soft tissue enlargement
	   4. Aberrant frenum/muscle position
	   5. Decreased vestibular depth
	   6. Abnormal color

• Occlusal trauma	D. Occlusal trauma
	   1. Primary occlusal trauma
	   2. Secondary occlusal trauma

[a]Can be further classified on the basis of extent and severity.
Data from Armitage GC. Development of a classification system for periodontal disease and conditions. (Used with permission from *Ann Periodontol.* 1999; (4):1–6.)

Chapter Summary Statement

The two basic diagnostic categories of periodontal disease are (1) gingivitis and (2) periodontitis. It is important to be thoroughly familiar with the terms *periodontal disease, gingivitis,* and *periodontitis* and the precise definition of each term.

Classification systems, like the one for periodontal diseases and conditions, group similar diseases and conditions into general categories. Classification systems provide a tool to study the etiology, pathogenesis, and treatment of periodontal diseases in an orderly manner. From the clinician's point of view, the classification system provides a starting point for formulating a diagnosis and individualized treatment plan. In addition, periodontal disease classifications assist the dental hygienist in communicating with other dental healthcare providers, patients, and dental insurance providers.

Section 4
Focus on Patients

Clinical Patient Care

CASE 1

During the assessment of the periodontium, you note the following: apical migration of the junctional epithelium and attachment loss. The patient's medical history is normal; he takes no medications. According to the 1999 AAP Classification of Periodontal Diseases and Conditions, would this patient be classified as having plaque-induced gingivitis, non–plaque-induced gingivitis, plaque-induced gingival disease modified by systemic factors or periodontitis?

CASE 2

During the assessment of the periodontium, you note the following: bleeding, redness, and swelling of the tissue; abundant plaque biofilm, no apical migration of the junctional epithelium, and no attachment loss. The patient's medical history is normal; he takes no medications. According to the 1999 AAP Classification of Periodontal Diseases and Conditions, would this patient be classified as having plaque-induced gingivitis, non–plaque-induced gingivitis, plaque-induced gingival disease modified by systemic factors or periodontitis?

CASE 3

During the assessment of the periodontium, you note the following: bleeding, redness, and swelling of the tissue; abundant plaque biofilm, no apical migration of the junctional epithelium, and no attachment loss. The patient has a history of diabetes mellitus for which he takes daily insulin injections. According to the 1999 AAP Classification of Periodontal Diseases and Conditions, would this patient be classified as having plaque-induced gingivitis, non–plaque-induced gingivitis, plaque-induced gingival disease modified by systemic factors or periodontitis?

References

1. Nevins M, Becker W, Kornman KS. *American Academy of Periodontology.* Proceedings of the World Workshop in Clinical Periodontics, Princeton, New Jersey, July 23–27, 1989. Chicago, IL: American Academy of Periodontology; 1989.
2. Armitage GC. Development of a classification system for periodontal diseases and conditions. *Ann Periodontol.* 1999;4(1):1–6.
3. Armitage GC. Classifying periodontal diseases—a long-standing dilemma. *Periodontol 2000.* 2002;30:9–23.

 STUDENT ANCILLARY RESOURCES

A wide variety of resources to enhance your learning and understanding of this chapter are available on thePoint®.

- Visit thePoint to access:
  - Audio Glossary
  - Animations
  - Suggested Readings
  - Answers to Review Questions
  - Case Studies

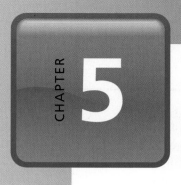

Clinical Features of the Gingiva

Clinical Application. A dental hygienist's ability to recognize the clinical features of both healthy and diseased gingiva plays a part in nearly every patient care visit. Knowledge of these clinical features continuously will be expanded throughout the hygienist's career. The outline of these features presented in this chapter provides a fundamental framework for recognition of clinical features and will allow a new clinician to enter a clinical setting with confidence.

Learning Objectives

• Describe characteristics of the gingiva in health.

• List clinical signs of gingival inflammation.

• Compare and contrast clinical features of healthy and inflamed gingival tissue.

• Explain the difference in color between acute and chronic inflammation.

• Differentiate between bulbous, blunted, and cratered papilla.

• Write a description of gingival inflammation that includes descriptors of duration, extent, and distribution of inflammation.

Key Terms

Stippling
Inflammation
Gingivitis

Bulbous papilla
Blunted papilla
Cratered papilla

Extent of inflammation

Section 1
Clinical Features of Healthy Gingiva

It is important for clinicians to recognize the appearance of healthy gingiva and to recognize all of its variations in health. In addition, clinicians must be able to describe gingiva accurately when documenting the findings from a periodontal assessment. Careful choice of verbal descriptors documents the state of gingival health, or lack of it, and allows the clinician to focus on areas that may need additional treatment.

1. **Tissue Color and Contour in Health**
    A. **Tissue Color**
        1. Healthy gingival tissue has a uniform, pink color. The precise color depends on the number and size of blood vessels in the connective tissue and the thickness of the gingival epithelium.
        2. The shade of pink usually is lighter in blondes with fair complexions and darker in brunettes with dark complexions (Fig. 5-1).
        3. The coral pink of the gingiva is easily distinguished from the darker alveolar mucosa.
        4. Healthy tissue also can be pigmented. The pigmented areas of the attached gingiva may range from light brown to black.
    B. **Tissue Contour (Size and Shape)**
        1. In health, the gingival tissue lies snugly around the tooth and firmly against the alveolar bone (Fig. 5-2).
        2. The gingival margin is smoothly scalloped in an arched form as the gingiva margin flows across the tooth surface from papilla to papilla.
        3. The gingival margin meets the tooth with a tapered (knife-edge), flat, or slightly rounded edge.
        4. Papillae come to a point and fill the space between teeth (Fig. 5-2).
        5. Teeth with a diastema—no contact between adjacent teeth—or large spaces between teeth will have flat papillae.
2. **Tissue Consistency and Texture in Health**
    A. **Tissue Consistency**
        1. The attached gingiva is firmly connected to the underlying cementum and bone.
        2. The tissue is resilient (elastic). If gentle pressure is applied to the gingiva with the side of a probe, the tissue resists compression and springs back almost immediately.
        3. The attached gingiva will not pull away from the tooth when air is blown into the sulcus.

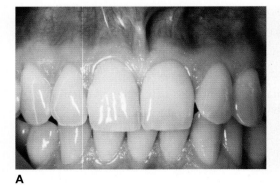
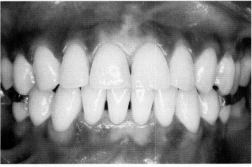

A   **B**

Figure 5-1. Tissue Color in Health. **A:** Periodontal health showing coral pink gingiva. Note the distinct difference in appearance between the keratinized gingiva and the nonkeratinized alveolar mucosa. **B:** Pigmentation of the gingiva showing how the gingiva can vary in color in some patients.

B. **Surface Texture of the Tissue**
1. In health, the surface of the attached gingiva is firm and may have a dimpled appearance similar to the skin of an orange peel (Fig. 5-3).
2. This dimpled appearance is known as **stippling**, appearing as minute elevations and depressions of the surface of the gingiva due to connective tissue projections within the epithelial tissue (connective tissue papillae). Stippling varies greatly from individual to individual and in some patients healthy tissue may not exhibit a stippled appearance. The presence of stippling is best viewed by drying the tissue with compressed air.
3. Healthy tissue may or may not exhibit a stippled appearance as the presence of stippling varies greatly from individual to individual.
3. **Position of Gingival Margin in Health.** Ideally, the gingival margin is slightly coronal to the cementoenamel junction (CEJ) (Figs. 5-4 and 5-5). Patients with a previous history of bone loss, but healthy gingival tissue, may have a gingival margin that is apical to the CEJ (Fig. 5-6).
4. **Absence of Bleeding in Health.** Healthy tissue does not bleed when disturbed by clinical procedures such as gentle probing of the sulcus.

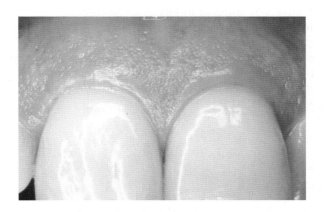

Figure 5-2. Contours of Healthy Gingiva. This tissue on the facial aspect of the maxillary anteriors exhibits all the characteristics of health, including a smoothly scalloped gingival margin, a tapered margin slightly coronal to the CEJ, and pointed papillae that completely fill the space between the teeth. (Courtesy of Dr. Don Rolfs, Wenachee, WA.)

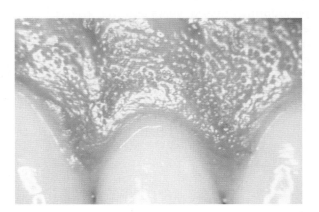

Figure 5-3. Stippling of Gingival Tissue. Healthy gingival tissue showing a stippled appearance. Stippling varies greatly from individual to individual and in some patients healthy tissue may not exhibit a stippled appearance.

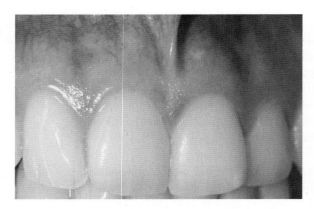

Figure 5-4. Position of the Margin in Health. In health, the gingival margin is slightly coronal to the cementoenamel junction. In anterior sextants, the margin is characterized by pronounced scalloping of the margin and pointed interdental papillae.

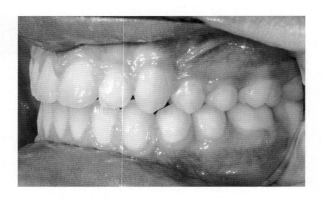

Figure 5-5. Gingiva in Posterior Sextants in Health. In posterior sextants, the tissue is characterized by a gently scalloped margin and papillae that fill the interdental embrasure spaces. (Used with permission from Langlais RP. *Color Atlas of Common Oral Diseases*. Philadelphia, PA: Wolters Kluwer; 2003.)

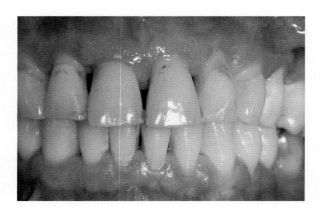

Figure 5-6. Health or Disease? This individual received periodontal treatment for chronic periodontitis several years ago. The assessment at today's appointment reveals no inflammation and no additional attachment loss since the beginning of periodontal maintenance several years ago. Therefore, this tissue is considered healthy. The attachment loss is simply an indicator of previous disease activity. (Courtesy of Dr. Ralph Arnold.)

Section 2
Clinical Features of Gingival Inflammation

Gingival **inflammation** is the body's reaction to the bacterial infection of the gingival tissues by periodontal pathogens. The inflammatory response to this bacterial infection results in clinical changes in the gingival tissue involving the free and attached gingiva as well as the papillae. Inflammation that is confined to gingival tissue with no effect on attachment level is called **gingivitis**, and is the mildest form of periodontal disease. Most patients are unaware they have a gingival infection because there usually is no discomfort.

A clinician with a trained eye can discern subtle differences in color, contour, and consistency even in gingival tissues that appear relatively healthy at first glance. The phrase "tissue talks" is a good phrase to remember when assessing the gingival tissue. Indications that the tissue is not healthy include such clinical observations as red, swollen tissue or papillae that do not fill the interdental space. Table 5-1 contrasts the characteristics of healthy versus inflamed gingival tissue.

TABLE 5-1. CHARACTERISTICS OF HEALTHY VERSUS INFLAMED GINGIVAL TISSUE

	Healthy Tissue	Gingivitis
Color	Uniform pink color Pigmentation may be present	Acute: bright red Chronic: bluish red to purplish red
Contour	Marginal gingiva 　Meets the tooth in a tapered or slightly 　rounded edge Interdental papillae 　Pointed papilla fills the space between 　the teeth	Marginal gingiva 　Meets the tooth in a rolled, thickened 　edge Interdental papillae 　Bulbous, blunted, cratered
Consistency	Firm Resilient under compression	Spongy, flaccid Indents easily when pressed lightly Compressed air deflects the tissue
Texture	Smooth and/or stippled	Tissue shiny in appearance Stretched appearance
Margin	Slightly coronal to the CEJ	Coronal to the CEJ
Bleeding	No bleeding upon probing	Bleeding upon probing

1. **Characteristics of Gingivitis**
   A. **Tissue Color in Gingivitis**
      1. Gingivitis is an inflammation of the gingiva often causing the tissue to become red and swollen, to bleed easily, and sometimes to become slightly tender. There is also an increased flow of crevicular fluid (sulcular fluid) from the sulcus, corresponding to the severity of inflammation (1).
      2. Inflammation results in increased blood flow to the gingiva causing the tissue to appear bright red. Figures 5-7 and 5-8 show examples of common clinical presentations of gingivitis.

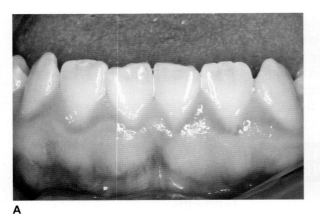
A

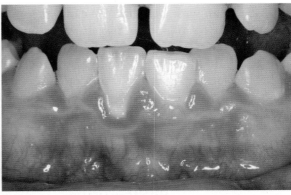
B

Figure 5-7. Color Changes in Gingivitis. A: Slight marginal redness is a clinical sign of early gingivitis. **B:** This gingival tissue shows more inflammation than seen in photograph **A**. The marginal and papillary gingival tissues are bright red in color. Note, also, the swelling of the marginal gingiva and papillae in this example. (Courtesy of Dr. Richard Foster, Guilford Technical Community College, Jamestown, NC.)

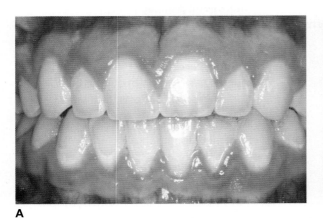
A

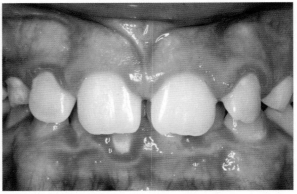
B

Figure 5-8. Color Changes in Gingivitis. A: This example shows subtle color changes in the marginal and papillary gingival tissues. **B:** In this example, the color changes are pronounced with fiery red marginal gingiva and papillae. (Courtesy of Dr. Richard Foster, Guilford Technical Community College, Jamestown, NC.)

B. **Tissue Contour (Size and Shape) in Gingivitis**
1. An increase of fluid within the tissue spaces—edema—causes enlargement of the gingival tissues. The normal scalloped appearance of the gingiva is lost if the gingival papillae are swollen.
2. Examples of types of changes in the appearance of the papillae are listed below.
   a. Bulbous papilla—a papilla that is enlarged and appears to bulge out of the interproximal space (Fig. 5-9).
   b. Blunted papilla—a papilla that is flat and does not fill the interproximal space (Fig. 5-10).
   c. Cratered papillae—a papilla that appears to have been "scooped out" leaving a concave depression in the midproximal area. Cratered papillae are associated with necrotizing ulcerative gingivitis (Fig. 5-11).

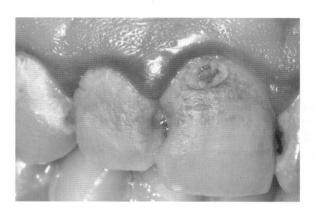

Figure 5-9. Bulbous Papillae. In gingivitis, the papillae may be enlarged and appear to bulge out of the interproximal space as seen in the papilla between the central and lateral incisors in this clinical photograph. (Courtesy of Dr. Ralph Arnold, San Antonio, TX.)

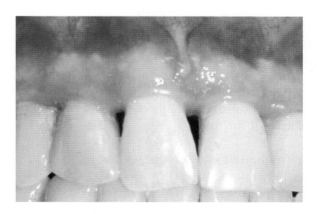

Figure 5-10. Blunted Papillae. In gingivitis, the papillae may be blunted and missing as seen in the papillae between the central and lateral incisors. (Courtesy of Dr. Don Rolfs, Wenachee, WA.)

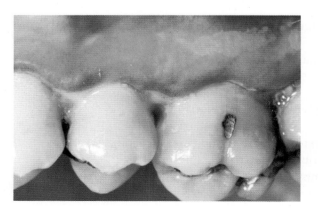

Figure 5-11. Cratered Papillae. The papillae may have a concave appearance in the midproximal area as seen in the papillae between second premolar and molar in this clinical photo. (Courtesy of Dr. Don Rolfs, Wenachee, WA.)

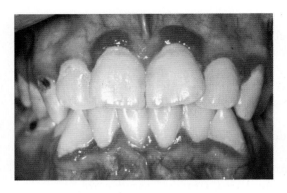

Figure 5-12. Soft, Spongy Tissue. Inflamed gingival tissue may be soft and spongy. The inflammatory fluids can cause the gingival tissues to feel somewhat like a moist sponge. (Courtesy of Dr. Ralph Arnold, San Antonio, TX.)

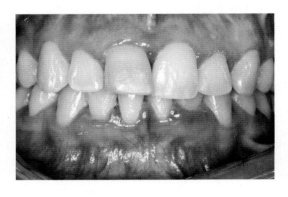

Figure 5-13. Smooth, Shiny Tissue. In gingivitis, fluid in the tissue can cause the tissue to appear smooth and shiny with a stretched appearance. (Courtesy of Dr. Richard Foster, Guilford Technical Community College, Jamestown, NC.)

2. **Tissue Consistency and Texture in Gingivitis**
   A. **Tissue Consistency in Gingivitis**
      1. Increased fluid in the inflamed tissue also causes the gingiva to be soft, spongy, and nonelastic (Fig. 5-12).
      2. When pressure is applied to the inflamed gingiva with the side of a probe, the tissue is easily compressed and can retain an imprint of the probe for several seconds.
      3. Inflamed gingival tissue loses its firm consistency becoming flaccid (soft, movable). When compressed air is directed into the sulcus, it readily deflects the gingival margin and papillae away from the neck of the tooth.
   B. **Surface Texture in Gingivitis**
      1. The increase in fluid due to the inflammatory response can cause the gingival tissues to appear smooth and very shiny (Fig. 5-13).
      2. The tissue almost has a "stretched" appearance that resembles plastic wrap that has been pulled tightly.
3. **Position of Margin in Gingivitis**
   A. In gingivitis, the position of the gingival margin may move more coronally (further above the CEJ).
   B. This change in the position of the gingival margin is due to tissue swelling and enlargement (Fig. 5-14).
4. **Presence of Bleeding in Gingivitis**
   A. Bleeding upon gentle probing is seen clinically before changes in color are clinically detectable (Fig. 5-15).
   B. In gingivitis, the sulcus lining becomes ulcerated and the blood vessels become engorged. The tissues bleed easily during probing or instrumentation.
   C. There is a direct relationship between inflammation and bleeding: The more severe the inflammation, the heavier the bleeding.

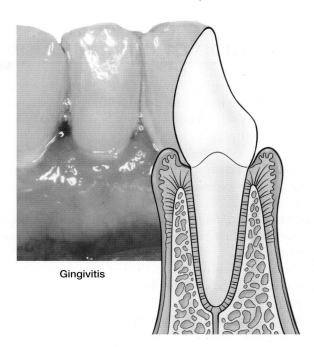

Gingivitis

Figure 5-14. Tissue Margin in Gingivitis. The tissue swelling in gingivitis may cause the position of the gingival margin to move coronally—further above the CEJ—than in health. There is no destruction of periodontal ligament fibers or alveolar bone in gingivitis.

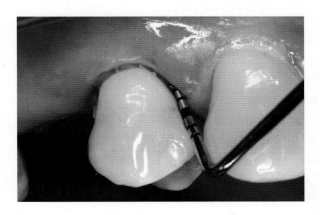

Figure 5-15. Bleeding on Probing. Bleeding is an important clinical indicator of inflammation. Inflammation results in ulceration of the sulcus/pocket wall causing the gingival tissues to bleed easily during gentle probing.

Section 3
Extent and Distribution of Inflammation

In documenting inflammation of the gingival tissues it is useful to note both the extent and distribution of the inflammation. Just documenting the presence of gingival inflammation is too vague, and does not identify severity of inflammation accurately enough to help establish a treatment plan.

1. **Gingival Inflammation**
   A. **Extent of Inflammation.** The extent of inflammation is the area of tissue that is affected by inflammation. The extent of inflammation is described as localized or generalized in the mouth.
      1. Localized inflammation is confined to the gingival tissue of a single tooth—such as the maxillary right first molar—or to a group of teeth—such as the mandibular anterior sextant.
      2. Generalized inflammation involves all or most of the tissue in the mouth.
   B. **Distribution of Inflammation.** The distribution of inflammation describes the area where the gingival tissue is inflamed.
      1. The inflammation may affect only the interdental papilla, the gingival margin and the papilla, or the gingival margin, papilla, and the attached gingiva.
      2. Table 5-2 summarizes how to describe the extent and distribution of inflammation of the gingival tissue. Figures 5-16 to 5-20 illustrate the use of this descriptive terminology.

TABLE 5-2. GINGIVAL INFLAMMATION	
Extent	• **Localized**—inflammation confined to the tissue of a single tooth or a group of teeth • **Generalized**—inflammation of the gingival tissue of all or most of the mouth
Distribution	• **Papillary**—inflammation of the interdental papilla only • **Marginal**—inflammation of the gingival margin and papilla • **Diffuse**—inflammation of the gingival margin, papilla, and attached gingiva
Descriptions	Descriptive terms may be combined to create a verbal picture of the inflammation, such as the following: • "Localized marginal inflammation in the mandibular anterior sextant" • "Localized papillary inflammation on the maxillary right canine" • "Generalized marginal inflammation" • "Generalized diffuse inflammation"

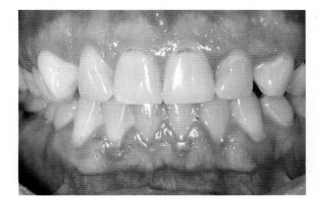

Figure 5-16. Localized Marginal Inflammation.
Note the redness and swelling of the marginal and papillary gingival tissues that is localized to the mandibular anterior sextant. (Courtesy of Dr. Ralph Arnold.)

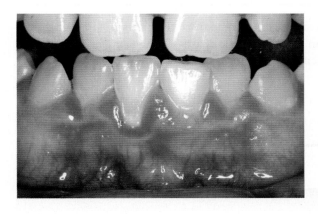

Figure 5-17. Localized Diffuse Inflammation.
Redness and edema of the gingival margin, papillae, and attached gingiva in the mandibular anterior sextant. (Courtesy of Dr. Richard Foster, Guilford Technical Community College, Jamestown, NC.)

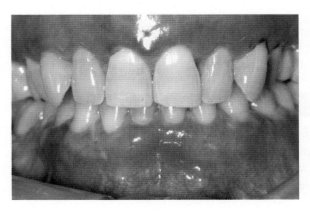

Figure 5-18. Generalized Diffuse Inflammation.
Diffuse inflammation of the gingival margin, papillae, and attached gingiva throughout the entire mouth. (Courtesy of Dr. Ralph Arnold.)

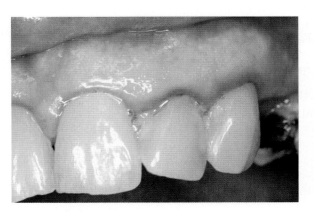

Figure 5-19. Localized Marginal Inflammation.
Note the reddened tissue color along the gingival margin, extending down into the papillae on these maxillary anterior teeth. (Courtesy of Dr. Richard Foster, Guilford Technical Community College, Jamestown, NC.)

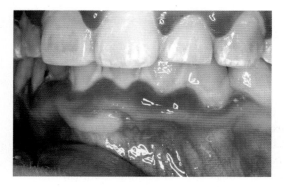

Figure 5-20. Localized Diffuse Inflammation. Inflammation involving the gingival margin, papillae, and attached gingiva of the mandibular anterior sextant. (Courtesy of Dr. Richard Foster, Guilford Technical Community College, Jamestown, NC.)

Chapter Summary Statement

Clinicians must have a clear mental image of gingival health to recognize the signs of gingival inflammation when it occurs. Inflammation in the gingiva causes changes in the color, contour, and consistency of the gingiva that can be recognized even in the earliest stages by the trained clinician.

Section 4
Focus on Patients

Clinical Patient Care

CASE 1

A patient new to your dental team has been appointed with you for a dental prophylaxis. The patient has just relocated to your town. The patient tells you that he saw a dentist just before moving who told him that he has gingivitis. During your discussion with the patient, he asks if there is some way he can tell at home if he has gingivitis. How might you reply to this patient's question?

CASE 2

Reading through your patient's treatment notes from the previous visit, you notice the clinician documented "presence of gingival inflammation." Explain why this statement is not adequate in order to provide quality patient treatment. What would you add to the description to provide another clinician with a clear verbal description of the clinical features of the patient's gingival tissues?

Reference

1. Himani GS, Prabhuji ML, Karthikeyan BV. Gingival crevicular fluid and interleukin-23 concentration in systemically healthy subjects: their relationship in periodontal health and disease. *J Periodontal Res.* 2014;49(2):237–245.

 STUDENT ANCILLARY RESOURCES

A wide variety of resources to enhance your learning and understanding of this chapter are available on thePoint®.

- Visit thePoint to access:
  - Audio Glossary
  - Animations
  - Suggested Readings
  - Answers to Review Questions
  - Case Studies

CHAPTER

6

Diseases of the Gingiva

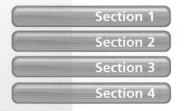
Clinical Application. Examination of the gingiva is part of every patient visit. The dynamic nature of the gingival tissue allows these tissues to show signs of disease in early stages. The dental hygienist often is the first member of the dental team to be able to note these early signs of periodontal disease. This chapter outlines the numerous conditions that can affect the gingiva and can serve as a foundation reference for organizing knowledge about these conditions.

Learning Objectives

- Define the two major subdivisions of gingival disease as established by the American Academy of Periodontology.
- Compare and contrast dental plaque–induced gingival diseases and non–plaque-induced gingival lesions.
- Describe the clinical signs of inflammation you would expect to find in a patient with moderate plaque-induced gingivitis.
- List systemic factors that may modify gingival disease.
- Name three types of medications that may cause gingival enlargement.
- Explain how the use of certain medications and malnutrition can modify gingival disease.
- Develop a list of suggestions for managing patients with primary herpetic gingivostomatitis.

Key Terms

Gingival diseases
Dental plaque–induced gingival diseases
Acute gingivitis
Chronic gingivitis

Gingival diseases associated with modifying factors
Pregnancy-associated pyogenic granuloma
Non–plaque-induced gingival lesions

Section 1
Classification of Gingival Diseases

Gingival diseases usually involve inflammation of the gingival tissues, most often in response to bacterial plaque biofilm. Certain characteristics must be present for a periodontal disease to be classified as a gingival disease (Box 6-1). The 1999 AAP Classification of Periodontal Diseases and Conditions subdivides the major diagnostic category of gingivitis into specific types of diseases: (1) dental plaque–induced gingival diseases and (2) non–plaque-induced gingival lesions. Each gingivitis disease type has two or more subcategories (Fig. 6-1).

Box 6-1. Characteristics Common to Gingival Diseases

1. Signs or symptoms of inflammation are confined to the gingiva.
2. No loss of attachment (no destruction of periodontal ligament fibers or alveolar bone) is associated with the inflammation of the gingival tissues.
3. The presence of dental plaque biofilm initiates and/or aggravates the inflammation.
4. Clinical signs of inflammation include changes such as enlarged gingival contours, color transition to a red and/or bluish-red hue, bleeding upon stimulation, increased crevicular fluid flow.

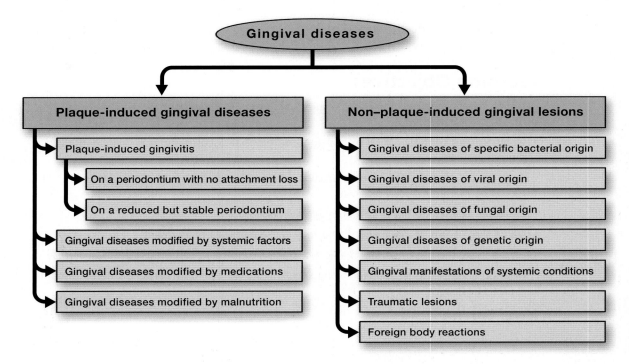

Figure 6-1. Two Major Subdivisions of Gingival Diseases. The two major subdivisions of gingival diseases are (1) dental plaque–induced gingival diseases and (2) non–plaque-induced gingival lesions. These two major subdivisions are further subdivided into types.

Section 2
Dental Plaque–Induced Gingival Diseases

Dental plaque–induced gingival diseases are periodontal diseases involving inflammation of the gingiva in response to plaque biofilm. Ineffective plaque biofilm control triggers the body's immune response. As long as bacteria remain in contact with the gingival tissue, inflammation continues. Certain species of bacteria that are elevated during times of gingival inflammation are listed in Table 6-1.

TABLE 6-1. BACTERIA ASSOCIATED WITH HEALTH AND GINGIVITIS

	Bacterial Species Associated with Health	Bacterial Species Elevated in Gingivitis
Gram-Positive Rods	Actinomyces israelii Actinomyces naeslundii Actinomyces odontolyticus Rothia dentocariosa Actinomyces gerencseriae	Actinomyces naeslundii III
Gram-Positive Cocci	Streptococcus mitis Streptococcus oralis Peptostreptococcus micros Streptococcus sanguis Streptococcus gordonii	Streptococcus anginosus Streptococcus sanguis
Gram-Negative Rods	Selenomonas sputigena Capnocytophaga gingivalis Prevotella intermedia Fusobacterium nucleatum	Campylobacter concisus Porphyromonas gingivalis
Gram-Negative Diplococci		Neisseria gonorrhoeae
Spirochete		Treponema pallidum

1. Gingivitis Associated with Dental Plaque Biofilm Only
   A. Characteristics
      1. *Gingivitis associated with plaque biofilm* is by far the most common type of periodontal disease.
      2. The clinical signs of gingivitis may vary between individuals and also within the dentition of an individual.
      3. Three separate stages of gingivitis mark the progression of disease:
         a. Initial lesion—develops within 4 days of plaque biofilm accumulation; sulcus heavily populated with gram-positive cocci.
         b. Early lesion—inflammation can be detected clinically after 7 days; gram-negative bacteria begin to flourish.
         c. Established lesion—bleeding upon probing; spirochetes and gram-negative rods are detected microscopically.
      4. Incidence of gingivitis differs between children and adults.
         a. Inflammation is not as intense in children versus young adults with the same quantity of plaque biofilm (1–3).
         b. Adolescents may have elevated levels of certain bacteria: Actinomyces, Capnocytophaga, Leptotrichia, and Selenomonas species (4).

    c. Children may have fewer pathogenic bacteria in their plaque biofilm, a thicker junctional epithelium, and a less developed immune response (5,6).

    d. Gingival inflammation in senior adults is more pronounced even when similar amounts of plaque biofilms are present, perhaps attributed to age-related differences in cellular inflammatory response to plaque biofilm (7,8).

  5. Local factors—such as dental restorations, appliances, root fractures, and tooth anatomy—act as a site for plaque biofilm retention and may contribute to the disease.

B. Clinical Signs of Gingivitis Associated with Dental Plaque Only

  1. Clinical signs of gingival inflammation include changes in gingival color, contour, and consistency. Common clinical signs include redness (erythema), swelling (edema), bleeding, and tenderness (Box 6-2, Figs. 6-2A, 2B).

  2. The disease process begins at the gingival margin—the site of plaque biofilm accumulation—and is characterized clinically by red, swollen, tender gums that bleed easily.

C. Duration of Gingivitis

  1. *Acute gingivitis*—gingivitis of a short duration, after which professional care and patient self-care returns the gingiva to a healthy state.

  2. *Chronic gingivitis*—long-lasting gingivitis; gingivitis may exist for years without ever progressing to periodontitis.

Box 6-2. Gingivitis Associated with Dental Plaque Only

- Most common form of periodontal disease
- Plaque biofilm present at the gingival margin
- Gingival redness; tenderness
- Increase in sulcular temperature
- Bleeding upon probing
- Stable attachment levels
- Condition reversible with plaque biofilm removal

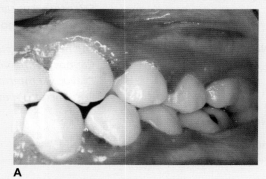

A

Figure 6-2A. Plaque-Induced Gingivitis. Plaque-induced gingivitis in this patient has resulted in rolled gingival margins and enlarged papillae.

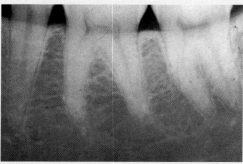

B

Figure 6-2B. Radiograph Reveals No Bone Loss. The dental radiographs of an individual with plaque-induced gingivitis do not reveal any changes in either the alveolar bone height or the character of the alveolar bone.

2. Plaque-Associated Gingival Diseases with Modifying Factors. The category **gingival diseases associated with modifying factors** includes the less common types of plaque-induced gingivitis. There are three main subcategories of gingival diseases with modifying factors: (1) gingival diseases modified by systemic factors, (2) gingival diseases modified by medications, and (3) gingival diseases modified by malnutrition.

A. Gingival Diseases Modified by Systemic Factors. In this form of gingival disease, plaque biofilm initiates the disease; then, specific systemic factors found in the host will modify the disease process (9).

1. *Gingival diseases associated with the endocrine system and fluctuations in sex hormones.* In this subcategory, changes in the endocrine system or levels of sex hormones result in an exaggerated response to the presence of plaque biofilm. Gingival tissues may appear bright red, soft, friable (easily damaged; thinly stretched), smooth, and exhibit bleeding from slight provocation.

   a. *Puberty-associated gingivitis* is an exaggerated inflammatory response of the gingiva to a relatively small amount of plaque biofilm and hormones during puberty.
      1. Although severity is directly related to the amount of plaque biofilm, gingivitis will manifest with a very small amount of plaque biofilm.
      2. Puberty-associated gingivitis is found in both male and female adolescents.
      3. Clinical features are inflamed gingiva with prominent bulbous papillae on the facial aspect (Fig. 6-3). Bulbous papillae are rarely seen on the lingual gingival tissue.

   b. *Menstrual cycle–associated gingivitis* is an exaggerated inflammatory response of the gingiva to plaque biofilm and hormones estrogen and progesterone before ovulation.

   c. *Oral contraceptive–associated gingivitis* is an exaggerated inflammatory response of the gingiva to plaque biofilm and in patients taking oral contraceptives.
      1. A recent study by Taichman and Eklund (10) found no association between the use of oral contraceptives and increased gingival inflammation in young women.
      2. Long-term use of oral contraceptives may affect periodontal attachment levels. A study of 50 women aged 20 to 35 years, found that current pill users had deeper mean probing depths compared to nonusers (3.3 vs. 2.7 mm) and more severe attachment loss (2.6 vs. 1.7 mm). Pill users had more sites with bleeding on probing (44.0% vs. 31.1%) (11).

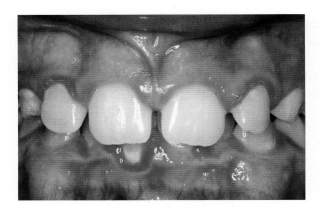

Figure 6-3. Puberty-Associated Gingivitis. Puberty-associated gingivitis is an exaggerated inflammatory response of the gingiva to a relatively small amount of plaque biofilm. The exaggerated response is modulated by hormones released during puberty. (Courtesy of Dr. Richard Foster, Guilford Technical Community College, Jamestown, NC.)

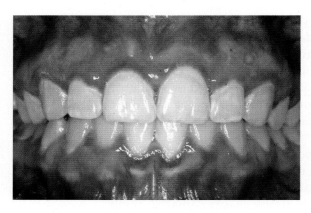

Figure 6-4. Pregnancy-Associated Gingivitis. Note the red gingiva and bulbous interdental papilla on this patient with pregnancy-associated gingivitis. (Courtesy of Dr. Richard Foster, Guilford Technical Community College, Jamestown, NC.)

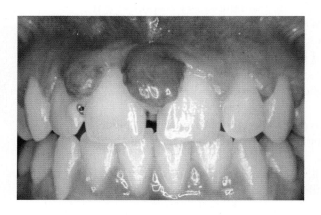

Figure 6-5. Pregnancy-Associated Pyogenic Granuloma. This mushroom-like mass of the gingiva bleeds easily if disturbed.

d. *Pregnancy-associated gingivitis* is an exaggerated inflammatory response of the gingiva to plaque biofilm and hormone changes usually occurring during the second and third trimesters of pregnancy (12–15). During pregnancy, the levels of estrogen and progesterone continue to rise and reach their peak in the eighth month of gestation. High levels in both blood and saliva cause an exaggerated tissue response to plaque biofilm. Increased quantities of hormones also trigger gingival crevicular fluid flow, which may precipitate gingival inflammation.

1. Pregnancy-associated gingivitis can manifest in response to even small amounts of plaque biofilm.
2. The gingival tissue may be edematous and dark red, with bulbous interdental papillae (Fig. 6-4).
3. Pregnancy-associated gingivitis can spontaneously resolve postpartum.
4. In some cases, a gingival papilla can react so strongly to plaque biofilm that a large, localized overgrowth of gingival tissue called a **pregnancy-associated pyogenic granuloma** (pregnancy tumor), may form on the interdental gingiva or on the gingival margin.

e. *Pregnancy-associated pyogenic granuloma ("pregnancy tumor")* is a localized, mushroom-shaped gingival mass projecting from the gingival margin or more commonly from a gingival papilla during pregnancy.
   1. This condition is the result of an exaggerated tissue response to plaque biofilm or other irritants that usually occurs after the first trimester of pregnancy.
   2. The gingival mass is characterized by a mushroom-like tissue mass that most commonly occurs in the maxilla and interproximally (Fig. 6-5).
   3. A pregnancy-associated pyogenic granuloma is painless and noncancerous.
   4. The tissue mass bleeds easily if disturbed and may appear to be covered with dark red pinpoint markings.
   5. The growth usually resolves after childbirth.

f. *Diabetes-associated gingivitis* is an inflammatory response of the gingiva to plaque biofilm that is aggravated by poorly controlled blood glucose levels (16–19).
   1. This condition is often seen in children with poorly controlled type I diabetes mellitus.
   2. Reduction in gingival inflammation in adults with diabetes may reduce the amount of insulin needed to control blood glucose levels. Diabetes mellitus is discussed in more detail in Chapter 15.

2. *Gingival diseases associated with blood dyscrasias*
   a. *Leukemia-associated gingivitis* is an exaggerated inflammatory response of the gingiva to plaque biofilm resulting in increased bleeding and tissue enlargement. Oral lesions may be the first clinical signs of leukemia; therefore, dental healthcare providers can be the first to suspect that a patient may have leukemia.
      1. Gingival tissues appear swollen, spongy, shiny, and red to deep purple in appearance (Fig. 6-6).
      2. Tissues are very friable (tear easily) and have a tendency to hemorrhage with slight provocation.
      3. The presence of plaque biofilm is NOT a prerequisite for gingivitis in patients with leukemia.
      4. Typically, leukemia-associated gingivitis begins in the papillae and spreads to the marginal and then, the attached gingiva.
   b. *Blood dyscrasias–associated gingivitis* is gingivitis associated with abnormal function or number of blood cells.

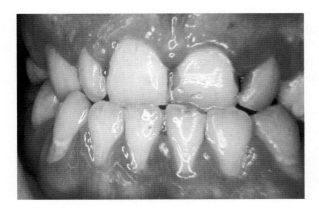

Figure 6-6. Leukemia-Associated Gingivitis. Note the red, swollen appearance of the gingiva in this patient with leukemia. (Courtesy of Dr. Ralph Arnold.)

3. **Plaque-Associated Gingival Diseases Modified by Medications**
   A. *Drug-influenced gingivitis* is an exaggerated inflammatory response of the gingiva to plaque biofilm and a systemic medication.
   B. *Drug-influenced gingival enlargement* is an increase in size of the gingiva resulting from systemic medications, most commonly anticonvulsants, calcium channel blockers, and immunosuppressants. Plaque biofilm accumulation is not necessary for the initiation of gingival enlargement, but it will exacerbate the gingival disease. Meticulous plaque biofilm control can reduce but will not eliminate gingival overgrowth.
      1. Medications Associated with Gingival Enlargement
         a. Anticonvulsants (e.g., phenytoin, Celontin, zerontin, Paganone, sodium valproate). Anticonvulsants are a diverse group of pharmaceuticals used in the treatment of epileptic seizures. In addition, anticonvulsants are now used in the treatment of bipolar disorder.
         b. Immunosuppressants (e.g., cyclosporine). Immunosuppressant drugs suppress the natural immune responses. Immunosuppressants are given to transplant patients to prevent organ rejection or to patients with autoimmune diseases. The immunosuppressant stimulates fibroblast proliferation with excessive extracellular matrix accumulation in gingival tissues (20).
         c. Calcium Channel Blocking Agents (e.g., amlodipine, nifedipine, verapamil). Calcium channel blocking agents relax the blood vessels and increase the supply of blood and oxygen to the heart while reducing its workload. Some of the calcium channel blocking agents are used to relieve and control angina pectoris (chest pain). Some are also used to treat high blood pressure (hypertension). These drugs affect gingival connective tissues by stimulating an increase of fibroblasts and increasing the production of connective tissue matrix.
      2. Clinical Appearance of Gingival Enlargement
         a. Tissue enlargement is an exaggerated inflammatory response in relation to the amount of plaque biofilm present.
         b. The onset of tissue enlargement usually occurs within 3 months of taking medication.
         c. The pattern of tissue enlargement is irregular, first observed in papillae. Begins as a painless area of enlargement on the papilla and then proceeds to the marginal gingiva.
         d. Gingiva in anterior sextants is most commonly affected, however, can occur in posterior sextants (Figs. 6-7 and 6-8).
         e. The severity of overgrowth is directly affected by level of self-care; scrupulous homecare can reduce the severity of the overgrowth.
         f. Gingival overgrowth appears more frequently in the maxillary and mandibular anterior sextants.
         g. Gingival enlargement is characterized by an increased flow of crevicular fluid from the sulcus and bleeding upon probing with no attachment loss.
         h. Drug-influenced gingival enlargement is more commonly seen in children.
4. **Plaque-Associated Gingival Diseases Modified by Malnutrition.** Even with our adequate food supply in North America, infants, institutionalized elderly, and alcoholics are all at risk for vitamin deficiencies.
   A. *Ascorbic acid–deficiency gingivitis* is an inflammatory response of the gingiva to plaque biofilm aggravated by chronically low ascorbic acid (vitamin C) levels. Ascorbic acid–deficiency gingivitis manifests as bright red, swollen, ulcerated gingival tissue that bleeds with the slightest provocation (Fig. 6-9) (21,22).

B. **Other.** Specific nutrient deficiencies can decrease the efficiency of the immune system and exacerbate the response of the gingival tissues to plaque biofilm. In animal studies, a deficiency in vitamin A and B-complex vitamins has had an effect on the gingival tissues. Vitamin A helps maintain healthy sulcular epithelium. B-complex vitamins help maintain healthy mucosal tissues.

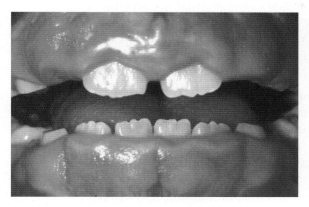

Figure 6-7. Phenytoin-Induced Gingival Enlargement. Massive tissue overgrowth may be seen in phenytoin-induced gingival enlargement.

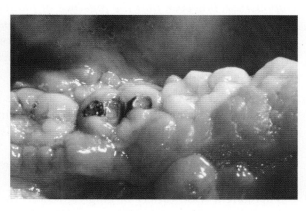

Figure 6-8. Cyclosporine-Induced Gingival Enlargement. Gingival changes seen in cyclosporine-induced gingival enlargement.

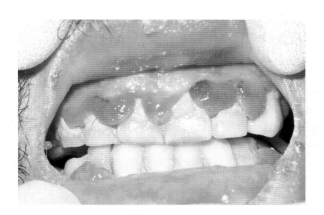

Figure 6-9. Ascorbic Acid–Deficiency Gingivitis. A photograph of a patient with scurvy. Scurvy is the clinical state arising from dietary deficiency of vitamin C (ascorbic acid). Note the bright red, swollen, and ulcerated gingival tissue. (Courtesy of Mediscan Company.)

Section 3
Non–Plaque-Induced Gingival Lesions

A small percentage of gingival diseases—non–plaque-induced gingival lesions—are not caused by plaque biofilm and do not disappear after plaque biofilm removal. *It should be emphasized, however, that the presence of plaque biofilm could increase the severity of the gingival inflammation in noninduced lesions.*

Non–plaque-induced gingivitis can result from such varied causes as bacterial, viral, or fungal infections; genetic origin; dermatological (skin) diseases; allergic reactions; and mechanical trauma.

- Specific bacteria can infect the gingival tissues and cause a form of gingivitis (23).
- Some types of gingivitis can be caused by an infection with a specific virus (24–27). Although rare in otherwise healthy individuals, gingival lesions can be caused by fungal infections (24,28,29).
- There are some gingival lesions that are not infections at all, but rather have a genetic etiology (30).
- There are a wide variety of gingival lesions that occur as manifestations of systemic conditions such as mucocutaneous disorders or allergic reactions (24,31).

This section presents some examples of this small percentage of gingival disease in which plaque biofilm does not have an etiologic role. Of the non–plaque-induced gingival lesions, the two most commonly seen in the dental office are primary herpetic gingivostomatitis and allergic reactions.

1. Gingival Diseases of Specific Bacterial Origin
   A. **Definition.** Gingival diseases in this category are characterized by a bacterial infection of the gingiva by a specific bacterium that is *not a common component* of the bacterial plaque biofilm.
   B. **Characteristics of Gingival Diseases of Specific Bacterial Origin**
      1. Gingival diseases of specific bacterial origin occur on rare occasions when a bacterial infection overwhelms the host resistance. In these cases, the gingivitis is due to an infection by a specific bacterium that is usually not considered a periodontal pathogen. Examples include infections with *Neisseria gonorrhea, Treponema pallidum,* and streptococcal species (32–34).
      2. The gingival lesions manifest as painful ulcerations, chancres or mucous patches, or atypical highly inflamed gingivitis (Fig. 6-10).
      3. Lesions may not be present elsewhere on the body.

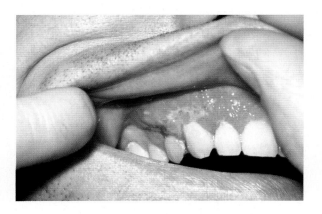

Figure 6-10. Atypical Mycobacterial Infection.
This patient has an atypical bacterial infection of the gingiva. The fingers shown in this photograph are the patient's own. (Courtesy of Mediscan Company.)

2. **Primary Herpetic Gingivostomatitis (PHG)** is a severe reaction to the initial infection with—first exposure of an individual to—the herpes simplex type-I virus (HSV-1).
   A. **Disease Characteristics**
   1. By the time individuals reach middle age about 70% have been infected with HSV-1.
      a. In most cases, the virus never causes symptoms during this primary HSV-1 infection. This is known as a subclinical—symptom free—infection.
      b. In some individuals, however, this initial infection presents with intensely painful gingivitis and multiple vesicles that easily rupture to form painful ulcers. This severe reaction to the initial HSV-1 infection is known as primary herpetic gingivostomatitis (Fig. 6-11).
      c. Once infected, most individuals develop immunity to the virus. In certain individuals, the herpes simplex virus type-1 can remain latent in the trigeminal ganglion and is responsible for recurrent oral herpetic lesions (cold sores).
   2. The initial infection with the HSV-1 usually affects young children—with heightened incidence from 1 to 3 years of age—but may affect adolescents and adults.
      a. Of children with primary infections, 99% are symptom free or the symptoms are attributed to teething.
      b. The remaining 1% develops significant gingival inflammation and ulceration of the lips and mucous membranes (35).
   3. The infection is contagious during the vesicular stage as the virus is contained in the clear fluid in the vesicles. The virus may be easily spread through close personal contact.
   4. PHG is associated with severe pain that makes eating and drinking difficult.
   5. Associated symptoms of PHG are headache, swollen lymph nodes, and sore throat. Because this condition is a viral infection, there may be a low-grade fever usually not above 101°F.
   6. Regresses spontaneously within 10 to 20 days without scarring.
   B. **Clinical Manifestations of PHG.** PHG may occur anywhere on the free or the attached gingiva or in the alveolar mucosa.
   1. PHG is characterized by widespread inflammation of the marginal and attached gingiva.
   2. The gingiva will demonstrate intense gingivitis and pain.
   3. Small clusters of vesicles rapidly erupt throughout the mouth.
   4. Later, these vesicles burst, forming yellowish ulcers that are surrounded by a red halo. Ulcers may occur on the lips, tongue, palate, and buccal mucosa (Fig. 6-12).
   5. Headache, fever, swollen lymph nodes, and sore throat usually are present.

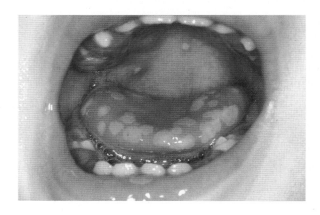

Figure 6-11. Primary Herpetic Gingivostomatitis. This photograph shows an initial HSV-1 infection in a young child. (Courtesy of Mediscan Company.)

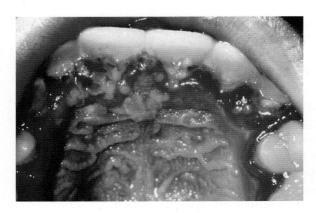

Figure 6-12. Primary Herpetic Gingivostomatitis.
Primary herpetic gingivostomatitis is seen on the palate of this patient. Note the fiery red gingival margins and ulcers surrounded by red halos.

C. Treatment for Primary Herpetic Gingivostomatitis
  1. Encourage the intake of fluids to prevent dehydration that can result from fever. Athletic drinks, such as Gatorade , can be consumed to replenish electrolytes lost due to dehydration.
  2. A dietary replacement drink, such as PediaSure or Ensure, can be a good source of nutrition since eating will be difficult. The patient may be able to eat foods processed in a blender.
  3. Counsel the patient that adequate intake of fluids is important. Since eating and drinking are painful, dehydration is a major concern with these individuals.
  4. An antimicrobial mouthwash like Listerine or Peridex should be recommended to prevent a secondary infection.
  5. Precautions should be taken to prevent the spread of the virus to the patient's eyes or from the infected individual to other persons. The infected patient should wash with soap and water frequently. Wash toys that an infected child puts in his or her mouth before and after play time. Do not let an infected child share contaminated items, such as eating utensils with another person.

3. Linear Gingival Erythema (LGE)
  A. Disease Characteristics
    1. LGE is a gingival manifestation of immunosuppression (36–38).
    2. It is characterized by inflammation that is exaggerated for the amount of plaque biofilm present.
    3. LGE does not respond well to improved oral self-care or professional therapy.
    4. For a diagnosis of LGE, the condition must persist after removal of plaque biofilms (39).
  B. Clinical Manifestations of LGE
    1. LGE is characterized by a distinct red band that is limited to the free gingiva (Fig. 6-13).
    2. There is no evidence of attachment loss in LGE.
    3. A key feature of LGE is a lack of bleeding on probing (40).
    4. LGE is often associated with HIV infection.
    5. LGE usually does not respond well to therapy.

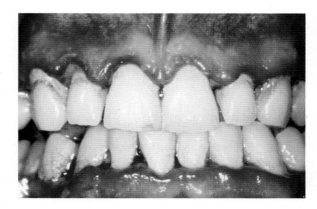

Figure 6-13. Linear Gingival Erythema. This patient has linear gingival erythema associated with HIV infection. Note the distinct red band along the free gingiva.

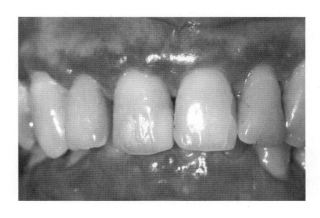

Figure 6-14. Oral Lichen Planus. Oral lichen planus of the maxillary gingiva. The gingival tissues are erythematous, ulcerated, and painful. (Courtesy of Dr. Ralph Arnold, San Antonio, TX.)

4. Lichen Planus
   A. Disease Characteristics
      1. Lichen planus is a disease of the skin and mucous membranes in which there is an itchy, swollen rash on the skin or in the mouth. Both the skin and mucous membranes may be affected; however, oral involvement or skin involvement alone is common. The exact cause of lichen planus is unknown. However, it is likely to be related to an allergic or immune reaction.
      2. Lichen planus is the most common mucocutaneous disease affecting the gingiva (41).
      3. Oral lichen planus may affect persons of any age although it is rarely seen in children (26).
      4. An initial episode of oral lichen planus may last for weeks or months. Unfortunately, oral lichen planus is usually a chronic condition and can last for many years.
      5. Good patient self-care can relieve the painful symptoms of the gingival lesions (42).
   B. Clinical Manifestations
      1. Oral manifestations include intense erythema of the gingiva (Fig. 6-14).
      2. Ulcerations of the gingiva may be present and are associated with pain.
      3. Interlacing white lines (Wickham striae) may be present on the buccal mucosa and gingiva.
      4. Raised white lesions may be present as individual papules or in plaque-like configurations.

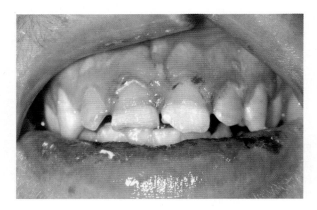

Figure 6-15. Erythema Multiforme. Erythema multiforme with ulcerations of the gingiva and crust formation of the lower lip. (Courtesy of Dr. Ralph Arnold, San Antonio, TX.)

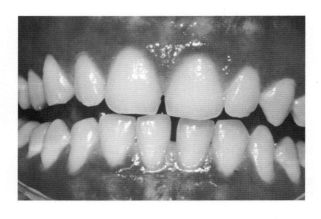

Figure 6-16. Allergic Reaction. Clinical signs of allergic reactions in the gingival tissues include redness extending from the gingival margin to the mucogingival junction.

5. **Erythema Multiforme**
   A. **Disease Characteristics**
      1. Erythema multiforme is a disorder of the skin and mucous membranes due to an allergic reaction or infection. Large, symmetrical red blotches, resembling a target, appear all over the skin in a circular pattern.
      2. On mucous membranes, it begins as blisters and progresses to ulcers. Oral involvement occurs in as many as 25% to 60% of cases and is sometimes the only involved site (43,44).
      3. The exact cause is unknown, though may involve a hypersensitivity reaction.
   B. **Clinical Manifestations**
      1. Oral manifestations include swollen lips often with extensive crust formation.
      2. Lesions on the gingiva involve bullae that rupture and leave ulcers (Fig. 6-15).
6. **Allergic Reactions.** Allergic reactions can occur to ingredients in toothpastes, mouthwashes, or chewing gum (45). These reactions are usually the result of a flavor additive or preservatives in the product. Flavor additives known to cause gingival reactions are cinnamon and carvone (45–47).
   A. **Occurrence of Allergic Reactions**
      1. Allergic reactions occur most commonly in patients who have a history of allergic conditions such as hay fever, allergic skin rashes, or asthma.
      2. Allergic patients seem to be particularly sensitive to the flavoring agent. The most secret part of the formulation of toothpastes and mouthwashes is the flavoring agent, and this is usually the most allergenic component.

B. **Clinical Manifestations.** The clinical manifestations of allergy are a diffuse fiery red gingivitis sometimes with ulcerations (Fig. 6-16).

C. **Recognition and Treatment of Allergic Reaction**

1. The hygienist might suspect this problem in a patient with good self-care who previously has had healthy gingiva (especially if the patient has a history of allergies). Inquire if the patient is using a new toothpaste or mouthwash or chewing gum.

2. Advise the patient to change brands or flavors of gum, toothpaste, or mouthwash. Cessation of the allergen-containing product should result in a resolution of the gingivitis.

3. If necessary, the diagnosis of allergic response can be confirmed by a biopsy with a diagnosis of plasma cell gingivitis.

4. When the manufacturer becomes aware of allergic reactions, the flavoring agent or additive causing the problem is usually altered. For this reason, the patient sometimes can switch back to the original product (after 6 to 12 months) and use it without problem.

Chapter Summary Statement

Gingival diseases are the mildest form of periodontal disease. Plaque-induced gingivitis is the most common of the periodontal diseases. Clinically, plaque-induced gingivitis is characterized by gingiva that is red, swollen, bleeds easily, and is slightly tender. Plaque-induced gingivitis may be modified by systemic factors, medications, or malnutrition.

Non–plaque-induced gingival lesions are a group of uncommon gingival lesions that are not caused by plaque biofilm. Non–plaque-induced gingivitis can result from such diverse causes as infection, skin diseases, allergic reactions, or trauma.

Section 4
Focus on Patients

Clinical Patient Care

CASE 1

You are scheduled to do a dental prophylaxis on a patient with a diagnosis of localized severe plaque-induced gingivitis. At the time of the appointment the patient informs you that she has just received notice that lab results indicate that she is pregnant. How might this pregnancy alter the periodontal diagnosis?

CASE 2

A patient who has been cared for by your dental team suddenly exhibits poor self-care with quite a bit of plaque biofilm accumulation. This is unusual for this patient. Discussions reveal that the patient is having difficulty with brushing and flossing due to soreness of the mouth. Examination reveals numerous small mucosal ulcers. Further discussions reveal that the patient has been experiencing this soreness since she began using tartar control toothpaste. How might your dental team manage this patient's diminished effectiveness of self-care?

CASE 3

Your patient is a 12-year-old male, who in spite of good oral hygiene practices, presents with generalized marginal redness and bleeding upon probing. His demonstration of tooth brushing and flossing indicates high dexterity and ability to remove plaque biofilm and in talking with his mother, she confirms that he practices daily oral hygiene. How would you explain the presence of gingival disease to this patient and what would you recommend to improve his gingival health?

CASE 4

Your patient reports a change in his medical history from last visit; he is now taking Depakote as a mood stabilizer. The PDR states it is an anticonvulsant and may cause gingival enlargement. How will this new information alter your plan for dental hygiene care and patient education?

CASE 5

During the oral exam, you see a localized area of marginal redness and edema on the distofacial of the mandibular right first molar. While exploring in that area, there is a restoration with an overhanging margin. How does the overhang contribute to the presence of gingival inflammation, how can it be treated, and what will happen if the overhang remains?

Ethical Dilemma

Lily E, a 17-year-old high school senior, who is a routine 6-month recall patient, is your first patient of the afternoon. She received her driver's license 3 months ago, and has driven herself to today's appointment. You review her medical history, and she states there are "no changes," and she has no "chief complaint."

As you are performing your intraoral examination, you notice that the tissue between the maxillary central incisors does not appear to be normal. You observe a mushroom-shaped gingival mass, projecting from the gingival papilla. It appears red, and bleeds easily upon digital palpation. You ask Lily if it bothers her, and she denies any discomfort. She also states that she was not aware of any problem.

You are concerned that the lesion may be a pyogenic granuloma associated with pregnancy. You would like to discuss the possible implication of this lesion with Lily, but you are not sure how to proceed.

1. What is the best way for you to handle this ethical dilemma?
2. What is the best way to address/discuss Lily's treatment plan with her?
3. Under the ethical principle of confidentiality, can you discuss this with your employer dentist, without violating Lily's confidentiality?
4. Do you have the right to divulge your findings and concerns to her parents?
5. Can a 17-year-old consent to treatment, or must you receive parental consent?

References

1. American Academy of Periodontology-Research, Science and therapy Committee. Periodontal diseases of children and adolescents. *Pediatr Dent.* 2008;30(7 suppl):240–247.
2. Hamadneh N, Khan WA, Sathasivam S, et al. Design optimization of pin fin geometry using particle swarm optimization algorithm. *PloS One.* 2013;8(5):e66080.
3. Matsson L, Goldberg P. Gingival inflammatory reaction in children at different ages. *J Clin Periodontol.* 1985;12(2):98–103.
4. Yang NY, Zhang Q, Li JL, et al. Progression of periodontal inflammation in adolescents is associated with increased number of Porphyromonas gingivalis, Prevotella intermedia, Tannerella for sythensis, and Fusobacterium nucleatum. *Int J Paediatr Dent.* 2014;24(3):226–233.
5. Bimstein E, Matsson L. Growth and development considerations in the diagnosis of gingivitis and periodontitis in children. *Pediatr Dent.* 1999;21(3):186–191.
6. Gafan GP, Lucas VS, Roberts GJ, et al. Prevalence of periodontal pathogens in dental plaque of children. *J Clin Microbiol.* 2004;42(9):4141–4146.
7. Fransson C, Berglundh T, Lindhe J. The effect of age on the development of gingivitis. Clinical, microbiological and histological findings. *J Clin Periodontol.* 1996;23(4):379–385.
8. Fransson C, Mooney J, Kinane DF, et al. Differences in the inflammatory response in young and old human subjects during the course of experimental gingivitis. *J Clin Periodontol.* 1999;26(7):453–460.
9. Trombelli L, Farina R. A review of factors influencing the incidence and severity of plaque-induced gingivitis. *Minerva Stomatol.* 2013;62(6):207–234.
10. Taichman LS, Eklund SA. Oral contraceptives and periodontal diseases: rethinking the association based upon analysis of National Health and Nutrition Examination Survey data. *J Periodontol.* 2005;76(8):1374–1385.
11. Mullally BH, Coulter WA, Hutchinson JD, et al. Current oral contraceptive status and periodontitis in young adults. *J Periodontol.* 2007;78(6):1031–1036.
12. Armitage GC. Bi-directional relationship between pregnancy and periodontal disease. *Periodontol 2000.* 2013;61(1):160–176.
13. Gursoy M, Gursoy UK, Sorsa T, et al. High salivary estrogen and risk of developing pregnancy gingivitis. *J Periodontol.* 2013;84(9):1281–1289.
14. Markou E, Eleana B, Lazaros T, et al. The influence of sex steroid hormones on gingiva of women. *Open Dent J.* 2009;3:114–119.
15. Xie Y, Xiong X, Elkind-Hirsch KE, et al. Change of periodontal disease status during and after pregnancy. *J Periodontol.* 2013;84(6):725–731.
16. Botero JE, Yepes FL, Roldan N, et al. Tooth and periodontal clinical attachment loss are associated with hyperglycemia in patients with diabetes. *J Periodontol.* 2012;83(10):1245–1250.
17. Chang PC, Chien LY, Yeo JF, et al. Progression of periodontal destruction and the roles of advanced glycation end products in experimental diabetes. *J Periodontol.* 2013;84(3):379–388.
18. Chapple IL, Genco R, working group 2 of the joint EFP/AAP workshop. Diabetes and periodontal diseases: consensus report of the Joint EFP/AAP Workshop on Periodontitis and Systemic Diseases. *J Periodontol.* 2013;84(4 suppl):S106–S112.
19. Mealey BL, Oates TW. Diabetes mellitus and periodontal diseases. *J Periodontol.* 2006;77(8):1289–1303.
20. Lin YT, Yang FT. Gingival enlargement in children administered cyclosporine after liver transplantation. *J Periodontol.* 2010;81(9):1250–1255.
21. Bacci C, Sivolella S, Pellegrini J, et al. A rare case of scurvy in an otherwise healthy child: diagnosis through oral signs. *Pediatr Dent.* 2010;32(7):536–538.
22. Chapman JM, Marley JJ. Scurvy and the ageing population. *Br Dent J.* 2011;211(12):583–584.
23. Siegel MA. Syphilis and gonorrhea. *Dent Clin North Am.* 1996;40(2):369–383.
24. Holmstrup P. Non-plaque-induced gingival lesions. *Ann Periodontol.* 1999;4(1):20–31.
25. Miller CS, Redding SW. Diagnosis and management of orofacial herpes simplex virus infections. *Dent Clin North Am.* 1992;36(4):879–895.
26. Scully C, de Almeida OP, Welbury R. Oral lichen planus in childhood. *Br J Dermatol.* 1994;130(1):131–133.
27. Scully C, Epstein J, Porter S, et al. Viruses and chronic disorders involving the human oral mucosa. *Oral Surg Oral Med Oral Pathol.* 1991;72(5):537–544.
28. Loh FC, Yeo JF, Tan WC, et al. Histoplasmosis presenting as hyperplastic gingival lesion. *J Oral Pathol Med.* 1989;18(9):533–536.
29. Machado FC, de Souza IP, Portela MB, et al. Use of chlorhexidine gel (0.2%) to control gingivitis and candida species colonization in human immunodeficiency virus-infected children: a pilot study. *Pediatr Dent.* 2011;33(2):153–157.
30. Hart TC, Zhang Y, Gorry MC, et al. A mutation in the SOS1 gene causes hereditary gingival fibromatosis type 1. *Am J Hum Genet.* 2002;70(4):943–954.
31. Cohen DM, Bhattacharyya I. Cinnamon-induced oral erythema multiformelike sensitivity reaction. *J Am Dent Assoc.* 2000;131(7):929–934.
32. Littner MM, Dayan D, Kaffe I, et al. Acute streptococcal gingivostomatitis. Report of five cases and review of the literature. *Oral Surg Oral Med Oral Pathol.* 1982;53(2):144–147.
33. Ramirez-Amador V, Madero JG, Pedraza LE, et al. Oral secondary syphilis in a patient with human immunodeficiency virus infection. *Oral Surg Oral Med Oral Pathol Oral Radiol Endod.* 1996;81(6):652–654.
34. Rivera-Hidalgo F, Stanford TW. Oral mucosal lesions caused by infective microorganisms. I. Viruses and bacteria. *Periodontol 2000.* 1999;21:106–124.
35. King DL, Steinhauer W, Garcia-Godoy F, et al. Herpetic gingivostomatitis and teething difficulty in infants. *Pediatr Dent.* 1992;14(2):82–85.
36. Lugo RI, Fornatora ML, Reich RF, et al. Linear gingival erythema in an HIV-seropositive man. *AIDS Read.* 1999;9(2):97–99.
37. Thaler R, Ojha J, Bhola M. Oral pathology quiz #19. Linear gingival erythema. *J Mich Dent Assoc.* 2009;91(4):44, 46–47.
38. Velegraki A, Nicolatou O, Theodoridou M, et al. Paediatric AIDS–related linear gingival erythema: a form of erythematous candidiasis? *J Oral Pathol Med.* 1999;28(4):178–182.

39. Umadevi M, Adeyemi O, Patel M, et al. (B2) Periodontal diseases and other bacterial infections. *Adv Dent Res.* 2006;19(1):139–145.

40. Robinson PG, Winkler JR, Palmer G, et al. The diagnosis of periodontal conditions associated with HIV infection. *J Periodontol.* 1994;65(3):236–243.

41. Camacho-Alonso F, Lopez-Jornet P, Bermejo-Fenoll A. Gingival involvement of oral lichen planus. *J Periodontol.* 2007;78(4):640–644.

42. Salgado DS, Jeremias F, Capela MV, et al. Plaque control improves the painful symptoms of oral lichen planus gingival lesions. A short-term study. *J Oral Pathol Med.* 2013;42(10):728–732.

43. Barrett AW, Scully CM, Eveson JW. Erythema multiforme involving gingiva. *J Periodontol.* 1993;64(9):910–913.

44. Huff JC, Weston WL, Tonnesen MG. Erythema multiforme: a critical review of characteristics, diagnostic criteria, and causes. *J Am Acad Dermatol.* 1983;8(6):763–775.

45. Skaare A, Kjaerheim V, Barkvoll P, et al. Skin reactions and irritation potential of four commercial toothpastes. *Acta Odontol Scand.* 1997;55(2):133–136.

46. Calapai G, Miroddi M, Mannucci C, et al. Oral adverse reactions due to cinnamon-flavoured chewing gums consumption. *Oral Dis.* 2013;20(7):637–643.

47. Drake TE, Maibach HI. Allergic contact dermatitis and stomatitis caused by a cinnamic aldehyde-flavored toothpaste. *Arch Dermatol.* 1976;112(2):202–203.

 STUDENT ANCILLARY RESOURCES

A wide variety of resources to enhance your learning and understanding of this chapter are available on thePoint®.

- Visit thePoint to access:
  - Audio Glossary
  - Animations
  - Suggested Readings
  - Answers to Review Questions
  - Case Studies

CHAPTER

7

Chronic Periodontitis

Clinical Application. Chronic periodontitis is the most frequently encountered form of periodontitis. All dental hygienists will participate in helping to diagnose this disease and in providing care designed to bring this rather common disease under control. An understanding of the features of behavior of chronic periodontitis is absolutely essential for every member of the dental team.

Learning Objectives

- In a clinical setting for a patient with chronic periodontitis, describe to your clinical instructor the clinical signs of disease present in the patient's mouth.

- Define the term *clinical attachment loss* and explain its significance in the periodontal disease process.

- In the clinical setting, explain to your patient the warning signs of chronic periodontal disease.

- Recognize and describe clinical and radiographic features of chronic periodontitis.

- Contrast the extent of periodontal destruction typically seen in localized chronic periodontitis with that of generalized chronic periodontitis.

- Describe the change or advancement—disease progression—typically seen in chronic periodontitis.

- According to the AAP 1999 classification system, define the meaning of the descriptors *recurrent chronic periodontitis* and *refractory chronic periodontitis.*

Key Terms

Periodontitis
Chronic periodontitis
Clinical attachment loss
Peri-implantitis
Extent
Localized chronic periodontitis

Generalized chronic
  periodontitis
Disease progression
Site-specific
Severity
Slight (mild) periodontitis

Moderate periodontitis
Severe periodontitis
Recurrent disease
Refractory disease
Refractory chronic
  periodontitis

Section 1
Chronic Periodontitis—The Most Common Form

Periodontitis is a bacterial infection that affects all parts of the periodontium including the gingiva, periodontal ligament, bone, and cementum. It is the result of complex interaction between the plaque biofilm that accumulates on tooth surfaces and the body's efforts to fight this infection. Periodontitis is the number one cause of tooth loss in adults. There are also some individuals who are genetically predisposed to developing periodontitis.

   Chronic periodontitis is a complex infection resulting in inflammation within the supporting tissues of the teeth, progressive destruction of the periodontal ligament, and loss of supporting alveolar bone (1,2). Chronic periodontitis begins as plaque-induced gingivitis. Plaque-induced gingivitis is a reversible condition that if left untreated may develop into chronic periodontitis (3–10). *Chronic periodontitis involves irreversible loss of attachment and bone and is the most frequently occurring form of periodontitis.*

GENERAL CHARACTERISTICS OF CHRONIC PERIODONTITIS

1. **Alternative Terminology.** Chronic periodontitis was previously known as adult periodontitis. The name adult periodontitis, however, is misleading as this type of periodontitis can occur in individuals of any age: children, adolescents, and adults.
2. **Signs and Symptoms of Chronic Periodontitis.** Signs and symptoms of chronic periodontitis include swelling, redness, gingival bleeding, periodontal pockets, bone loss, tooth mobility, suppuration (pus), moderate or heavy deposits of plaque biofilms, and dental calculus (2).
   A. **Alterations in Color, Texture, and Size of the Marginal Gingiva**
      1. Red or Purplish Tissue. In chronic periodontitis, the gingival tissue may appear bright red or purplish.
         a. In such cases, the clinical signs of chronic periodontitis are very evident at the initial examination of the oral cavity. The gingiva appears swollen with the color ranging from pale red to magenta. Alterations in contour and form are evident such as rolled gingival margins, blunted or flattened papillae.
         b. An example of chronic periodontitis exhibiting this type of appearance is shown in Box 7-1, Figure 7-1A,B,C.
      2. Pale Pink Tissue. In chronic periodontitis, the gingival tissue may be pale pink and have an almost normal-looking appearance.
         a. *The clinical appearance of the tissues is not a reliable indicator of the presence or severity of chronic periodontitis* (Figs. 7-2–7-4).
         b. In many patients, the changes in color, contour, and consistency may not be visible on inspection. At first glance, an inexperienced clinician may mistake the clinical appearance of chronic periodontitis for one of health. Closer examination will reveal firm, rigid (fibrotic) tissue, the presence of pocketing, and bleeding upon probing. Chronic periodontitis exhibiting this type of appearance is shown in Figure 7-2.
   B. **Bleeding, Crevicular Fluid, and Exudate**
      1. Gingival bleeding is common, either spontaneous bleeding or bleeding in response to probing.
      2. Increased flow of gingival crevicular fluid or suppuration (pus) from periodontal pockets is common.

C. Plaque Biofilm and Calculus Deposits
   1. Chronic periodontitis is characterized by mature supra- and subgingival plaque biofilms and calculus deposits. Teeth with chronic periodontitis usually have very complex and thick deposits of plaque biofilm on affected root surfaces (11).
   2. Although chronic periodontitis is initiated and sustained by plaque biofilms, host factors determine the pathogenesis and rate of progression of the disease (12–17).

D. Loss of Attachment
   1. **Clinical attachment loss** is an estimate of the extent that the tooth-supporting structures have been destroyed around a tooth. Loss of attachment occurs in periodontitis and is characterized by (1) relocation of the junctional epithelium to the tooth root (2), destruction of the fibers of the gingiva (3), destruction of the periodontal ligament fibers (4), and loss of alveolar bone support around the tooth (Figs. 7-5 and 7-6). The changes that occur in the alveolar bone in periodontal disease are significant because loss of bone height eventually can result in tooth loss.
   2. Clinical attachment loss of 1 to 2 mm at one or several sites can be found in nearly all members of the adult population.
   3. Clinical characteristics of attachment loss may include the following:
      a. Loss of alveolar bone support to the teeth
      b. Periodontal pockets or recession of the gingival margin
      c. Furcation involvement in multirooted teeth (Fig. 7-6)
      d. Tooth mobility and/or drifting
   4. It has been established that the extent of probe penetration is influenced by the inflammatory status of the periodontal tissues (Fig. 7-7) (18–32).

E. Localized or Generalized Inflammation. In chronic periodontitis, there is no consistent pattern to the number and types of teeth involved (2,33).
   1. Localized inflammation may involve one site on a single tooth, several sites on a tooth, or several teeth. Generalized inflammation may involve the entire dentition.
   2. A patient may simultaneously have areas of health and areas with chronic periodontitis with tissue destruction.
   3. Chronic periodontitis is classified as localized when less than 30% of sites are affected and generalized when greater than 30% of sites are affected.

F. Contributing Factors
   1. Chronic periodontitis may be modified by and/or associated with local factors. It can be modified by other factors, especially cigarette smoking.
   2. Individuals affected by chronic periodontitis have no known medical or general health considerations that might contribute to the development of their periodontitis (2). According to the 1999 classification system, if an individual has a systemic disease that can profoundly modify the initiation and clinical course of periodontal infections, the resulting periodontitis is classified as "periodontitis as a manifestation of systemic disease" (34).

G. Symptoms
   1. Chronic periodontitis usually is painless. Therefore, an individual with chronic periodontitis may be totally unaware of the disease, not seek treatment, and be unlikely to accept treatment recommendations.
   2. Individuals may first become aware that something is wrong when they notice that their gums bleed when brushing; that spaces occur between the teeth; or that teeth have become loose.
   3. Patients may complain of food impaction, sensitivity to hot or cold due to exposed roots, or dull pain radiating into the jaw.

H. **Chronic Periodontitis in Dental Implant Tissues.** Peri-implantitis is the term for chronic periodontitis in the tissues surrounding a dental implant. Peri-implantitis is discussed in more detail in Chapter 31.

3. **Onset and Progression of Chronic Periodontitis**
   A. **Gingivitis as a Risk Factor for Chronic Periodontitis**
      1. Plaque-induced gingivitis precedes the onset of chronic periodontitis. Plaque-induced gingivitis may remain stable for many years and never progress to become periodontitis.
      2. Bacterial plaque biofilms will induce gingivitis, but the host susceptibility and other contributing factors determine whether or not chronic periodontitis will develop.
      3. Gingivitis manifests after only days or weeks of plaque biofilm accumulation. In most cases, chronic periodontitis requires longer periods (years) of plaque biofilm and calculus exposure to develop (2,20,35).
      4. Findings from epidemiologic studies and clinical trials indicate that the presence of gingivitis may be regarded as a risk factor for chronic periodontitis (36,37).
   B. **Age of Onset.** The onset of chronic periodontitis may be at any age (2). It is most commonly detected in adults older than age 35 but can occur in children and adolescents. The prevalence and severity of chronic periodontitis increases with age.
   C. **Rate of Disease Progression.** The rate of disease progression is considered an important characteristic by which chronic and aggressive forms of periodontitis can be clinically distinguished (2). In most cases, chronic periodontitis progresses in a slow to moderate pace (2,33).
   D. **Patient Education: The Warning Signs of Chronic Periodontitis**
      1. The warning signs of periodontitis are red or swollen gingiva, bleeding during brushing, a bad taste in the mouth, persistent bad breath, sensitive teeth, loose teeth, and pus around teeth and gingiva (Figs. 7-8 to 7-13).
      2. Pain usually is not a symptom of periodontitis. This absence of pain may explain why periodontitis is often advanced before the patient seeks treatment and why a patient may avoid treatment even after receiving a diagnosis of periodontitis.
      3. Tools such as oral health self-evaluations distributed at health fairs or other events can be helpful in increasing the public's awareness of the signs and symptoms of periodontal disease.

Box 7-1. Chronic Periodontitis

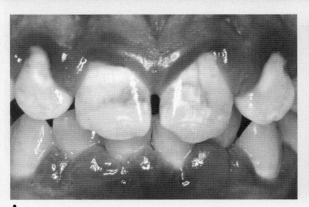

A

Figure 7-1A. Highly Visible Changes in the Gingiva. Chronic periodontitis may exhibit many clinically visible signs, such as changes in the contour of the tissue.

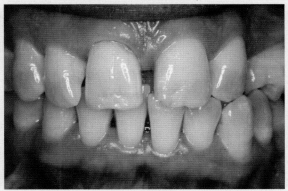

B

Figure 7-1B. Minimal Visible Changes in Gingiva. In this example of chronic periodontitis, there are minimal visible tissue changes. Since periodontitis is a disease affecting the deeper tissues of the periodontium, the appearance of the surface tissue often is not a reliable indicator of disease severity.

Characteristics of Chronic Periodontitis

- Most commonly seen in adults over 35 years of age but can occur in children and adolescents
- Initiated and continued by plaque biofilms but host response plays an essential role in disease progression
- Occurs in individuals with no known medical or general health considerations that might contribute to the development of periodontitis
- Signs and symptoms of inflammation include swelling, redness, gingival bleeding, periodontal pockets, bone loss, tooth mobility, suppuration (pus), moderate or heavy deposits of plaque biofilms, and dental calculus
- Bone loss may be evident on radiographs
- Untreated chronic periodontitis progresses slowly over time
- Attachment loss may occur in one area of a tooth's attachment, on several teeth, or the entire dentition
- It can be modified by other factors, especially cigarette smoking

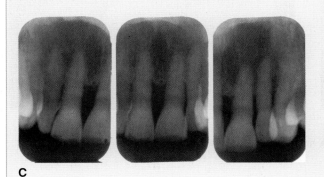

C

Figure 7-1C. Radiographic Evidence of Chronic Periodontitis. Dental radiographs of patients with chronic periodontitis usually reveal horizontal patterns of alveolar bone loss.

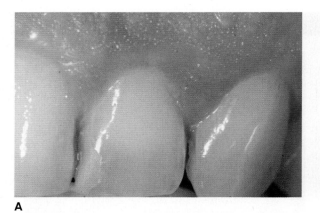

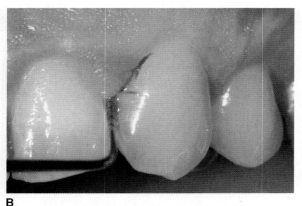

A **B**

Figure 7-2. Health or Disease? **A:** The clinical appearance of the tissue in this photograph suggests health. **B:** When assessed with a probe, however, a deep 7-mm pocket reveals bone loss on the mesiofacial of the canine. This example underscores the importance of a thorough periodontal assessment. (Courtesy of Dr. Don Rolfs, Wenachee, WA.)

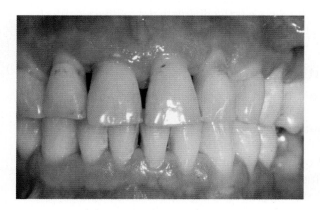

Figure 7-3. Health or Disease? This individual received periodontal treatment for chronic periodontitis several years ago. The assessment at today's appointment reveals meticulous patient self-care and no additional attachment loss since beginning periodontal maintenance several years ago. Therefore, this tissue is considered healthy. The attachment loss is simply an indicator of previous disease. (Courtesy of Dr. Ralph Arnold.)

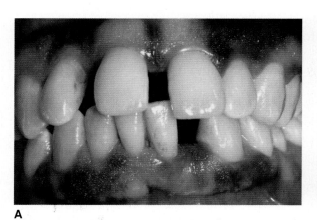

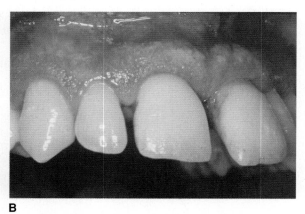

A **B**

Figure 7-4. Chronic Periodontitis. Two examples, **A** and **B**, of chronic periodontitis showing firm, nodular (fibrotic) tissue changes.

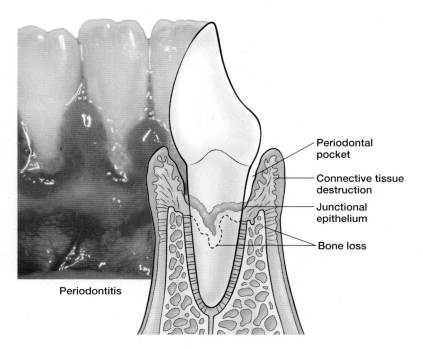

Periodontal pocket

Connective tissue destruction

Junctional epithelium

Bone loss

Periodontitis

Figure 7-5. Clinical Changes in Chronic Periodontitis. Chronic periodontitis is characterized by inflammation within the supporting tissues of the teeth, progressive destruction of the periodontal ligament, and loss of supporting alveolar bone.

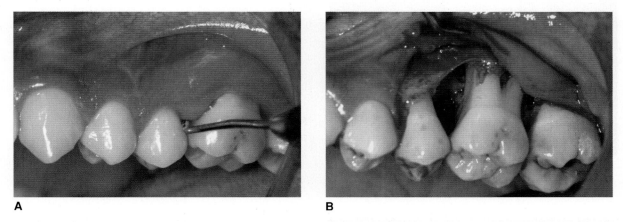

A

B

Figure 7-6. Attachment Loss. A: Assessment with a periodontal probe indicates severe loss of attachment on this molar tooth. **B:** The gingival tissue is lifted away from the molar during periodontal surgery to reveal the severe loss of alveolar bone and connective tissue attachment. (Courtesy of Dr. Ralph Arnold.)

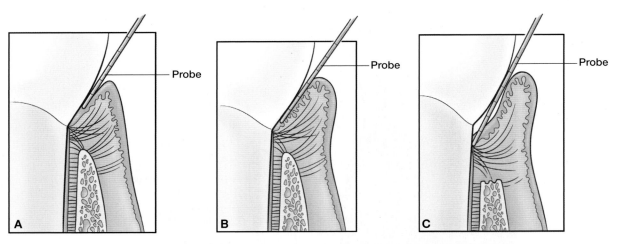

Figure 7-7. Diagrammatic Representation of Probe Tip Penetration Relative to the Periodontal Tissues. It has been established that the extent of probe penetration is influenced by the inflammatory status of the periodontal tissues (18–32). **A:** In a normal sulcus, the probe penetrates about one-third of the length of the junctional epithelium. **B:** With moderate inflammation within the tissues, the probe tip penetrates approximately half the length of the junctional epithelium. **C:** Severe inflammation within the tissues, the probe tip penetrates through the length of the junctional epithelium, and only stops when it encounters the collagen fibers of the gingival connective tissue.

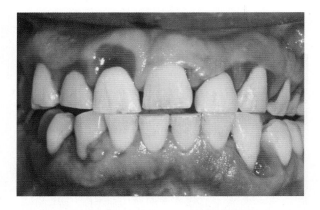

Figure 7-8. Chronic Periodontitis. Chronic periodontitis showing pronounced changes in the appearance of the gingiva.

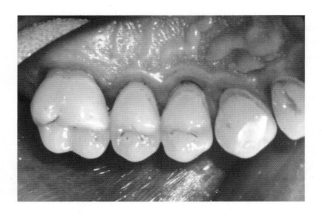

Figure 7-9. Chronic Periodontitis. Palatal gingiva in a patient with chronic periodontitis. Note the calculus deposits on the tooth surfaces and the rolled gingival margins. Clinical signs on the lingual aspect usually are not as evident as those seen on the facial aspect of the gingiva.

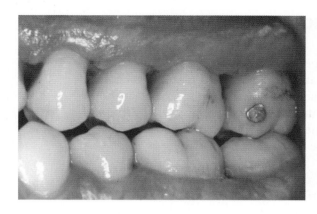

Figure 7-10. Chronic Periodontitis. Chronic periodontitis showing blunting of the interdental papillae and recession of the gingival margin.

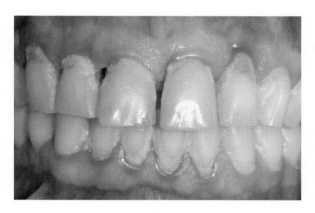

Figure 7-11. Chronic Periodontitis. Heavy accumulation of bacterial plaque biofilms in an individual with chronic periodontitis. (Courtesy of Dr. Ralph Arnold, San Antonio, TX.)

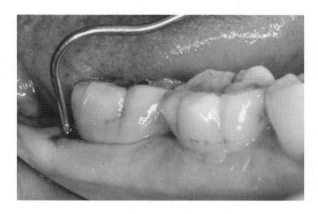

Figure 7-12. Chronic Periodontitis. Chronic periodontitis case with periodontal probe inserted in a pocket showing attachment loss.

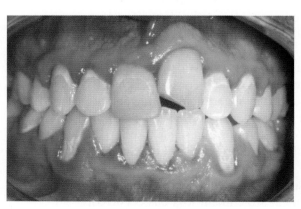

Figure 7-13. Chronic Periodontitis. Chronic periodontitis showing pronounced changes in the appearance of the gingiva. (Courtesy of Dr. Ralph Arnold.)

SEVERITY, EXTENT, AND PROGRESSION OF CHRONIC PERIODONTITIS

1. Extent of Destruction in Chronic Periodontitis
   A. Overview. Extent is the degree or amount of periodontal destruction and can be characterized based on the number of sites that have experienced tissue destruction.
      1. Localized inflammation may involve one site on a single tooth, several sites on a tooth, or several teeth. A patient may simultaneously have areas of health and areas with chronic periodontitis with tissue destruction.
      2. Generalized inflammation may involve the entire dentition.
   B. Localized or Generalized Extent
      1. Localized chronic periodontitis is chronic periodontitis in which 30% or less of the sites in the mouth have experienced attachment loss and bone loss.
      2. Generalized chronic periodontitis is chronic periodontitis in which more than 30% of the sites in the mouth have experienced attachment loss and bone loss.
2. Disease Progression
   A. Overview. Disease progression refers to the change or advancement of periodontal destruction. For example, how does the amount of attachment loss and bone destruction seen today compare with that seen several months ago? Is it the same, somewhat worse, or much worse?
   B. Progression of Chronic Periodontitis. In most cases, untreated chronic periodontitis progresses in a slow to moderate pace.
      1. The current view is that the progression of untreated chronic periodontitis in most individuals and at most disease sites is a continuous slow process but that periods of exacerbation occasionally may occur.
      2. Tissue destruction in untreated chronic periodontitis does not affect all teeth evenly but rather is a site-specific disease. That is, in the same dentition some teeth may have severe tissue destruction while other teeth are almost free of signs of attachment and bone loss.
         a. Some disease sites may remain unchanged for long periods of time (35,38,39).
         b. Other disease sites may progress more rapidly. More rapidly progressing disease sites occur most frequently in interproximal areas, and may be associated with areas of greater plaque biofilm accumulation and inaccessibility to plaque biofilm control measures (e.g., sites of malposed teeth, restorations with overhanging margins, areas of food impaction, deep periodontal pockets, furcation areas) (40).
      3. The desired outcome of periodontal therapy for chronic periodontitis is to stop the progression of the disease to prevent further attachment loss. Figures 7-14 to 7-16 show the clinical features before and after treatment for three different patients.
      4. The number of sites of attachment loss, bone loss, and/or deep pockets is a good predictor of future disease occurrence in an individual patient. The best predictor of disease progression is an individual's previous disease experience.
3. Disease Severity
   A. Overview. The severity, or seriousness, of the tissue destruction is determined by the rate of disease progression over time and the response of the tissues to treatment.
   B. Tissue Destruction. Disease severity may be described as slight (mild), moderate, or severe. These terms may be used to describe the disease severity of the entire dentition, part of the mouth (sextant or quadrant), or the disease status of a single tooth.
      1. Slight (mild) periodontitis—no more than 1 to 2 mm of clinical attachment loss.
      2. Moderate periodontitis—3 to 4 mm of clinical attachment loss has occurred.
      3. Severe periodontitis—5 mm or more of clinical attachment loss has occurred.

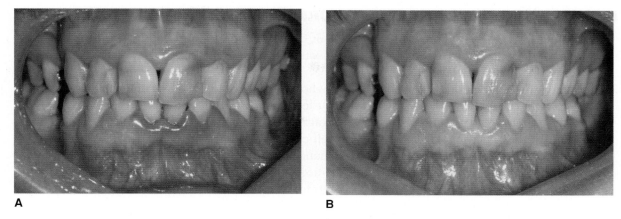

Figure 7-14. Chronic Periodontitis: Before and After Periodontal Therapy. A: Note the tissue changes before periodontal therapy. Clinical changes are particularly pronounced on the lower anterior sextant. **B:** The same individual after treatment. (Courtesy of Dr. Ralph Arnold, San Antonio, TX.)

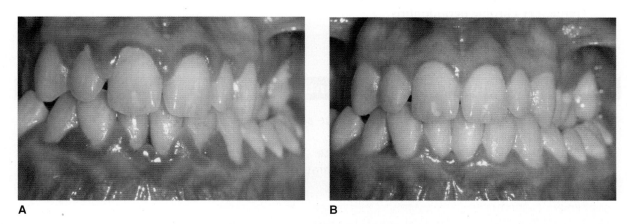

Figure 7-15. Chronic Periodontitis: Before and After Periodontal Therapy. A: Very pronounced tissue changes are evident prior to therapy. **B:** Much improved clinical picture at 3-month follow-up appointment. (Courtesy of Dr. Ralph Arnold, San Antonio, TX.)

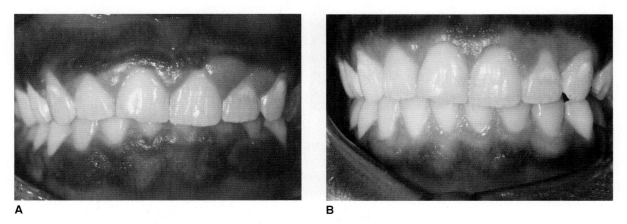

Figure 7-16. Chronic Periodontitis: Before and After Periodontal Therapy. A: Very swollen gingival tissues pretreatment. **B:** The same individual after treatment. (Courtesy of Dr. Ralph Arnold, San Antonio, TX.)

RECURRENT AND REFRACTORY FORMS OF CHRONIC PERIODONTITIS

1. **Recurrent disease**—new signs and symptoms of destructive periodontitis that reappear after periodontal therapy because the disease was not adequately treated and/or the patient did not practice adequate self-care.
2. **Refractory disease**—periodontitis in a patient who has been monitored over time and who continues to exhibit additional attachment loss in spite of the following conditions: (a) The patient has received appropriate and continuous professional periodontal therapy, (b) the patient practices satisfactory self-care, and (c) the patient follows the recommended program of periodontal maintenance visits (Box 7-2, Fig. 7-17 A,B,C).
   A. Under the 1989 classification system, "refractory periodontitis" was a separate disease category. It is now believed that refractory periodontitis is not a single disease entity, but rather that a small percentage of all forms of periodontitis may not respond to treatment.
   B. *In the new 1999 classification system, the designation "refractory" can be applied to all types of periodontal diseases that do not respond to treatment.* Cases of chronic periodontitis that do not respond to periodontal therapy are designated as refractory chronic periodontitis.

Box 7-2. Refractory Chronic Periodontitis

Additional attachment loss in a patient despite all of the following:
* Appropriate periodontal therapy
* A patient who practices satisfactory self-care
* An appropriate program of periodontal maintenance visits

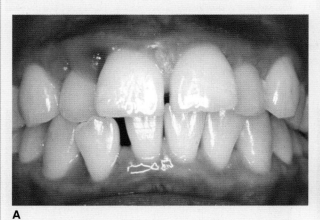
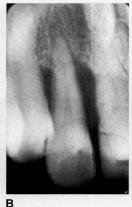
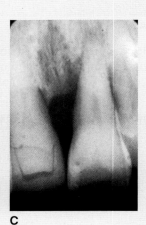

A B C

Figure 7-17. A–C: Refractory Chronic Periodontitis. Chronic periodontitis is considered refractory when the disease is not controlled by the conventional periodontal therapy normally recommended for patients with chronic periodontitis. In a refractory case, the patient experiences additional attachment loss despite appropriate periodontal therapy and satisfactory self-care. The dental radiographs of a patient with refractory periodontitis reveal *continuing evidence of bone loss over time despite appropriate therapy.*

Chapter Summary Statement

Chronic periodontitis is a bacterial infection resulting in inflammation within the supporting tissues of the teeth, progressive destruction of the periodontal ligament, and loss of supporting alveolar bone.

- Chronic periodontitis involves *irreversible* loss of attachment and bone and is the most frequently occurring form of periodontitis.
- Chronic periodontitis may involve one area of a tooth's attachment, several teeth, or the entire dentition. A patient can simultaneously have areas of health and areas with periodontitis.
- Untreated chronic periodontitis usually is characterized by slow to moderate rates of disease progression and a favorable response to periodontal therapy.
- The desired outcome of periodontal therapy for chronic periodontitis is to stop the progression of the disease to prevent further attachment loss.

Section 2
Focus on Patients

Clinical Patient Care

CASE 1

A new patient has a diagnosis of severe generalized chronic periodontitis. The patient tells you that it is hard for him to believe he has serious periodontal problems since he has never had any discomfort and has never even noticed any dental problems. How could you respond to this patient's comments?

CASE 2

A patient who has recently moved to your city has an appointment with you regarding self-care instructions. The periodontal diagnosis is severe chronic periodontitis. In your discussion with the patient you learn that the patient is upset because she has been treated for periodontitis twice during the past decade in other dental offices. She is upset because now apparently she needs periodontal treatment again, and she states she is confused about how this might be possible. How could you respond to this patient's concerns?

Ethical Dilemma

Your next patient, Josiah S, has recently relocated to your town, approximately 6 months ago, and is a new patient in your practice. He is a 45-year-old divorced male, who admits to smoking approximately 15 cigarettes per day, and drinks a nightly alcoholic cocktail. He works in sales, and due to his hectic travel schedule, tells you that he has had to cancel his last few dental hygiene appointments.

   Your intraoral exam reveals that Josiah presents with moderate calculus and plaque biofilm. His gingival tissues appear red and swollen, have blunted papillae, and bleed readily upon palpation. You take a full mouth series of radiographs that show generalized horizontal bone loss throughout his mouth. You begin to probe his mouth, to determine his pocket readings when he sits up in the dental chair and demands that you stop. He states that he has always refused periodontal probing, as he just "can't stand the pain" and the last dental office abided by his wishes. He refuses to let you continue "poking around his gums" and asks that you just proceed to cleaning his teeth, so he can be on time for his 11:00 AM business appointment.

1. How would you classify Josiah's periodontal condition?
2. What ethical principles are in conflict in this dilemma?
3. Do you have an ethical obligation to treat this patient?
4. What is the best way to address/discuss Josiah's treatment plan with him?
5. What, if any alternatives, can you offer Josiah in terms of his treatment plan?

References

1. Armitage GC. Classifying periodontal diseases–a long-standing dilemma. *Periodontol 2000*. 2002;30:9–23.
2. Armitage GC. Comparison of the microbiological features of chronic and aggressive periodontitis. *Periodontol 2000*. 2010;53:70–88.
3. Loe H, Theilade E, Jensen SB. Experimental gingivitis in man. *J Periodontol*. 1965;36:177–187.
4. Loesche WJ, Syed SA. Bacteriology of human experimental gingivitis: effect of plaque and gingivitis score. *Infect Immun*. 1978;21(3):830–839.
5. Moore LV, Moore WE, Cato EP, et al. Bacteriology of human gingivitis. *J Dent Res*. 1987;66(5):989–995.
6. Moore WE, Holdeman LV, Smibert RM, et al. Bacteriology of experimental gingivitis in young adult humans. *Infect Immun*. 1982;38(2):651–667.
7. Seymour GJ, Powell RN, Aitken JF. Experimental gingivitis in humans. A clinical and histologic investigation. *J Periodontol*. 1983;54(9):522–528.
8. Seymour GJ, Powell RN, Cole KL, et al. Experimental gingivitis in humans. A histochemical and immunological characterization of the lymphoid cell subpopulations. *J Periodontal Res*. 1983;18(4):375–385.
9. Theilade E, Wright WH, Jensen SB, et al. Experimental gingivitis in man. II. A longitudinal clinical and bacteriological investigation. *J Periodontal Res*. 1966;1:1–13.
10. van der Velden U, Abbas F, Hart AA. Experimental gingivitis in relation to susceptibility to periodontal disease. (I.) Clinical observations. *J Clin Periodontol*. 1985;12(1):61–68.
11. Listgarten MA. Structure of the microbial flora associated with periodontal health and disease in man. A light and electron microscopic study. *J Periodontol*. 1976;47(1):1–18.
12. Haffajee AD, Teles RP, Socransky SS. The effect of periodontal therapy on the composition of the subgingival microbiota. *Periodontol 2000*. 2006;42:219–258.
13. Ledder RG, Gilbert P, Huws SA, et al. Molecular analysis of the subgingival microbiota in health and disease. *Appl Environ Microbiol*. 2007;73(2):516–523.
14. Paster BJ, Boches SK, Galvin JL, et al. Bacterial diversity in human subgingival plaque. *J Bacteriol*. 2001;183(12):3770–3783.
15. Socransky SS, Haffajee AD. Dental biofilms: difficult therapeutic targets. *Periodontol 2000*. 2002;28:12–55.
16. Socransky SS, Haffajee AD, Teles R, et al. Effect of periodontal therapy on the subgingival microbiota over a 2-year monitoring period. I. Overall effect and kinetics of change. *J Clin Periodontol*. 2013;40(8):771–780.
17. Waerhaug J. Subgingival plaque and loss of attachment in periodontosis as evaluated on extracted teeth. *J Periodontol*. 1977;48(3):125–130.
18. Anderson GB, Caffesse RG, Nasjleti CE, et al. Correlation of periodontal probe penetration and degree of inflammation. *Am J Dent*. 1991;4(4):177–183.
19. Armitage GC. Periodontal diseases: diagnosis. *Ann Periodontol*. 1996;1(1):37–215.

20. Carranza FA, Newman MG, Takei HH, et al. *Carranza's Clinical Periodontology.* 10th ed. St. Louis, MO: Saunders Elsevier; 2006; xxxvi:1286.

21. Caton J, Greenstein G, Polson AM. Depth of periodontal probe penetration related to clinical and histologic signs of gingival inflammation. *J Periodontol.* 1981;52(10):626–629.

22. Fowler C, Garrett S, Crigger M, et al. Histologic probe position in treated and untreated human periodontal tissues. *J Clin Periodontol.* 1982;9(5):373–385.

23. Hancock EB, Wirthlin MR. The location of the periodontal probe tip in health and disease. *J Periodontol.* 1981;52(3): 124–129.

24. Hefti AF. Periodontal probing. *Crit Rev Oral Biol Med.* 1997;8(3):336–356.

25. Khan S, Cabanilla LL. Periodontal probing depth measurement: a review. *Compend Contin Educ Dent.* 2009;30(1):12–14, 16, 18–21; quiz 22, 36.

26. Lindhe J, Lang NP, Karring T. *Clinical Periodontology and Implant Dentistry.* 5th ed. Oxford; Ames, Iowa: Blackwell Munksgaard; 2008.

27. Listgarten MA, Mao R, Robinson PJ. Periodontal probing and the relationship of the probe tip to periodontal tissues. *J Periodontol.* 1976;47(9):511–513.

28. Magnusson I, Listgarten MA. Histological evaluation of probing depth following periodontal treatment. *J Clin Periodontol.* 1980;7(1):26–31.

29. Moriarty JD, Hutchens LH Jr, Scheitler LE. Histological evaluation of periodontal probe penetration in untreated facial molar furcations. *J Clin Periodontol.* 1989;16(1):21–26.

30. Robinson PJ, Vitek RM. The relationship between gingival inflammation and resistance to probe penetration. *J Periodontal Res.* 1979;14(3):239–243.

31. Spray JR, Garnick JJ, Doles LR, et al. Microscopic demonstration of the position of periodontal probes. *J Periodontol.* 1978;49(3):148–152.

32. Tessier JF, Ellen RP, Birek P, et al. Relationship between periodontal probing velocity and gingival inflammation in human subjects. *J Clin Periodontol.* 1993;20(1):41–48.

33. Lindhe J, Haffajee AD, Socransky SS. Progression of periodontal disease in adult subjects in the absence of periodontal therapy. *J Clin Periodontol.* 1983;10(4):433–442.

34. Armitage GC. Development of a classification system for periodontal diseases and conditions. *Ann Periodontol.* 1999;4(1):1–6.

35. Armitage GC. Learned and unlearned concepts in periodontal diagnostics: a 50-year perspective. *Periodontol 2000.* 2013;62(1):20–36.

36. Schatzle M, Loe H, Lang NP, et al. The clinical course of chronic periodontitis. *J Clin Periodontol.* 2004;31(12):1122–1127.

37. Suda R, Cao C, Hasegawa K, et al. 2-year observation of attachment loss in a rural Chinese population. *J Periodontol.* 2000;71(7):1067–1072.

38. Armitage GC, Cullinan MP. Comparison of the clinical features of chronic and aggressive periodontitis. *Periodontol 2000.* 2010;53:12–27.

39. Lindhe J, Okamoto H, Yoneyama T, et al. Longitudinal changes in periodontal disease in untreated subjects. *J Clin Periodontol.* 1989;16(10):662–670.

40. Lindhe J, Okamoto H, Yoneyama T, et al. Periodontal loser sites in untreated adult subjects. *J Clin Periodontol.* 1989;16(10):671–678.

 STUDENT ANCILLARY RESOURCES

A wide variety of resources to enhance your learning and understanding of this chapter are available on thePoint®.

- Visit thePoint to access:
  - Audio Glossary
  - Animations
  - Suggested Readings
  - Answers to Review Questions
  - Case Studies

Aggressive Periodontitis

Clinical Application.   Aggressive periodontitis can destroy a dentition in a relatively short time frame. All members of the dental team must remain on continuous alert for this highly destructive condition since delay in its diagnosis can prove disastrous for a patient. Familiarity with the characteristics of both localized and generalized aggressive periodontitis is a valuable tool to help insure that members of the dental team make a timely diagnosis of this condition.

Learning Objectives

- Compare and contrast the clinical and radiographic features of chronic periodontitis and aggressive periodontitis.

- In the clinical setting, explain to your patient the signs and symptoms of aggressive periodontal disease.

- In a clinical setting for a patient with aggressive periodontitis, describe to your clinical instructor the primary clinical signs of disease present in the patient's mouth.

- Compare and contrast the clinical and radiographic features of localized aggressive periodontitis and generalized periodontitis.

- Given the clinical and radiographic features for a patient with a history of aggressive periodontitis, determine if the disease is localized or generalized aggressive periodontitis.

Key Terms

Aggressive periodontitis (AgP)
Episodic disease progression

Localized aggressive periodontitis (LAP)
Generalized aggressive periodontitis (GAP)

Section 1
Aggressive Periodontitis—Highly Destructive Form

Periodontitis is a bacterial infection that may have many different clinical presentations. This chapter discusses aggressive periodontitis. **Aggressive periodontitis** (AgP) is a complex bacterial infection characterized by a rapid destruction of the periodontal ligament, rapid loss of supporting bone, high risk for tooth loss, and a poor response to periodontal therapy in an otherwise healthy individual. Fortunately, aggressive periodontitis is less common than chronic periodontitis.

Drs. Armitage and Cullinan (1) identified a number of significant clinical differences between chronic periodontitis and aggressive periodontitis including (a) age of onset of disease, (b) clinical signs of inflammation, (c) amount of plaque biofilm and calculus present, and (d) rates of progression (Table 8-1).

TABLE 8-1. SIGNIFICANT CLINICAL DIFFERENCES BETWEEN CHRONIC AND AGGRESSIVE FORMS OF PERIODONTITIS

Clinical Characteristic	Chronic Periodontitis	Aggressive Periodontitis
Age of Onset	Onset at any age; most commonly detected in adults over 35 y of age	Onset at any age; most commonly detected in adults under the age of 30 y; given similar amounts of periodontal destruction, affected individuals are significantly younger than individuals with chronic periodontitis (1)
Inflammation	Redness, swelling, bleeding on probing; however, clinical appearance is not a reliable indicator of the presence or severity of disease	Minimal signs of clinical inflammation in early stages
Plaque Biofilm	Moderate to heavy amounts of plaque biofilm and calculus	Relatively small amounts of plaque biofilm and calculus
Rates of Progression	Slow rate of disease progression	Rapid rate of disease progression

GENERAL CHARACTERISTICS OF AGGRESSIVE PERIODONTITIS

1. **Alternative Terminology.** Until recently, aggressive periodontitis was defined as occurring in individuals under the age of 30 years and was known as *early-onset periodontitis* (EOP). Features of aggressive periodontitis can present at any age and is not confined to individuals under the arbitrarily chosen age of 30 years.
2. **Characteristics**
   A. **Primary Features.** The primary features of aggressive periodontitis are the following (1–5):
      1. Rapid destruction of the attachment and rapid loss of supporting bone. Baer estimated that the loss of attachment in aggressive periodontitis patients progressed three or four times faster than in cases of chronic periodontitis (1,6–10).
      2. No obvious signs or symptoms of systemic disease

3. Other family members (parents, siblings) with aggressive periodontitis

B. **Secondary Features.** Secondary features that are generally but not always present are

1. Relatively small amounts of bacterial plaque biofilm; the disease severity seems to be exaggerated given the light amount of plaque biofilm

2. Elevated proportions of *Aggregatibacter actinomycetemcomitans* (*Aa*)

3. Phagocyte abnormalities

4. Elevated production of prostaglandin E2 (PGE2) and interleukin-1β (IL-1β) in response to bacterial endotoxins

5. A lack of clinical signs of disease
   a. Affected tissue may have a normal clinical appearance
   b. Probing reveals deep periodontal pockets on affected teeth

6. A poor response to periodontal therapy

7. **Episodic disease progression** (Fig. 8-1)
   a. Chronic periodontitis is a very slowly progressing disease.
   b. In aggressive periodontitis, attachment loss is **episodic**, occurring in a succession of acute destructive phases with intermittent inactive phases.

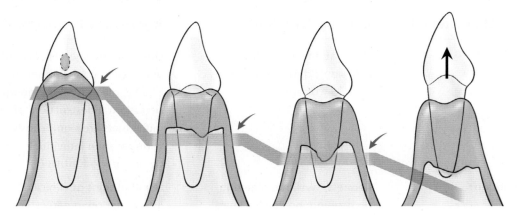

Figure 8-1. Episodic Disease Progression in Untreated Aggressive Periodontitis. Aggressive periodontitis progresses in a series of acute phases of tissue destruction followed by periods of disease inactivity.

LOCALIZED AND GENERALIZED AGGRESSIVE PERIODONTITIS

1. Localized Aggressive Periodontitis (LAP)
   A. **Features of Localized Aggressive Periodontitis** (Box 8-1, Figs. 8-2A, 2B, 2C)
      1. Onset of localized aggressive periodontitis is around the time of puberty.
      2. Localized attachment loss affecting the first molars and/or incisors and involving no more than two teeth other than first molars and incisors (1,6–10)
      3. There is a lack of tissue inflammation and minimal amounts of plaque biofilm that seem inconsistent with the amount of periodontal destruction (1,11). Most patients with LAP exhibit some clinical inflammation at affected sites, such as slight redness and swelling of the gingival margin and bleeding upon gentle probing (1).
      4. Frequently associated with *Aa* (*A. actinomycetemcomitans*)
      5. Vertical bone loss around the first molars and incisors, beginning around puberty is a classic radiographic sign of LAP.
   B. **Alternative Terminology.** LAP was previously known as localized juvenile periodontitis (LJP).

Box 8-1. Localized Aggressive Periodontitis (LAP)

- Onset around the time of puberty
- Minimal signs of inflammation
- Localized attachment loss involving the first molars and incisors
- Thin, unimpressive biofilm on affected teeth
- Frequently associated with *Aa*
- Previously called localized juvenile periodontitis

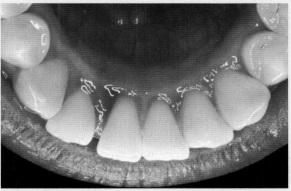

A

Figure 8-2A. Localized Aggressive Periodontitis. The photograph shows a patient with LAP. Note that there are not any supragingival calculus deposits evident.

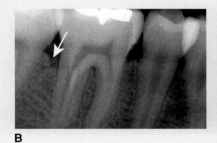

B

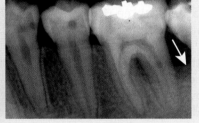

C

Figure 8-2B-C. Radiographic Characteristics of Localized Aggressive Periodontitis. Patients with LAP have bone loss on the *first molar and incisor teeth*. The radiographs shown here reveal a pattern of bone loss on the first molars that is similar on both sides of the mandibular arch.

2. Generalized Aggressive Periodontitis (GAP)
   A. Features of Generalized Aggressive Periodontitis (Box 8-2, Figs. 8-2A, 2B, 2C)
      1. Generalized aggressive periodontitis usually occurs in persons younger than 30 years of age, but patients may be older (1,12).
      2. Generalized interproximal attachment loss affecting at least three permanent teeth other than the first molars and incisors. In most cases of generalized aggressive periodontitis, most permanent teeth are affected (1,9,13).
      3. Destruction of attachment and alveolar bone is very episodic, occurring in a succession of acute phases rather than in a gradual progression.

4. Small amounts of bacterial plaque biofilm that seem inconsistent with the amount of periodontal destruction.
5. The appearance of the gingival tissues varies in GAP.
   a. The gingival tissues may be acutely inflamed, ulcerated, and fiery red (1). This tissue response is believed to occur in the destructive phase of disease progression.
   b. The gingival tissues may appear pink and free of inflammation. Deep pockets can be detected, however, with periodontal probing. This tissue response may coincide with periods of disease inactivity (14).
B. **Alternative Terminology.** GAP was previously known as generalized juvenile periodontitis (GJP) or early-onset periodontitis (G-EOP).
3. **Clinical Appearance of Aggressive Periodontitis.** Figures 8-4 to 8-7 illustrate the clinical appearance of patients with a diagnosis of aggressive periodontitis.

Box 8-2. Generalized Aggressive Periodontitis (GAP)

- Disease onset usually occurs in persons under 30 years of age, but patients may be older
- Generalized interproximal attachment loss affecting at least three permanent teeth other than the first molars and incisors
- Associated with *Aa*
- Family history of GAP (1,15)
- Previously known as generalized juvenile periodontitis

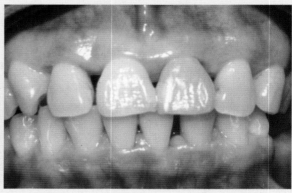

A

Figure 8-3A. Generalized Aggressive Periodontitis. The rate of attachment loss and bone loss is rapid in GAP compared to chronic periodontitis.

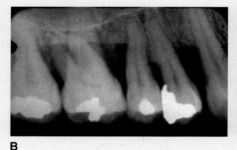

B

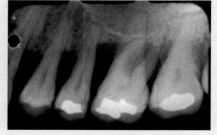

C

Figure 8-3B-C. Radiographic Characteristics of Generalized Aggressive Periodontitis. Radiographs of patients with GAP reveal severe alveolar bone loss *around most teeth*.

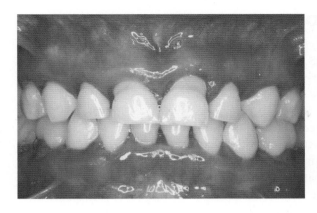

Figure 8-4. Child with Aggressive Periodontitis. Aggressive periodontitis in a 5-year-old child with attachment loss on all teeth.

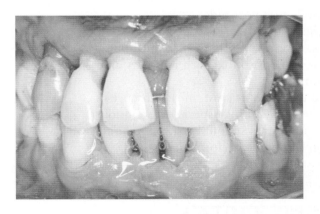

Figure 8-5. Aggressive Periodontitis. Aggressive periodontitis in a patient with good self-care (plaque biofilm control). In aggressive periodontitis, the disease severity typically seems exaggerated given the amount of bacterial plaque biofilm.

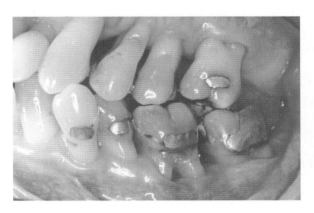

Figure 8-6. Aggressive Periodontitis. An example of aggressive periodontitis with continued disease progression despite good daily self-care by the patient. (Courtesy of Dr. John S. Dozier)

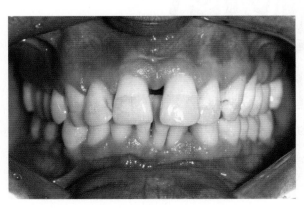

Figure 8-7. Aggressive Periodontitis. Aggressive periodontitis in a 30-year-old male with good daily self-care.

SCREENING FOR AGGRESSIVE PERIODONTITIS

A small but significant proportion of children and young adults are thought to be affected by aggressive periodontitis. A survey of U.S. adolescents aged 14 to 17 reports that 0.13% had aggressive periodontitis (1,12). Early detection is important given the severity and progression of aggressive periodontitis.

1. **Screening of Adolescents and Adults**
    A. Periodontal probing is the most accurate screening method for detecting attachment loss currently available. The measurement of attachment by probing is the screening method of choice for adolescents and adults.
    B. If aggressive periodontitis is suspected, the patient's medical history should be updated and reviewed to rule out possible systemic contributing factors. Periodontitis as a manifestation of systemic disease is the disease category used when the systemic condition is the major predisposing factor for periodontitis.

2. **Screening of Primary and Mixed Dentitions**
    A. The measurement of attachment loss on primary teeth or partially erupted teeth may be difficult.
    B. Measurement of the distance between the CEJ and the alveolar bone crest on bitewing radiographs is a useful screening approach with children (Fig. 8-8). Bitewing radiographs routinely are taken on children for caries screening and these radiographs also should be screened for the presence of marginal alveolar bone loss.
    C. The "normal" distance between the CEJ and the alveolar bone crest has been evaluated by recent investigations (11,16).
        1. The median distances between the CEJ and the alveolar crest of primary molars in 7- to 9-year-old children is 0.8 to 1.4 mm. The CEJ of permanent molars is 0 to 0.5 mm coronal to the alveolar crest in 7- to 9-year-olds.
        2. Greater distances between the CEJ and the alveolar crest are seen at sites with caries, restorations, or open contacts. These local conditions may contribute to localized bone loss in children in a similar manner to that seen in adults and are not indicative of aggressive periodontitis.
        3. A distance of 2 mm between the CEJ and the alveolar crest, in the absence of local contributing factors, should cause the clinician to suspect periodontitis. If the measurement exceeds this value, periodontitis should be suspected and a comprehensive periodontal examination should be performed.

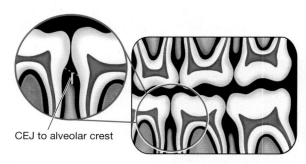

CEJ to alveolar crest

Figure 8-8. Use of Bitewing Radiographs in Screening for LAP in Children. The distance from the CEJ and the alveolar bone crest is measured from a line connecting the CEJs of the two adjacent teeth. Measurements are taken for each mesial and distal surface. Normal CEJ to alveolar bone crest distances for 7- to 9-year-olds are less than 2 mm.

Chapter Summary Statement

Periodontitis is a bacterial infection of all parts of the periodontium that results in irreversible destruction of the periodontal ligament fibers and alveolar bone. Periodontitis is a bacterial infection that may have many different clinical presentations. The 1999 AAP Classification of Periodontal Diseases and Conditions reclassified the forms of periodontitis into chronic periodontitis, aggressive periodontitis, and less common types of periodontal diseases.

Aggressive periodontitis is a bacterial infection characterized by a rapid destruction of the periodontal ligament, rapid loss of supporting bone, high risk for tooth loss, and a poor response to periodontal therapy. Features of aggressive periodontitis can present at any age. The primary features of aggressive periodontitis are (1) rapid destruction of the attachment and rapid loss of supporting bone, (2) no obvious signs or symptoms of systemic disease, and (3) other family members (parents, siblings) with aggressive periodontitis.

Section 2
Focus on Patients

Clinical Patient Care

CASE 1

While reading a journal article you find a reference to a periodontal disease called localized juvenile periodontitis (LJP). Since this is not a disease category in the currently accepted disease classification system, how does this terminology relate to modern periodontal diagnoses?

Ethical Dilemma

Your small private dental practice, which is within an urban city, has many long-standing patients. A number of patients within the practice are on public assistance and struggle with money issues. Dr. Gordon is very generous and understanding about her patients' limitations and often provides free dental services.

Your next patient of the morning is Jason S, a 14-year-old junior high school soccer player. His mother has made an emergency appointment, as he was hit in the mouth during a soccer game yesterday. His mother is concerned that Jason's front teeth may be loose as a result. His mother reports that Jason had a thorough "cleaning" in another dental office 4 months ago. Clinical examination reveals no trauma but some mobility, so you take radiographs. Clinically, Jason presents with no obvious signs or symptoms of disease, with lack of tissue inflammation and minimal amounts of plaque biofilm. Jason's radiographs, however, show moderate vertical bone loss around the maxillary central incisors and mandibular central incisors. Bitewing radiographs also indicate moderate bone loss around the maxillary and mandibular first molars. Probe readings on his incisors and molars are in the 4 to 6 mm range.

continued on next page

You present your findings to Dr. Gordon, who asks you to perform thorough periodontal instrumentation on Jason. You remind Dr. Gordon, that Jason had a dental hygiene appointment in another office 4 months ago and that his insurance only allows for periodontal instrumentation every 6 months. Dr. Gordon states that Jason is in dire need of this treatment and asks you to instruct the office manager to hold off on submitting Jason's insurance claim until it is within the 6-month time frame.

1. How would you classify Jason's periodontal condition?
2. What ethical principles are in conflict in this dilemma?
3. What is the best way for you to handle this ethical dilemma?
4. What should you do when treating future patients?

References

1. Armitage GC, Cullinan MP. Comparison of the clinical features of chronic and aggressive periodontitis. *Periodontol 2000*. 2010;53:12–27.
2. American Academy of Periodontology. *Annals of Periodontology*. Chicago, IL: American Academy of Periodontology; 1996:v.
3. Armitage GC. Periodontal diseases: diagnosis. *Ann Periodontol*. 1996;1(1):37–215.
4. Lang NP, Bartold PM, Cullinam M, et al. International classification workshop. Consensus report: Aggressive periodontitis. In: Lang NP, Bartold PM, Cullinam M, eds. *Annals of periodontology*. Chicago, IL: American Academy of Periodontology; 1999;4:53.
5. Armitage GC, Cullinan MP, Seymour GJ. Comparative biology of chronic and aggressive periodontitis: introduction. *Periodontol 2000*. 2010;53:7–11.
6. Baer PN. The case for periodontosis as a clinical entity. *J Periodontol*. 1971;42(8):516–520.
7. Manson JD, Lehner T. Clinical features of juvenile periodontitis (periodontosis). *J Periodontol*. 1974;45(8):636–640.
8. Liljenberg B, Lindhe J. Juvenile periodontitis. Some microbiological, histopathological and clinical characteristics. *J Clin Periodontol*. 1980;7(1):48–61.
9. Burmeister JA, Best AM, Palcanis KG, et al. Localized juvenile periodontitis and generalized severe periodontitis: clinical findings. *J Clin Periodontol*. 1984;11(3):181–192.
10. Saxen L, Murtomaa H. Age-related expression of juvenile periodontitis. *J Clin Periodontol*. 1985;12(1):21–26.
11. Needleman HL, Ku TC, Nelson L, et al. Alveolar bone height of primary and first permanent molars in healthy seven- to nine-year-old children. *ASDC J Dent Child*. 1997;64(3):188–196, 65.
12. Loe H, Brown LJ. Early onset periodontitis in the United States of America. *J Periodontol*. 1991;62(10):608–616.
13. Armitage GC. Development of a classification system for periodontal diseases and conditions. *Ann Periodontol*. 1999; 4(1):1–6.
14. Page RC, Baab DA. A new look at the etiology and pathogenesis of early-onset periodontitis. Cementopathia revisited. *J Periodontol*. 1985;56(12):748–751.
15. Griffiths GS, Ayob R, Guerrero A, et al. Amoxicillin and metronidazole as an adjunctive treatment in generalized aggressive periodontitis at initial therapy or re-treatment: a randomized controlled clinical trial. *J Clin Periodontol*. 2011;38(1):43–49.
16. Sjodin B, Matsson L. Marginal bone level in the normal primary dentition. *J Clin Periodontol*. 1992;19(9 Pt 1):672–678.

 ## STUDENT ANCILLARY RESOURCES

A wide variety of resources to enhance your learning and understanding of this chapter are available on thePoint®.

- Visit thePoint to access:
  - Audio Glossary
  - Animations
  - Suggested Readings
  - Answers to Review Questions
  - Case Studies

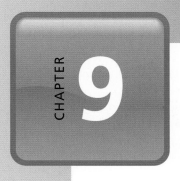

CHAPTER

9

Other Periodontal Conditions

Clinical Application. This chapter outlines the interesting array of conditions that can affect the periodontium in addition to the common varieties of periodontal diseases. Familiarity with these other conditions is critical for all clinicians, since failure to recognize them may have a profound impact on the well-being of some patients. The importance of study of these conditions by the student and experienced clinician cannot be overrated.

Learning Objectives

- Name and explain systemic or genetic factors that may contribute to the initiation and progression of periodontitis.
- Describe the impact of PMN (neutrophil) dysfunction and hematologic disorders on the periodontium.
- Describe clinical signs of periodontitis that may be associated with HIV infection.
- Describe the tissue destruction that occurs in necrotizing periodontal diseases.
- Compare and contrast the clinical findings of necrotizing ulcerative gingivitis and necrotizing ulcerative periodontitis.
- Compare and contrast the tissue destruction in chronic periodontitis with that seen in necrotizing ulcerative periodontitis.
- Name several local factors, such as tooth-related or mucogingival deformities, that may contribute to the initiation and progression of periodontitis.
- Define secondary occlusal trauma and explain how it can lead to rapid bone loss.

Key Terms

Periodontitis as a manifestation of systemic disease
Neutropenia
Linear gingival erythema (LGE)

Necrotizing periodontal disease (NPD)
Tissue necrosis
Necrotizing ulcerative gingivitis

Necrotizing ulcerative periodontitis
Pseudomembrane
Secondary occlusal trauma

LESS COMMON FORMS OF PERIODONTITIS

This group is composed of uncommon types of periodontitis including (1) periodontitis as a manifestation of systemic diseases (2), necrotizing periodontal diseases (NPDs) (3), abscesses of the periodontium (4), periodontitis associated with endodontic lesions (5), developmental or acquired deformities and conditions, and (6) occlusal trauma. *Abscesses of the periodontium are discussed in the chapter on periodontal emergencies.*

Section 1
Periodontitis as a Manifestation of Systemic Diseases

A number of systemic diseases and conditions are a contributing factor in the development of periodontitis. Several hematologic (blood disorders) and genetic disorders are associated with the development of periodontitis (Box 9-1) (1,2). *Refer to Chapter 15 for a detailed discussion of systemic disease as a contributing factor to periodontitis.* Periodontitis as a manifestation of systemic disease is the diagnosis used when the systemic condition is the major contributing factor for periodontitis and local factors such as heavy accumulations of dental plaque biofilm and calculus deposits are not evident.

Box 9-1. Periodontitis as a Manifestation of Systemic Diseases

1. **Associated with Hematological Disorders**
   A. Acquired neutropenia
   B. Leukemias
   C. Other
2. **Associated with Genetic Disorders**
   A. Familial and cyclic neutropenia
   B. Down syndrome
   C. Leukocyte adhesion deficiency syndromes
   D. Papillon–Lefèvre syndrome
   E. Chédiak–Higashi syndrome
   F. Histiocytosis syndromes
   G. Glycogen storage disease
   H. Infantile genetic agranulocytosis
   I. Cohen syndrome
   J. Ehlers–Danlos syndrome (Types IV and VIII)
   K. Hypophosphatasia
   L. Other
3. **Not Otherwise Specified (NOS)**

1. **Hematologic Disorders.** Hematologic disorders are abnormalities in the structure or function of the blood and blood-forming tissues such as: red cells, white cells, platelets, or clotting factors. There are numerous rare hematologic disorders that may affect the periodontium (Box 9-3, Fig. 9-2).
   A. **Acquired Neutropenia**
      1. Neutropenia is a blood disorder characterized by abnormally low levels of neutrophils (polymorphonuclear leukocytes [PMNs]) in the blood.
      2. Neutropenia has numerous causes. It may be genetic or may be seen with viral infections and after radiotherapy and chemotherapy. It affects as many as one in three patients receiving chemotherapy for cancer.
      3. Neutropenia lowers the immunologic barrier to bacterial and fungal infection.
      4. Neutrophil disorders that affect the production or function of PMNs may result in severe periodontal destruction (Box 9-2, Fig. 9-1).
      5. Reported periodontal manifestations include either a localized or generalized pattern of periodontitis (3–5). Professional dental hygiene care and meticulous daily self-care, in combination with systemic antibiotics to supplement therapy for the underlying disease, have been successful in many cases (4).
   B. **Leukemia**
      1. Leukemia is cancer that begins in blood cells. In people with leukemia, the bone marrow produces a large number of abnormal white blood cells, that don't function properly.
      2. At first, leukemia cells function almost normally. In time, they may crowd out normal white blood cells, red blood cells, and platelets.
      3. Periodontal manifestations of leukemia frequently include gingival enlargement, mucosal bleeding and ulceration, petechiae, and opportunistic infections of the gingiva (6–9).

Box 9-2. Periodontitis Associated with PMN Dysfunction

- Occurs in patients of any age
- Seen in young children beginning with the eruption of primary teeth
- Characterized with severe bone loss and tooth loss
- Associated with systemic conditions that interfere with the body's resistance to bacterial infection

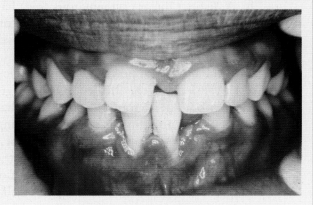

Figure 9-1. Periodontitis Associated with Immune Dysfunction. This photo shows the dentition of a young patient with PMN deficiency. Note the primary dentition is being lost and the permanent dentition is being exfoliated as soon as the permanent teeth erupt.

Box 9-3. Hemorrhagic Periodontitis–Associated Blood Disorder

- Characterized by soft, swollen gingival tissue. Bleeding occurs spontaneously or on the slightest provocation.

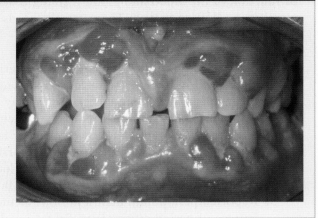

Figure 9-2. Periodontitis Associated with a Blood Disorder. This male patient has a rare blood disorder. His soft, swollen gingiva bleeds easily. (Courtesy of Dr. Ralph Arnold, San Antonio, TX)

C. AIDS/HIV Infection
1. Since the early 1990s, the death rate from AIDS among adults has declined in most developed countries, largely because of newer antiretroviral therapies and improved access to these therapies. In addition, from 2006 to 2011, the total number of new cases of human immunodeficiency virus (HIV) infection worldwide has declined somewhat and has remained relatively constant (10).
2. The periodontal conditions most closely associated with HIV infection are linear gingival erythema (LGE) and necrotizing periodontal diseases (NPD) are the most common HIV-associated periodontal conditions reported in the literature (Box 9-4, Fig. 9-3A,B,C) (10).
   a. Linear gingival erythema (LGE) is a gingival manifestation of immunosuppression.
   b. A distinct linear erythematous (red) band that is limited to the free gingiva characterizes the clinical appearance of LGE (Box 9-4).
   c. LGE does not respond well to improved self-care or periodontal instrumentation.
3. With the advent of newer pharmacological approaches to the treatment of HIV infection, the incidence and progression of both atypical and conventional periodontal diseases are changing. The incidence of necrotizing periodontitis and gingival diseases of fungal origin appears to be on the decline as a result of these therapies that have led to increased life spans for HIV patients. However, in cases where these therapies lose their effectiveness and HIV patients relapse into an immunosuppressed state, these conditions may recur. Recent evidence has shown that HIV patients with more conventional periodontal diseases such as chronic periodontitis may have increased attachment loss and gingival recession when compared to their HIV-negative counterparts (11,12).

Box 9-4. Periodontitis Associated with HIV Infection

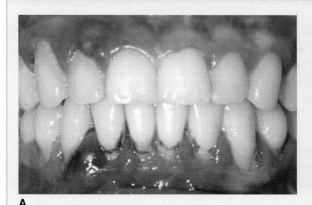

A

Figure 9-3A. Periodontitis Associated with HIV Infection. This HIV-positive individual exhibits a severe form of necrotizing ulcerative periodontitis with tissue necrosis of the gingival tissues combined with loss of attachment. Clinical signs are visible on the mandibular anterior sextant.

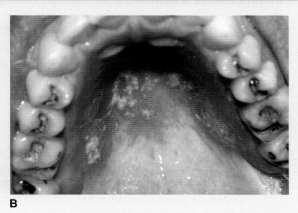

B

Figure 9-3B. Periodontitis Associated with HIV Infection. Palatal candidiasis on the palatal mucosa of an HIV-positive individual. (Courtesy of Dr. Ralph Arnold).

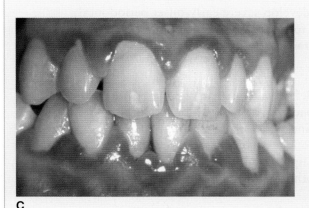

C

Figure 9-3C. Linear Gingival Erythema. Linear gingival erythema in an HIV-infected patient.

- The periodontal conditions most closely associated with HIV infection are linear gingival erythema (LGE) and necrotizing periodontal diseases (NPDs).
- HIV-infected patients with more conventional periodontal diseases such as chronic periodontitis may have increased attachment loss and gingival recession when compared to their HIV-negative counterparts.
- Oral manifestations of HIV infection include oral candidiasis, oral hairy Leukoplakia, oral hyperpigmentation, oral ulcers; red, purple, or blue edematous soft tissue lesions; and Kaposi sarcoma and other oral malignancies.

2. **Genetic Disorders.** A genetic disorder is a disease caused by the absence of a gene or by-products of a defective gene. Genetic diseases are passed from one generation to the next but do not necessarily appear in each generation.
   A. **Familial and Cyclic Neutropenia**
      1. Hereditary and congenital disorders that affect the bone marrow, resulting in abnormally low level of neutrophils (PMNs) in the blood.
      2. Individuals with cyclic neutropenia may experience severe periodontal destruction. Periodontal manifestations of this disease appear at a young age (13).
   B. **Down Syndrome**
      1. A common birth defect caused by an error in cell division results in the presence of an additional third chromosome. One in every 691 babies in the United States is born with Down syndrome, making Down syndrome the most common genetic condition.
      2. Most people with Down syndrome have cognitive delays that are mild to moderate. A few of the common physical traits of Down syndrome are low muscle tone, small stature, an upward slant to the eyes, and a single deep crease across the center of the palm. People with Down syndrome have an increased risk for certain medical conditions such as congenital heart defects, respiratory and hearing problems, Alzheimer disease, childhood leukemia, and thyroid conditions.
      3. Individuals with Down syndrome often develop severe early-onset periodontal diseases (14). Substantial plaque biofilm formation, deep periodontal pockets, and extensive gingival inflammation characterize periodontal disease in Down syndrome (Box 9-5, Fig. 9-4).
   C. **Leukocyte Adhesion Deficiency Syndromes**
      1. An inherited disorder in which there is defective leukocyte chemotaxis. Affected individuals are susceptible to recurrent bacterial and fungal infections, impaired pus formation, delayed wound healing, and periodontitis (15).
      2. Cases of periodontal disease attributed to leukocyte adhesion deficiency syndromes are rare. Periodontitis begins upon eruption of the primary teeth with rapid attachment loss and early tooth loss (16).
   D. **Papillon–Lefèvre Syndrome**
      1. An inherited disorder characterized by hyperkeratosis of the palms of the hands and soles of the feet and severe periodontitis affecting both primary and secondary dentitions (17).
      2. Periodontitis causes bone loss and exfoliation of the teeth. Primary teeth may be lost by 5 or 6 years of age. The permanent teeth erupt but are lost due to bone destruction. By age 15 some individuals are edentulous.
   E. **Chédiak–Higashi Syndrome**
      1. A rare, inherited disorder of the immune and nervous systems characterized by pale-colored hair, eyes, and skin. Impairment of neutrophil chemotaxis is a characteristic of this disease (18).
      2. Patients with Chédiak–Higashi Syndrome are prone to severe periodontitis (19).
   F. **Glycogen Storage Disease**
      1. One of the 14 recognized diseases that interfere with the storage of carbohydrates as glycogen in the body; characterized by neutropenia.
      2. Periodontal manifestations of this disease appear at a young age with the potential for early tooth loss (20).

Box 9-5. Periodontitis-Associated Down Syndrome

- Characterized by substantial biofilm formation, deep periodontal pockets, and extensive gingival inflammation

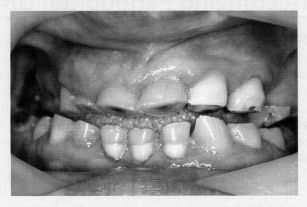

Figure 9-4. Periodontitis Associated with Down Syndrome. (Courtesy of Dr. Richard Foster, Guilford Technical Community College, Jamestown, NC)

G. **Infantile Genetic Agranulocytosis (Kostmann syndrome)**
1. A rare inherited form of severe chronic neutropenia usually detected soon after birth (21).
2. Individuals with infantile genetic agranulocytosis experience severe periodontal disease (22).

H. **Cohen Syndrome**
1. An inherited disorder that affects many parts of the body and is characterized by neutropenia, developmental delay, mental retardation, small head size, and weak muscle tone (23).
2. Individuals with Cohen syndrome have increased susceptibility to early periodontal breakdown, which is likely to be associated with neutropenia.

I. **Ehlers–Danlos Syndrome (Types IV and VIII)**
1. A heritable disorder of connective tissue with easy bruising, joint hypermobility (loose joints), skin laxity, and weakness of tissues (24).
2. Early-onset generalized periodontitis is one of the most significant oral manifestations of the syndrome. This can lead to the premature loss of deciduous and permanent teeth (25–27).

J. **Hypophosphatasia**
1. A genetic metabolic disorder of bone mineralization caused by a deficiency in alkaline phosphatase in serum and tissues; characterized by skeletal defects resembling those of rickets (28).
2. Periodontal manifestations include severe loss of alveolar bone and premature loss of primary and permanent teeth in the absence of an inflammatory response (29). Early exfoliation particularly affects the anterior teeth. Children with hypophosphatasia are at risk of developing oral complications during adolescent and adult life (30).

Section 2
Necrotizing Periodontal Diseases

Necrotizing periodontal diseases include necrotizing ulcerative gingivitis (NUG) and necrotizing ulcerative periodontitis (NUP). To date, there is insufficient evidence to establish if NUG and NUP are two unique diseases or different stages of the same disease that progresses from NUG to NUP. Until a distinction between NUG and NUP can be clarified, NUG and NUP are classified together under the category of necrotizing periodontal diseases. Both NUG and NUP appear to be related to diminished systemic resistance to bacterial infection. Treatment of necrotizing periodontal diseases is discussed in Chapter 28, Periodontal Emergencies.

1. **Necrotizing periodontal disease (NPD)** is an inflammatory destructive infection of periodontal tissues that involve **tissue necrosis** (localized tissue death). Both NUG and NUP are painful infections with ulceration, swelling, and sloughing off of dead epithelial tissue from the gingiva.
   A. **Necrotizing ulcerative gingivitis (NUG)**—tissue necrosis that is limited to the gingival tissues (Box 9-6, Fig. 9-5).
   B. **Necrotizing ulcerative periodontitis (NUP)**—tissue necrosis of the gingival tissues combined with loss of attachment and alveolar bone loss (Box 9-7, Fig. 9-6).
      1. NUP is a painful infection characterized by necrosis of gingival tissues, periodontal ligament, and alveolar bone.
      2. NUP is an extremely rapid and destructive form of periodontitis that can produce loss of periodontal attachment within days.
2. **Alternative Terminology.** These conditions previously have been known as trench mouth, Vincent infection, acute ulcerative necrotizing gingivitis (ANUG), and necrotizing ulcerative gingivostomatitis.
3. **Signs and Symptoms of Necrotizing Periodontal Disease**
   A. **Oral Signs and Symptoms.** The clinical appearance of NPD is noticeably different than that of any other periodontal disease (31,32).
      1. NPD is a painful infection, primarily involving the interdental and marginal gingiva.
      2. NPD is characterized by ulcerated and necrotic papillae and gingival margins, giving the appearance that the papillae and gingival margins have been "punched-out" or "cratered" (Fig. 9-7). The ulcerated margin is bounded by a red halo.

Box 9-6. Necrotizing Ulcerative Gingivitis (NUG)

- Sudden onset
- Pain
- Necrosis of interdental papillae (cratered, punched-out papillae)
- Yellowish white or grayish tissue slough
- Fiery red gingiva with spontaneous bleeding

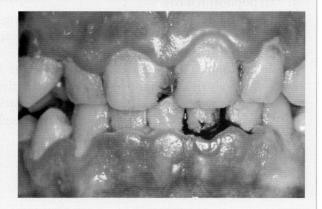

Figure 9-5. Necrotizing Ulcerative Gingivitis.

Box 9-7. Necrotizing Ulcerative Periodontitis (NUP)

- The same signs and symptoms of NUG
- Attachment loss

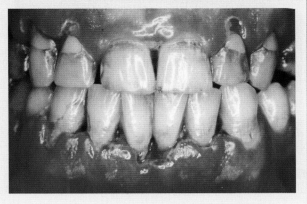

Figure 9-6. Necrotizing Ulcerative Periodontitis.

3. The necrotic areas of the gingiva are covered by a yellowish white or grayish tissue slough, which is termed a **pseudomembrane**.
   a. The pseudomembrane consists primarily of fibrin and necrotic tissue with leukocytes, erythrocytes, and masses of bacteria. (Fibrin is stringy protein formed during the process of blood clot formation.)
   b. The term, pseudomembrane, however, is misleading since the slough has no coherence and is not similar to a true membrane. It is easily wiped off with gauze, exposing an area of fiery red, shiny gingiva.
   c. The pseudomembrane may involve the gingiva of several teeth or it may cover the entire gingiva.
   d. The sloughing off of dead gingival epithelial tissue exposes the underlying connective tissue.
4. Fiery red gingiva with spontaneous gingival bleeding or bleeding to gentle touch.
5. *The **necrotizing lesions develop rapidly and are painful.*** Intense oral pain that causes affected patients to seek dental treatment. This symptom is unusual since gingivitis and periodontitis normally are *not* painful.
6. The first lesions often are seen interproximally in the mandibular anterior sextant but may occur in any interproximal papilla. Usually, the papillae swell rapidly and develop a rounded contour (Fig. 9-8).
7. A pronounced, fetid oral odor (bad breath) may be present but can vary in intensity and in some cases is not very noticeable.
   a. The pain associated with NPDs usually causes the individual to stop brushing.
   b. Materia alba, plaque biofilm, sloughed tissue, blood, and stagnant saliva collect in the oral cavity causing the oral odor.
8. NPDs may be associated with excessive salivation.

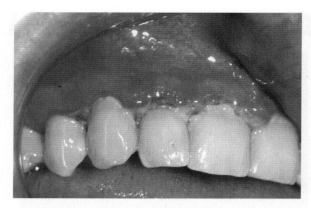
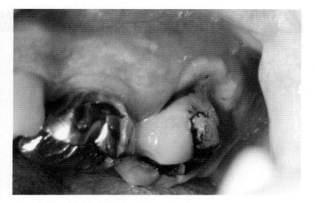

Figure 9-7. Necrotic Papillae and Gingival Margins. This patient with NPD exhibits the characteristic ulcerated, necrotic papillae and gingival margins. (Courtesy of Dr. Ralph Arnold)

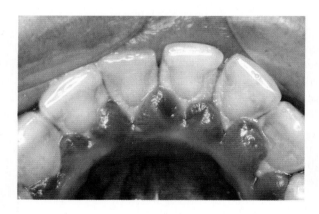

Figure 9-8. Swollen Papillae. Swollen papillae in the anterior regions of the mouth are characteristic of NPD. (Courtesy of Dr. Richard Foster, Guilford Technical Community College, Jamestown, NC)

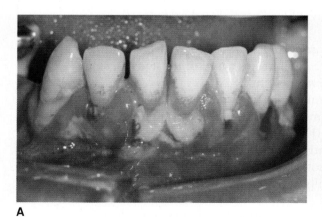
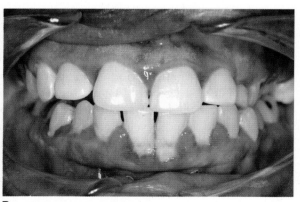

A   **B**

Figure 9-9. Necrotizing Ulcerative Periodontitis. NUP is characterized by loss of attachment. (**A:** Courtesy of Dr. Ralph Arnold; **B:** Courtesy of Dr. Richard Foster, Guilford Technical Community College, Jamestown, NC)

9. As tissue necrosis progresses, interproximal craters are formed.
   a. Within a few days the involved papillae are often separated into one facial and one lingual portion with a necrotic depression between them.
   b. This central tissue destruction between the facial and lingual portions of a papilla results in a crater.
   c. Once interproximal craters are formed, the disease process usually involves the periodontal ligament and alveolar bone, resulting in loss of attachment.
   d. Deep craters in the interdental alveolar bone characterize NUP.
   e. The deep periodontal pockets seen in other forms of periodontitis are not common in NUP because the tissue necrosis destroys the marginal epithelium and connective tissue, resulting in gingival recession (Fig. 9-9). Progression of the interproximal disease process often results in destruction of most of the interdental bone.
10. As the result of pain it is often difficult for patients to eat.
B. Systemic Signs and Symptoms
   1. Swelling of the lymph nodes, especially the submandibular and cervical lymph nodes, may occur in NPDs.
   2. Fever and malaise is not a consistent characteristic of NPDs. Investigations indicate that fever is not common (33,34).
4. **Etiology of Necrotizing Periodontal Diseases**
   A. **Microorganisms.** NPDs are associated with *Treponema* species, *Selenomonas* species, *Fusobacterium* species, *and Bacteroides melaninogenicus ss. intermedius* (*Provotella intermedia*).
   B. **Predisposing Factors for Necrotizing Periodontal Diseases**
      1. Systemic diseases, which impair immunity, including HIV infection, leukemia, measles, chicken pox, tuberculosis, herpetic gingivostomatitis, and malaria
      2. Poor self-care (plaque control)
      3. Emotional stress (35,36)
      4. Inadequate sleep, fatigue
      5. Alcohol use
      6. Caucasian background
      7. Cigarette smoking—most patients who experience NPDs are smokers (34,37)
      8. Increased levels of personal stress
      9. Poor nutrition
         a. In North America, NUG is associated with poor eating habits of young adults, such as college students.
         b. In developing countries, NUG occurs in very young children and appears to be related to poor nutritional status, especially a low protein intake.
      10. Pre-existing gingivitis or tissue trauma
      11. Young age—this disease can occur at any age, however, the reported mean age for NPDs in industrialized countries is between 22 and 24 years (38).

Section 3
Developmental or Acquired Deformities and Conditions

In general, this classification comprises local factors that contribute to the initiation and progression of periodontal disease. These factors fall into four subgroups (Table 9-1).

TABLE 9-1. DEVELOPMENTAL OR ACQUIRED DEFORMITIES AND CONDITIONS

1. Localized tooth-related factors that modify or predispose to plaque-induced gingival diseases or periodontitis
   A. Tooth anatomic factors
   B. Dental restorations/appliances
   C. Root fractures
   D. Cervical root resorption and cemental tears

2. Mucogingival deformities and conditions around teeth
   A. Recession of the gingival margin
     1. Facial or lingual surfaces
     2. Interproximal (papillary)
   B. Lack of keratinized gingiva
   C. Decreased vestibular depth
   D. Aberrant frenum/muscle position
   E. Gingival excess
     1. Pseudopocket
     2. Inconsistent gingival margin
     3. Excessive gingival display
     4. Gingival enlargement
   F. Abnormal color

3. Mucogingival deformities and conditions on edentulous ridges
   A. Vertical and/or horizontal ridge deficiency
   B. Lack of gingiva/keratinized tissue
   C. Gingival/soft tissue enlargement
   D. Aberrant frenum/muscle position
   E. Decreased vestibular depth
   F. Abnormal color

4. Occlusal trauma
   A. Primary occlusal trauma
   B. Secondary occlusal trauma

TOOTH-RELATED FACTORS

Tooth anatomic factors that predispose to plaque-related gingival diseases or periodontitis include tooth anatomic factors, such as cervical enamel projections and enamel pearls, palatolingual grooves, or tooth malalignment (Figs. 9-10 and 9-11). Local factors such as orthodontic appliances (braces) or faulty dental restorations can lead to plaque biofilm retention (Figs. 9-12 and 9-13) and may impinge on the biologic width.

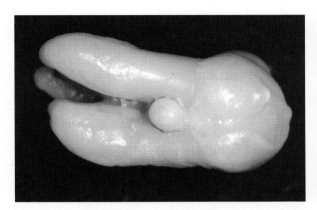
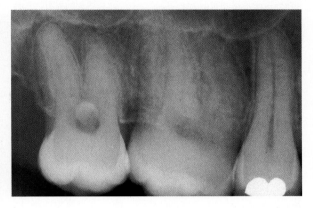

Figure 9-10. Enamel Pearl as Predisposing Factor. This maxillary second molar exhibits enamel pearl. Although not clear on the radiograph, this tooth experienced alveolar bone loss on the facial aspect. (Courtesy of Dr. Ralph Arnold)

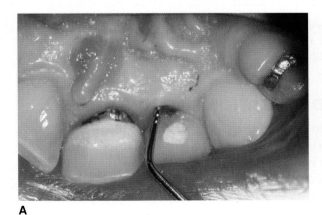
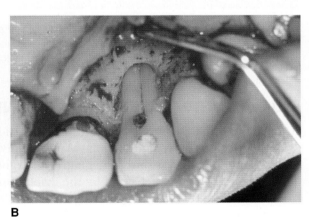

A   **B**

Figure 9-11. Palatolingual Groove. **A:** This patient has a deep periodontal pocket on the lingual of the maxillary lateral incisor. **B:** Periodontal surgery reveals a palatolingual groove as the predisposing factor for bone loss at this site. (Courtesy of Dr. Ralph Arnold)

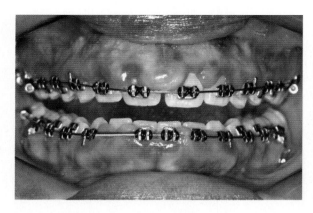

Figure 9-12. Orthodontic Appliances as a Predisposing Factor. Infrequent self-care and plaque biofilm accumulation results in periodontitis in this individual with orthodontic appliances. (Courtesy of Dr. Richard Foster, Guilford Technical Community College, Jamestown, NC)

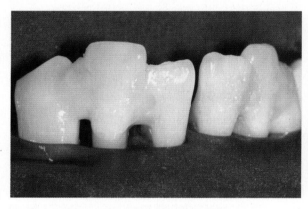

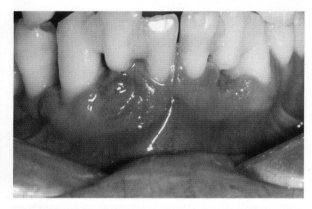

Figure 9-13. Dentistry as Predisposing Factor. The photo to the left shows anterior teeth with a rubber dam in place. The splinting of these mandibular anterior teeth leads to plaque biofilm accumulation and is a predisposing factor for periodontitis. (Courtesy of Dr. Ralph Arnold)

MUCOGINGIVAL DEFORMITIES AND CONDITIONS AROUND TEETH

A mucogingival deformity is a significant alteration of the morphology, size, and interrelationships between the gingiva and the alveolar mucosa that may involve the underlying bone. Recession of the gingival margin is the most common mucogingival deformity and it is characterized by the displacement of the gingival margin apically from the cementoenamel junction (Figs. 9-14 to 9-17).

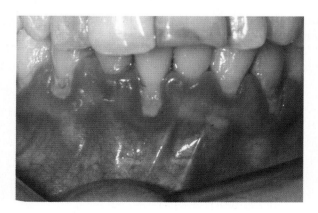

Figure 9-14. Recession of the Gingival Margin. Recession on the mandibular central incisor extending to the mucogingival junction. (Courtesy of Dr. Ralph Arnold)

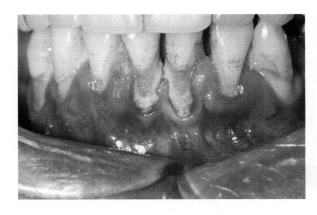

Figure 9-15. Recession of the Gingival Margin. Recession on the mandibular central incisors extending to the mucogingival junction. (Courtesy of Dr. Ralph Arnold)

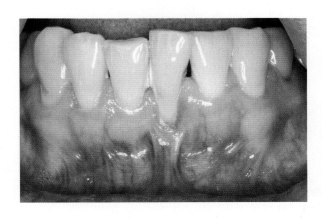

Figure 9-16. Frenum Attachments. Tension of the frenum may pull the gingiva away from the tooth and may be conducive to plaque biofilm accumulation and recession of the gingival margin. (Fig. 9-16 courtesy of Dr. Richard Foster, Guilford Technical Community College, Jamestown, NC)

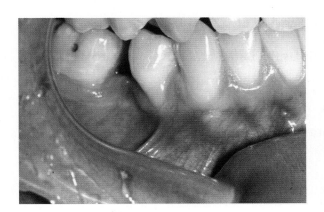

Figure 9-17. Frenum Attachments. Tension of a frenum may pull the gingiva away from the tooth and may be conducive to plaque biofilm accumulation and recession of the gingival margin. (Fig. 9-17 courtesy of Dr. Ralph Arnold)

OCCLUSAL TRAUMA IN PATIENTS WITH PERIODONTITIS

1. **Secondary occlusal trauma** is injury as the result of occlusal forces applied to a tooth or teeth that have previously experienced attachment loss and/or bone loss.
2. *In this type of occlusal trauma, the periodontium was unhealthy before experiencing excessive occlusal forces* (Box 9-8, Figs. 9-18A, 18B).
3. Rapid bone loss and pocket formation may result when excessive occlusal forces are applied to a tooth that has previously experienced attachment loss and/or bone loss.

Box 9-8. Secondary Occlusal Trauma

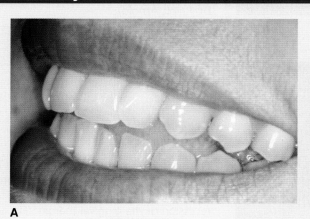 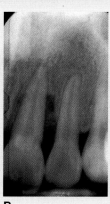

A   B

Figure 9-18. Secondary Occlusal Trauma. A: The woman pictured above puts repeated heavy pressure against her central incisor tooth. **B:** A dental radiograph of her central incisor shows severe bone loss around the central incisor that is subjected to the heavy pressure.

Clinical indicators of occlusal trauma may include one or more of the following:
- Tooth mobility (progressive)
- Fremitus (vibration felt when palpating a tooth, as the patient taps the teeth together)
- Tooth migration
- Fractured tooth
- Thermal sensitivity on chewing or percussion

Radiographic indicators may include one or more of the following:
- Widened periodontal ligament space
- Bone loss
- Root resorption

Chapter Summary Statement

The 1999 AAP Classification of Periodontal Diseases and Conditions includes several less common types of periodontitis as well as other periodontal conditions. These are divided into the following subcategories:

- Periodontitis as manifestation of systemic disease
- Necrotizing periodontal diseases
- Abscesses of the periodontium
- Periodontitis associated with endodontic lesions
- Developmental or acquired deformities and conditions.

Section 4
Focus on Patients

Clinical Patient Care

CASE 1

A new patient comes to the dental office on an emergency basis. The patient complains of severe pain in his gums and reports that he was unable to eat over the weekend due to the pain. A clinical examination reveals necrotic papillae and gingival margins, cratered papillae, a yellowish tissue slough, spontaneous bleeding, and no loss attachment or bone loss. Which type of periodontal disease does this patient exhibit?

Ethical Dilemma

Your last patient of the day is Luana G., a 16-year-old girl, who has Down Syndrome. She presents with moderate mental retardation. This is the first dental appointment in her life, as she has a fear of clinical settings, and her parents have not wanted to frighten or upset her. Your clinical exam reveals substantial plaque, biofilm and calculus formation, deep periodontal pockets, and extensive gingival inflammation. Radiographs show severe alveolar bone loss around most of her teeth. There is furcation involvement and some mobility present. There is also extensive cervical decay present on all of her mandibular anterior teeth. Due to Luana's mental deficits, it is difficult to determine if she is experiencing oral discomfort. Half way through your appointment, however, Luana refuses to open her mouth, starts to cry, and rocks back and forth. Her parents say this is her typical behavior when she is upset.

1. How would you classify Luana's periodontal condition?
2. What ethical principles are in conflict in this dilemma?
3. What is the best way for you to handle this ethical dilemma?

References

1. Kinane D. Blood and lymphoreticular disorders. *Periodontol 2000.* 1999;1:84–93.
2. Kinane DF. Periodontitis modified by systemic factors. *Ann Periodontol.* 1999;4(1):54–64.
3. Okada M, Kobayashi M, Hino T, et al. Clinical periodontal findings and microflora profiles in children with chronic neutropenia under supervised oral hygiene. *J Periodontol.* 2001;72(7):945–952.
4. Schmidt JC, Walter C, Rischewski JR, et al. Treatment of periodontitis as a manifestation of neutropenia with or without systemic antibiotics: a systematic review. *Pediatr Dent.* 2013;35(2):E54–E63.
5. Zaromb A, Chamberlain D, Schoor R, et al. Periodontitis as a manifestation of chronic benign neutropenia. *J Periodontol.* 2006;77(11):1921–1926.
6. Gillette WB. Re: oral manifestations of acute myelomonocytic leukemia: a case report and review of the classification of leukemias. Wu J, Fantasia Je, Kaplan R. (2002;73:664–668). *J Periodontol.* 2002;73(10):1228.
7. Haytac MC, Antmen B, Dogan MC, et al. Severe alveolar bone loss and gingival hyperplasia as initial manifestation of Burkitt cell type acute lymphoblastic leukemia. *J Periodontol.* 2003;74(4):547–551.
8. Soga Y, Saito T, Nishimura F, et al. Appearance of multidrug-resistant opportunistic bacteria on the gingiva during leukemia treatment. *J Periodontol.* 2008;79(1):181–186.
9. Wu J, Fantasia JE, Kaplan R. Oral manifestations of acute myelomonocytic leukemia: a case report and review of the classification of leukemias. *J Periodontol.* 2002;73(6):664–668.
10. Ryder MI, Nittayananta W, Coogan M, et al. Periodontal disease in HIV/AIDS. *Periodontol 2000.* 2012;60(1):78–97.
11. Ryder MI. An update on HIV and periodontal disease. *J Periodontol.* 2002;73(9):1071–1078.
12. Vastardis SA, Yukna RA, Fidel PL Jr., et al. Periodontal disease in HIV-positive individuals: association of periodontal indices with stages of HIV disease. *J Periodontol.* 2003;74(9):1336–1341.
13. Rylander H, Ericsson I. Manifestations and treatment of periodontal disease in a patient suffering from cyclic neutropenia. *J Clin Periodontol.* 1981;8(2):77–87.
14. Amano A, Kishima T, Kimura S, et al. Periodontopathic bacteria in children with Down syndrome. *J Periodontol.* 2000;71(2):249–255.
15. Dababneh R, Al-Wahadneh AM, Hamadneh S, et al. Periodontal manifestation of leukocyte adhesion deficiency type I. *J Periodontol.* 2008;79(4):764–768.
16. Cox DP, Weathers DR. Leukocyte adhesion deficiency type 1: an important consideration in the clinical differential diagnosis of prepubertal periodontitis. A case report and review of the literature. *Oral Surg Oral Med Oral Pathol Oral Radiol Endod.* 2008;105(1):86–90.
17. Cagli NA, Hakki SS, Dursun R, et al. Clinical, genetic, and biochemical findings in two siblings with Papillon-Lefevre Syndrome. *J Periodontol.* 2005;76(12):2322–2329.
18. Delcourt-Debruyne EM, Boutigny HR, Hildebrand HF. Features of severe periodontal disease in a teenager with Chediak-Higashi syndrome. *J Periodontol.* 2000;71(5):816–824.
19. Bailleul-Forestier I, Monod-Broca J, Benkerrou M, et al. Generalized periodontitis associated with Chediak-Higashi syndrome. *J Periodontol.* 2008;79(7):1263–1270.
20. Salapata Y, Laskaris G, Drogari E, et al. Oral manifestations in glycogen storage disease type 1b. *J Oral Pathol Med.* 1995;24(3):136–139.
21. Saglam F, Atamer T, Onan U, et al. Infantile genetic agranulocytosis (Kostmann type). A case report. *J Periodontol.* 1995;66(9):808–810.
22. Carlsson G, Andersson M, Putsep K, et al. Kostmann syndrome or infantile genetic agranulocytosis, part one: celebrating 50 years of clinical and basic research on severe congenital neutropenia. *Acta Paediatr.* 2006;95(12):1526–1532.
23. Alaluusua S, Kivitie-Kallio S, Wolf J, et al. Periodontal findings in Cohen syndrome with chronic neutropenia. *J Periodontol.* 1997;68(5):473–478.
24. Perez LA, Al-Shammari KF, Giannobile WV, et al. Treatment of periodontal disease in a patient with Ehlers-Danlos syndrome. A case report and literature review. *J Periodontol.* 2002;73(5):564–570.
25. Karrer S, Landthaler M, Schmalz G. Ehlers-Danlos type VIII. Review of the literature. *Clin Oral Investig.* 2000;4(2):66–69.
26. Letourneau Y, Perusse R, Buithieu H. Oral manifestations of Ehlers-Danlos syndrome. *J Can Dent Assoc.* 2001;67(6):330–334.
27. Moore MM, Votava JM, Orlow SJ, et al. Ehlers-Danlos syndrome type VIII: periodontitis, easy bruising, marfanoid habitus, and distinctive facies. *J Am Acad Dermatol.* 2006;55(2 suppl):S41–S45.
28. McKee MD, Hoac B, Addison WN, et al. Extracellular matrix mineralization in periodontal tissues: noncollagenous matrix proteins, enzymes, and relationship to hypophosphatasia and X-linked hypophosphatemia. *Periodontol 2000.* 2013;63(1):102–122.
29. Watanabe H, Umeda M, Seki T, et al. Clinical and laboratory studies of severe periodontal disease in an adolescent associated with hypophosphatasia. A case report. *J Periodontol.* 1993;64(3):174–180.
30. Olsson A, Matsson L, Blomquist HK, et al. Hypophosphatasia affecting the permanent dentition. *J Oral Pathol Med.* 1996;25(6):343–347.
31. Loesche WJ, Syed SA, Laughon BE, et al. The bacteriology of acute necrotizing ulcerative gingivitis. *J Periodontol.* 1982;53(4):223–230.
32. Proctor DB, Baker CG. Treatment of acute necrotizing ulcerative gingivitis with metronidazole. *J Can Dent Assoc (Tor).* 1971;37(10):376–380.
33. Shields WD. Acute necrotizing ulcerative gingivitis. A study of some of the contributing factors and their validity in an Army population. *J Periodontol.* 1977;48(6):346–349.
34. Stevens AW Jr., Cogen RB, Cohen-Cole S, et al. Demographic and clinical data associated with acute necrotizing ulcerative gingivitis in a dental school population (ANUG-demographic and clinical data). *J Clin Periodontol.* 1984;11(8):487–493.
35. da Silva AM, Newman HN, Oakley DA. Psychosocial factors in inflammatory periodontal diseases. A review. *J Clin Periodontol.* 1995;22(7):516–526.

36. Hildebrand HC, Epstein J, Larjava H. The influence of psychological stress on periodontal disease. *J West Soc Periodontol Periodontal Abstr.* 2000;48(3):69–77.
37. Gaggl AJ, Rainer H, Grund E, et al. Local oxygen therapy for treating acute necrotizing periodontal disease in smokers. *J Periodontol.* 2006;77(1):31–38.
38. Horning GM, Cohen ME. Necrotizing ulcerative gingivitis, periodontitis, and stomatitis: clinical staging and predisposing factors. *J Periodontol.* 1995;66(11):990–998.

 STUDENT ANCILLARY RESOURCES

A wide variety of resources to enhance your learning and understanding of this chapter are available on thePoint®.

- Visit thePoint to access:
  - Audio Glossary
  - Animations
  - Suggested Readings
  - Answers to Review Questions
  - Case Studies

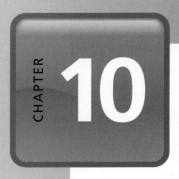

10 Guidelines for Periodontal Decision Making

Clinical Application. Members of the dental team are equipped with a broad array of skills that can be called upon when caring for patients with periodontal disease. The dental hygienist is superbly trained to provide many of the therapies that are required during this care, and the hygienist needs to understand how to make decisions related to this care to be an effective member of the dental team. This chapter outlines guidelines for decision making including those related to arriving at a periodontal diagnosis, sequencing periodontal treatment, obtaining consent for treatment, and the ongoing need for decision making.

Learning Objectives

- List the three fundamental diagnostic questions used when assigning a periodontal diagnosis.
- Explain how to arrive at appropriate answers to each of the fundamental diagnostic questions.
- Explain the difference between the terms signs of a disease and symptoms of a disease.
- Explain the term silent disease.
- Describe what is meant by the term clinical attachment loss.
- Describe the elements of a well-written diagnosis for periodontitis.
- List the phases of treatment.
- Describe the importance of informed consent to treatment planning.
- List guidelines for obtaining informed consent.
- Describe two formats for documenting informed consent.
- Describe the ADPIE nursing process.
- Explain how the ADPIE nursing process might apply to periodontal decision making

Key Terms

Signs of periodontal disease
Symptoms of periodontal
  disease
Silent disease
Overt signs
Hidden signs
Natural level of gingival
  attachment

Clinical attachment loss
Disease sites
Master treatment plan
Assessment and preliminary
  therapy phase
Nonsurgical periodontal
  therapy phase
Surgical therapy phase

Restorative phase
Periodontal maintenance
  phase
Informed consent
Informed refusal
ADPIE

Section 1
Guidelines Related to Arriving at a Periodontal Diagnosis

The first step in planning periodontal treatment is assigning a correct periodontal diagnosis (or correct diagnoses). Determination of a periodontal diagnosis can be simplified by asking and answering three fundamental clinical questions in a systematic manner (Fig. 10-1).

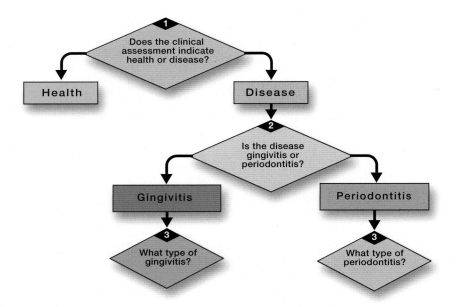

Figure 10-1. Decision Tree. A decision tree illustrating the three fundamental questions for determining an initial periodontal diagnosis.

These three fundamental questions can be used to guide the dental team through the diagnostic process. Many decisions, including assigning a periodontal diagnosis and planning nonsurgical therapy, revolve around the answers to these fundamental questions.

1. **Answering Fundamental Diagnostic Questions when Assigning a Periodontal Diagnosis**
    A. **The First Fundamental Diagnostic Question is:** *"Does the clinical assessment indicate health or inflammatory disease in the periodontium?"*
        1. The answer to the first question should be based on the signs of inflammation that are noted and recorded during the clinical assessment, and by its very nature is not usually difficult for members of the dental team to answer.
            a. Signs of Periodontal Disease. The dental team should be familiar with the difference between the *signs* of a disease and the *symptoms* of a disease. **Signs of periodontal disease** are the features of a disease that can be observed or are measurable by clinicians.
                1. Examples of periodontal disease signs might include gingival erythema (redness), gingival edema (swelling), bleeding on gentle probing, loss of attachment, tooth mobility, or loss of alveolar bone support.
                2. Some of these signs are easy to detect by the clinician (i.e., gingival erythema or gingival redness); some of these signs require careful assessment by the dental team (i.e., loss of attachment).
            b. Symptoms of Periodontal Disease. **Symptoms of periodontal disease** are features of a disease that are noticed by the patient.

1. Examples of symptoms of moderate to severe periodontitis might include difficulty chewing, itching gums, blood on the bed pillow, or a bad taste in the mouth.
2. It should be noted that in many patients, periodontitis does not cause much in the way of obvious symptoms to the patients, and some clinicians refer to periodontitis as a **silent disease** because of this lack of or "silence" of symptoms that are obvious to the patient.
3. Calling periodontitis a silent disease underscores the frequent clinical observation that periodontitis can exist in patients who are totally unaware of its presence.

c. It is critical for members of the dental team to realize that signs of inflammation in the periodontium include both **overt signs** of inflammation (i.e., those signs that are readily visible) and **hidden signs** of inflammation (i.e., those signs that not readily visible) (Table 10-1).
1. Examples of overt signs of inflammation are changes in the color, contour, and consistency of the gingival tissue.
2. Examples of hidden signs of inflammation are alveolar bone loss, bleeding on probing, and sometimes purulence or exudate.

2. Health as an answer to the first diagnostic question
a. If the clinical periodontal assessment reveals no signs of inflammation in the periodontium, then the answer to Question #1 is health (i.e., an inflammation-free periodontium).
b. This means that inflammatory disease is not present and, though other problems in the periodontium *may well be present*, the patient certainly does not have either gingivitis or periodontitis.

3. Inflammatory disease as an answer to the first diagnostic question
a. If the clinical periodontal assessment reveals either overt or hidden signs of inflammation in the periodontium, then the answer to Question #1 is, of course, inflammatory disease.
b. This means that some type of inflammatory disease is present (i.e., some type of gingivitis or periodontitis) and that further diagnostic decisions related to this inflammatory disease will need to be made by the team.

4. Additional Diagnostic Measures
a. Note that even in the absence of any inflammatory disease in the periodontium, some patients will require additional diagnostic measures.
b. For example, a patient with no inflammation in the periodontium at all but with severe gingival recession accompanied by cervical abrasion of the teeth may need to be evaluated for possible use of traumatic toothbrushing techniques.

TABLE 10-1. SIGNS OF INFLAMMATION IN THE PERIODONTIUM

Overt (Readily Visible) Signs	Hidden Signs
• Color changes in the gingiva	• Bone loss
• Contour changes in the gingiva	• Purulence (exudate)
• Changes in consistency in the gingiva	• Bleeding on probing

B. The Second Fundamental Diagnostic Question is: *"If the clinical assessment indicates inflammatory disease, is the disease gingivitis or is it periodontitis?"*

   1. Using Attachment Loss to Answer Fundamental Diagnostic Question 2
      a. The answer to this second fundamental question is based on clinical evidence of attachment loss as determined from the findings recorded during the clinical assessment.
         1. The **natural level of gingival attachment** to the tooth is slightly coronal to (or in a sense above) the level of the cementoenamel junction (CEJ).
         2. **Clinical attachment loss** or attachment loss refers to migration of the junctional epithelium to a position apical to (or in a sense below) the level of the CEJ (Fig. 10-2).
      b. Gingivitis. If the clinical assessment reveals no attachment loss in the presence of inflammation, then the answer to Question #2 is gingivitis.
      c. Periodontitis. If the clinical assessment revealed attachment loss in the presence of inflammation, then the answer to Question #2 is periodontitis.
   2. It is important for the dental team to use dental radiographs as well as the clinical findings during the clinical assessment process.
      a. In most patients with moderate to severe periodontitis, alveolar bone loss will be evident on the radiographs.
      b. However, even before radiographic changes occur, attachment loss will normally be detectable by alert clinicians.
      c. The members of the dental team must make every effort to detect periodontitis before there is obvious radiographic evidence of alveolar bone loss.

C. The Third Fundamental Diagnostic Question is: *"If the patient has gingivitis, what type of gingivitis?"* or *"If the patient has periodontitis, what type of periodontitis?"*

   1. The classification of various types of gingival disease and the various types of periodontitis will be discussed in many other chapters in this textbook (Chapters 5, 6, 7, 8, and 9).
   2. The dentist will use these disease classifications to assign a specific periodontal diagnosis based on the clinical features outlined in those chapters.

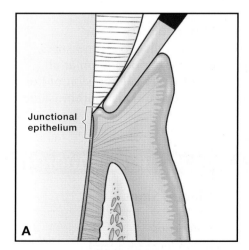
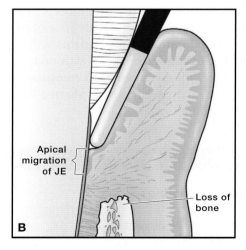

Figure 10-2. Level of Attachment. A: Natural level of attachment. The natural level of the junctional epithelium is at *the same level as* the cementoenamel junction (CEJ). Note that the probe tip does not reach the CEJ if the attachment is at its natural level. **B:** Attachment loss. In attachment loss, the junctional epithelium is *apical* to the level of the CEJ. Note that the probe tip extends beyond the CEJ if the attachment apparatus has migrated apically.

2. **Recognizing the Need for Flexibility When Assigning a Periodontal Diagnosis.**
   A. **Flexibility.** The members of the dental team must be aware of the need for some flexibility when assigning a periodontal diagnosis since more than one periodontal condition may be found in a patient.
      1. *Flexibility* in this case refers to a realization that the important fundamental decision as to the presence of either gingivitis or periodontitis in a patient may not describe the total periodontal condition of that patient.
      2. Other periodontal conditions may indeed be present, and this finding must be noted when documenting a periodontal diagnosis in addition to any fundamental decision about the presence of gingivitis or periodontitis.
   B. **Other Findings.** Examples of some of these other periodontal conditions might be recession of the gingival margin, occlusal trauma, or aberrant frenum position. (Many of these other conditions will be discussed in Chapter 9.)
3. **Thorough Documentation of the Periodontal Diagnosis.** Documenting the periodontal diagnosis is a critical skill for the dental team, and adhering to a standard format for such documentation is helpful. The following are some guidelines for documenting periodontal diagnoses.
   A. **Diagnostic Term.** As part of the diagnosis, include the correct diagnostic term as outlined in the classification scheme, such as chronic periodontitis or aggressive periodontitis (as discussed in Chapters 7 and 8).
   B. **Disease Severity.** When assigning a diagnosis, add descriptive modifiers such as slight (mild), moderate, or severe to describe the *severity* of the disease.
      1. Table 10-2 shows how the terms slight, moderate, and severe should be used as part of documentation of a periodontitis diagnosis.
      2. Note that the term *clinical attachment loss* (CAL) is used to underscore that these measurements are clinical measurements and may not coincide exactly with precise histologic measurements.
   C. **Disease Extent.** When assigning a diagnosis, also include descriptive modifiers such as localized or generalized to describe the *extent* of the disease.
      1. Table 10-2 also shows how the terms localized and generalized should be used as part of documentation of the extent of periodontal disease.
      2. Note that the term **disease sites** refers to the individual teeth or specific surfaces of a tooth that are experiencing periodontal destruction.
      3. Examples of appropriate periodontal diagnoses might be *generalized moderate chronic periodontitis* or *localized severe aggressive periodontitis*. Table 10-3 provides some examples of well-written periodontal diagnoses.
4. **Using the Case Type System for Periodontal Patients**
   A. **Case Types**
      1. Although the case type system is somewhat limited in value, it has been standard practice in the United States to assign a periodontal case type to all periodontal patients. These case types are sometimes used in insurance reporting and in communication with third-party payers.
      2. Assigning a periodontal case type is included in the initial decision-making process in most dental offices and is included here as additional information related to assigning a periodontal diagnosis.
         a. Case Type I.   Patients with gingivitis only
         b. Case Type II. Patients with slight (mild) periodontitis
         c. Case Type III. Patients with moderate periodontitis
         d. Case Type IV. Patients with severe periodontitis

B. **Limited Value of Case System.** The value of the case type system is very limited because the case type alone does not specify the precise periodontal disease classification.

1. For example, a Case Type III patient could be a patient with either chronic periodontitis or a patient with aggressive periodontitis since the Case Type system does not specify the precise type of periodontitis.

2. Note that a designation of Case Type III only signifies that the disease is of moderate severity.

3. It is important for all members of the dental team to use the written periodontal diagnosis (e.g., generalized moderate chronic periodontitis) when describing the periodontal status of a patient and to use the case type only as a supplemental description if called for.

TABLE 10-2. USE OF MODIFIERS IN DOCUMENTING DISEASE SEVERITY AND EXTENT

	Descriptive Modifier	**Definition**
Disease Severity	Slight	1–2 mm clinical attachment loss
	Moderate	3–4 mm clinical attachment loss
	Severe	5 mm or more of clinical attachment loss
Disease Extent	Localized	30% or less of the sites in the mouth are involved
	Generalized	More than 30% of the sites in the mouth are involved

TABLE 10-3. EXAMPLES OF A WELL-WRITTEN PERIODONTAL DIAGNOSIS

Extent	**Severity**	**Name of Disease**
Localized	Slight	Chronic periodontitis
Localized	Moderate	Chronic periodontitis
Generalized	Moderate	Chronic periodontitis
Generalized	Severe	Chronic periodontitis
Localized	Moderate	Aggressive periodontitis

Section 2
Guidelines Related to Periodontal Treatment Sequencing

1. **The Periodontal Master Treatment Plan.** The **master treatment plan** is a sequential outline of the measures to be carried out by the dentist, the dental hygienist, or the patient to eliminate disease and restore a healthy periodontal environment.
   - The master treatment plan can be used to coordinate and to sequence all treatment and educational measures employed.
   - Although some of the treatment included in the master treatment plan may not involve the dental hygienist directly, it is important that the hygienist understand how all phases of treatment contribute to the goal of restoring a healthy periodontal environment.

2. **Understanding the Phases of Periodontal Treatment.** The master treatment plan can be sequenced into phases. An overview of the sequence of phases of treatment is presented in Figure 10-3 as well as in the discussion below. Refer to Table 10-4 for examples of components of each of the phases in the management of periodontal patients. It should be noted that much overlap in these phases is required in the management of some patients, but understanding these basic phases can help the members of the dental team understand the entire scope of therapy needed for many patients.

   A. **Assessment and Preliminary Therapy Phase**
      1. The **assessment and preliminary therapy phase** includes (1) assessment data collection and (2) needed care for any immediate treatment needs such as emergency dental care. Details of the clinical periodontal assessment are discussed in Chapters 19 and 20, and periodontal emergencies are discussed in Chapter 28.
      2. This phase of care also has been referred to as emergency therapy by some authors.

   B. **Nonsurgical Periodontal Therapy Phase**
      1. The **nonsurgical periodontal therapy phase** of treatment includes all the *nonsurgical* measures used to control gingivitis and periodontitis.
         a. This phase includes intensive dental hygiene care and comprehensive patient educational measures.
         b. This phase can also include measures to minimize the impact of local contributing factors.
      2. The nonsurgical periodontal therapy phase has also been called *initial periodontal therapy, Phase I therapy, bacterial control,* and *anti-infective therapy.*

   C. **Surgical Therapy Phase**
      1. The **surgical therapy phase** of treatment includes any needed periodontal surgery and placement of dental implants.
      2. The surgical therapy phase of care has also been called *Phase II* therapy. Periodontal surgical procedures are discussed in Chapter 27 of this book.
      3. Note that this phase of treatment is not needed for all patients.

   D. **Restorative Therapy Phase**
      1. The **restorative therapy phase** of treatment may include placement of dental restorations and replacement of missing teeth by fixed or removable prostheses.
      2. The restorative therapy phase of care has also been called *Phase III* therapy.

   E. **Periodontal Maintenance Phase**
      1. The **periodontal maintenance phase** of treatment includes all measures used by the dental team and by the patient to keep periodontitis from recurring once the inflammatory disease is brought under control.

2. The objective of the periodontal maintenance phase is to maintain the teeth functioning throughout the life of the patient and may actually be needed for the rest of the patient's life.
3. The periodontal maintenance phase of care has also been called *Phase IV* therapy. Periodontal maintenance is discussed in detail in Chapters 30 and 31.

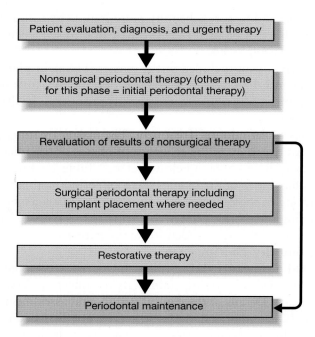

Figure 10-3. Sequencing of Treatment Phases. This flow chart provides an overview of the sequence of the normal phases of treatment for a patient.

TABLE 10-4. EXAMPLES OF COMPONENTS OF THE PHASES IN THE MANAGEMENT OF PATIENTS WITH PERIODONTITIS

Phase	Measures and Procedures
Assessment Phase and Preliminary Therapy	Health history
	Comprehensive oral examination
	Assessment data collection
	Radiographs as indicated
	Diagnosis of oral conditions
	Treatment of urgent conditions
	Planning of nonsurgical therapy
	Referral for care of medical conditions
	Extraction of hopeless teeth
Nonsurgical Periodontal Therapy	Self-care education
	Nutritional counseling
	Smoking cessation counseling
	Periodontal debridement (instrumentation)
	Antimicrobial therapy
	Correction of local risk factors
	Fluoride therapy
	Caries control and temporary restorations
	Occlusal therapy
	Minor orthodontic treatment
	Reevaluation of Phase I therapy
Surgical Therapy	Periodontal surgery
	Endodontic surgery
	Dental implant placement
Restorative Therapy	Dental restorations, Fixed and removable prostheses
	Reevaluation of overall response to treatment
Periodontal Maintenance	Ongoing care at specified intervals

Section 3
Guidelines Related to Consent for Periodontal Treatment

Periodontal treatment is always based upon the best available scientific evidence, but many times there will be more than a single course of treatment that could benefit an individual patient. An appropriate plan for any individual patient must include input from that patient and requires some detailed discussions with the patient. During dental hygiene treatment, it is frequently the role of the dental hygienist to provide patients with the information necessary to make informed decisions about their oral health. One important decision in patient care is how to manage these discussions with a patient prior to treatment.

According to the American Dental Hygienists' Association (ADHA) code of Ethics, a patient has the right to informed consent prior to treatment, and they have the right to full disclosure of all relevant information, so that they can make informed choices about their care (1). *This makes the patient a critical participant in any plan involving periodontal therapy, and communications with the patient are vital as the treatment plan is developed.*

Studies demonstrate that patients who believe that they have been well informed regarding their condition and who have had their questions answered by members of the dental team are more compliant with treatment recommendations, have a higher trust in their healthcare providers, and are more satisfied with their care. These factors lead to better treatment outcomes and reduced malpractice risk.

1. **Informed Consent for Periodontal Treatment. Informed consent** is a patient's voluntary agreement to proposed treatment. A patient can only give informed consent to treatment after achieving an understanding of the relevant facts, benefits, and risks involved (2). Informed consent requires that recommended treatment, alternate treatment options, and the likely consequences of declining treatment have been explained in language understood by the patient.
   A. **What Constitutes Informed Consent?**
      1. An individual's consent is informed only if the recommended treatment, alternate treatment options, and the benefits and risks of treatment have been thoroughly described to the person in language understood by the patient (3).
      2. Informed consent must be voluntary, and this informed consent originates from (a) a person's legal right to direct what happens to his or her body and (b) the ethical duty of the dental healthcare provider to involve the individual in his or her own dental care.
      3. Informed consent is more than simply getting a patient to agree to a procedure or to sign a written consent form. It is *a process of communication between a patient and healthcare provider* that allows the patient to make a knowledgeable decision about his or her own dental care.
   B. **What are the Goals of Informed Consent?** The most important goal of informed consent is to provide an individual an opportunity to be an informed participant in healthcare decisions, and it is generally accepted that complete informed consent includes a discussion of the following elements:
      1. The diagnosis and an explanation of the periodontal condition that warrants the proposed treatment.
      2. An explanation of the purpose of the proposed periodontal treatment.
      3. A description of the proposed treatment and the individual patient's role and responsibilities during and after periodontal treatment.
      4. A discussion of the known risks and benefits of the proposed periodontal treatment.

5. An assessment of the likelihood that the proposed treatment will accomplish the desired objectives.
   a. Note that when discussing treatment outcomes it is important not to appear to guarantee treatment outcomes to the patient.
   b. Dental healthcare providers should remember that individual patients may well respond differently to similar treatments.
6. A presentation of alternative treatment options, if any, and the known risks and benefits of these options.
7. The risks and benefits of not receiving the proposed periodontal treatment.
8. A discussion of the prognosis (or outcomes expected) if no treatment is provided.
9. A discussion of the actual costs associated with the proposed treatment.
10. Reinforcement of the individual's right to refuse consent to the proposed treatment.
    a. Keep in mind that patients often feel powerless when dealing with healthcare providers.
    b. To encourage the patient's voluntary consent, the dental healthcare provider should make it clear to the patient that she or he is participating in a decision, not merely signing a consent form.

2. **Informed Refusal for Periodontal Treatment.** Informed refusal is a person's right to refuse all or a portion of the proposed treatment. Informed refusal requires that recommended treatment, alternate treatment options, and the likely consequences of declining treatment have been explained in language understood by the patient. A patient always has a legal right to refuse proposed periodontal care.

3. **Obtaining Informed Consent from Patients.** The doctrine of informed consent reminds dental healthcare providers to respect patients by fully and accurately providing information relevant to their healthcare decisions. The following are some guidelines to use when obtaining informed consent from a patient.
   A. **Use Understandable Language.** Information should be provided in language that is easily understood by the patient.
      1. Use simple, straightforward sentences.
      2. Use commonly recognizable terms.
      3. Avoid the use of professional jargon or technical terms, and explain any terms that may not be readily understood.
      4. Use a translator if the patient does not speak English or speaks English with little understanding.
   B. **Provide Opportunities for Patient Questions.** An opportunity should be provided for the patient to ask questions. Foster an open exchange of information and encourage the patient to ask questions. Using open-ended and nondirective questions such as those below can simplify this process.
      1. *"What more would you like to know?"*
      2. *"What are your concerns?"*
      3. *"What is your next question?"*
   C. **Assess Patient Understanding.** An assessment should be made of the patient's understanding of information provided.
      1. A simple strategy to assess understanding is to let patient know that *"many people have difficulty understanding the information that I give them or have questions that they need answered. So, please let's discuss anything you do not understand."*
      2. Another strategy is to make a comment such as: *"Most of my patients want to explain my treatment suggestions to another family member. What additional information can I give you to help you explain this treatment to your spouse?"*

4. **Legal Responsibilities Related to the Consent Process**
   A. **The Dental Hygienist's Legal Responsibility Related to Consent**
      1. The dental hygienist has a legal responsibility for the services that he or she provides. Failure to obtain consent from the patient for services can have serious legal consequences.
      2. A patient could claim "battery" (i.e., unconsented touching) for dental services provided without the patient's consent.
      3. Patients also can claim "negligence" (i.e., lack of reasonable and prudent care resulting in harm) for failure to provide sufficient information for the patient to make an informed decision. This type of negligence also is called malpractice.
   B. **Basic Legal Requirement to Demonstrate Informed Consent.** Basic requirements for demonstrating that informed consent has been obtained are listed below. If any element were missing, it would indicate that informed consent is not complete.
      - Patient's periodontal diagnosis presented in language that is easily understood by the patient
      - Discussion of proposed periodontal treatment and benefits diagnosis presented in language that is easily understood by the patient
      - Discussion of the risks and likelihood of success of the proposed periodontal therapy
      - Discussion of alternative treatments
      - Documentation that the patient was encouraged to ask questions and that answers were provided in language that is easily understood by the patient
      - Patient's signature on the consent form
   C. **Legal Requirements Necessary for a Patient to Give Informed Consent.** There are certain legal requirements necessary for a patient to give informed consent. These legal requirements are listed below.
      - The patient is fully informed (as discussed in point "B" above).
      - The patient is of legal age. Legal age is determined by state law—not federal law—and so may vary from state to state. Dental healthcare providers should know the legal age for the state in which they practice.
      - The patient is mentally competent (understands information presented and is able to make a decision about the proposed treatment).
      - The patient is able to give voluntary consent (without coercion from care providers, family members, or others).
5. **Format for the Consent Process.** The format for the consent process may be either verbal or written. Some states have statutes or regulations requiring dentists to secure written informed consent from patients (1). Dentists should ensure that they are familiar with and in compliance with the informed consent laws in their states.
   A. **Written Consent.** Most dental healthcare providers prefer to have the patient sign and date a written consent form for documentation of the consent process. Figure 10-4 shows an example of a written informed consent/informed refusal form.
      1. In addition, the written consent document should be signed and dated by the dentist and a witness (generally, another staff member).
      2. Once signed, a written consent document becomes part of the individual's permanent dental record.
   B. **Verbal Consent.** If a written consent document is not used, the patient's verbal consent should be documented in the patient chart. An example of documentation of verbal consent would be a written entry in the patient's chart that says, "*Discussed the diagnosis; purpose, description, benefits, and risks of the proposed treatment; alternative treatment options; the prognosis of no treatment; and costs.*

The patient asked questions and demonstrated that he understood all information presented during the discussion. Informed consent was obtained for the attached treatment plan."

Sample Informed Consent/Informed Refusal Form

1. I _____ , (name) agree to the proposed periodontal treatment by _____ , (name) RDH.

2. I fully understand the importance of the proposed treatment. ___Yes ___No

3. I understand that _____ is the expected outcome of the proposed periodontal treatment.

4. I understand that the possible risks and/or unanticipated outcomes of the proposed periodontal treatment are _____.

5. The possible treatment alternatives to the proposed treatment are _____.

6. I have been informed of the costs of the proposed and alternative treatments. ___Yes ___No

7. I understand the possible consequence(s) of refusal of the proposed periodontal treatment is/are_____.

8. I have the capacity to consent to the proposed treatment. ___Yes ___No

9. I refuse the proposed treatment. ___Yes ___No

10. I am refusing the proposed periodontal treatment for the following reason(s):

_____ _____ _____
Patient Signature   Date   RDH Signature

_____
Witness Signature

Figure 10-4. Sample Informed Consent/Informed Refusal Form for Periodontal Therapy.

Section 4
Guidelines Related to the Need for Ongoing Decision Making

1. The Ongoing Nature of the Decision-Making Process
   A. Since most patients are monitored for many years or even decades by the members of the dental team, clinical decision making and treatment planning is best described as an ongoing, evolving process over time.
   B. In addition, the periodontium consists of dynamic and continuously changing tissues (even in the absence of disease), and an individual's plan for periodontal care frequently requires adjustment over time because of these changes.
   C. The dental team must be aware that a perfectly sensible periodontal diagnosis and plan for therapy at one point in time may require modification at a later date, and this fact must be communicated to the patient.
2. Applying Principles from the ADPIE Nursing Process to Periodontal Decisions
   A. Some nurses are trained to use a nursing process referred to as **ADPIE**. ADPIE is an acronym for Assess, Diagnose, Plan, Implement, and Evaluate.
   B. In many ways, the ADPIE nursing process can be a helpful tool for members of the dental team to adopt. The process parallels most of the periodontal decision-making principles and underscores the need for constant reevaluation of the results of any therapy provided.
   C. Table 10-5 outlines the steps in the ADPIE process and shows an example of each step related as it might be related to the management of patients with periodontal disease.
   D. It can be helpful for members of the dental team to understand the principles of the ADPIE nursing process when dealing with patients with periodontal disease since this process seems to be ideally suited to the kinds of decisions the team must make when dealing with most patients with periodontal conditions.

TABLE 10-5. THE ADPIE NURSING PROCESS

Acronym	Meaning	Example of Parallel in Dentistry
A	Assess	Performing a comprehensive periodontal evaluation
D	Diagnose	Arriving at periodontal diagnosis or diagnoses
P	Plan	Establishing a master plan for periodontal therapy
I	Implement	Performing the periodontal therapy by the members of the team
E	Evaluate	Reevaluating the response to any periodontal therapy provided

Table 10-1. **ADPIE Nursing Process.** Table 10-5 provides an example of how the ADPIE process might be applied to the management of patients with periodontal disease.

Chapter Summary Statement

This chapter outlines guidelines that can be helpful to the members of the dental team during the management of patients with periodontal diseases. These guidelines include those related to arriving at a periodontal diagnosis, periodontal treatment sequencing, consent for treatment, and the need for ongoing decision making.

Section 5
Focus on Patients

Clinical Patient Care

CASE 1

Periodontal assessment of a new patient reveals generalized bleeding on probing but very little gingival erythema (redness) and very little gingival edema (swelling). How would you answer the first fundamental diagnostic question for this patient?

CASE 2

Periodontal assessment of a new patient reveals definite signs of inflammation in the periodontium. Explain how to answer the second diagnostic question for this patient.

CASE 3

Periodontal assessment of a new patient reveals localized signs of gingival inflammation but no attachment loss. The findings also include a site of gingival recession and toothbrush abrasion on the facial surface of a canine tooth. At this site of recession, there is no sign of inflammation of the gingiva. How should this site of gingival recession due to traumatic brushing affect the basic diagnostic questions?

CASE 4

Following thorough clinical assessment of the periodontal condition of a patient, you are convinced that the patient has periodontitis. Explain how you would determine the severity of the periodontitis?

Ethical Scenario

Mrs. E is the first patient of the afternoon in your periodontal office. She is new to the practice. She is a 50-year-old lady who has only lived in the United States for the last 3 years. Her English skills are minimal, but she works as a medical researcher, so you assume that she understands medical terminology.

Mrs. E has generalized moderate chronic periodontitis with generalized horizontal bone loss on her posterior teeth. You determine that periodontal instrumentation using local anesthesia is indicated. The next phase of treatment will be based on the findings at the time of the reevaluation, and will be determined by Dr. Evans, one of the periodontists in the office.

You review your dental hygiene treatment plan with her. She asks no questions and signs at the bottom of the consent for treatment form, on the signature line. You tell her that you will begin the recommended treatment at today's appointment. You prepare the anesthesia syringe and as you approach Mrs. E, she becomes very agitated, screaming and covering her mouth with her hands. She refuses to allow any further treatment today. She gets up abruptly, and leaves the office.

1. What could the hygienist have done differently, to avoid the above situation?
2. What ethical principles are in conflict in this dilemma?
3. Now, that Mrs. E's experience has been a negative one for her; what is the best way to handle this ethical dilemma?
4. What changes might the hygienist make when explaining proposed treatment to future patients?

References

1. *Bylaws and Code of Ethics*. Chicago, IL: American Dental Hygienists' Association; 2009.
2. McCombs G. Protect yourself with informed consent. *Dimensions Dent Hyg*. 2010;8(11):60–63.
3. Sfikas PM. A duty to disclose. Issues to consider in securing informed consent. *J Am Dent Assoc*. 2003;134(10): 1329–1333.

Suggested Readings

SC: Suit for malpractice & lack of consent: directed verdict-malpractice: trial on consent. Fletcher v. Medical University of South Carolina, 4732 SCCA (9/1/2010)-SC. *Nurs Law Regan Rep*. 2011;51(8):3.

Baker JN, Leek AC, Salas HS, et al. Suggestions from adolescents, young adults, and parents for improving informed consent in phase 1 pediatric oncology trials. *Cancer*. 2013;119(23):4154–4161.

Brands WG, van der Ven JM, Brands-Bottema GW. [Dental and health law 4. The treatment of minors and of adults who are unable to give informed consent]. *Ned Tijdschr Tandheelkd*. 2013;120(7–8):394–398.

Brands WG, van der Ven JM, Eijkman MA. [Dentistry and healthcare legislation 3: informed consent]. *Ned Tijdschr Tandheelkd*. 2013;120(6):327–332.

Coulter A. International standards on informed patient consent are available. *BMJ*. 2013;347:f5454.

Eyal N. Informed consent, the value of trust, and hedons. *J Med Ethics*. 2014;40(7):447.

Fullbrook S, Sanders K. Consent and capacity 2: the Mental Capacity Act 2005 and 'living wills'. *Br J Nurs*. 2007;16(8): 474–475.

Glick M. Informed consent: a delicate balance. *J Am Dent Assoc*. 2006;137(8):1060.

Govan P. Dental ethics case 5. Child consent and the Children's Act (2005) as amended. *SADJ*. 2010;65(8):382.

Greco PM. Informed consent or informed refusal? *Am J Orthod Dentofacial Orthop*. 2013;143(5):598.

Hodgson J, Mendenhall T, Lamson A. Patient and provider relationships: consent, confidentiality, and managing mistakes in integrated primary care settings. *Fam Syst Health*. 2013;31(1):28–40.

Hudgins C, Rose S, Fifield PY, et al. Navigating the legal and ethical foundations of informed consent and confidentiality in integrated primary care. *Fam Syst Health*. 2013;31(1):9–19.

Ingravallo F, Gilmore E, Vignatelli L, et al. Factors associated with nurses' opinions and practices regarding information and consent. *Nurs Ethics*. 2014;21(3):299–313.

Jenkins VA, Anderson JL, Fallowfield LJ. Communication and informed consent in phase 1 trials: a review of the literature from January 2005 to July 2009. *Support Care Cancer*. 2010;18(9):1115–1121.

Lamont S, Jeon YH, Chiarella M. Assessing patient capacity to consent to treatment: an integrative review of instruments and tools. *J Clin Nurs*. 2013;22(17–18):2387–2403.

Lamont S, Jeon YH, Chiarella M. Health-care professionals' knowledge, attitudes and behaviours relating to patient capacity to consent to treatment: an integrative review. *Nurs Ethics*. 2013;20(6):684–707.

McQuoid Mason D. Provisions for consent by children to medical treatment and surgical operations, and duties to report child and aged persons abuse: 1 April 2010. *S Afr Med J*. 2010;100(10):646–648.

Nijhawan LP, Janodia MD, Muddukrishna BS, et al. Informed consent: issues and challenges. *J Adv Pharm Technol Res*. 2013;4(3):134–140.

Paasche-Orlow MK, Brancati FL, Taylor HA, et al. Readability of consent form templates: a second look. *IRB*. 2013;35(4):12–19.

Rait JL. Informed consent in 2012. *Clin Experiment Ophthalmol*. 2012;40(9):835–837.

Richardson V. Patient comprehension of informed consent. *J Perioper Pract*. 2013;23(1–2):26–30.

Robertson CG, Verco CJ. The quality of consent - what is the evidence? *Aust N Z J Obstet Gynaecol*. 2013;53(5):502–504.

Sand K, Eik-Nes NL, Loge JH. Readability of informed consent documents (1987–2007) for clinical trials: a linguistic analysis. *J Empir Res Hum Res Ethics*. 2012;7(4):67–78.

Stoopler ET. The importance of informed consent. *J Can Dent Assoc.* 2013;79:d81.

Taylor JS. Introduction: children and consent to treatment. *HEC Forum.* 2013;25(4):285–287.

Toumba KJ. Children and consent/assent to treatment. *Eur Arch Paediatr Dent.* 2013;14(4):195–196.

 STUDENT ANCILLARY RESOURCES

A wide variety of resources to enhance your learning and understanding of this chapter are available on thePoint°.

- Visit thePoint to access:
  - Audio Glossary
  - Animations
  - Suggested Readings
  - Answers to Review Questions
  - Case Studies

CHAPTER

Etiologic Factors: Risk for Periodontitis

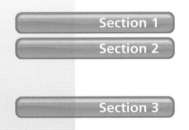

Clinical Application.
It is always a challenge to explain why periodontal disease affects some patients while others seem so resistant to its development. This chapter organizes information about the risk factors for periodontal disease, information about the biologic equilibrium involved with this disease, and the possible alterations to this equilibrium that can help clarify this perplexing issue. This information is useful when developing recommendations for a course of treatment for patients with periodontal diseases, as well as, when explaining the nature of these diseases to patients and other healthcare providers.

Learning Objectives

- Define the term biologic equilibrium and discuss factors that can disrupt the balance between health and disease in the periodontium.
- Define and give examples of the term "contributing risk factors."
- Discuss the importance of a periodontal risk assessment in periodontal treatment planning.
- For a patient in your care with periodontitis, explain to your clinical instructor the factors that may have contributed to your patient's disease progression.

Key Terms

Multifactorial etiology
Biologic equilibrium

Homeostasis
Risk Assessment

Section 1
Risk Factors for Periodontal Disease

Research studies have clearly demonstrated that periodontal disease is a bacterial infection of the periodontium and that bacteria are the primary etiologic agents in the initiation of periodontal disease (1–4). The presence of pathogenic bacteria, however, does not necessarily mean that an individual will experience periodontitis.

Periodontitis has a **multifactorial etiology**, that is, periodontitis is a disease that results from the interaction of many factors (Fig. 11-1). Some persons with abundant biofilm exhibit only mild disease while others with sparse amounts of biofilm suffer severe disease. Untreated gingivitis does not always lead to periodontitis and everyone infected with periodontal pathogens does not experience periodontitis.

These findings suggest that additional factors, other than the mere presence of bacteria, must play a significant role in determining why some individuals are more susceptible to periodontal disease than others (1,2,4–15). Many contributing factors help to determine the initiation and progression of periodontal disease. Table 11-1 lists some risk factors that may be involved in the etiology of periodontitis. Contributing etiologic factors negatively influence the periodontium as well as the host immune response. It is critical for the dental team to recognize contributing factors for periodontal disease during a periodontal assessment. Whenever possible, the dental team should eliminate or minimize the impact of contributing factors during the nonsurgical periodontal treatment (Table 11-2).

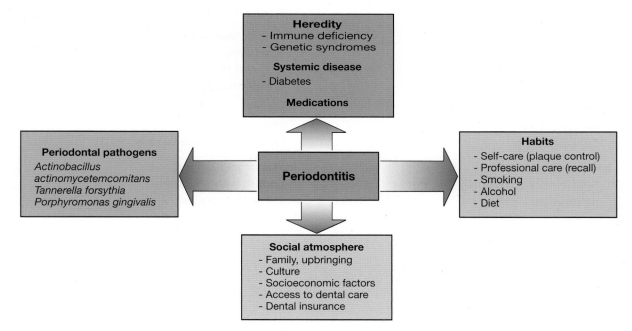

Figure 11-1. Risk Factors for Periodontal Disease. Periodontitis has a multifactorial etiology. Additional factors—other than the presence of bacteria—play a significant role in determining why some individuals are more susceptible to periodontal disease than others.

TABLE 11-1. RISK FACTORS FOR PERIODONTAL DISEASE

Poor Self-Care
  Plaque biofilm
  Calculus deposits

Faulty Dentistry
  Overhangs
  Subgingival margins

Smoking/Tobacco
  Frequency
  Current history
  Past history

Nutrition
  Diet high in fast foods, junk foods

Medications
  Dilantin
  Calcium channel blockers
  Cyclosporin
  Drugs known to cause xerostomia

Diabetes
  Duration
  Poor glycemic control

Hormonal Variations
  Puberty
  Pregnancy
  Menopause

Heredity
  Family history
  Genetic testing

Immunocompromised
  Neutropenia (abnormally low levels of
  neutrophils)

TABLE 11-2. MANAGEMENT OF RISK FACTORS

Poor Self-Care
  Improved biofilm control
  Frequent professional care

Faulty Dentistry
  Corrective dentistry

Smoking/Tobacco
  Cessation counseling
  Chemotherapeutics

Nutrition
  Diet high in fruits/vegetables

Medications
  Change medications
  Work with physician
  Good daily self-care
  Frequent professional care

Diabetes
  Good glycemic control
  Work with physician
  Good daily self-care
  Frequent professional care

Hormonal Variations
  Good daily self-care
  Frequent professional care
  Chemotherapeutics

Heredity
  Chemotherapeutics
  Frequent professional care

Immunocompromised
  Consult with physician
  Chemotherapeutics

Section 2
Balance Between Periodontal Health and Disease

BIOLOGIC EQUILIBRIUM

1. Biologic Equilibrium. The human body is continually working to maintain a state of balance in the internal environment of the body, known as biologic equilibrium or homeostasis.
   A. Periodontal Health
      1. In the oral cavity, most of the time, things are in a state of balance between the biofilm bacteria and the host.
      2. For the periodontium to remain healthy, the bacterial challenge must be contained at a level that can be tolerated by the host (2).
      3. The situation can be thought of as a balance scale, with the disease-promoting factors on one side of the scale and the health-promoting factors on the other (Fig. 11-2). As long as the two sides of the scale are in balance, there will be no disease progression.
   B. Periodontal Disease
      1. The intermittent pattern of disease activity seen in periodontitis is believed to result from the changing balance between the pathogenic bacteria and the host's inflammatory and immune responses.
      2. This balance also can be affected by other risk factors, such as local or systemic variables.
2. The Delicate Balance Between Health and Disease. When active periodontal disease sites are present in the mouth, the goal is to return the oral cavity to a state of biologic equilibrium.

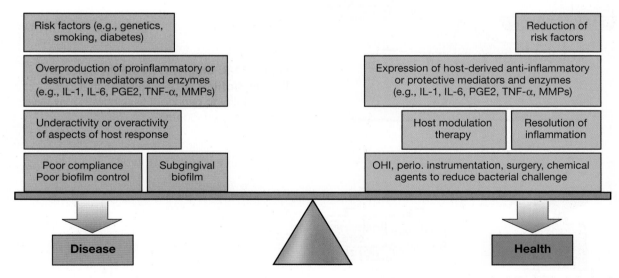

Figure 11-2. Periodontal Equilibrium. Equilibrium occurs when there is a balance between disease-promoting factors and health-promoting factors.

A. Periodontal Equilibrium and Dental Plaque Biofilm
   1. Experienced dental hygienists will attest to the fact that major differences exist in the way that individuals respond to the plaque biofilm.
      a. Many patients return to the dental office year after year with generalized plaque biofilm. These patients exhibit gingivitis and yet, year after year, show no clinical signs of progression to periodontitis. For some reason, in these individuals, gingivitis never progresses to periodontitis. Perhaps these individuals have no systemic or acquired risk factors that add stress to the biologic equilibrium. Basically, if an individual's immune system can effectively deal with a mouthful of periodontal pathogens, there will be no destructive periodontal disease (Fig. 11-3).
      b. In a few individuals, gingivitis progresses to periodontitis. It is theorized that in these individuals the body's immune response (host response) is responsible for the tissue destruction seen in periodontitis (Fig. 11-4). In addition, some individual possess systemic risk factors (such as genetic variables or systemic disease) that significantly increase their susceptibility to periodontitis (13).
   2. There are many patients who are unable or unwilling to perform the thorough self-care necessary to control plaque biofilm. For these patients, it is necessary to increase the frequency of professional care to compensate for the inadequate level of self-care. Professional care at frequent intervals can be effective in restoring the balance between health and disease (Fig. 11-5).

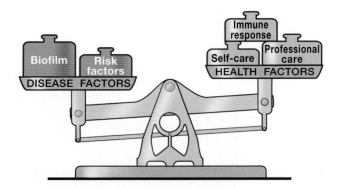

Figure 11-3. Gingivitis in the Presence of Plaque Biofilms. In individuals with a low susceptibility to periodontitis, gingivitis may never progress to periodontitis.

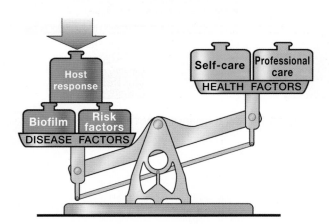

Figure 11-4. Periodontitis in the Presence of Plaque Biofilm. In susceptible individuals, the body's immune response (host response) results in damage to the periodontal tissues and progression from gingivitis to periodontitis.

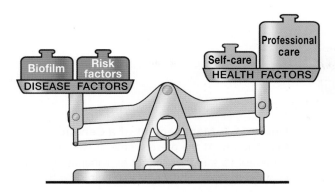

Figure 11-5. Frequent Professional Care. An individual who is unwilling or unable to obtain adequate biofilm control on a daily basis. More frequent periodontal instrumentation can help to control the development of mature plaque biofilms.

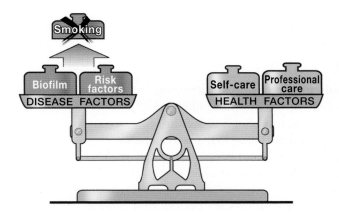

Figure 11-6. Eliminating a Systemic Risk Factor. Smoking cessation, combined with adequate self-care and professional care, restores the balance.

B. Local Contributing Factors
1. It is possible to totally eliminate a local risk factor in many cases. A faulty restoration is a good example of a local factor that can be corrected, restoring the balance between local disease-promoting and health-promoting factors at the site.
2. In other cases, it is possible to compensate for a local risk factor by improving the patient's self-care and/or increasing the frequency of professional care. For example, the patient may need to use tufted dental floss to clean around the abutment teeth of a fixed bridge. This situation can be compared to adding more weight on the health side of the balance scale to equal or exceed the weight on the disease side of the scale.
C. Systemic or Genetic Contributing Factors
1. Certain systemic or acquired risk factors are possible to control or eliminate if the patient is willing to do so (14). For example, the individual can work with a physician to keep diabetes well controlled. A smoker may decide to stop smoking. In both cases the individual has made a change that is health promoting, both systemically and for the periodontium (Fig. 11-6).
2. In the case of a contributing risk factor that cannot be controlled, it is necessary to add weight to the health side of the scale. For example, some individuals have a genetic risk factor—such as abnormal neutrophil function—that causes them to be susceptible to severe periodontitis. At the present time, we are unable to eliminate or control genetic risk factors. It is possible, however, to assist the patient in maintaining health by increasing the extent of professional care. Frequent professional care will increase the weight on the health side of the scale (Fig. 11-7).

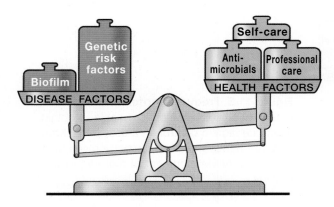

Figure 11-7. Management of a Genetic Risk Factor. At the present time, there are some risk factors that cannot be eliminated or controlled. Professional care can help slow disease progression.

PERIODONTAL RISK ASSESSMENT

Dental healthcare providers are interested not only in diagnosing and treating periodontal disease but also in predicting which individuals are more likely to develop periodontitis. The process of identifying risk factors that increase an individual's probability of disease is called **risk assessment** (8,16–19). The American Academy of Periodontology (AAP) describes the risk assessment process as "increasingly important in periodontal treatment planning and should be part of every comprehensive dental and periodontal evaluation" (16).

It is becoming possible to consider an individual's risk factors for periodontal disease (systemic disease, genetic information, personal habits, and characteristics) and to classify patients into high- or low-risk groups (19). For example, individuals who smoke have a higher risk of periodontitis than nonsmokers (12). Clinicians also use the risk assessment process to prevent disease (such as, identifying smokers and offering smoking cessation counseling).

Information concerning individual risk for developing periodontal disease is obtained through careful evaluation of the individual's demographic data, medical history, dental history, and comprehensive periodontal clinical examination (Table 11-3).

Risk assessment questionnaires are practical tools that can be helpful in identifying individuals who are at a high risk for periodontal disease (19). Figure 11-8A,B shows an example of a simple two-page periodontal risk questionnaire that can elicit the presence of common periodontal risk factors. Dental hygienists can use risk questionnaires to initiate discussion with patients about periodontal risk factors.

TABLE 11-3. CLINICAL RISK ASSESSMENT FOR PERIODONTAL DISEASE

Demographic Data	Age
	Duration of exposure to contributing risk factors
	Self-care (plaque control)
	Frequency of professional care
	Male gender
	Dental awareness
	Socioeconomic status
Medical History	Tobacco use
	Diabetes
	Osteoporosis
	HIV/AIDS
	Genetic predisposition to aggressive disease
Dental History	Frequency of professional care
	Family history of early tooth loss
	Previous history of periodontal disease
Clinical Examination	Plaque biofilm accumulation and microbial composition
	Calculus deposits
	Bleeding on probing
	Loss of attachment
	Plaque retentive areas
	Anatomic contributing factors
	Restorative contributing factors

PERIODONTAL ASSESSMENT QUESTIONNAIRE FOR _____

TOBACCO USE

Tobacco use is the most significant risk factor for gum disease.

Do you now or have you ever used the following?

	Amount per day?	How many years?	If you quit, what year?
❏ Cigarette	_____	_____	_____
❏ Cigar	_____	_____	_____
❏ Pipe	_____	_____	_____
❏ Chew	_____	_____	_____
❏ Snuff	_____	_____	_____

HEART ATTACK AND STROKE

Untreated gum disease can increase your risk for heart attack and stroke.

Do you have any other risk factors for heart disease or stroke?

❏ Family history of heart disease   ❏ Tobacco use
❏ High cholesterol   ❏ High blood pressure

If you have any of these other risk factors it is especially important for you to always keep your gums as healthy and inflammation free as possible to reduce your overall risk for heart attack and stroke.

MEDICATIONS

A side effect of some medications can cause changes in your gums.

Have you ever taken any of the following medications?

❏ Dilantin antiseizure medication

❏ Calcium channel blocker blood pressure medicine
  (such as Procardia, Cardizem, Norvasc, Verapamil, etc.)

❏ Cyclosporin immunosuppressant therapy

GENETIC

The tendency for gum disease to develop can be inherited.

Has anyone on your side of the family had gum problems (e.g., your mother, father, or siblings)?

❏ Yes

❏ No

CONTAGIOUS

The bacteria, which cause gum disease may be spread to other family members.

Has anyone in your immediate family been tested or treated for gum problems? If so, whom?

❏ Spouse

❏ Children

FEMALES

Females can be at increased risk for gum disease at different points in their life.

The following can adversely affect your gums. Please check all that apply

❏ Pregnant   ❏ Nursing   ❏ Osteoporosis
❏ Taking birth control pills
❏ Taking hormone supplements
❏ Infrequent care during previous pregnancies

over

A

Figure 11-8A. Side 1 of Periodontal Risk Questionnaire. Risk assessment questionnaires are practical tools that can be helpful in identifying individuals who have a high susceptibility to periodontitis. Side one of a risk assessment questionnaire is shown here. See Figure 11-8B for side two of this questionnaire. (Courtesy of Timothy G. Donley, DDS, MSD, Bowling Green, KY.)

DIABETES

Gum disease is a common complication of diabetes. Untreated gum disease makes it more difficult for individuals with diabetes to control their blood sugar.

If you *ARE* diabetic...

For how many years? _____

Is your diabetes well controlled? ❑ Yes ❑ No

Who is your physician for diabetes? _____

If you *ARE NOT* diabetic...

Any family history of diabetes? ❑ Yes ❑ No

Have you had any of these warning signs of diabetes?

❑ Frequent urination ❑ Excessive thirst
❑ Excessive hunger ❑ Tingling or numbness in extremities
❑ Weakness and fatigue ❑ Slow healing of cuts
❑ Unexplained weight loss ❑ Any change of vision

 HEART MURMUR, ARTIFICIAL JOINT PROSTHESIS

With the slightest amount of gum inflammation, bacteria from the mouth can enter the bloodstream and cause a serious infection of the heart muscle or your artificial joint.

Do you have a heart murmur or artificial joint?
❑ Yes ❑ No

If so, does your physician recommend antibiotics prior to dental visits? ❑ Yes ❑ No

Name of physician: _____

It is especially important in your case to always keep your gums as healthy and inflammation free as possible to reduce the chance of bacterial infection originating in the mouth.

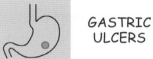 GASTRIC ULCERS

When your gums are inflamed, bacteria from the mouth can travel to the gut and cause ulcers to become active.

Have you been treated for ulcers?
❑ Yes ❑ No

Is the ulcer active now?
❑ Yes ❑ No

Ulcers are caused by bacteria. If you have been treated for ulcers you should make sure your gums are as inflammation free as possible.

ALL PATIENTS PLEASE COMPLETE THE FOLLOWING:

Have you noticed any of the following signs of gum disease?
❑ Bleeding gums during toothbrushing ❑ Pus between the teeth and gums
❑ Red, swollen, or tender gums ❑ Loose or separating teeth
❑ Gums that have pulled away from the teeth ❑ Change in the way your teeth fit together
❑ Persistent bad breath ❑ Food catching between teeth

Is it important to you to keep your teeth as long as possible? ❑ Yes ❑ No
Any particular reason why missing teeth have not been replaced?

_____

Do you like the appearance of your smile? ❑ Yes ❑ No
Do you like the color of your teeth? ❑ Yes ❑ No
Do your teeth keep you from eating any specific food? ❑ Yes ❑ No

B

Figure 11-8B. Side 2 of Periodontal Risk Questionnaire. Side 2 of a two-page risk assessment questionnaire. (Courtesy of Timothy G. Donley, DDS, MSD, Bowling Green, KY.)

Chapter Summary Statement

In the oral cavity, most of the time, things are in a state of balance between the bacteria in plaque biofilms and the host.

- For the periodontium to remain healthy, the bacterial challenge must be contained at a level that can be tolerated by the host.
- The situation can be thought of as a balance scale, with the disease-promoting factors on one side of the scale and the health-promoting factors on the other.
- As long as the two sides of the scale are in balance, there will be no disease progression.
- The intermittent pattern of disease activity seen in periodontitis is believed to result from the changing balance between the pathogenic bacteria and the host's inflammatory and immune responses.

Periodontal disease is a bacterial infection of the periodontium. The presence of pathogenic bacteria, however, does not necessarily mean that an individual will experience periodontitis.

- Additional factors play a role in determining why some individuals are more susceptible to periodontitis than others.
- Contributing factors are factors that increase an individual's susceptibility to periodontitis by modifying the host response to bacterial infection.
- Contributing factors such as systemic disease, smoking, and genetic factors can play a significant role in determining the onset and progression of periodontitis.

Thorough daily self-care (plaque control) by the patient and routine professional care are the best methods for prevention of periodontal disease. Other risk factors must be evaluated, however, to develop the best treatment plan for each individual.

Section 3
Focus on Patients

Ethical Dilemma

Your first patient on Monday morning is Joyce Robbins. She is new to your practice. She has filled out a Periodontal Assessment Questionnaire to assist you in determining her risk assessment. She states that she has never filled one out before, and is concerned that she has received poor quality dental work as a result. As she enters your operatory, you notice that she is a very petite, well-dressed woman. Her medical history and Periodontal Assessment Questionnaire reveal the following:

Joyce is a 58-year-old college professor. She has stage 1 hypertension, and takes 20 mg of Lisinopril daily as a result. She has a family history of cardiac disease (from both her mother and father), and her father developed type II diabetes at age 50. She takes Simvastatin for high cholesterol. She is a borderline diabetic, and her blood sugar levels have been rising at each primary care visit. She suffers from osteoporosis of the spine and hip. She is presently a nonsmoker but did smoke while she was in college. Her oral exam and radiographs reveal that she has generalized slight recession, generalized horizontal bone loss, generalized 3-mm pockets, with some 4- and 5-mm pockets on the posterior teeth, little plaque biofilm, but generalized slight to moderate supragingival and subgingival calculus deposits. She flosses daily but hasn't had her teeth cleaned in 5 years. She frequently gets food stuck between her teeth, and is increasingly becoming concerned about "the way her teeth look and feel." She wants to know what she can do to maintain her "pretty smile," and why no other office was as thorough with her care.

1. What do you think have may caused the patient's generalized recession?
2. What factors may have contributed to the patient's disease progression?
3. How will you discuss the balance between periodontal health and disease?
4. Is there an ethical dilemma involved?

Clinical Patient Care

CASE 1

Mr. Archie Newcomer is a new patient in your dental office. Mr. Newcomer is 35 years of age and reports that this is his first dental checkup in 5 or 6 years. *Mr. Newcomer's completed Periodontal Assessment Questionnaire is shown in Figure 11-9A,B on the next two pages of this module.* Review Mr. Newcomer's questionnaire, make a list of periodontal risk factors, and suggest strategies for managing these risk factors.

QUESTIONNAIRE

PERIODONTAL ASSESSMENT QUESTIONNAIRE FOR _Mr. Newcomer_

TOBACCO USE

Tobacco use is the most significant risk factor for gum disease.

Do you now or have you ever used the following?

	Amount per day?	How many years?	If you quit, what year?
☒ Cigarette	2 packs	15 yrs.	
☐ Cigar			
☐ Pipe			
☐ Chew			
☐ Snuff			

HEART ATTACK AND STROKE

Untreated gum disease can increase your risk for heart attack and stroke.

Do you have any other risk factors for heart disease or stroke?

☐ Family history of heart disease   ☒ Tobacco use
☐ High cholesterol   ☐ High blood pressure

If you have any of these other risk factors it is especially important for you to always keep your gums as healthy and inflammation free as possible to reduce your overall risk for heart attack and stroke.

MEDICATIONS

A side effect of some medications can cause changes in your gums.

Have you ever taken any of the following medications?

☐ Dilantin antiseizure medication

☐ Calcium channel blocker blood pressure medicine (such as Procardia, Cardizem, Norvasc, Verapamil, etc.)

☐ Cyclosporin immunosuppressant therapy

GENETIC

The tendency for gum disease to develop can be inherited.

Has anyone on your side of the family had gum problems (e.g., your mother, father, or siblings)?

☒ Yes

☐ No

CONTAGIOUS

The bacteria, which cause gum disease may be spread to other family members.

Has anyone in your immediate family been tested or treated for gum problems? If so, whom?

☒ Spouse

☐ Children

FEMALES

Females can be at increased risk for gum disease at different points in their life.

The following can adversely affect your gums. Please check all that apply

☐ Pregnant   ☐ Nursing   ☐ Osteoporosis
☐ Taking birth control pills
☐ Taking hormone supplements
☐ Infrequent care during previous pregnancies

over

A

Figure 11-9A. Page 1 of Mr. Newcomer's Risk Questionnaire.

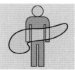 DIABETES

Gum disease is a common complication of diabetes. Untreated gum disease makes it more difficult for individuals with diabetes to control their blood sugar.

If you *ARE* diabetic...
For how many years? ___ 20 yrs. ___
Is your diabetes well controlled? ☒ Yes ☐ No
Who is your physician for diabetes? ___ Dr. Samuel Burlington ___

If you *ARE NOT* diabetic...
Any family history of diabetes? ☐ Yes ☐ No
Have you had any of these warning signs of diabetes?

☐ Frequent urination   ☐ Excessive thirst
☐ Excessive hunger   ☐ Tingling or numbness in extremities
☐ Weakness and fatigue   ☐ Slow healing of cuts
☐ Unexplained weight loss   ☐ Any change of vision

 HEART MURMUR, ARTIFICIAL JOINT PROSTHESIS

With the slightest amount of gum inflammation, bacteria from the mouth can enter the bloodstream and cause a serious infection of the heart muscle or your artificial joint.

Do you have a heart murmur or artificial joint?
☐ Yes ☒ No

If so, does your physician recommend antibiotics prior to dental visits? ☐ Yes ☐ No

Name of physician: _____

It is especially important in your case to always keep your gums as healthy and inflammation free as possible to reduce the chance of bacterial infection originating in the mouth.

 GASTRIC ULCERS

When your gums are inflamed, bacteria from the mouth can travel to the gut and cause ulcers to become active.

Have you been treated for ulcers?
☐ Yes ☒ No

Is the ulcer active now?
☐ Yes ☐ No

Ulcers are caused by bacteria. If you have been treated for ulcers you should make sure your gums are as inflammation free as possible.

ALL PATIENTS PLEASE COMPLETE THE FOLLOWING:

Have you noticed any of the following signs of gum disease?
☒ Bleeding gums during toothbrushing   ☐ Pus between the teeth and gums
☐ Red, swollen, or tender gums   ☐ Loose or separating teeth
☐ Gums that have pulled away from the teeth ☐ Change in the way your teeth fit together
☐ Persistent bad breath   ☒ Food catching between teeth

Is it important to you to keep your teeth as long as possible? ☐ Yes ☐ No
Any particular reason why missing teeth have not been replaced?

_____

Do you like the appearance of your smile? ☒ Yes ☐ No
Do you like the color of your teeth? ☒ Yes ☐ No
Do your teeth keep you from eating any specific food? ☐ Yes ☒ No

B

Figure 11-9B. Page 2 of Mr. Newcomer's Risk Questionnaire.

References

1. Armitage GC. Learned and unlearned concepts in periodontal diagnostics: a 50-year perspective. *Periodontol 2000*. 2013;62(1):20–36.
2. Bartold PM, Van Dyke TE. Periodontitis: a host-mediated disruption of microbial homeostasis. Unlearning learned concepts. *Periodontol 2000*. 2013;62(1):203–217.
3. Dick DS, Shaw JR. The infectious and transmissible nature of the periodontal syndrome of the rice rat. *Arch Oral Biol*. 1966;11(11):1095–1108.
4. Wade WG. The oral microbiome in health and disease. *Pharmacol Res*. 2013;69(1):137–143.
5. Berezow AB, Darveau RP. Microbial shift and periodontitis. *Periodontol 2000*. 2011;55(1):36–47.
6. Cullinan MP, Seymour GJ. Understanding risk for periodontal disease. *Ann R Australas Coll Dent Surg*. 2010;20:86–87.
7. Ebersole JL, Dawson DR 3rd, Morford LA, et al. Periodontal disease immunology: 'double indemnity' in protecting the host. *Periodontol 2000*. 2013;62(1):163–202.
8. Genco RJ, Borgnakke WS. Risk factors for periodontal disease. *Periodontol 2000*. 2013;62(1):59–94.
9. Hajishengallis G, Lamont RJ. Beyond the red complex and into more complexity: the polymicrobial synergy and dysbiosis (PSD) model of periodontal disease etiology. *Mol Oral Microbiol*. 2012;27(6):409–419.
10. Marsh PD, Devine DA. How is the development of dental biofilms influenced by the host? *J Clin Periodontol*. 2011;38 (suppl 11):28–35.
11. Marsh PD, Moter A, Devine DA. Dental plaque biofilms: communities, conflict and control. *Periodontol 2000*. 2011;55(1):16–35.
12. Matthews JB, Chen FM, Milward MR, et al. Effect of nicotine, cotinine and cigarette smoke extract on the neutrophil respiratory burst. *J Clin Periodontol*. 2011;38(3):208–218.
13. Mealey BL, Ocampo GL. Diabetes mellitus and periodontal disease. *Periodontol 2000*. 2007;44:127–153.
14. Michalowicz BS, Diehl SR, Gunsolley JC, et al. Evidence of a substantial genetic basis for risk of adult periodontitis. *J Periodontol*. 2000;71(11):1699–1707.
15. Peruzzo DC, Benatti BB, Ambrosano GM, et al. A systematic review of stress and psychological factors as possible risk factors for periodontal disease. *J Periodontol*. 2007;78(8):1491–1504.
16. American Academy of Periodontology. American Academy of Periodontology statement on risk assessment. *J Periodontol*. 2008;79(2):202.
17. Douglass CW. Risk assessment and management of periodontal disease. *J Am Dent Assoc*. 2006;137 Suppl:27S–32S.
18. Koshi E, Rajesh S, Koshi P, et al. Risk assessment for periodontal disease. *J Indian Soc Periodontol*. 2012;16(3):324–328.
19. Thyvalikakath TP, Padman R, Gupta S. An integrated risk assessment tool for team-based periodontal disease management. *Stud Health Technol Inform*. 2013;192:1150.

 STUDENT ANCILLARY RESOURCES

A wide variety of resources to enhance your learning and understanding of this chapter are available on the**Point**.

- Visit thePoint to access:
  - Audio Glossary
  - Animations
  - Suggested Readings
  - Answers to Review Questions
  - Case Studies

Oral Biofilms and Periodontal Infections

Clinical Application. Caring for patients with periodontal diseases requires a comprehensive understanding of the concept of oral biofilms and how individual types of bacteria interact as residents in these biofilms. This chapter discusses what is currently known about oral biofilms and sets the stage for the inevitable expansion of our knowledge about these biofilms as the results of additional research become available.

Learning Objectives

- Explain the difference in the cell membrane of a gram-positive versus a gram-negative bacterium.
- Define the term biofilm and explain the advantages of a bacterium living in a biofilm.
- Describe the life cycle of a biofilm.
- Given a drawing of a mature biofilm, label the following: bacterial microcolonies, fluid channels, extracellular slime layer, acquired pellicle, and tooth surface.
- Explain the significance of the extracellular slime layer and fluid channels of a biofilm.
- Define coaggregation and explain its significance in bacterial colonization of the tooth surface.
- Explain why systemic antibiotics and antimicrobial agents are not effective in eliminating dental plaque biofilms.

- State the most effective ways to control dental plaque biofilms.

- Name several reasons why newer microbe detection methods have brought Socransky's microbial complexes and the specific plaque hypothesis model into question.

- Discuss the hypothesis that plaque biofilm is necessary but not sufficient for periodontal destruction (microbial homeostasis–host response hypothesis).

- Name the three bacteria designated by The World Workshop in Periodontology (1996) as periodontal pathogens.

Key Terms

Bacterium/Bacteria
Cell membrane
Gram staining
Gram-positive bacteria
Gram-negative bacteria
Biofilm
Acquired pellicle

Fimbriae
Bacterial blooms
Mushroom-shaped
  microcolonies
Extracellular slime layer
Fluid channels
Coaggregation

Tooth-associated plaque
  biofilms
Tissue-associated plaque
  biofilms
Unattached bacteria
Transmission
Commensal organisms

Section 1
Bacterial Biofilms

One human mouth is home to more microorganisms than there are people on the planet Earth. It is currently estimated that some 650 to 1,000 microbial species reside in the oral cavity (1–3). These microorganisms have evolved to survive in the environment of the tooth surface, gingival epithelium, and oral cavity. Though this is not a microbiology textbook, knowledge of several characteristics of bacteria is fundamental to understanding many of the ideas presented in this chapter. The bacterial characteristics discussed in this section include cell membrane structure, Gram staining of bacteria, and the environments in which bacteria live.

CHARACTERISTICS OF BACTERIA

1. Characteristics of Bacteria
   A. Description
      1. **Bacterium** (plural, **bacteria**). Bacteria are the simplest organisms and can be seen only through a microscope.
      2. There are thousands of kinds of bacteria, most of which are harmless to humans.
      3. Bacteria have existed on earth for longer than any other organisms and are still the most abundant type of cell.
      4. Bacteria can replicate quickly. This ability to divide quickly enables populations of bacteria to adapt rapidly to changes in their environment.
   B. Structure of the Bacterial Cell Membrane. A tough protective layer called a **cell membrane** encloses nearly all bacteria.
      1. The composition of the cell membrane is an important characteristic used in identifying and classifying bacteria. **Gram staining** is a laboratory method that reveals differences in the chemical and physical properties of bacterial cell membranes. Depending on their permeability, the bacterial cell membranes appear either purple or red in color under a light microscope.
      2. Gram staining divides bacteria into gram-positive (purple color) and gram-negative (red color) bacterial cell membrane types.
         a. Gram-positive bacteria (purple stain)
            1. Have a single, thick cell membrane
            2. Retain a purple color when stained with a dye known as crystal violet and so, the bacterial cell membranes show a purple stain under a light microscope
         b. Gram-negative bacteria (red stain)
            1. Have double cell membranes
            2. Do not stain purple with crystal violet and therefore, show a red stain under a light microscope

BACTERIAL COMMUNITIES

Until recently, bacteria were studied as they grew on culture plates in a laboratory. Recent advances in research technology have allowed researchers to study bacteria in their natural environment. These studies have revealed that most bacteria live in complex communities called biofilms and that biofilms are found everywhere in nature.

1. **Where Bacteria Live.** Bacteria live almost everywhere, even in environments where other life forms cannot survive. Bacteria are always present on the skin and in the digestive and respiratory systems of humans.
   A. **Free-Floating Bacteria**
      1. Bacteria may be free floating. These free-floating bacteria are also known as planktonic bacteria.
      2. Until recently, most research done on bacteria was conducted on free-floating bacteria.
   B. **Attached Bacteria**
      1. Bacteria can attach to surfaces and to one another. *Communities of bacteria that attach to each other and to a surface are described as living in a biofilm.*
      2. Once a bacterium attaches to a surface, it activates a whole different set of genes that give the bacterium different characteristics from those it had as a free-floating organism.
      3. It has been estimated that more than 99% of all bacteria on earth live as attached bacteria.
2. **Biofilms and Where They Form**
   A. **Description**
      1. A **biofilm** is a living film—containing a well-organized community of microorganisms—that grows on a surface. Usually biofilms consist of many species of bacteria as well as other organisms and debris.
      2. By some estimates 65% of all diseases may be biofilm induced. Biofilm-induced diseases include tuberculosis, cystic fibrosis, subacute bacterial endocarditis, and periodontal disease.
   B. **Biofilm Environments**
      1. Biofilms are everywhere in nature (Fig. 12-1). "Biofilm" may seem like a new term, but everyone encounters biofilms on a regular basis. The plaque biofilm that forms on teeth, the slime in fish tanks, and the slime deposit that clogs the sink drain are all examples of biofilms. The slimy rocks in a stream are biofilm coated.
      2. *Biofilms can exist on any solid surface that is exposed to a bacteria-containing fluid.*
      3. Biofilms thrive in dental unit water and suction lines and have been shown to be the primary source of contaminated water delivered by dental units. Stagnant fluid flow allows free-floating bacteria to attach to the tubing walls in the dental unit and form intricate biofilms.

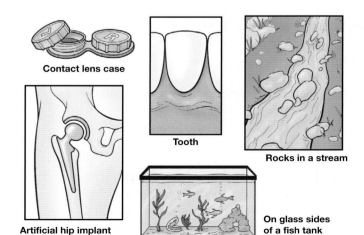

Contact lens case

Tooth

Rocks in a stream

Artificial hip implant

On glass sides of a fish tank

Figure 12-1. Biofilm Environments. Biofilms are found nearly everywhere in nature. They have a major impact on human health.

3. Life Cycle of a Biofilm. The biofilm life cycle has three stages: attachment, growth, and detachment (Fig. 12-2).
   A. Attachment. Bacteria attach to a surface.
   B. Growth
      1. The attached bacteria begin releasing substances that attract other free-floating bacteria to join the biofilm community.
      2. The attached bacteria secrete a film known as the extracellular slime layer. This slimy film helps to keep the bacteria attached to the surface and acts as a protective shield for the bacteria.
      3. The bacteria multiply rapidly and grow away from the surface to form three-dimensional mushroom-shaped mature biofilms that attach to a surface at a narrow base.
      4. Movement of the fluid surrounding the mature biofilms results in extensions that stream from the main body of the biofilm.
   C. Detachment
      1. Clumps of the main biofilm break off and are carried away by the fluid surrounding the biofilm.
      2. These detached clumps can attach to other portions of a surface and form new bacterial colonies.

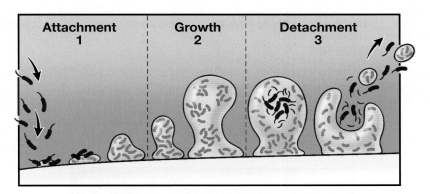

Figure 12-2. Biofilm Life Cycle. The three major stages in the life cycle of a biofilm: attachment, growth, and detachment in clumps.

Section 2
Structure and Colonization of Dental Plaque Biofilms

The pattern of dental plaque biofilm development can be divided into five phases:
(1) formation of acquired pellicle, (2) attachment of early bacterial colonizers, (3) coaggregation of additional bacterial colonizers, and (4) formation of an extracellular slime layer and microcolony formation (Fig. 12-3). Phase 5 is a mature biofilm characterized by the bacterial microcolonies that form complex groups with a primitive communication system and fluid channels (Fig. 12-4).

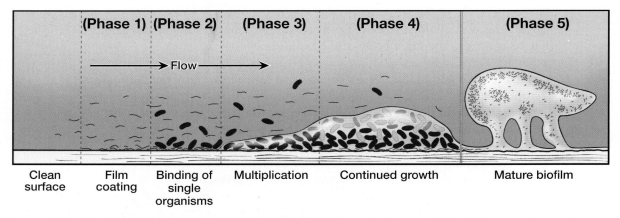

(Phase 1)	(Phase 2)	(Phase 3)	(Phase 4)	(Phase 5)
Clean surface	Film coating	Binding of single organisms	Multiplication Continued growth	Mature biofilm

Figure 12-3. Five Phases in the Formation of a Biofilm. Phase 1, the acquired pellicle coats the tooth surface. Phase 2, initial colonizers attach to the tooth surface. Additional bacteria coaggregate with the initial colonizers in Phase 3. Phase 4 is signaled by the formation of the extracellular slime layer. Phase 5 is a mature biofilm.

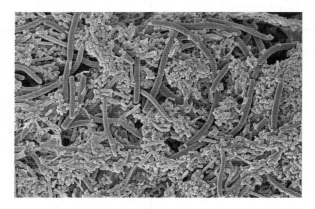

Figure 12-4. Dental Plaque Biofilm. Scanning electron micrograph of dental plaque biofilm showing bacteria (*red and yellow stain*) and extracellular matrix (*orange stain*). (Courtesy of Getty Images.)

SPECIES CAPABLE OF COLONIZING THE MOUTH

Many different species and subspecies are capable of colonizing the mouth. Figure 12-5 lists some examples of over 600 cultivable species.

	Gram positive ⊕		Gram negative ⊖	
	Facultative anaerobes	**Obligate anaerobes**	**Facultative anaerobes**	**Obligate anaerobes**
Cocci	**Streptococcus** –S. anginosus (S. milleri) –S. mutans –S. sanguis • Ss –S. oralis –S. mitis –S. intermedius	**Peptostreptococcus** –P. micros • Pm **Peptococcus**	**Neisseria** **Branhamella**	**Veillonella** –V. parvula
Rods	**Actinomyces** –A. naeslundii • An –A. viscosus • Av –A. odontolyticus –A. israelii **Propionibacterium** **Rothia** –R. dentocariosa **Lactobacillus** –L. oris –L. acidophilus –L. salivarius –L. buccalis	**Eubacterium** –E. nodatum • En –E. saburreum –E. timidum –E. brachy –E. alactolyticum **Bifidobacterium** –B. dentium	**Aggregatibacter** –A. actinomycetem- comitans • Aa **Capnocytophaga** –C. ochracea –C. gingivalis –C. sputigena **Campylobacter** –C. rectus • Cr –C. curvus –C. showae **Eikenella** –E. corrodens • Ec **Haemophilus** –H. aphrophilus –H. segnis	**Porphyromonas** –P. gingivalis • Pg –P. endodontalis **Prevotella** –P. intermedia • Pi –P. nigrescens –P. denticola –P. loescheii –P. oris –P. oralis **Tannerella** –T. forsythia • Tf **Fusobacterium** –F. nucleatum • Fn –F. periodonticum **Selenemonas** –S. sputigena –S. noxia
Spirochetes and mycoplasms	**Mycoplasm** –M. orale –M. salivarium –M. hominis		**Spirochetes of ANUG** **Treponema sp.** –T. denticola • Td –T. socranskii –T. pectinovorum –T. vincentii	
Eukaryotes	**Candida** –C. albicans	**Entamoeba**		**Trichomonas**

Figure 12-5. Examples of Microorganisms Capable of Colonizing the Mouth.

THE COMPLEX STRUCTURE OF DENTAL PLAQUE BIOFILMS

1. Pattern of Plaque Biofilm Development
    A. Phase 1—Film Coating
        1. Within minutes after cleaning the tooth surface, a film forms over the tooth surface. This film, the acquired pellicle, is composed of a variety of salivary glycoproteins (mucins) and antibodies.
            a. The purpose of the acquired pellicle is to protect the enamel from acidic activity.
            b. Unfortunately, in addition to providing protection from acids, the acquired pellicle also alters the charge and energy of the tooth surface, facilitating bacterial adhesion.
            c. A helpful analogy in understanding the role of acquired pellicle in plaque biofilm formation is to think of the pellicle as "double-sided adhesive tape." The double-sided tape adheres to the tooth surface on one side and provides a sticky surface on the other side that facilitates attachment by bacteria to the tooth surface.
    B. Phase 2—Initial Attachment of Bacteria to Pellicle
        1. Within a few hours after pellicle formation, bacteria begin to attach to the outer surface of the pellicle.
        2. Some bacteria possess attachment structures, such as extracellular substances and hundreds of hair-like structures, which enable them to attach rapidly upon contact with the tooth surface. The hair-like structures are termed fimbriae.
    C. Phase 3—New Bacteria Join In. Once bacteria stick to the tooth, they begin producing substances that stimulate other free-floating bacteria to join the community.
    D. Phase 4—Extracellular Slime Layer and Microcolony Formation
        1. Production of an Extracellular Slime Layer
            a. It appears that the act of attaching to the tooth surface stimulates the bacteria to excrete a slimy, glue-like substance, called the extracellular slime layer.
            b. This extracellular slime layer helps to anchor bacteria to the tooth surface and provides protection for the attached bacteria.
        2. Microcolony Formation
            a. Once the surface of the tooth has been covered with attached bacteria, the biofilm grows primarily through cell division of the adherent bacteria (rather than through the attachment of new bacteria).
            b. Next, the proliferating bacteria begin to grow away from the tooth.
            c. Bacterial blooms are periods when specific species or groups of species grow at rapidly accelerated rates.
    E. Phase 5—Mature Biofilm: Mushroom-Shaped Microcolonies
        1. The bacteria cluster together to form mushroom-shaped microcolonies that are attached to the tooth surface at a narrow base.
        2. The result is the formation of complex collections of different bacteria linked to one another.
2. The Complex Structure of Mature Dental Plaque Biofilms
    A. Bacterial Microcolonies
        1. The bacteria in a biofilm are not distributed evenly. As the bacteria attach to a surface and to each other, they cluster together to form microcolonies (Fig. 12-6).
        2. Each microcolony is a tiny independent community containing thousands of compatible bacteria. Different microcolonies may contain different combinations of bacterial species.

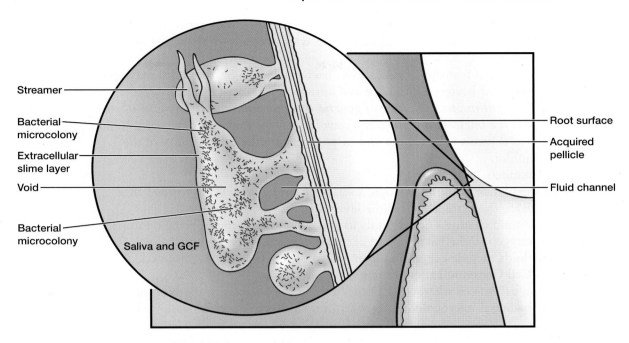

Figure 12-6. Structure of Plaque Biofilm. The complex structure of dental plaque biofilm includes clusters of bacterial microcolonies, streamers, and fluid channels.

a. Environmental conditions within each microcolony of bacteria vary radically. The environmental conditions among several microcolonies may include differences in oxygen concentration, pH, and temperature.

b. The differing environmental conditions within a biofilm mean that the bacterial population is very diverse—with each different bacterial species preferring a certain environment within the biofilm.

1. This bacterial diversity helps to ensure the survivability of the plaque biofilm in widely varying oral conditions.

2. If the plaque biofilm had only one species of bacteria, it would be much more likely that a toxic agent or condition would destroy the biofilm.

B. Extracellular Slime Layer

1. The **extracellular slime layer** is a dense protective barrier that surrounds the bacterial microcolonies (Fig. 12-6).

2. *The slime layer acts like a shield protecting the bacterial microcolonies from antibiotics, antimicrobials, and the body's immune system.*

C. Fluid Forces

1. The fluid forces of the saliva surrounding the biofilm influence the shape of the plaque biofilm, as well as the spatial arrangement of the bacteria inside.

2. These fluid forces result in the development of extensions from the main body of the biofilm. These biofilm extensions can break free and be swallowed, expectorated, or form new biofilm colonies in other areas of the mouth.

3. Fluid forces also result in cell-to-cell collisions of the bacteria within the biofilm.

  a. Bacterial cell collisions lead to a more rapid spread of genes among the bacteria than there would be if there were no fluid forces acting on the biofilm.

  b. This rapid transfer of genes from bacterial cell to bacterial cell may result in enhanced bacterial virulence and antimicrobial resistance.

  c. ***The continuous exchange of genetic information among bacteria means that the bacteria are constantly evolving.*** This makes the bacterial biofilm very difficult to eradicate and helps to ensure the survivability of the biofilm.

D. Fluid Channels

 1. As the plaque biofilm develops, a series of **fluid channels** are formed that penetrate the extracellular slime layer (Fig. 12-6).

 2. These fluid channels direct fluids in and around the biofilm bringing nutrients and oxygen to the bacteria and carrying bacterial waste products away.

 3. The fluids include everything from saliva to any beverages consumed.

E. Cell-to-Cell Communication System

 1. Direct cell-to-cell interaction occurs among the bacteria in the biofilm.

 2. The bacterial microcolonies use chemical signals to communicate with each other.

 3. This cell-to-cell communication also results in the transfer of genes among bacteria.

F. Bacterial Signaling

 1. Bacterial communication occurs when bacteria within the biofilm release and sense small proteins (signaling molecules). This type of communication among bacteria is termed quorum sensing.

 2. Bacteria in the biofilm use quorum sensing to trigger events such as adhesion of additional bacteria to the biofilm and formation of the extracellular slime layer that surrounds the bacteria.

BACTERIAL COLONIZATION AND SUCCESSION

1. Microbial Complexes

A. Internal Organization

 1. The internal structure of plaque biofilm has been examined in a number of studies by light and electron microscopy (4–8).

 2. The organization of bacteria within biofilms is not random; rather there are specific associations among bacterial species (9). The bacteria within a biofilm no longer work as single entities, but rather, act as a functioning system of interdependent parts.

B. Bacterial Colonization of the Tooth Surface

 1. **Layers and Layers of Bacteria.** The biofilm develops by stacking one bacterial species on top of another bacterial species. A mature dental biofilm does not consist of only one species of bacteria.

 2. Coaggregation of Bacteria

  a. **Coaggregation** is the cell-to-cell adherence of one oral bacterium to another (Fig. 12-7).

  b. ***Coaggregation is not random; rather, each bacterial strain only has a limited set of bacteria to which they are able to adhere.***

  c. The ability to adhere and coaggregate is an important determinant in the development of the bacterial biofilm.

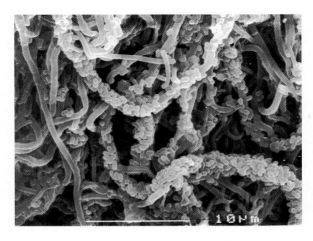

Figure 12-7. Bacterial Coaggregation. One example of coaggregation of bacteria has a corncob appearance that is created when a central rod-shaped bacterium becomes surrounded by many round cocci. (Courtesy of Ziedonis Skobe, PhD, Head, Biostructure Core Facility, The Forsyth Institute.)

2. Sequence of Colonization
    A. Early Bacterial Colonizers: Important to Bacterial Succession
        1. The first bacteria to colonize the tooth surface are nonpathogenic (Fig. 12-8). The ability of these species to attach to the tooth surface lays the foundation for the growth of dental plaque biofilms.
        2. Early bacterial colonizers of the tooth surface include many streptococcal species, such as *Streptococcus mitis* and *Streptococcus oralis* that have the ability to attach to the tooth pellicle, as well as, to each other (10,11). Another early colonizer is *Actinomyces viscosus*.
        3. The early bacterial colonizers release chemical signals that indicate to the next group of bacteria that conditions are favorable for them to join the biofilm.
        4. The early streptococcal colonizers are able to coaggregate with many of the other early colonizing bacteria and intermediate species. Many early and intermediate colonizing species are **unable** to attach to the tooth pellicle but have the ability to coaggregate with the streptococcal species.
        5. Free-floating bacteria cannot join the biofilm until the conditions are favorable (Box 12-1). The succession of bacteria joining the biofilm is comparable to elementary school students who are asked to line up in alphabetical order as their teacher calls out their names. Students whose last names start with the letter "O" cannot get in line until all the students whose last names start with "M and N" have taken their place in the line.
    B. Intermediate and Late Colonizers
        1. As is the case with the early bacterial colonizers, the intermediate and late colonizers must join the biofilm in the proper sequence.
        2. The intermediate species, such as *Fusobacterium nucleatum*, in turn coaggregate with the last colonizers.
        3. A mature plaque biofilm is a very complex collection of multiple bacterial species (Fig. 12-9).

Box 12-1. The Importance of Early Colonizers in Biofilm Succession

1. Free-floating bacteria cannot initiate periodontal disease.
2. If the biofilm is adequately disrupted by daily self-care and routine professional care, the biofilm will always be reforming. Every time the biofilm is disrupted, the entire process of bacterial succession starts over beginning with the early colonizers.

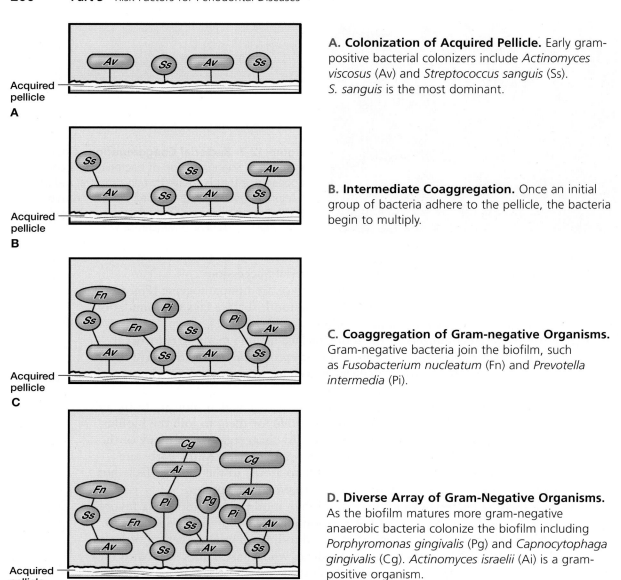

A. Colonization of Acquired Pellicle. Early gram-positive bacterial colonizers include *Actinomyces viscosus* (Av) and *Streptococcus sanguis* (Ss). *S. sanguis* is the most dominant.

B. Intermediate Coaggregation. Once an initial group of bacteria adhere to the pellicle, the bacteria begin to multiply.

C. Coaggregation of Gram-negative Organisms. Gram-negative bacteria join the biofilm, such as *Fusobacterium nucleatum* (Fn) and *Prevotella intermedia* (Pi).

D. Diverse Array of Gram-Negative Organisms. As the biofilm matures more gram-negative anaerobic bacteria colonize the biofilm including *Porphyromonas gingivalis* (Pg) and *Capnocytophaga gingivalis* (Cg). *Actinomyces israelii* (Ai) is a gram-positive organism.

Figure 12-8. Stages of Bacterial Colonization of the Tooth Surface.

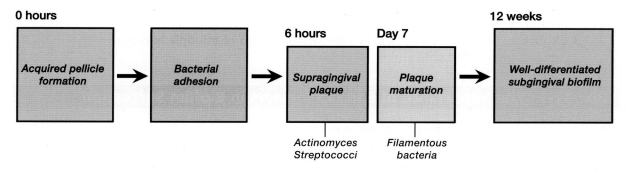

Figure 12-9. Sequence of Bacterial Attachment. Dental plaque biofilm development always begins supragingivally and progresses subgingivally.

3. **Bacterial Attachment Zones.** The zones of *sub*gingival bacterial attachment (Fig. 12-10) are the tooth surface and the epithelial lining of the periodontal pocket. Bacteria also may attach to other bacteria that are attached to one of these surfaces.
   A. **Tooth-Associated Plaque Biofilms**—bacteria that are attached to the tooth surface.
      1. Bacteria attach to an area of the tooth surface that extends from the gingival margin almost to the junctional epithelium at the base of the pocket.
      2. Subgingival bacteria appear to have the ability to invade the dentinal tubules of the cementum.
      3. Filamentous microorganisms, cocci, and rods—including *S. mitis, S. sanguis,* and *A. viscosus*—dominate the tooth-associated plaque biofilms.
   B. **Tissue-Associated Plaque Biofilms**—bacteria that adhere to the epithelium.
      1. The bacteria that adhere loosely to the epithelium of the pocket wall are distinctly different from those of the tooth-associated plaque biofilms.
      2. The layers closest to the soft tissue wall contain large numbers of spirochetes and flagellated bacteria. Gram-negative cocci and rods are also present. There is a predominance of species such as *S. oralis, Streptococcus intermedius, Porphyromonas gingivalis, Prevotella intermedia, Tannerella forsythia,* and *F. nucleatum.*
      3. Bacteria from the tissue-attached plaque biofilms can invade the gingival connective tissue and be found within the periodontal connective tissues and on the surface of the alveolar bone.
   C. **Unattached Bacteria.** In addition to the attached bacteria, the periodontal pocket also contains many free-floating bacteria that are not part of the biofilm.

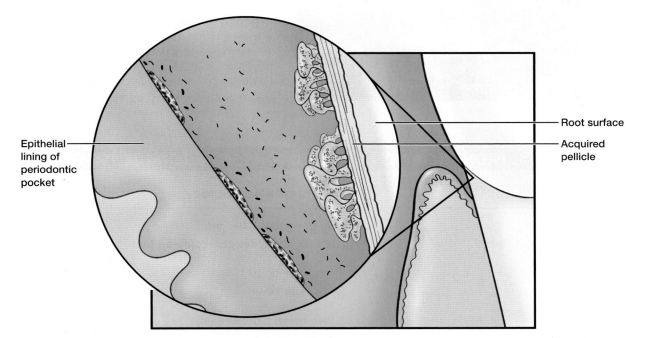

Epithelial lining of periodontic pocket

Root surface

Acquired pellicle

Figure 12-10. Subgingival Plaque Biofilm Attachment Zones. Within a periodontal pocket, bacteria attach to the tooth surface or the epithelial lining of the pocket.

4. Transmission of Periodontal Bacteria
   A. Molecular epidemiology techniques that isolate DNA provide evidence that bacteria in the biofilm are transmissible. **Transmission** is the transfer of bacteria from the oral cavity of one person to another.
   B. Transmission should not be confused with contagion. There is little or no evidence that periodontal infections are communicable. The term communicable refers to a disease that may be passed from one person to another by direct or indirect contact via substances such as inanimate objects.
   C. Studies demonstrate that *A. actinomycetemcomitans* (Fig. 12-11) and *P. gingivalis* strains isolated from parents and children within the same family exhibited identical restriction endonuclease DNA fragment patterns (12–15). Kissing is the primary means by which saliva and its bacterial contents are transmitted (14,16,17).
   D. Table 12-1 provides a pronunciation guide to bacteria commonly associated with plaque biofilms.

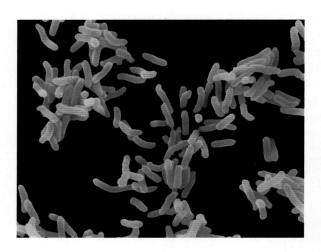

Figure 12-11. *Aggregatibacter actinomycetemcomitans* (Aa). A three-dimensional image of *A. actinomycetemcomitans* taken with a scanning electron microscope (SEM). (Used with permission from Dennis Kunkel Microscopy, Inc.)

TABLE 12-1. PRONUNCIATION GUIDE TO BACTERIAL TONGUE TWISTERS

Name	Pronunciation Guide
Aggregatibacter *actinomycetemcomitans*	ag-gre-gat-eee-bac-ter act-tin-oh-my-see-tem-comb-ah-tans
Tannerella *forsythia*	tann-er-ella fawr-**sith**-ee-uh
Fusobacterium *nucleatum*	fuse-so-back-tier-EEE-um nu-klee-ah-tum
Porphyromonas *gingivalis*	pour-fy-roh-mo-nas ging-jih-val-lis

Section 3
Control of Plaque Biofilms

1. **Mechanisms of Bacterial Survival.** The biofilm provides the bacteria with an advantage that permits long-term survival within the sulcus or pocket environment. *The protective extracellular slime layer makes bacteria extremely resistant to antibiotics, antimicrobial agents, and the body's immune response.* It is likely that several mechanisms are responsible for biofilm resistance to systemic antibiotics, antimicrobial agents, and the immune system.
   A. **Resistance to Systemic Antibiotics and Antimicrobial Agents**
      1. Bacteria living in a biofilm are unusually resistant to systemic antibiotics (in dentistry, usually administered in pill form) and antimicrobials (placed locally in the oral cavity).
      2. *Antibiotic doses that kill free-floating bacteria, for example, need to be increased as much as 1,500 times to kill plaque biofilm bacteria* (and at these high doses, the antibiotic would kill the patient before the biofilm bacteria!) (18).
      3. Antimicrobial agents work best when used in conjunction with mechanical cleaning that removes or disrupts the dental plaque biofilm (19).
   B. **Protective Mechanisms of Biofilms**
      1. Extracellular Slime Layer
         a. The extracellular slime layer is very dense and may prevent the drugs from penetrating fully into the depth of the biofilm.
         b. The thick slime layer may protect the bacteria against leukocytes (defensive cells of the body's immune system). The dense slime layer may block substances released by leukocytes. As a result the leukocyte substances end up causing more damage to the surrounding body tissue than to the biofilm bacteria.
      2. Enzymes. Some bacteria produce enzymes that degrade antibiotics faster than the drug can penetrate into the biofilm.
      3. Dormant Bacteria
         a. The biofilm is very thick and bacteria in the deepest layers become dormant—not dead—because they are cut off from the sources of nutrients. **Dormant bacteria** are in an inactive state in order to survive adverse environmental conditions.
         b. Antibiotics only work on bacteria that are active and reproducing.
         c. When the course of antibiotics is finished, the dormant active bacteria within the biofilm reactivate.

2. **Physical Removal of Dental Plaque Biofilms is Essential**
   A. *Control of bacteria in dental plaque biofilms is best achieved by the physical disruption (such as brushing, flossing, and periodontal instrumentation).*
      1. It takes some time for the complex structure of a mature plaque biofilm to form.
      2. Mechanical cleaning forces the bacteria to start over with initial attachment, initial colonization, secondary colonization, and finally to become a mature biofilm.
      3. In areas that are cleaned regularly, a mature biofilm will not be able to develop. The cleaner the tooth surface, the less complex the bacterial formation.
   B. Toothbrushes and floss cannot reach the subgingival plaque biofilm located within pockets. For this reason, frequent periodontal instrumentation of subgingival root surfaces by a dental hygienist or dentist is an essential component in the treatment of periodontitis.

Section 4
The Role of Bacteria in Periodontitis

CHANGING EVIDENCE FOR THE ROLE OF BACTERIA

In 1683, Antonie van Leeuwenhoek, using a homemade microscope, first described oral microorganisms. Despite 330 years of scientific investigation in the field of oral microbiology, researchers have failed to identify bacterial pathogens that cause periodontitis (20). Over the years, three main hypotheses have been proposed to explain the etiology of periodontal disease: (1) accumulation of bacterial biofilms leads to periodontal destruction, (2) specific pathogenic bacteria and their products in the biofilm lead to periodontal destruction, and (3) bacterial plaque biofilm is necessary but not sufficient for periodontal destruction.

1. Historical Perspective: Accumulation of Bacterial Biofilms Lead to Periodontal Destruction (Nonspecific Plaque Hypothesis)
   A. Hypothesis. This theory proposed that the accumulation of plaque biofilm adjacent to the gingival margin led to gingival inflammation and subsequent periodontal destruction (21–23).
   B. Problems with the Nonspecific Plaque Hypothesis
      1. A failing of the nonspecific hypothesis is that it fails to explain why most cases of gingivitis never progress to periodontitis. Some individuals with heavy amounts of plaque biofilm fail to develop periodontitis. Yet, ironically other individuals with very light amounts of biofilm suffer from aggressive forms of periodontitis (24).
      2. This hypothesis cannot clarify why some sites in a particular individual's periodontium experience considerable periodontal destruction while other sites are unaffected.

2. Historical Perspective: Specific Pathogenic Bacteria Lead to Periodontal Destruction (Specific Plaque Hypothesis)
   A. Hypothesis. This theory proposed that specific pathogenic bacteria present in subgingival biofilms and their toxic products resulted in destruction of the periodontal tissues (22,23).
      1. An increase in the number of specific pathogens was thought to be associated with periodontitis.
      2. This model postulates that a microbial shift occurs in which the bacteria in the biofilm change from a predominantly gram-positive aerobic community to one consisting mainly of groups of gram-negative anaerobes (25).
   B. Socransky's Microbial Complexes. As a result of the specific plaque hypothesis, research efforts, over many years, focused on identifying specific microorganisms associated with various periodontal diseases and conditions.
      1. These studies identified specific groups of bacteria—*T. forsythia, P. gingivalis,* and *Treponema denticola*—that were significantly associated with periodontitis. It was noted that these bacteria were interdependent and often could not exist without the presence of the others (9,26).
      2. Socransky grouped microorganisms into complexes and assigned each complex a color (Fig. 12-12) (9). The yellow, green, and orange complexes were thought to be compatible with gingival health. The orange and red complexes comprise the species that were thought to be the major etiologic agents of periodontal disease.

3. *The appeal of the concept of red and other color-coded complexes led to the theory's widespread adoption until molecular-based approaches to microbe detection brought its validity into question.*

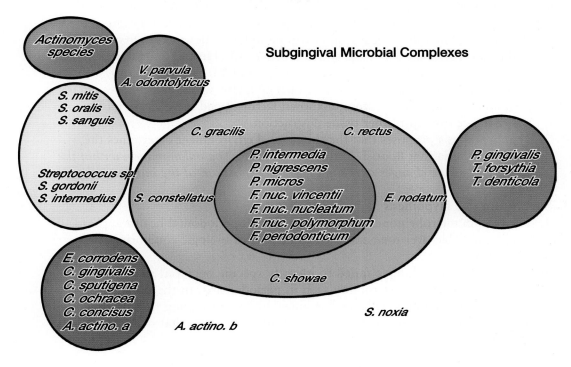

Figure 12-12. Socransky's Microbial Complexes. Socransky organized bacteria into complexes and assigned each complex a color. (Data from Socransky SS, Haffajee AD, Cugini MA, et al. Microbial complexes in subgingival plaque. *J Clin Periodontol.* 1998;25(2):134–144.)

C. **Problems with the Specific Plaque Hypothesis**
   1. Recently the development of newer microbe detection methods brought the model of the specific plaque hypothesis into question. First, it is established that red complex organisms can be found in the absence of periodontal disease (27,28). The fact that *P. gingivalis* and *T. forsythia* frequently are found in healthy periodontal sites brings into question whether these bacteria are true periodontal pathogens (29).
   2. Second, the periodontal microbe population is more heterogeneous and diverse than previously thought (30–32). Over 600 organisms are recognized as possible oral inhabitants, of which around 200 can be present in any one individual and about 50 present at any one site (33). Many of these newly recognized organisms show as good or better correlation with disease as the classical red complex (34–36). The identification of so many more bacterial species in the oral cavity makes the concept of specific bacteria causing periodontitis even more unlikely (37).
   3. Contrary to the doctrine that gram-negative bacteria dominate disease sites in periodontitis, numbers of gram-positive anaerobic bacteria species are shown to exhibit a significant increase in deep periodontal pockets relative to healthy sites and can be detected in greater numbers than gram-negative species in some studies (35).
   4. It is evident that the concept of a three-species red complex as representing the primary etiologic unit in periodontitis requires refinement (38).

3. Current Perspective: Plaque Biofilm is Necessary but not Sufficient for Periodontal Destruction (Microbial Homeostasis–Host Response Hypothesis)
   A. **Hypothesis.** This theory proposes that while plaque biofilms are the cause of the initial inflammatory response leading to gingivitis, *it is the host response, not the type of bacteria, which determines whether periodontal destruction progresses* (39).
      1. Evidence for the role of host response in periodontal destruction first emerged in the landmark paper by Page and Schroeder (40). Host and inflammatory response is discussed in detail in Chapters 13 and 14.
      2. Page and Schroeder noted that established gingivitis would not progress to periodontitis unless some other unknown factor tipped the delicate biofilm–host balance toward further tissue destruction.
      3. This hypothesis proposes that the subgingival environment determines the specific bacteria that flourish in the environment. *The inflammation within the tissues drives the changes in the microbial composition of the biofilm* and not vice versa.
   B. **Support for this Hypothesis**
      1. The biofilm microbe population associated with periodontal health appears to remain stable over time and exists in a state of biologic equilibrium or homeostasis.
      2. Decades of research have failed to identify specific bacterial pathogens that cause the tissue destruction seen in periodontitis. In the same time period, overwhelming evidence has amassed demonstrating that it is the uncontrolled host inflammatory and immune responses that drive the tissue destruction (41).

IS THERE SUCH A THING AS A PERIODONTAL PATHOGEN?

Most organisms that colonize the human body are commensal. Commensalism is a relationship between individuals of two species in which one species—the commensal organisms—obtains benefits from the other species without either harming or helping the host species. The commensal organism may obtain nutrients, shelter, or locomotion from the host species. The commensal relation often is between a larger host (the human body) and a smaller commensal organism. As with the human body as a whole, most organisms that colonize the oral cavity are commensal (3,42,43).

A. What is a Bacterial Pathogen? How Do We Define the Term "Periodontal Pathogen"?
   1. A pathogen usually is defined as a microorganism that causes or can cause a disease; a microbe that can cause damage in a host.
   2. It is generally accepted that bacteria can cause disease in humans through three different pathways: (1) as a true pathogen that generally is not found in humans and causes disease upon first exposure, (2) as part of the indigenous (natural) flora in one site—but when moved to another site in the body—cause disease, and (3) as a commensal organism, which can only cause disease if a change occurs in the host body that allows it to flourish and cause disease (44).

B. How do we define the term "periodontal pathogen"?
   1. There is little evidence to support the concept that periodontal bacteria are true pathogens.
      a. Periodontal plaque biofilms are found in the oral cavities throughout the general population and yet, not all individuals infected with biofilms develop periodontitis. On the contrary, most individuals do not develop periodontitis.

      b. Studies have shown the inoculation of gingival sulci with periodontal pathogens from periodontitis sites failed to induce a successful colonization and periodontitis at the recipient site (45).

2. The plaque biofilm community is an association of commensal organisms (3,42). Under certain circumstances, which are not fully understood, commensal organisms can transform to being pathogenic in nature (37).

      a. Under appropriate environmental conditions, commensal organisms in the plaque biofilm can become pathogenic and be associated with disease. Hajishengallis and Lamont (38) postulate that some organisms become what he terms "keystone pathogens." Hajishengallis suggests that the keystone pathogens—a minor constituent of the plaque biofilm—have the ability to tip the balance in favor of disease progression (1,38,46).

      b. Hajishengallis contends that key pathogens only can become virulent within a synergistic microbial biofilm community. The biofilm community has both gram-negative and gram-positive bacteria that can tolerate inflammation or provide other useful service to the biofilm community.

3. No definitive evidence exists in the literature that specific bacteria are responsible for the progression and manifestation of periodontitis.

      a. In 1996, the World Workshop in Periodontology (Consensus Report, 1996) designated *A. actinomycetemcomitans, P. gingivalis,* and *T. forsythia* as periodontal pathogens (47).

      b. It seems possible that these bacteria that have been noted to date as "periodontal pathogens" are present as the result of the periodontal disease but did not cause the disease (20).

4. Despite the presence of plaque biofilms, bacteria do not appear to be the major determining factor in the progression of gingivitis to periodontitis.

Chapter Summary Statement

More than 600 bacterial strains have been identified in dental plaque biofilm. The recognition that dental plaque is a biofilm helps to explain why periodontal diseases have been so difficult to prevent and to treat. Bacteria within a biofilm environment behave very differently from free-floating bacteria. The protective extracellular slime matrix makes bacteria extremely resistant to systemic antibiotics, antimicrobial agents, and the body's immune system. Mechanical removal is the most effective treatment for the control of dental plaque biofilms.

    To date, there is no definitive evidence that specific bacteria are responsible for the progression of periodontal disease. One theory suggests that the specific bacteria noted to date are present as the result of the disease but do not cause the disease. Considerable evidence indicates that it is more likely to be the host response to plaque biofilm that leads to the tissue destruction seen in periodontitis. It seems that it is the host inflammatory and immune responses that determine whether gingivitis progresses to periodontitis.

Section 5
Focus on Patients

Clinical Patient Care

CASE 1

You have just completed a thorough cleaning of a tooth surface. Describe what deposits you might expect to form on the tooth surface over the next few days if the patient does absolutely no further cleaning of the tooth surface.

CASE 2

Imagine that you are holding an "interview" of bacteria living in an oral biofilm. How might the bacteria respond to your question about advantages of living in a biofilm?

Evidence in Action

Mr. and Mrs. Jones have been patients in the dental office for several years. Mr. Jones has mild gingivitis while Mrs. Jones has chronic periodontitis that is slowly progressive.

Today you are seeing Mrs. Jones for her 3-month maintenance visit. You show Mrs. Jones areas of her mouth that exhibit increased attachment loss. Mrs. Jones begins to cry and asks: "My husband only comes every 6 months and only gives his teeth a quick brush. I come every 3 months and spend a lot of time on every single day flossing, using that tiny brush (interdental brush) and carefully brushing. You tell me that I have more bone loss and yet, my husband has *NO* bone loss. How can this be?!!"

How would you answer Mrs. Jones?

References

1. Jenkinson HF, Lamont RJ. Oral microbial communities in sickness and in health. *Trends Microbiol.* 2005;13(12):589–595.
2. Paster BJ, Olsen I, Aas JA, et al. The breadth of bacterial diversity in the human periodontal pocket and other oral sites. *Periodontol 2000.* 2006;42:80–87.
3. Wade WG. The oral microbiome in health and disease. *Pharmacol Res.* 2013;69(1):137–143.
4. Eastcott AD, Stallard RE. Sequential changes in developing human dental plaque as visualized by scanning electron microscopy. *J Periodontol.* 1973;44(4):218–224.
5. Lie T. Ultrastructural study of early dental plaque formation. *J Periodontal Res.* 1978;13(5):391–409.
6. Ronstrom A, Attstrom R, Egelberg J. Early formation of dental plaque on plastic films. 1. Light microscopic observations. *J Periodontal Res.* 1975;10(1):28–35.
7. Saxton CA. Scanning electron microscope study of the formation of dental plaque. *Caries Res.* 1973;7(2):102–119.
8. Theilade E, Theilade J, Mikkelsen L. Microbiological studies on early dento-gingival plaque on teeth and Mylar strips in humans. *J Periodontal Res.* 1982;17(1):12–25.
9. Socransky SS, Haffajee AD, Cugini MA, et al. Microbial complexes in subgingival plaque. *J Clin Periodontol.* 1998;25(2):134–144.
10. Bradshaw DJ, Marsh PD, Watson GK, et al. Role of Fusobacterium nucleatum and coaggregation in anaerobe survival in planktonic and biofilm oral microbial communities during aeration. *Infect Immun.* 1998;66(10):4729–4732.
11. Li J, Helmerhorst EJ, Leone CW, et al. Identification of early microbial colonizers in human dental biofilm. *J Appl Microbiol.* 2004;97(6):1311–1318.
12. Alaluusua S, Saarela M, Jousimies-Somer H, et al. Ribotyping shows intrafamilial similarity in Actinobacillus actinomycetemcomitans isolates. *Oral Microbiol Immunol.* 1993;8(4):225–229.
13. DiRienzo JM, Slots J. Genetic approach to the study of epidemiology and pathogenesis of Actinobacillus actinomycetemcomitans in localized juvenile periodontitis. *Arch Oral Biol.* 1990;(35 suppl):79S–84S.

14. Petit MD, van Steenbergen TJ, Scholte LM, et al. Epidemiology and transmission of Porphyromonas gingivalis and Actinobacillus actinomycetemcomitans among children and their family members. A report of 4 surveys. *J Clin Periodontol.* 1993;20(9):641–650.

15. Slots J, Feik D, Rams TE. Actinobacillus actinomycetemcomitans and Bacteroides intermedius in human periodontitis: age relationship and mutual association. *J Clin Periodontol.* 1990;17(9):659–662.

16. Petit MD, van Steenbergen TJ, Timmerman MF, et al. Prevalence of periodontitis and suspected periodontal pathogens in families of adult periodontitis patients. *J Clin Periodontol.* 1994;21(2):76–85.

17. Petit MD, van Winkelhoff AJ, van Steenbergen TJ, et al. Porphyromonas endodontalis: prevalence and distribution of restriction enzyme patterns in families. *Oral Microbiol Immunol.* 1993;8(4):219–224.

18. Elder MJ, Stapleton F, Evans E, et al. Biofilm-related infections in ophthalmology. *Eye.* 1995;9(Pt 1):102–109.

19. Costerton JW, Lewandowski Z, Caldwell DE, et al. Microbial biofilms. *Annu Rev Microbiol.* 1995;49:711–745.

20. Bartold PM, van Dyke TE. Periodontitis: a host-mediated disruption of microbial homeostasis. Unlearning learned concepts. *Periodontol 2000.* 2013;62(1):203–217.

21. Loe H, Theilade E, Jensen SB. Experimental gingivitis in man. *J Periodontol.* 1965;36:177–187.

22. Loesche WJ. Chemotherapy of dental plaque infections. *Oral Sci Rev.* 1976;9:65–107.

23. Theilade E. The non-specific theory in microbial etiology of inflammatory periodontal diseases. *J Clin Periodontol.* 1986;13(10):905–911.

24. Socransky SS, Haffajee AD. Evidence of bacterial etiology: a historical perspective. *Periodontol 2000.* 1994;5:7–25.

25. Marsh PD. Microbial ecology of dental plaque and its significance in health and disease. *Adv Dent Res.* 1994;8(2):263–271.

26. Socransky SS, Haffajee AD. Dental biofilms: difficult therapeutic targets. *Periodontol 2000.* 2002;28:12–55.

27. Mayanagi G, Sato T, Shimauchi H, et al. Detection frequency of periodontitis-associated bacteria by polymerase chain reaction in subgingival and supragingival plaque of periodontitis and healthy subjects. *Oral Microbiol Immunol.* 2004;19(6):379–385.

28. Ximenez-Fyvie LA, Haffajee AD, Socransky SS. Comparison of the microbiota of supra- and subgingival plaque in health and periodontitis. *J Clin Periodontol.* 2000;27(9):648–657.

29. Papapanou PN. Population studies of microbial ecology in periodontal health and disease. *Ann Periodontol.* 2002;7(1):54–61.

30. Curtis MA, Zenobia C, Darveau RP. The relationship of the oral microbiota to periodontal health and disease. *Cell Host Microbe.* 2011;10(4):302–306.

31. Dewhirst FE, Chen T, Izard J, et al. The human oral microbiome. *J Bacteriol.* 2010;192(19):5002–5017.

32. Griffen AL, Beall CJ, Firestone ND, et al. CORE: a phylogenetically-curated 16 S rDNA database of the core oral microbiome. *PLoS One.* 2011;6(4):e19051.

33. Aas JA, Paster BJ, Stokes LN, et al. Defining the normal bacterial flora of the oral cavity. *J Clin Microbiol.* 2005;43(11):5721–5732.

34. Griffen AL, Beall CJ, Campbell JH, et al. Distinct and complex bacterial profiles in human periodontitis and health revealed by 16 S pyrosequencing. *ISME J.* 2012;6(6):1176–1185.

35. Kumar PS, Griffen AL, Moeschberger ML, et al. Identification of candidate periodontal pathogens and beneficial species by quantitative 16 S clonal analysis. *J Clin Microbiol.* 2005;43(8):3944–3955.

36. Kumar PS, Leys EJ, Bryk JM, et al. Changes in periodontal health status are associated with bacterial community shifts as assessed by quantitative 16 S cloning and sequencing. *J Clin Microbiol.* 2006;44(10):3665–3673.

37. Avila M, Ojcius DM, Yilmaz O. The oral microbiota: living with a permanent guest. *DNA Cell Biol.* 2009;28(8):405–411.

38. Hajishengallis G, Lamont RJ. Beyond the red complex and into more complexity: the polymicrobial synergy and dysbiosis (PSD) model of periodontal disease etiology. *Mol Oral Microbiol.* 2012;27(6):409–419.

39. Page RC, Kornman KS. The pathogenesis of human periodontitis: an introduction. *Periodontol 2000.* 1997;14:9–11.

40. Page RC, Schroeder HE. Pathogenesis of inflammatory periodontal disease. A summary of current work. *Lab Invest.* 1976;34(3):235–249.

41. Page RC, Offenbacher S, Schroeder HE, et al. Advances in the pathogenesis of periodontitis: summary of developments, clinical implications and future directions. *Periodontol 2000.* 1997;14:216–248.

42. Darveau RP. The oral microbial consortium's interaction with the periodontal innate defense system. *DNA Cell Biol.* 2009;28(8):389–395.

43. Feng Z, Weinberg A. Role of bacteria in health and disease of periodontal tissues. *Periodontol 2000.* 2006;40:50–76.

44. Hirsch RS, Clarke NG. Infection and periodontal diseases. *Rev Infect Dis.* 1989;11(5):707–715.

45. Christersson LA, Slots J, Zambon JJ, et al. Transmission and colonization of Actinobacillus actinomycetemcomitans in localized juvenile periodontitis patients. *J Periodontol.* 1985;56(3):127–131.

46. Hansen SK, Rainey PB, Haagensen JA, et al. Evolution of species interactions in a biofilm community. *Nature.* 2007;445(7127):533–536.

47. American Academy of Periodontology. *Annals of Periodontology.* Chicago, IL: The Academy; 1996.

 STUDENT ANCILLARY RESOURCES

A wide variety of resources to enhance your learning and understanding of this chapter are available on thePoint®.

- Visit thePoint to access:
  - Audio Glossary
  - Animations
  - Suggested Readings
  - Answers to Review Questions
  - Case Studies

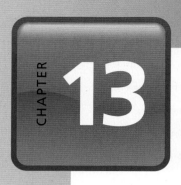

Basic Concepts of Immunity and Inflammation

Clinical Application. Periodontal diseases are in part the result of the body's defense mechanism reacting to a bacterial challenge in the oral cavity. It is critical for healthcare providers caring for patients with periodontal disease to have a basic understanding of immunity and inflammation. This chapter presents a brief outline of this complex topic that can prove invaluable during further study of periodontal diseases and in understanding the fundamental behavior of these diseases.

Learning Objectives

- Define the term immune system and describe its function.
- Describe the role of polymorphonuclear leukocytes, macrophages, B lymphocytes, and T lymphocytes in the immune system.
- Contrast the terms macrophage and monocyte.
- Describe the three ways that antibodies participate in the host defense.
- Define complement system and explain its principle functions in the immune response.
- Describe the steps in the process of phagocytosis.
- Give an example of a type of injury or infection that would result in inflammation in an individual's arm. Describe and contrast the symptoms of inflammation that the individual would experience due to acute inflammation versus chronic inflammation.
- Define the term inflammatory mediator and give several examples of inflammatory mediators of importance in periodontitis.

Key Terms

Immune system
Host
Host response
Leukocyte
Polymorphonuclear leukocytes (PMNs)
Neutrophil
Chemotaxis
Lysosome
Neutropenia
Macrophage

Monocyte
Lymphocyte
B lymphocyte
Antibody
Immunoglobulin
T lymphocyte
Cytokine
Complement system
Membrane attack complex
Opsonization
Endothelium

Transendothelial migration
Phagocytosis
Phagosome
Phagolysosome
Inflammation
Inflammatory biochemical mediator
Chemokines
Acute Inflammation
C-reactive protein (CRP)
Chronic Inflammation

Section 1
The Body's Defense System

Humans are surrounded by millions of microorganisms, many of which may prove to be deadly. Our hands, alone, harbor up to two million microorganisms. The only reason that the human body survives is that it has a protective defense system that is remarkably effective in recognizing and fighting disease-causing microorganisms. The immune system is a complex system that is responsible for defending the body against millions of bacteria, viruses, fungi, toxins, and parasites.

INTRODUCTION TO THE IMMUNE SYSTEM

1. Description
   A. A Complex System of Responses
      1. The immune system is a collection of responses that protects the body against infections by bacteria, viruses, fungi, toxins, and parasites.
      2. Bacteria, viruses, and other disease-causing microorganisms attack the human body over 100 million times a day. For this reason, the human immune system attempts to control quickly the spread of invading microorganisms.
      3. The immune system is composed of two major subdivisions—the innate and adaptive immune systems (Table 13-1) (1).
         a. The innate immune system—which humans are born with—is the first line of defense against invading organisms while the adaptive immune system acts as a second line of defense and also affords protection against reexposure to the same pathogen.
         b. The adaptive immune system—which develops throughout life—requires some time to react to an invading organism, whereas the innate immune system includes defenses that, for the most part, are present and ready to be mobilized upon infection.
         c. The adaptive immune system demonstrates immunological memory. It "remembers" that it has encountered an invading organism and reacts more rapidly on subsequent exposure to the same organism. In contrast, the innate immune system does not demonstrate immunological memory.

TABLE 13-1. INNATE AND ADAPTIVE IMMUNITY	
Innate Immunity	**Adaptive Immunity**
Present at birth	Develops throughout life
Not antigen specific (exposure results in no immunologic memory)	Antigen specific (exposure results in immunologic memory)
Present at all times (immediate response to infection)	Lag time between infection and response (develops in response to infection)
Does not improve with repeated exposure to an infectious agent	Memory develops, which may provide lifelong immunity to reinfection to the same infectious agent

B. **Self Versus Nonself.** When the immune system encounters cells or molecules, it must determine whether these are *self* (part of the body) or foreign substances. Molecules might be harmless substances, such as pollen, or constitute part of a microorganism. Microorganisms, in turn, might be innocuous or pathogenic.

2. **Function**

A. **Prime Purpose**

1. The prime purpose of the human immune system is to defend the life of the individual (**host**) by identifying foreign substances in the body (bacteria, viruses, fungi, or parasites) and developing a defense against them (Fig. 13-1) (1,2).

2. The body recognizes bacteria, viruses, fungi, and parasites as something foreign to itself and ***responds by*** (1) ***sending certain types of cells to the infection site and*** (2) ***producing biochemical substances to counteract the foreign invaders.***

B. The way that an individual's body responds to an infection is known as the **host response.**

3. **Consequences of Loss of Immune Function.** Loss of immune function is deadly to the body. An example is the human immunodeficiency virus (HIV), the virus that causes acquired immune deficiency syndrome (AIDS). HIV disables a specific group of immune system cells responsible for coordinating immune responses. People infected with HIV may develop infections from microorganisms that rarely cause infection in individuals with normal, healthy immune systems.

4. **Consequences of an Overzealous Immune Response.** The immune system can sometimes become confused or so intense in its response ***that it begins to harm the body it is trying to protect***. Rheumatic heart disease is an example of a confused immune response to infection. The problem begins as an infection of the skin or pharynx with streptococcal bacteria. Unfortunately, there are similarities between certain molecules of the streptococcal bacteria and molecules of human heart tissue. As a result of this molecular similarity, immune responses against the streptococcal bacteria also attack and damage the heart tissue of the infected individual.

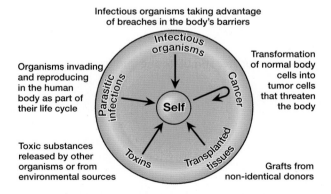

Figure 13-1. The Immune Defense System. The immune system defends the body against invading microorganisms, as well as toxins in the environment. This includes protection against infectious organisms, parasitic infections, toxins, and cancerous cells. Unfortunately, cells of transplanted tissues are recognized as "nonself" or invaders. For this reason, strong drugs are needed to keep the body's immune system from rejecting a transplant.

COMPONENTS OF THE IMMUNE SYSTEM

Components of the immune system that play an important role in combating periodontal disease are the (1) cellular defenders (phagocytes, lymphocytes) and (2) the complement system (Fig. 13-2A–F in Table 13-2) (1,2).

TABLE 13-2. SUMMARY: COMPONENTS OF THE IMMUNE SYSTEM	
Component	**Function**
Polymorphonuclear leukocyte (PMN) **Figure 13-2A**	• Phagocytosis • Release of lysosomes • Release of powerful regulatory proteins (cytokines) that signal the immune system to send additional phagocytic cells to the site of an infection
Macrophage **Figure 13-2B**	• Phagocytosis • Release of lysosomes • Release of powerful regulatory proteins (cytokines) that signal the immune system to send additional phagocytic cells to the site of an infection
B-lymphocyte/ Plasma cell **Figure 13-2C**	• Production of immunoglobulins
T-lymphocytes **Figure 13-2D**	• Further stimulate the immune response
Immunoglobulins IgG, IgM, IgA, IgD, IgE **Figure 13-2E**	• Neutralize bacteria or bacterial toxins • Coat bacteria to facilitate phagocytosis • Activate the complement system
Complement system **Figure 13-2F**	• Lysis of cell membranes of certain bacteria • Phagocytosis • Recruitment of additional phagocytic cells to the infection site and clearance of immune complexes from circulation

CELLS OF THE IMMUNE SYSTEM

1. **Leukocytes.** Leukocytes are white blood cells that act much like independent single-cell organisms able to move and capture microorganisms on their own (Fig. 13-3).

   A. **Polymorphonuclear leukocytes.** Polymorphonuclear leukocytes (PMNs) are phagocytes that play a vital role in combating the bacteria in plaque biofilms (Fig. 13-4).

      1. PMNs, also known as **neutrophils**, are phagocytic cells that actively engulf and destroy microorganisms.
      2. These cells are the *rapid responders* and provide the first line of defense against many common microorganisms and are essential for the control of bacterial infections.
      3. Once in the blood stream, PMNs can move through capillary walls and into the tissue. PMNs are attracted to bacteria by a process called **chemotaxis**.
      4. The cytoplasm of a PMN contains many granules filled with strong bactericidal and digestive enzymes. These granules (called **lysosomes**) can kill and digest bacterial cells after phagocytosis.
      5. PMNs are *short-lived cells* that die when they become engorged with the bacteria they phagocytize. The pus formed at sites of inflammation contains many dead and dying PMNs. PMNs have a short life span, generally less than 1 day.
      6. The bacteria associated with periodontal disease are most effectively phagocytized by PMNs.
      7. Normally, each milliliter of blood contains between 3,000 and 6,000 PMNs. A PMN count of less than 1,000 cells/mL is called **neutropenia** and indicates an increased risk of infection.

   B. **Monocytes/Macrophages.** Macrophages are large phagocytes with one kidney-shaped nucleus and some granules (Figs. 13-5 and 13-6).

      1. These leukocytes are called **monocytes** when found in the bloodstream and macrophages when they are located in the tissues.

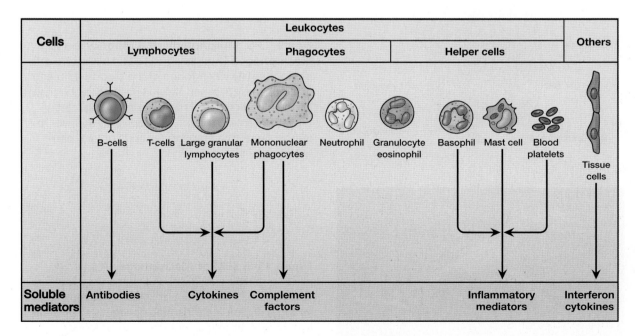

Figure 13-3. Cells and Chemical Mediators of the Immune System. Immune system cells and the chemical mediators are closely related since the cells produce most of the mediators.

2. Macrophages are highly phagocytic cells that actively engulf and destroy microorganisms. Macrophages contain a few lysosomes that are filled with bactericidal and digestive enzymes.

3. Macrophages are slower to arrive at the infection site than PMNs. The **slower, long-lived** macrophages are often the most numerous cells in chronic inflammation.

4. Macrophages present antigen to T cells. Together macrophages and T lymphocytes play an important role in chronic inflammation.

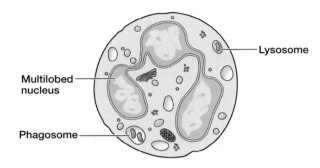

Figure 13-4. Morphology of a Polymorphonuclear Leukocyte. PMNs contain granules called lysosomes that are used to digest bacteria.

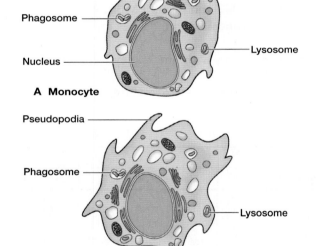

Figure 13-5. Morphology of a Monocyte and a Macrophage. These phagocytic leukocytes are called monocytes **(A)** when found in the bloodstream and macrophages **(B)** when they are located in the tissues. Of the blood cells, macrophages are the largest—thus, the name "macro." Macrophages are five- to tenfold larger than monocytes and contain more lysosomes.

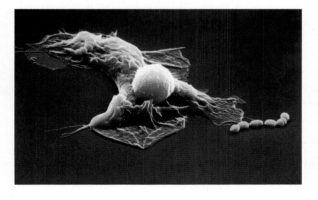

Figure 13-6. SEM of Macrophage. A scanning electron micrograph (SEM) of a human macrophage (*gray*) approaches a chain of Streptococcus pyogenes (*orange*). Riding atop the macrophage is a spherical lymphocyte. Both macrophages and lymphocytes are important in eliminating infection.
(SEM courtesy of Cells Alive.)

2. **Lymphocytes.** Lymphocytes are small white blood cells that play an important role in recognizing and controlling foreign invaders. The two main types of lymphocytes that are important in defense against the bacteria in plaque biofilm are B lymphocytes (B cells) and T lymphocytes (T cells).
A. B Lymphocytes
   1. Description
      a. B lymphocytes are small leukocytes that help in the defense against bacteria, viruses, and fungi.
      b. B lymphocytes can further differentiate into one of the two types of B cells: plasma B cells and memory B cells.
      c. The principal functions of B lymphocytes are to **make antibodies.** Once a B cell has been activated, it manufactures millions of antibodies and pours them into the bloodstream (Fig. 13-7).
   2. Antibodies
      a. Antibodies are Y-shaped proteins. One end of the Y binds to the outside of the B cell. The other end binds to a microorganism and helps to kill it.
      b. Antibodies are known collectively as **immunoglobulins.** The five major classes of immunoglobulin are immunoglobulin M (IgM), immunoglobulin D (IgD), immunoglobulin G (IgG), immunoglobulin A (IgA), and immunoglobulin E (IgE).
      c. Antibodies participate in host defense in three main ways:
         1. Neutralize bacteria or bacterial toxins to prevent bacteria from destroying host cells.
         2. Coat bacteria making them more susceptible to phagocytosis.
         3. Activate the complement system.
B. T lymphocytes
   1. T lymphocytes are small leukocytes whose main function is to intensify the response of other immune cells—such as B lymphocytes and macrophages—to the bacterial invasion.
   2. T cells can produce substances called cytokines, such as the interleukins (ILs), that further stimulate the immune response. Cytokine is a general name for any protein that is secreted by cells and affects the behavior of nearby cells.

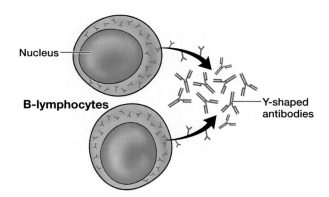

Figure 13-7. B lymphocytes. Diagram of a B cell showing the Y-shaped antibody protein attached to the cell wall.

THE COMPLEMENT SYSTEM

In addition to the cellular defenders, the other major component of the immune response is the complement system. The cellular defenders only respond after they encounter a microorganism. Pathogens, however, can avoid contact with the immune cells. If this happens, the complement system provides a second means of defense.

1. **Definition.** The **complement system** is a complex series of proteins circulating in the blood that works to facilitate phagocytosis or kill bacteria directly by puncturing bacterial cell membranes. The complement proteins are activated by and work with (complement) the antibodies, hence the name.

2. **Three Principal Functions of Complement.** After activation, the complement proteins interact, in a highly regulated cascade, to carry out a number of defensive functions (Fig. 13-8):

   A. **Destruction of Pathogens.** Components of complement can destroy certain microorganisms directly by forming pores in their cell membranes. To accomplish this task, the complement system creates a protein unit called the **membrane attack complex** that is capable of puncturing the cell membranes of certain bacteria (lysis).

   B. **Opsonization of Pathogens.** The complement system facilitates the engulfment and destruction of microorganisms by phagocytes. This process, known as **opsonization** of pathogens, is the most important action of the complement system. Complement components coat the surface of the bacterium allowing the phagocytes to recognize, engulf, and destroy the bacterium.

   C. **Recruitment of Phagocytes.** The complement system recruits additional phagocytic cells to the site of the infection.

   D. **Immune Clearance.** Finally, the complement system performs a "housekeeping" function, the removal of immune complexes from circulation.

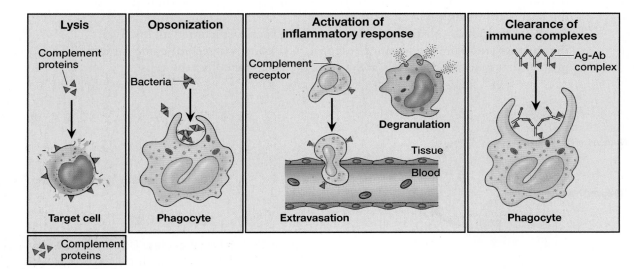

Figure 13-8. Activities of the Complement System. In this diagram, complement proteins are represented by small red triangles. Complement proteins facilitate a number of immune activities: puncturing the cell membranes of certain bacteria (lysis), phagocytosis of bacteria (opsonization), further activation of the inflammatory response by recruitment of additional phagocytic cells to the infection site, and clearance of immune complexes from circulation.

Section 2
Leukocyte Migration, Chemotaxis, and Phagocytosis

1. Leukocyte Migration from the Blood Vessels
   A. Transendothelial Migration
      1. In order to fight an infection, the cells of the immune system travel through the bloodstream and into the tissues (Fig. 13-9).
         a. Near the infection site, the immune cells push their way between the endothelial cells lining the blood vessels (extravasation) and enter the connective tissue (3).
         b. The thin layer of epithelial cells that line the interior surface of the blood vessels is called the endothelium. For this reason, the process of immune cells exiting the vessels and entering the tissues is called transendothelial migration.
      2. Defects in transendothelial migration are associated with aggressive periodontitis underscoring the importance of this process in the defense against the bacteria found in plaque biofilms.
   B. Leukocyte Migration to the Infection Site
      1. Once the leukocytes enter the connective tissue, the cells must migrate to the site of the infection.
      2. Chemotaxis is the process whereby leukocytes are attracted to the infection site in response to biochemical compounds released by the invading microorganisms.

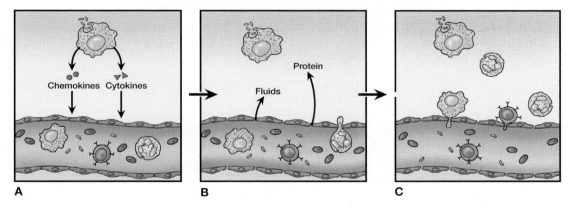

Figure 13-9. Leukocyte Migration to Connective Tissue. A: Leukocytes travel through the bloodstream to the site of infection. **B:** Leukocytes squeeze between the cells of the blood vessel wall. **C:** Leukocytes enter the connective tissue and are attracted to the invading bacteria.

2. Phagocytosis
   A. Description. Phagocytosis is the process by which leukocytes engulf and digest microorganisms (4).
      1. Steps in Phagocytosis
         a. First, the external cell wall of a phagocytic cell (such as a neutrophil or macrophage) adheres to the bacterium (Fig. 13-10). The phagocytic cell extends finger-like projections (pseudopodia) that surround the bacterium.
         b. Next, a phagocytic vesicle called a phagosome surrounds the bacterium.
         c. Lysosome granules fuse with the vesicle to form a phagolysosome.
         d. The bacterium is digested within the phagolysosome.
         e. Finally, the phagocytic cell discharges the contents of the phagolysosome into the surrounding tissue.

2. **Local Tissue Destruction from Phagocytosis**
   a. Lysosomal enzymes and other microbial products are released from a leukocyte after phagocytosis or when the leukocyte dies.
   b. Once released the lysosomal enzymes cause damage to tissue cells in the same manner that they destroy bacteria.

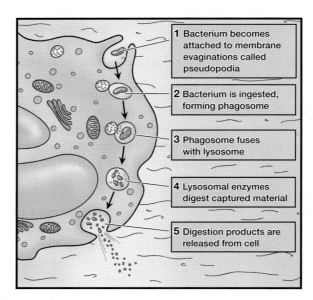

Figure 13-10. Phagocytosis. The steps involved in phagocytosis, the process by which leukocytes engulf and digest microorganisms.

Section 3
The Inflammatory Process

Inflammation is the body's reaction to injury or invasion by disease-producing organisms. The inflammatory response focuses on host defense components at the site of the infection to eliminate microorganisms and heal damaged tissue. Inflammation is part of the immune response. It is a process that depends both on the physical actions of leukocytes and the biochemical compounds that these cells produce (1,2).

MAJOR EVENTS IN THE INFLAMMATORY RESPONSE

1. The inflammatory response is triggered by the invasion of pathogens or tissue injury.
2. Immediately, mast cells (located in the connective tissues near to blood vessels) release chemicals that dilate the capillaries and increase vascular permeability (Fig. 13-11).
3. Minutes after tissue injury, there is an increase in blood flow to the area. Higher blood volume heats the tissue and causes it to redden. This increased blood flow is needed to deliver immune "cellular defenders" to the site.
4. Within hours, leukocytes pass through the walls of capillaries into the connective tissue. Plasma proteins leak from the capillaries and accumulate in the tissues.
5. The leukocytes phagocytose invading pathogens and release inflammatory mediators that contribute to the inflammatory response.
   A. **Inflammatory biochemical mediators** are biologically active compounds secreted by cells that activate the body's inflammatory response.
   B. Inflammatory mediators of importance in periodontitis are the cytokines, prostaglandins, and matrix metalloproteinases.
      1. Leukocytes secrete cytokines that play a major role in regulating the behavior of immune cells.
      2. Chemokines, a major subgroup of cytokines, cause additional immune cells to be attracted to the site of infection or injury (5).

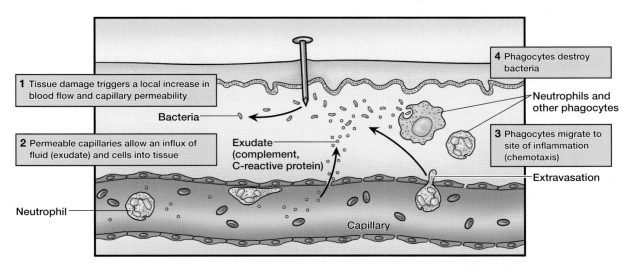

Figure 13-11. Inflammatory Response. In this illustration, bacteria have entered the body through a wound created by a nail puncture. The entry of bacteria initiates an inflammatory response that begins with the release of chemical substances that attract phagocytic cells to the site of the bacterial invasion.

TWO STAGES OF INFLAMMATION

1. Acute Inflammation
   A. Description
      1. **Acute inflammation** is a short-term, normal process that protects and heals the body following physical injury or infection (Fig. 13-12).
      2. In the absence of inflammation, wounds and infections would never heal and the progressive tissue destruction would threaten the life of the individual.
      3. The acute inflammatory process is achieved by the increased movement of plasma and leukocytes from the blood into the injured tissues.

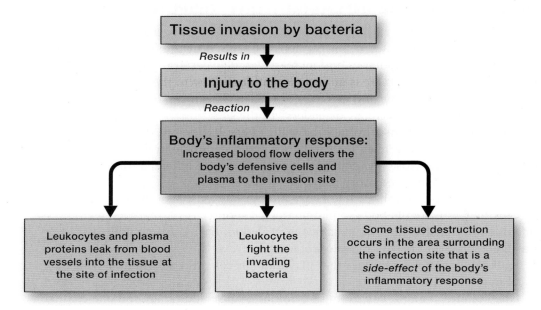

Figure 13-12. Major Events in the Body's Inflammatory Response. Inflammation is the body's response to injury or invasion by disease-producing organisms. This response focuses on the body's defense mechanisms at the site of an injury or infection.

   B. **Five Classic Symptoms of Acute Inflammation.** To inflame means "to set on fire," which makes us think of red, heat, and pain. Clinically, there are five classic symptoms of acute inflammation (Box 13-1, Fig. 13-13) at the site of infection or injury:
      1. **Heat**—a localized rise in temperature due to an increased amount of blood at the site.
      2. **Redness**—the result of increased blood in the area
      3. **Swelling**—the result of the accumulation of fluid at the site. The leukocytes and plasma that collect at the site cause the swelling (edema) associated with inflammation.
      4. **Pain**—the result of pressure from edema in the tissue. The excess fluid in the tissues puts pressure on sensitive nerve endings, causing pain.
      5. **Loss of function**—the result of swelling and pain. For example, inflammation of a finger (swelling and pain) would cause you to favor that finger and not use it in a normal manner.

Box 13-1. Everyday Example of Acute Inflammation

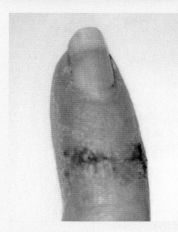

Figure 13-13.

Callie L sustained a deep cut to her little finger. She applied an antiseptic cream and covered the wound with an adhesive bandage. A few hours later, the injured finger is quite painful. When Callie applies pressure to the area near the wound, it feels warm and the pressure of her touch is quite painful. The finger looks red and swollen.

What is the source of the redness?
The redness is due to increased blood flow at the injury site.

What is the primary source of the swelling?
The primary source of the swelling is caused by the entry of fluid into the connective tissue. Cells entering the connective tissue also contribute to the swelling.

What is the cause of the warmth?
The warmth of an inflamed area results from increased blood flow to the area that brings with it the warmth.

C. The Acute Inflammatory Process
1. **Description.** The process of acute inflammation is initiated by the blood vessels, near the injured tissue, which alter to allow the release of plasma proteins and leukocytes into the surrounding tissue.
2. PMNs are the first leukocytes to arrive at the injured site.
   a. These cells phagocytose and kill invading microorganisms through the release of nonspecific toxins. These nonspecific toxins kill pathogens as well as adjacent host cells, sick and healthy alike.
   b. The PMNs release cytokines, including IL and tumor necrosis factor (TNF).
   c. Such inflammatory cytokines, in turn, induce the liver to synthesize various plasma proteins called acute phase reactant proteins.
      1. The liver produces **C-reactive protein (CRP)**, a type of acute phase protein, during episodes of acute inflammation. The levels of CRP increase up to 50,000-fold in acute inflammation.
      2. Periodontitis, as well as other systemic diseases—diabetes, hypertension, and cardiovascular disease—are associated with elevated levels of CRP (6,7).
      3. *A study published in the Journal of Periodontology, reports that the inflammatory effects from periodontal disease cause oral bacterial by-products to enter the bloodstream and trigger the liver to make CRP that inflames the arteries and promotes blood clot formation* (8).
3. PMNs are short lived and so are primarily involved in the early stages of inflammation.
4. If the body succeeds in eliminating all microorganisms, the tissue will heal and the inflammation will cease.
5. Inflammation is the body's first line of defense against injury and infection, but it's a double-edged sword. If the acute inflammatory responses are not effective in controlling the invading microorganisms, the inflammatory response becomes chronic (Fig. 13-14).

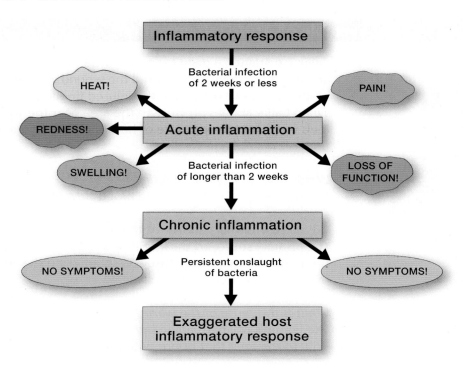

Figure 13-14. Two Stages of Inflammation. Acute inflammation is of short duration, whereas chronic inflammation is a long-lived inflammatory response.

2. Chronic inflammation
   A. Description
      1. **Chronic inflammation** is a long-lived, **out-of-control** inflammatory response that continues for more than a few weeks.
         a. It is a pathological condition characterized by active inflammation, tissue destruction, and attempts at repair.
         b. *The warning signs of acute inflammation are absent in chronic inflammation—such as periodontitis—and the problem may go unnoticed by the host (patient). Clinically, pain often is absent.*
      2. The inflammatory response has one all-important goal: respond immediately to destroy infectious microorganisms in the damaged tissue before they can spread to other areas of the body.
         a. Chronic inflammation occurs when the body is unable to eliminate the infection. In this stage, the invading microorganisms are persistent and stimulate an exaggerated response by the host's immune system.
         b. In its zeal to protect the body, the inflammatory response will destroy as much tissue as necessary to accomplish this goal.
         c. *In cases where inflammation becomes chronic, the inflammation can become so intense that it inflicts permanent damage to the body tissues.* This is the case in periodontitis.
   B. The Chronic Inflammatory Process
      1. The accumulation of macrophages characterizes chronic inflammation.
      2. Macrophages engulf and digest microorganisms.
      3. Leukocytes release several different inflammatory mediators, including IL-1, TNF-alpha, and prostaglandins that perpetuate the inflammatory response (Fig. 13-15).

a. One of the principle cytokines secreted by macrophages is TNF-alpha (9). Evidence indicates that TNF-alpha contributes to the tissue destruction that characterizes chronic inflammation (Table 13-3).

b. In fact, *tissue damage is the hallmark of chronic inflammation*.

4. If the infection persists, inflammation can last months or even years.

5. Chronic inflammation is abnormal and does not benefit the body. *Chronic inflammation is an out-of-control response that can destroy healthy tissue and cause more damage than the original problem.*

a. Left unchecked, a hyperactive inflammatory response can even start attacking healthy tissue.

b. Chronic inflammation is associated with a number of disease states, including asthma, rheumatoid arthritis, diabetes, atherosclerosis, gingivitis, and periodontitis.

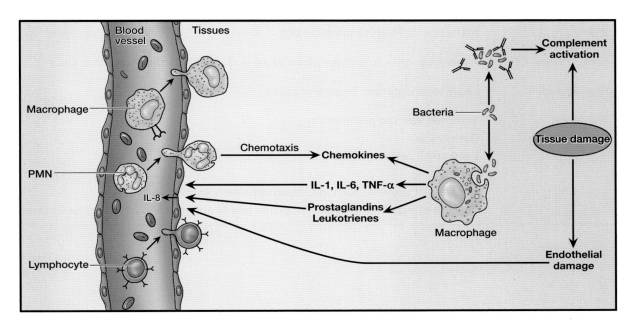

Figure 13-15. Cellular Defenders and Mediators in Inflammatory Response. The three primary cells involved in the inflammatory response are the polymorphonuclear leukocytes (PMNs), macrophages, and lymphocytes. The first of these cells to migrate into the tissues are the PMNs, followed by macrophages, and then the lymphocytes. In addition, this illustration shows some of the many chemical mediators that play a part in the inflammatory response. These include chemokines, IL-1, IL-6, TNF-alpha, prostaglandins, and leukotrienes.

TABLE 13-3. INFLAMMATORY BIOCHEMICAL MEDIATORS

Name	Effects
IL-1	Increased vascular permeability T cell and B cell activation Fever Synthesis of proteins, such as C-reactive protein, by liver
IL-6	Increased vascular permeability T cell and B cell activation Increased immunoglobulin synthesis Fever Synthesis of proteins, such as C-reactive protein, by liver
IL-8	Attraction of PMNs to infection site
Leukotrienes	Allow leukocytes to exit the blood vessel and move into the connective tissue
Prostaglandins	Cause vasodilatation, fever, and pain
TNF-alpha	Increased vascular permeability Chemotaxis T cell and B cell activation Fever Synthesis of proteins, such as C-reactive protein, by liver Systemic effects of inflammation such as loss of appetite and increased heart rate

Chapter Summary Statement

The immune system is a collection of responses that is responsible for defending the body against millions of bacteria, viruses, fungi, toxins, and parasites. The prime purpose of the human immune system is to defend the life of the individual (host) by identifying foreign substances and developing a defense against them. The way that an individual's body responds to infection is known as the host response. Without an effective immune system, human beings would not survive.

Components of the immune system that play an important role in combating periodontal disease are the cellular defenders and the complement system. In order to fight an infection, immune cells travel through the bloodstream and into the tissues (transendothelial migration). The process whereby leukocytes are attracted to the infection site in response to the invading microorganisms is known as chemotaxis. Phagocytosis is the process by which leukocytes engulf and digest microorganisms.

Inflammation is the body's reaction to injury or invasion by disease-producing organisms. The inflammatory response focuses on host immune components at the site of an infection to eliminate microorganisms and heal damaged tissue. It relies on both the physical actions of leukocytes and the biochemical compounds that these cells produce. Acute inflammation is a short-term, normal process that protects and heals the body. Chronic inflammation is a long-lived, out-of-control response that continues for more than a few weeks. In chronic inflammation, the immune system response can sometimes become so intense that it begins to harm the body that it is trying to protect. Tissue damage is the hallmark of chronic inflammation.

Periodontal disease is a bacterial infection that induces an inflammatory response in the periodontal tissues. Chapter 14 focuses on the host immune response in periodontal disease.

Section 4
Focus on Patients

Evidence in Action

CASE 1
You accidentally injure your arm by accidentally stabbing it with an ice pick. Within minutes following the injury, you note some changes in the tissues in the area of the injury. What changes in the tissues should you expect if your body responds with a typical inflammatory response?

CASE 2
A new patient in your office reports a history of rheumatic heart disease at a very early age on her health questionnaire. The patient explains that her physician at the time thought that the rheumatic heart disease was a result of a streptococcal skin infection that she developed a few months prior to the discovery of the heart disease, but the physician did not explain any of the details of these conditions to her. Explain how an infection of the skin could result in damage to the heart tissue.

References

1. Janeway C, Murphy KP, Travers P, et al. *Janeway's Immunobiology.* 7th ed. New York: Garland Science; 2008: p.xxi, 887.
2. Paul WE. *Fundamental Immunology.* 6th ed. Philadelphia, PA: Wolters Kluwer Health/Lippincott Williams & Wilkins; 2008. xviii, 1603.
3. Marshall D, Haskard DO. Clinical overview of leukocyte adhesion and migration: where are we now? *Semin Immunol.* 2002;14(2):133–140.
4. Greenberg S, Grinstein S. Phagocytosis and innate immunity. *Curr Opin Immunol.* 2002;14(1):136–145.
5. Van Haastert PJ, Devreotes PN. Chemotaxis: signalling the way forward. *Nat Rev Mol Cell Biol.* 2004;5(8):626–634.
6. Fitzsimmons TR, Sanders AE, Bartold PM, et al. Local and systemic biomarkers in gingival crevicular fluid increase odds of periodontitis. *J Clin Periodontol.* 2010;37(1):30–36.
7. Megson E, Fitzsimmons T, Dharmapatni K, et al. C-reactive protein in gingival crevicular fluid may be indicative of systemic inflammation. *J Clin Periodontol.* 2010;37(9):797–804.
8. Noack B, Genco RJ, Trevisan M, et al. Periodontal infections contribute to elevated systemic C-reactive protein level. *J Periodontol.* 2001;72(9):1221–1227.
9. Tieri P, Valensin S, Latora V, et al. Quantifying the relevance of different mediators in the human immune cell network. *Bioinformatics.* 2005;21(8):1639–1643.

 STUDENT ANCILLARY RESOURCES

A wide variety of resources to enhance your learning and understanding of this chapter are available on thePoint.

- Visit thePoint to access:
  - Audio Glossary
  - Animations
  - Suggested Readings
  - Answers to Review Questions
  - Case Studies

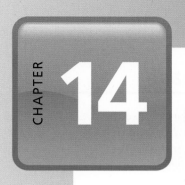
Host Immune Response to Plaque Biofilm

Clinical Application.   Members of the dental team will encounter many, many patients with gingivitis and periodontitis. Recognizing the clinical features of these conditions will become second nature to all clinicians. However, understanding the underlying body defense mechanisms that can both help protect patients and do damage to the periodontium will not always be so straightforward. This chapter focuses on the host response to plaque biofilm and the tissue destruction that ensues when bacteria present in plaque biofilm elicit a response in the host.

Learning Objectives

- Define the term host response and explain its primary function.
- Name factors that can enhance the microbial challenge to the periodontium.
- Define the term biochemical mediator and name three types of mediators.
- Describe the potential role of cytokines in the pathogenesis of periodontitis.
- Describe the potential role of prostaglandins in the pathogenesis of periodontitis.
- Describe the effect of increased levels of MMPs on periodontal tissues.
- Name three factors that can affect host immune response.
- For each of the histologic stages of gingivitis and periodontitis listed below name one change in the host immune response likely to be encountered:

  ✓ Bacterial Accumulation   ✓ Established Gingivitis

  ✓ Early Gingivitis   ✓ Periodontitis

Key Terms

Host response
Host
Virulence factor
Biochemical mediators

Cytokines
Prostaglandins
Prostaglandins of the E series
   (PGE)

Matrix metalloproteinases
   (MMPs)

Section 1
The Host Response in Periodontal Disease

Periodontal disease is a bacterial infection that induces an inflammatory response in the periodontal tissues (1–3). For the progression of disease from health to gingivitis to periodontitis, pathogenic bacteria must be present. Research findings indicate that although bacteria are essential for disease to occur, the presence of suspected periodontal pathogens alone is insufficient to cause the tissue destruction seen in periodontitis. Rather, it appears to be the body's response to the bacteria present in plaque biofilm that is the cause of nearly all the destruction seen in periodontal disease (1,3–8).

The body's response to bacteria is referred to as the **host response**. The prime purpose of the host response is to defend the life of the individual (i.e., the **host**). In the instance of periodontal disease, the immune system strives to defend the body against bacteria present in plaque biofilm. The body's defenses are activated to eliminate the potential pathogens and limit the spread of infection, not actually to preserve the tooth or its supporting periodontal tissues.

FACTORS ENHANCING THE MICROBIAL CHALLENGE

The presence of bacteria is essential for the initiation and progression of periodontal disease. It is known that bacteria can activate the human immune and inflammatory system, which can subsequently lead to damage of the periodontium (1,2). The term **virulence factor** refers to all of the mechanisms that enable biofilm bacteria to colonize and damage the tissues of the periodontium. Virulence factors may be either structural characteristics of the bacteria themselves or substances that are produced by the bacteria. The primary bacterial virulence factors that can enhance damage to the periodontium are:

1. **The presence of lipopolysaccharide (LPS):** Gram-negative bacteria are a component of mature plaque biofilm. LPS is an endotoxin that is present on the outer membrane of Gram-negative bacteria. LPS can be responsible for initiating inflammation in periodontal tissues.
2. **The ability to invade tissues:** Some of the periodontal bacteria—such as *Porphyromonas gingivalis* and *Aggregatibacter actinomycetemcomitans*—can invade host tissues. Penetration of tissues can to some degree allow the bacteria to escape host defense mechanisms.
3. **The ability to produce enzymes:** Several periodontal bacteria can produce enzymes such as collagenases and proteases that can directly degrade host proteins that are a basic part of the structure of the periodontium.

When pathogenic bacteria successfully infect the periodontium, the body responds by mobilizing defensive immune cells and releasing a series of biochemical mediators to combat the bacteria. Cells involved in immune and inflammatory processes include inflammatory cells, polymorphonuclear neutrophils (PMNs), antigen-presenting cells (macrophages and Langerhans cells), T and B lymphocytes, fibroblasts, and epithelial cells. These cellular components of the immune and inflammatory processes were discussed in Chapter 13.

INFLAMMATORY BIOCHEMICAL MEDIATORS

In response to a microbial challenge, host immune cells secrete biologically active compounds called **biochemical mediators**. These biochemical mediators are the "middlemen" sent by the host cells to activate the inflammatory response. Biochemical mediators of importance in periodontitis are cytokines, prostaglandins, and MMPs (Table 14-1).

1. Cytokines. Cytokines are powerful regulatory proteins released by host immune cells that influence the behavior of other cells. The cytokine (literally "cell protein") is a molecule that transmits information or signals from one cell to another. When released by host cells, cytokines signal the immune system to send additional phagocytic cells to the site of an infection.
   A. **Sources of Cytokines.** Many different cells including PMNs, macrophages, B lymphocytes, epithelial cells, gingival fibroblasts, and osteoblasts can produce cytokines in response to the bacterial challenge or in response to tissue injury.
   B. **Functions of Cytokines**
      1. Cytokines can recruit cells such as PMNs and macrophages to the infection site.
      2. Cytokines can increase vascular permeability allowing immune cells and complement to move into the tissues at the infection site.
      3. *Cytokines have the potential to initiate tissue destruction and bone loss in chronic inflammatory diseases, such as periodontitis.*
      4. Cytokines that play an important role in periodontitis include interleukin-1 (IL-1), interleukin-6 (IL-6), interleukin-8 (IL-8), and tumor necrosis factor-α (TNF-α) (5,9).
2. Prostaglandins. **Prostaglandins** are a group of powerful biochemical mediators derived from fatty acids. Biologically important prostaglandins are prostaglandin D, E, F, G, H, and I. **Prostaglandins of the E series (PGE) play an important role in the bone destruction seen in periodontitis.**
   A. **Sources of Prostaglandins.** Most cells can produce prostaglandins, but PMNs and macrophages are particularly important sources. The major source of PGE in inflamed periodontal tissues is the macrophage, although PMNs and gingival fibroblasts also produce them.
   B. **Functions of Prostaglandins**
      1. Prostaglandins can increase the permeability and dilation of the blood vessels, leading to redness and edema of the connective tissue.
      2. Prostaglandins can trigger osteoclasts (i.e., bone-resorbing cells) to destroy alveolar bone.
      3. Prostaglandins can promote the overproduction of destructive MMP enzymes.
      4. *Prostaglandins initiate most of the alveolar bone destruction in periodontitis.*
3. Matrix Metalloproteinases. **Matrix metalloproteinases (MMPs)** are a family of at least 12 different enzymes produced by various cells of the body. These enzymes can act together to break down the connective tissue matrix.
   A. **Sources of MMPs.** PMNs, macrophages, gingival fibroblasts, and junctional epithelial cells can produce MMPs. PMNs and gingival fibroblasts are the major source of MMPs in periodontitis.
   B. **Functions of MMPs**
      1. **MMPs Effects in Health.** In the absence of disease, MMPs facilitate the normal turnover of the periodontal connective tissue matrix.
      2. **MMPs Effects in Chronic Infection and Inflammation**

a. In the presence of chronic bacterial infection, large amounts of MMPs are released in what appears to be an attempt to kill the invading bacteria.

b. This overproduction of MMPs results in the enhanced breakdown of the connective tissue of the periodontium.

c. *In the presence of increased MMP levels, extensive collagen destruction occurs in the periodontal tissues.* It should be noted that collagen provides the structural framework of all periodontal tissues. Without collagen, the tissues of the gingiva, periodontal ligament, and supporting alveolar bone degrade, resulting in gingival recession, pocket formation, periodontal attachment loss, and tooth mobility.

TABLE 14-1. TISSUE DESTRUCTION BY BIOCHEMICAL MEDIATORS IN PERIODONTITIS

Mediators	Local Effects
Cytokine IL-1	Stimulates osteoclast activity resulting in bone resorption (5,10–12) Induces breakdown of collagen matrix in gingiva, periodontal ligament, and alveolar bone (10,13)
Cytokine IL-6	Stimulates bone resorption (5,14) Inhibits bone formation (5,15)
Cytokine IL-8	Stimulates connective tissue destruction (5,16) Stimulates bone resorption (5,11,17,18)
Cytokine TNF-α	Stimulates bone resorption (5,12) Induces breakdown of collagen matrix in gingiva, periodontal ligament, and alveolar bone (5,12)
Prostaglandin E_2	Stimulates MMP secretion (8,19) Stimulates bone resorption (12,20–22)
MMP Enzymes	Induce breakdown of collagen matrix in gingiva, periodontal ligament, and alveolar bone (13,23)

FACTORS AFFECTING THE HOST IMMUNE RESPONSE

Certain factors may have an effect on the host's susceptibility to periodontal disease by modifying the host response or modifying tissue metabolism (24,25). These factors include: genetic factors, environmental factors, and acquired factors—all of which can play important roles in periodontal disease pathogenesis (Fig. 14-1).

1. **Genetic Factors.** Genetic factors appear to contribute to periodontal disease. Studies in twins and families reported an association between periodontal disease and genetic factors (26). Diseases with genetic origin such as Papillon Lefevre Syndrome

or leucocyte adhesion deficiency (LAD) are associated with aggressive type of periodontal diseases. Also, variations in the genes controlling the formation of biochemical mediators can modify the immune response to the plaque biofilm enough to increase the susceptibility to periodontal disease (27–30).

2. **Environmental Factors.** Tobacco smoking is a known risk factor for periodontal diseases. It has a significant effect on the immune and inflammatory system. Smoking has been shown to decrease PMN phagocytic capacity, decrease vascularity of gingival tissues, and affect both T- and B lymphocyte response to periodontal pathogens (31–35).

3. **Acquired Factors.** Diabetes mellitus is a known risk factor for periodontal diseases and its progression (36–40). Diabetes mellitus affects the host response by reducing PMN function, increasing IL-1, TNF-α, and PGE$_2$ levels in gingival crevicular fluid and reducing growth and proliferation of periodontal ligament fibroblasts and osteoblasts in periodontium (25).

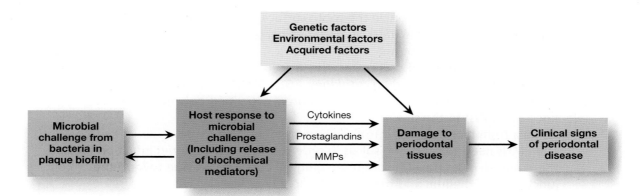

Figure 14-1. Theory of Pathogenesis. Periodontal disease may be the result of an imbalance between the microbial biofilm challenge and the resulting host response. The host response increases numbers of polymorphonuclear neutrophils (PMNs), produces cytokines, prostaglandins, and matrix metalloproteinases (MMPs) that mediate the destruction of connective tissue and alveolar bone.

Section 2
The Immune Response and Periodontitis

HISTOLOGIC STAGES IN DEVELOPMENT OF PERIODONTAL DISEASE

Researchers Page and Schroeder conducted the classic, landmark research on the histologic development of gingivitis and periodontitis (8,41,42). They described four distinct histologic stages in the development of periodontal disease: *initial lesion, early lesion, established lesion, and advanced lesion*. For clarity these terms appear in the discussion below, but more is understood today about the host immune response related to these stages than when these researchers initially published their descriptions (Boxes 14-1 to 14-4 and Figs. 14-2 to 14-5).

Box 14-1. Bacterial Accumulation (*Initial Lesion*) (Fig. 14-2)

1. **Bacterial Features.** Bacteria colonize the tooth surface near the gingival margin.
2. **Cellular Features.** The presence of Gram-negative bacteria and their metabolic products initiates the host immune response.
   A. In response to the bacterial pathogens, the junctional epithelial cells release various biochemical mediators, including **cytokines, PGE$_2$, MMPs,** and **TNF-α**.
   B. These mediators stimulate the immune response, recruiting polymorphonuclear leukocytes (PMNs) to the site.
   C. PMNs pass from blood vessels into the gingival connective tissue.
      1. The PMNs need to reach the sulcus in order to fight the bacterial infection located there and so must travel through the gingival connective tissue toward the junctional epithelium and the gingival sulcus.
      2. As they pass into the gingival connective tissue the PMNs release cytokines. ***Cytokines released by the PMNs destroy healthy gingival connective tissue creating a pathway that allows the PMNs to move quickly through the tissue.***
      3. The goal of the PMNs is to reach the bacteria in the sulcus and destroy them. The damage to the healthy connective tissue is not normally a concern. In a healthy body, this tissue destruction will be repaired after the bacterial infection is brought under control.
   D. PMNs migrate into sulcus and phagocytize bacteria.
   E. The presence of Gram-negative bacteria activates the complement system.
3. **Tissue Level Features**
   A. The plaque biofilm is initially located supragingivally.
   B. There is vascular dilatation of arterioles, capillaries, and venules in dentogingival complex.
   C. The gingival crevicular fluid increases in volume.
4. **Clinical Features**
   A. *At this stage the gingiva looks healthy clinically.*
   B. This initial lesion phase develops 2 to 4 days following plaque biofilm accumulation.
5. **Outcome of Host Response**
   A. The host response is successful if most of the bacteria are destroyed.
   B. If the bacterial infection is brought under control—through the efforts of the immune system and effective plaque biofilm control—the body is able to repair the destruction caused by the immune response.
   C. If the bacterial pathogens are not controlled, however, early gingivitis develops.

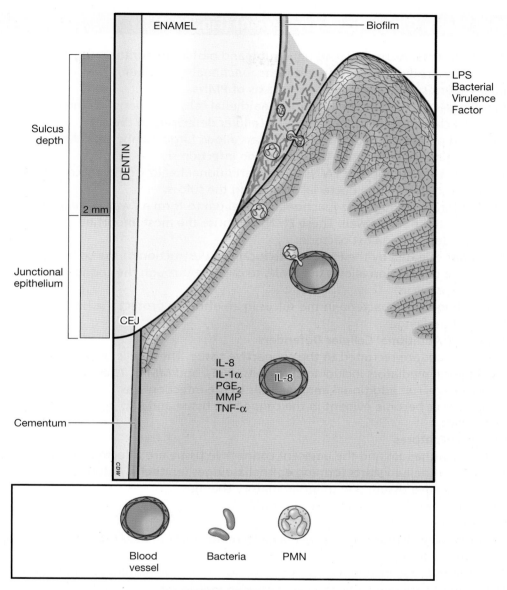

Figure 14-2. Bacterial Accumulation (*Initial Lesion*). This first phase is characterized by bacterial colonization near the gingival margin, increased vascular dilatation, and PMN migration to gingival sulcus. Although the host immune and inflammatory responses are activated, the gingival tissue looks clinically healthy in this phase.

Box 14-2. Early Gingivitis (*Early Lesion*) (Fig. 14-3)

1. **Bacterial Features.** As bacterial accumulation and biofilm maturation continues, bacterial toxins and by-products easily penetrate the junctional epithelium.
2. **Cellular Features: Migration and Chemotaxis of PMNs**
   A. *Cytokines*—released by the junctional epithelial cells in response to the increased bacterial challenge—attract additional cellular defenders to the site.
   B. Increased permeability of the blood vessels allows large numbers of PMNs to move to into the gingival connective tissue near the infection site.
   C. The increasing numbers of PMNs destroy additional healthy gingival connective tissue as they rush toward the bacterial invaders in the sulcus.
   D. PMNs migrate through the junctional epithelium to form a "wall of cells" between the biofilm and the sulcus wall. These PMNs comprise the most important component of the local defense against bacteria.
   E. *Cytokines* released by the PMNs cause localized destruction of the connective tissue. This tissue destruction allows the PMNs to migrate through the connective tissue toward the sulcus.
   F. PMNs phagocytize bacteria in the sulcus in an effort to protect the host tissues from the bacterial challenge.
3. **Migration of Additional Cellular Defenders**
   A. Macrophages are recruited to the connective tissue. These cells release many biochemical mediators including *cytokines, PGE₂,* and *MMPs*. These biochemical mediators recruit additional immune cells to the infection site.
   B. Lymphocytes become evident in the connective tissue and also produce *cytokines* and antibodies.
4. **Tissue Level Features**
   A. Sulcular epithelium and the adjacent connective tissue are affected the most.
   B. Sulcular epithelium starts forming epithelial ridges (epithelial extentions that protrude into connective tissue) due to inflammatory changes.
   C. Junctional epithelium cells start to proliferate.
5. **Clinical Features**
   A. *Inflammatory changes such as edema and redness of gingival marginal tissue can be observed clinically.*
   B. Early lesion phase develops 4 to 7 days following plaque biofilm accumulation.
   C. Duration of early gingivitis can vary between individuals.
6. **Outcome of Host Response**
   A. The large number of PMNs may control the bacterial pathogens.
   B. Initiation of good patient self-care can disrupt the plaque biofilm and result in a return to health. If the bacterial infection is brought under control—through the efforts of the immune system and effective plaque biofilm control—the body is able to repair the destruction caused by the immune response.
   C. If bacterial pathogens continue to proliferate, these early lesion changes will become established gingivitis—the next phase of disease progression.

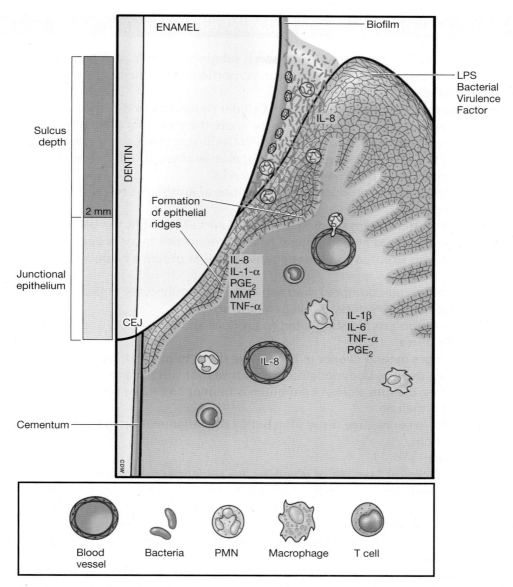

Figure 14-3. Early Gingivitis (*Early Lesion*). The biofilm overgrowth phase is characterized by subgingival plaque biofilm formation and intensified immune and inflammatory response compared to plaque biofilm accumulation phase. Early inflammatory changes are observed clinically as redness and swelling of the marginal gingiva.

Box 14-3. Established Gingivitis (*Established Lesion*) (Fig. 14-4)

1. **Bacterial Features.** The plaque biofilm extends subgingivally into the gingival sulcus, disrupting the attachment of the coronal most portion of the junctional epithelium from the tooth surface.
2. **Cellular Features: Migration of Additional Cellular Defenders to the Site**
   A. Large numbers of subgingival bacteria stimulate the epithelial cells to secrete *cytokines*, resulting in the recruitment of additional PMNs, macrophages, and lymphocytes.
   B. *Macrophages and lymphocytes* become the most numerous cells in the tissue. *PMNs, however, continue to fight bacteria in the sulcus.*
   C. Activated lymphocytes produce large quantities of antibodies to assist in controlling the bacterial challenge.
   D. The immune system keeps sending more immune cells to fight the bacteria. More toxic chemicals are released and additional healthy connective tissue is destroyed.
      1) Macrophages exposed to Gram-negative bacteria produce *cytokines*, *PGE*$_2$, and *MMPs*.
      2) *Cytokines* recruit additional macrophages and lymphocytes to the area.
      3) *PGE*$_2$ and the *MMPs* initiate collagen destruction.
      4) Gingival fibroblasts are stimulated to produce additional *PGE*$_2$ and *MMPs*.
3. **Tissue Level Features**
   A. Epithelial ridges extend deeper in connective tissue to maintain epithelial integrity.
   B. Junctional epithelium does not closely attach to root surface and starts to transform into pocket epithelium. Pocket epithelium is thinner and more permeable compared to junctional epithelium.
   C. Collagen loss in connective tissue affected by the inflammation extends in lateral and apical directions.
4. **Clinical Features**
   A. *All the usual clinical features of gingivitis are evident in this phase.*
   B. Established gingivitis is generally observed 21 days following plaque biofilm accumulation.
5. **Outcome of Host Response**
   A. In many individuals, the host response is adequate to contain the bacterial challenge during this phase.
   B. Periodontal instrumentation and patient education, at this point, can be helpful in controlling the bacterial challenge. The combination of professional treatment and good patient self-care can stop the bacterial challenge and return the periodontium to health.
   C. In certain susceptible individuals if the bacterial infection is not controlled, established gingivitis progresses to periodontitis. Unfortunately, no one can predict when and if established gingivitis will progress to periodontitis. Much current research is directed to trying to determine which individuals are at risk for developing periodontitis.

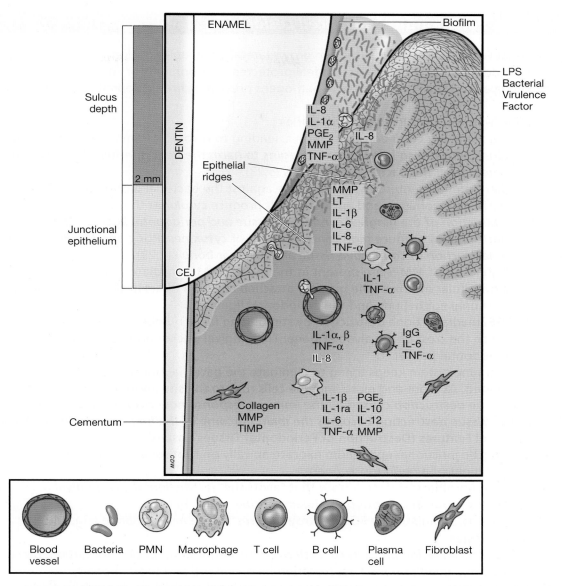

Figure 14-4. Established Gingivitis (*Established Lesion*): The Subgingival Plaque Phase. Subgingival plaque biofilm extends to junctional epithelium. Increased cellular infiltrate and collagen breakdown in connective tissue is observed. All clinical characteristics of gingivitis are evident in this phase.

Box 14-4. Periodontitis (*Advanced Lesion*) (Fig. 14-5)

1. **Bacterial Features.** The plaque biofilm grows laterally and apically along the root surface. The periodontal pocket provides an ideal protected environment for continued growth of subgingival bacteria. These bacterial pathogens present a chronic, repeated challenge to the host.

2. **Cellular Features: Host Response Intensifies**
   A. The bacterial infection becomes chronic, leading to chronic inflammation. *The immune response becomes so intense that it begins to harm the periodontium that it is trying to protect from the bacterial pathogens* (5,23).
   B. Cellular defenders intensify their defense against the bacterial pathogens.
      1. PMNs, macrophages, and epithelial cells produce **cytokines** that *cause the destruction of the gingival connective tissue and periodontal ligament fibers*.
      2. Macrophages produce high concentrations of **cytokines**, **PGE$_2$**, and **MMPs** that *result in destruction of connective tissue and alveolar bone* (12,23).
      3. High levels of **MMPs** are present in the tissues. MMPs mediate destruction of the extracellular matrix of the gingiva, attached collagen fibers at the apical edge of the junctional epithelium, and the periodontal ligament.
      4. **PGE$_2$** mediates bone destruction by stimulating large numbers of osteoclasts to resorb the crest of the alveolar bone. The gingival pocket progresses to become a periodontal pocket.
   C. The immune system keeps trying to eliminate the bacteria, but the bacteria are not eliminated. As more and more immune cells rush to the site, more tissue is damaged. *The tissue destruction caused by the immune response now overwhelms any tissue repair. Tissue destruction becomes the main outcome of the immune system response.*

3. **Tissue Level Features (Destruction of Periodontal Tissues Ensues)**
   A. Cells of the junctional epithelium migrate apically on root surface resulting in the development of a *periodontal pocket*.
   B. Gingival fibroblasts shift to a state that favors the *destruction of the gingival connective tissue and periodontal ligament fibers* (Fig. 14-5).
   C. Osteoclasts, stimulated by PGE$_2$ *destroy the crest of the alveolar bone* (Fig. 14-5).

4. **Clinical Features**
   A. *This advanced lesion phase is characterized by: periodontal pocket formation, bleeding on probing, alveolar bone loss, furcation involvement, and tooth mobility.*
   B. Tissue changes such as apical migration of junctional epithelium, connective tissue destruction, periodontal ligament destruction, and alveolar bone loss are not reversible.

5. **Outcome of Host Response**
   A. Chronic infection by the periodontal pathogens induces a chronic inflammatory response. *This chronic inflammation is an out-of-control response that destroys periodontal tissues and causes more damage to the periodontium than the bacterial infection. Tissue damage is the hallmark of periodontitis.*
   B. Factors influencing the host's failure to control the bacterial challenge may include:
      1) Abnormal PMN function.
      2) Persistence and virulence of bacteria in the biofilm.
      3) Acquired and environmental factors such as smoking and stress.
      4) Systemic factors such as uncontrolled diabetes mellitus or genetic factors.

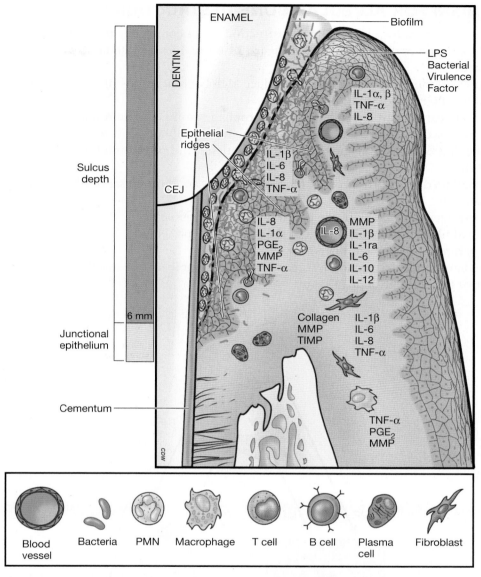

Figure 14-5. Periodontitis (*Advanced Lesion*). This phase is characterized by periodontal pocket formation, bleeding on probing, alveolar bone loss, furcation involvement, and tooth mobility.

MECHANISM FOR ALVEOLAR BONE DESTRUCTION

The precise mechanism for alveolar bone destruction is not completely understood, however, the cascade of events depicted in Figure 14-6 provides a reasonable explanation for this destruction.

1. In chronic periodontitis, macrophages produce high concentrations of cytokines (IL-L and TNF-α), PGE$_2$, and MMP (43).
2. The biochemical mediators produced by macrophages stimulate the resident fibroblasts to secrete both PGE$_2$ and MMP. Gingival fibroblasts shift to a state that favors the destruction of the gingival connective tissue and periodontal ligament fibers (44).
3. Biochemical mediators produced by the macrophages and fibroblasts result in destruction of:
   A. The extracellular matrix of the gingival connective tissue
   B. Gingival fibers at the apical edge of the junctional epithelium
   C. The periodontal ligament fibers.
4. PGE$_2$ mediates bone destruction by stimulating large numbers of osteoclasts to resorb the crest of the alveolar bone (12).

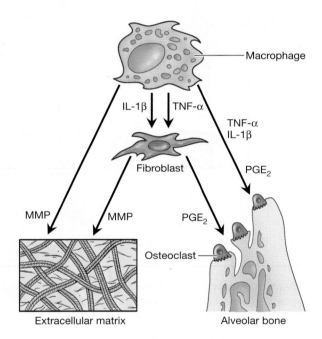

Figure 14-6. Destruction of Connective Tissue Matrix and Alveolar Bone. The cascade of events postulated to result in destruction of the gingival connective tissue matrix and supporting alveolar bone.

Chapter Summary Statement

The immune system provides the body with a strong defense against invading periodontal pathogens. In many cases, PMNs attracted to the site are able to contain the bacterial challenge and no tissue damage occurs. If the bacterial challenge is not contained, the plaque biofilm extends subgingivally and develops into a highly organized biofilm. In many cases, the host response still is able to contain the bacterial pathogens. In some individuals, however, the host resistance is insufficient to contain the bacterial challenge. *Biochemical mediators produced by immune cells are largely responsible for the tissue destruction seen in periodontitis. High levels of cytokines, MMPs, and PGE$_2$ characterize periodontitis. The unrelenting, chronic bacterial infection triggers immune responses that (1) destroy the connective tissue of the gingiva, (2) destroy the periodontal ligament, and (3) resorb the alveolar bone.*

Page and Schroeder described four distinct stages in histologic development of gingivitis and periodontitis: (1) bacterial accumulation (initial lesion), (2) early gingivitis (early lesion), (3) established gingivitis (established lesion), and periodontitis (advanced lesion).

Section 3
Focus on Patients

Clinical Patient Care

CASE 1

Mrs. Smith is a new patient in the dental office. Mrs. Smith is 45 years of age and has not received regular dental care in the past. Her new employer provides dental insurance for his employees and she has come to your office for oral health care. Mrs. Smith has chronic periodontitis. How will you explain inflammatory periodontal disease to Mrs. Smith?

CASE 2

Two unrelated individuals who have exactly the same level of daily self-care and exactly the same amount of plaque biofilm accumulation do not necessarily develop the same severity of periodontal disease. How do you explain this fact?

Evidence in Action

CASE 1

In reading a dental journal you find an article that describes a new medication that is reported to stop collagen destruction by one of the MMPs. If this new medication does indeed block such collagen destruction, what effect might this medication have on a patient with periodontitis? Can you think of another biochemical mediator target that could be inhibited would benefit a patient with periodontitis?

Ethical Dilemma

CASE 1

Your next two patients are identical twin sisters who are new to the practice, Mary and Katherine. They request that you review their health histories together. You learn that they are 68 years old, both widowed, and live together. They have received routine dental care from their longtime friend and dentist, Dr. Lipman, who just retired at 80, so they have decided to become patients in your dental office. They inform you that their mother is still alive at 90, but is edentulous, as she lost all of her teeth due to "gum disease." They both state that they are in good health, however, Mary was diagnosed with type II diabetes a few years back. She states that she hasn't paid much attention to it.

Your examination and radiographs of Katherine reveal that she has generally good oral health, with localized gingivitis on the mandibular anterior region. Her self-care appears to be more than adequate, and you compliment her on it.

Mary's examination is quite the opposite. She presents with generalized periodontitis, and vertical bone loss on her mandibular posterior teeth. She exhibits attachment loss in the 4- to 5-mm range, with localized posterior readings of 6 to 7 mm. Some of her mandibular posterior teeth are mobile. She too has good self-care but becomes very agitated when you present your findings to her. She states that she and Katherine "always" went to Dr. Lipman together and received the same treatments. She questions why her outcome is so different than that of her sister and asks if you think Dr. Lipman provided substandard dental care.

1. What factors may have contributed to the patient's disease progression?
2. How will you discuss the host immune response in periodontal disease and periodontitis with Katherine?
3. Are there any ethical dilemmas involved?

References

1. Bartold PM, Van Dyke TE. Periodontitis: a host-mediated disruption of microbial homeostasis. Unlearning learned concepts. *Periodontol 2000.* 2013;62(1):203–217.
2. Darveau RP. Periodontitis: a polymicrobial disruption of host homeostasis. *Nat Rev Microbiol.* 2010;8(7):481–490.
3. Ebersole JL, Dawson DR 3rd, Morford LA, et al. Periodontal disease immunology: 'double indemnity' in protecting the host. *Periodontol 2000.* 2013;62(1):163–202.
4. Deo V, Bhongade ML. Pathogenesis of periodontitis: role of cytokines in host response. *Dent Today.* 2010;29(9):60–62, 64–66.
5. Graves D. Cytokines that promote periodontal tissue destruction. *J Periodontol.* 2008;79(8 suppl):158S–161S.
6. Oringer RJ. Modulation of the host response in periodontal therapy. *J Periodontol.* 2002;73(4):460–470.
7. Page RC, Kornman KS. The pathogenesis of human periodontitis: an introduction. *Periodontol 2000.* 1997;14:9–11.
8. Page RC, Offenbacher S, Schroeder HE, et al. Advances in the pathogenesis of periodontitis: summary of developments, clinical implications and future directions. *Periodontol 2000.* 1997;14:216–248.
9. Page RC. The role of inflammatory mediators in the pathogenesis of periodontal disease. *J Periodontal Res.* 1991;26 (3 Pt 2):230–242.
10. McDevitt MJ, Wang HY, Knobelman C, et al. Interleukin-1 genetic association with periodontitis in clinical practice. *J Periodontol.* 2000;71(2):156–163.
11. Qwarnstrom EE, MacFarlane SA, Page RC. Effects of interleukin-1 on fibroblast extracellular matrix, using a 3-dimensional culture system. *J Cell Physiol.* 1989;139(3):501–508.
12. Schwartz Z, Goultschin J, Dean DD, et al. Mechanisms of alveolar bone destruction in periodontitis. *Periodontol 2000.* 1997;14:158–172.
13. Reynolds JJ, Meikle MC. Mechanisms of connective tissue matrix destruction in periodontitis. *Periodontol 2000.* 1997;14:144–157.
14. Roodman GD. Interleukin-6: an osteotropic factor? *J Bone Miner Res.* 1992;7(5):475–478.
15. Hughes FJ, Howells GL. Interleukin-6 inhibits bone formation in vitro. *Bone Miner.* 1993;21(1):21–28.
16. Meikle MC, Atkinson SJ, Ward RV, et al. Gingival fibroblasts degrade type I collagen films when stimulated with tumor necrosis factor and interleukin 1: evidence that breakdown is mediated by metalloproteinases. *J Periodontal Res.* 1989;24(3):207–213.

17. Bertolini DR, Nedwin GE, Bringman TS, et al. Stimulation of bone resorption and inhibition of bone formation in vitro by human tumour necrosis factors. *Nature*. 1986;319(6053):516–518.

18. Thomson BM, Mundy GR, Chambers TJ. Tumor necrosis factors alpha and beta induce osteoblastic cells to stimulate osteoclastic bone resorption. *J Immunol*. 1987;138(3):775–779.

19. Gemmell E, Marshall RI, Seymour GJ. Cytokines and prostaglandins in immune homeostasis and tissue destruction in periodontal disease. *Periodontol 2000*. 1997;14:112–143.

20. Dietrich JW, Goodson JM, Raisz LG. Stimulation of bone resorption by various prostaglandins in organ culture. *Prostaglandins*. 1975;10(2):231–240.

21. Offenbacher S, Farr DH, Goodson JM. Measurement of prostaglandin E in crevicular fluid. *J Clin Periodontol*. 1981;8(4):359–367.

22. Zubery Y, Dunstan CR, Story BM, et al. Bone resorption caused by three periodontal pathogens in vivo in mice is mediated in part by prostaglandin. *Infect Immun*. 1998;66(9):4158–4162.

23. Giannobile WV. Host-response therapeutics for periodontal diseases. *J Periodontol*. 2008;79(8 suppl):1592–1600.

24. Albandar JM. Global risk factors and risk indicators for periodontal diseases. *Periodontol 2000*. 2002;29:177–206.

25. Salvi GE, Lawrence HP, Offenbacher S, et al. Influence of risk factors on the pathogenesis of periodontitis. *Periodontol 2000*. 1997;14:173–201.

26. Cagli NA, Hakki SS, Dursun R, et al. Clinical, genetic, and biochemical findings in two siblings with Papillon-Lefevre Syndrome. *J Periodontol*. 2005;76(12):2322–2329.

27. Baker PJ. Genetic control of the immune response in pathogenesis. *J Periodontol*. 2005;76(11 suppl):2042–2046.

28. Hart TC, Kornman KS. Genetic factors in the pathogenesis of periodontitis. *Periodontol 2000*. 1997;14:202–215.

29. Michalowicz BS. Genetic and heritable risk factors in periodontal disease. *J Periodontol*. 1994;65(5 suppl):479–488.

30. Nibali L, O'Dea M, Bouma G, et al. Genetic variants associated with neutrophil function in aggressive periodontitis and healthy controls. *J Periodontol*. 2010;81(4):527–534.

31. Barbour SE, Nakashima K, Zhang JB, et al. Tobacco and smoking: environmental factors that modify the host response (immune system) and have an impact on periodontal health. *Crit Rev Oral Biol Med*. 1997;8(4):437–460.

32. Johnson GK, Guthmiller JM. The impact of cigarette smoking on periodontal disease and treatment. *Periodontol 2000*. 2007;44:178–194.

33. Kenney EB, Kraal JH, Saxe SR, et al. The effect of cigarette smoke on human oral polymorphonuclear leukocytes. *J Periodontal Res*. 1977;12(4):227–234.

34. Rezavandi K, Palmer RM, Odell EW, et al. Expression of ICAM-1 and E-selectin in gingival tissues of smokers and non-smokers with periodontitis. *J Oral Pathol Med*. 2002;31(1):59–64.

35. Tomar SL, Asma S. Smoking-attributable periodontitis in the United States: findings from NHANES III. National Health and Nutrition Examination Survey. *J Periodontol*. 2000;71(5):743–751.

36. Diabetes and periodontal diseases. Committee on Research, Science and Therapy. American Academy of Periodontology. *J Periodontol*. 2000;71(4):664–678.

37. Botero JE, Yepes FL, Roldan N, et al. Tooth and periodontal clinical attachment loss are associated with hyperglycemia in patients with diabetes. *J Periodontol*. 2012;83(10):1245–1250.

38. Deshpande K, Jain A, Sharma R, et al. Diabetes and periodontitis. *J Indian Soc Periodontol*. 2010;14(4):207–212.

39. Mealey BL, Oates TW; American Academy of Periodontology. Diabetes mellitus and periodontal diseases. *J Periodontol*. 2006;77(8):1289–1303.

40. Preshaw PM, Bissett SM. Periodontitis: oral complication of diabetes. *Endocrinol Metab Clin North Am*. 2013;42(4):849–867.

41. Page RC. The etiology and pathogenesis of periodontitis. *Compend Contin Educ Dent*. 2002;23(5 suppl):11–14.

42. Page RC, Schroeder HE. Pathogenesis of inflammatory periodontal disease. A summary of current work. *Lab Invest*. 1976;34(3):235–249.

43. McCauley LK, Nohutcu RM. Mediators of periodontal osseous destruction and remodeling: principles and implications for diagnosis and therapy. *J Periodontol*. 2002;73(11):1377–1391.

44. Dongari-Bagtzoglou AI, Ebersole JL. Gingival fibroblast cytokine profiles in Actinobacillus actinomycetemcomitans-associated periodontitis. *J Periodontol*. 1996;67(9):871–878.

 STUDENT ANCILLARY RESOURCES

A wide variety of resources to enhance your learning and understanding of this chapter are available on thePoint®.

- Visit thePoint to access:
  - Audio Glossary
  - Animations
  - Suggested Readings
  - Answers to Review Questions
  - Case Studies

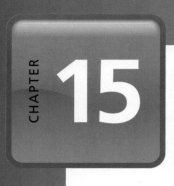

CHAPTER

15

Systemic Conditions that Amplify Susceptibility to Periodontal Disease

Clinical Application.
Plaque biofilm is the fundamental etiology for periodontal disease, but evaluating patients with periodontal disease often can be quite confusing. Frequently patients with minimal plaque biofilm challenge will be found to have advanced disease for no readily apparent reason. Some of these patients will have systemic conditions that can amplify their susceptibility to the periodontal disease, presenting a confusing clinical presentation. All members of the dental team must be alert for the possibility of systemic risk factors when evaluating patients with the signs of periodontal disease. This chapter presents an interesting outline of these systemic conditions.

Learning Objectives

- Name several systemic diseases/conditions that may modify the host response to periodontal pathogens.
- Discuss the potential implications of these systemic diseases on the periodontium: uncontrolled diabetes, leukemia, and acquired immunodeficiency syndrome.
- Discuss how hormone alterations may affect the periodontium.
- Define the term osteoporosis and discuss the link between skeletal osteoporosis and alveolar bone loss in the jaw.
- Discuss the implications of Down syndrome on the periodontium.

- Name three medications that can cause gingival enlargement.
- For a patient in your care with periodontitis who is amplified by a systemic condition, explain to your clinical instructor the risk factors that may have contributed to the severity of your patient's periodontitis.

Key Terms

Systemic risk factors
Diabetes mellitus
Well-controlled diabetes
Leukemia
Oral mucositis
Linear gingival erythema

Pregnancy gingivitis
Pregnancy-associated
  pyogenic granuloma
Menopausal
  gingivostomatitis

Drug-influenced gingival
  enlargement
Phenytoin
Cyclosporine
Nifedipine

Section 1
Systemic Risk Factors for Periodontitis

Additional factors, other than the presence of bacteria, play a significant role in determining why some individuals are more susceptible to periodontal disease than others. **Systemic risk factors** are conditions or diseases that increase an individual's susceptibility to periodontal infection by modifying or amplifying the host response to the bacterial infection. Proven systemic risk factors include diabetes mellitus, osteoporosis, hormone alteration, medications, tobacco use, and genetic influences. *Tobacco use as a risk factor for periodontal disease is discussed in Chapter 18.*

DIABETES MELLITUS

1. **Characteristics of Diabetes Mellitus. Diabetes mellitus** is a chronic disease in which the body does not produce or properly use insulin. Insulin is a hormone that is needed to convert sugar, starches, and other food into energy that the body uses to sustain life. The World Health Organization (WHO) estimates that the number of adults in the world with diabetes will rise to 366 million in the year 2030 (1).
2. **Diabetes as a Risk Factor for Periodontitis**
   A. **Incidence of Periodontitis**
      1. Patients with *well-controlled diabetes* have no more periodontal disease than persons without diabetes. Diabetes is **well controlled** if the blood glucose levels are stabilized within the recommended range. The response of individuals with *controlled diabetes* to nonsurgical periodontal therapy is similar to that of nondiabetic persons, with similar trends in improved probing depth and attachment gain (2).
      2. Individuals with *undiagnosed or poorly controlled diabetes* are at greater risk for severe periodontitis than are persons with controlled diabetes and nondiabetic individuals (Figs. 15-1–15-3). Periodontal disease is considered a complication of uncontrolled diabetes.
         a. Individuals with undiagnosed or poorly controlled diabetes have high blood glucose levels. There is a clear relationship between the degree of high blood sugar and the severity of periodontitis (3,4). As glucose levels increase, individuals with undiagnosed or poorly controlled diabetes experience a dramatic decline in periodontal health (4–7).
         b. A large number of epidemiologic studies demonstrate that periodontitis is more prevalent and severe in individuals with uncontrolled diabetes mellitus versus nondiabetic individuals. *People with uncontrolled or undiagnosed diabetes are approximately three times more likely to develop periodontitis* (3,4,8–12).
         c. Periodontal attachment loss (connective tissue destruction and bone loss) occurs more frequently in individuals with poorly controlled diabetes than in individuals with well-controlled diabetes (5,7,13–15). A person with diabetes who smokes, and who is age 45 or older, is 20 times more likely than a nondiabetic, nonsmoking individual to experience severe periodontitis.
         d. An unfavorable treatment outcome may occur in long-term maintenance therapy of individuals with poorly controlled diabetes (16). Individuals with *poorly controlled* diabetes have a poorer response to nonsurgical and surgical periodontal therapy, more rapid recurrence of deep pockets, and a less favorable long-term response to treatment.

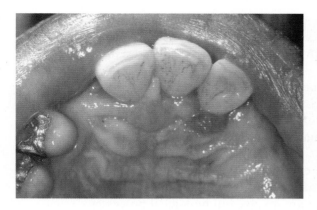

Figure 15-1. Inflammatory Reaction. Note the localized inflammatory swelling of the gingiva on the palatal surface of the maxillary lateral incisor. The patient has uncontrolled diabetes mellitus. This intense inflammatory reaction is typical for individuals with uncontrolled diabetes. (Courtesy of Dr. Ralph Arnold, San Antonio, TX.)

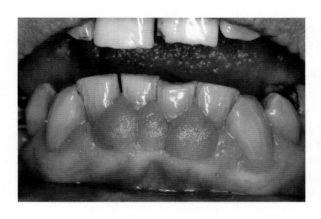

Figure 15-2. Periodontitis Associated with Poorly Controlled Diabetes. Marked tissue changes are evident in this individual with poorly controlled diabetes. (Courtesy of Dr. Richard Foster, Guilford Technical Community College, Jamestown, NC.)

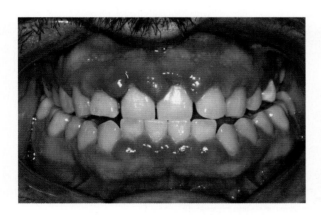

Figure 15-3. Periodontitis Associated with Uncontrolled Diabetes. Examination of this patient revealed pronounced tissue changes and loss of attachment. The patient stated that he has been diagnosed with diabetes but that he is not seeing a physician or taking any medications for diabetes. (Courtesy of Dr. Richard Foster, Guilford Technical Community College, Jamestown, NC.)

B. **Effects of Increased Glucose Blood Levels on the Periodontium.** An individual with uncontrolled or poorly controlled blood glucose levels has an increased risk for developing acute periodontal abscesses, more extensive attachment loss and progressive alveolar bone loss (Fig. 15-4).
   1. Hyperglycemia (high blood sugar) in uncontrolled diabetics results in increased glucose in the gingival crevicular fluid and blood. Since many bacteria thrive on sugars, this glucose-rich crevicular fluid may result in altered bacterial composition within the biofilm microcolonies and influence the development of periodontal disease (17). Periodontal status—as estimated by degree of attachment loss—deteriorates significantly with poor glycemic control in diabetes (5–7).

2. Reduced PMN function and defective chemotaxis in uncontrolled diabetics can contribute to impaired host defenses. Since PMNs are the first line of defense against periodontal pathogens, reduced PMN function allows the bacteria to increase greatly in number (16).

3. Individuals who have both diabetes and periodontitis have significantly higher levels of IL-1β and PGE2 in gingival crevicular fluid compared to nondiabetic controls with a similar degree of periodontal disease (18).

4. Hyperglycemia can affect the synthesis, maturation, and maintenance of collagen and extracellular matrix.

   a. The hyperglycemic state results in the excessive formation of accumulated glycation end-products (AGE). AGEs are derived from the reaction of glucose and proteins. These substances are involved in biological processes relating to collagen turnover.

   b. Collagen is cross-linked by AGE formation, making it less likely to be repaired or to be newly synthesized normally. Collagen in the gingival tissues of individuals with uncontrolled diabetes is aged and more susceptible to breakdown.

C. Other Oral Complications of Poorly Controlled Diabetes Mellitus

1. Reduced salivary flow and burning mouth or tongue are common complaints of patients with uncontrolled diabetes (19–21). Dental healthcare professionals should suspect undiagnosed diabetes as a likely cause of burning tongue and refer the patient to a physician for follow-up care.

2. Reduced salivary flow and xerostomia can encourage the growth of *Candida albicans* and the development of oral candidiasis (22).

3. Individuals with undiagnosed or poorly controlled diabetes frequently present with multiple periodontal abscesses, leading to rapid destruction of periodontal bone support.

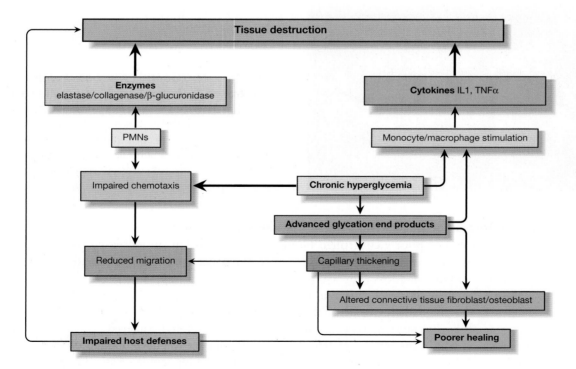

Figure 15-4. Postulated Effects of Uncontrolled Diabetes Mellitus on the Host Response.

D. Diabetes Mellitus: Implications for the Dental Hygienist

1. The dental team can act as an important point of contact for early screening and diagnosis of undiagnosed diabetes. In 2007, it was estimated that 24 million people in the United States have diabetes and 24% of those are undiagnosed (about 5.8 million undiagnosed diabetics). For every 1,000 adult dental patients, approximately 120 would have diabetes and about 40 would be undiagnosed (23,24). Knowledge about the association between diabetes and periodontal disease should be increased among dental and medical practitioners to prevent, manage, and control periodontal disease effectively (25).

2. The dental team is well placed to screen patients for diabetes since many people (70% of Americans) visit their dentist regularly (e.g., every 6 months) often more frequently than they visit their medical practitioner (23,26). The level of diabetic control and the health status should be carefully monitored for all individuals with diabetes.

3. Educating patients with diabetes about the importance of good oral self-care needs to become a priority for dental hygienists (27). Dental hygienists' role in periodontal care and regular, ongoing involvement with these individuals places hygienists in an optimal position to provide this education (28). Dental hygienists are very adept and experienced in instituting behavioral changes in their patients and represent an untapped resource for medical colleagues in this role.

4. Patients with diabetes often are poorly informed about the relationship between periodontitis and diabetes. Therefore, dental healthcare providers should be aware of this link and emphasize the importance of careful self-care at home and frequent professional care visits (27,29–31). People with poorly controlled diabetes (adults and children) must be considered at risk for periodontitis and should be informed of this risk.

5. Closer collaboration between medical and dental clinical teams is necessary for the joint management of people with diabetes and periodontitis (10,32). Collaboration of dental professionals with certified diabetes educators (CDEs) will improve the ability of CDEs to educate their clients about oral health topics (33).

6. Researchers at Columbia University reported on the largest study to date of 6- to 18-year-old individuals with diabetes and 350 individuals in the same age group without diabetes. The children and adolescents with diabetes showed significantly more periodontal disease than those without diabetes. Children and adolescents with diabetes had greater attachment loss than those without diabetes. Based on these findings, children with diabetes should be examined for signs of periodontal disease and receive early intervention and prevention (2,34).

LEUKEMIA

1. Characteristics of Leukemia
   A. Leukemia is cancer that begins in blood cells. In people with leukemia, the bone marrow produces a large number of abnormal white blood cells that don't function properly. At first, leukemia cells function almost normally. In time, they may crowd out normal white blood cells, red blood cells, and platelets. This makes it hard for blood to do its work. The National Cancer Institute estimates that there were 48,610 new cases and 23,720 deaths from leukemia in the United States in 2013. Leukemia is a disease of both children and adults and is more common in men and boys than girls and women.

B. **Types of Leukemia**
   1. Leukemia is classified on the duration (acute or chronic) and the type of cell involved (myeloid or lymphoid).
      a. Leukemia is either *chronic* (gets worse slowly) or *acute* (gets worse quickly).
      b. Leukemia that affects the lymphoid cells is called *lymphocytic*. Leukemia that affects the myeloid cells is called *myelogenous* leukemia.
   2. Leukemia is the most common cancer in children younger than 15 years old (35).
C. **Medical Treatment of Leukemia**
   1. Treatment for leukemia is complex and is not the same for all patients. It varies with the type of leukemia, extent of the disease, and also on the patient's age, symptoms, and general health. The physician plans the treatment to fit each patient's needs.
   2. Most patients with leukemia are treated with chemotherapy. Some also may have radiation therapy and/or bone marrow transplantation (BMT) or biological therapy.
   3. Chemotherapy causes patients to suffer from severe suppression of the immune system. Chemotherapy functions by suppressing the growth and spread of malignant cells; unfortunately, normal cells are also adversely affected. Normal cells with the highest rate of cell turnover (proliferation)—such as those of the mouth—are affected because chemotherapy interferes with cell production, maturation, and replacement.
   4. Dental care is a vital component of treatment. Anticancer treatments for leukemia can make the mouth sensitive, easily infected, and likely to bleed (35–40).
2. **Oral Complications of Leukemia**
   A. **Leukemia-Associated Gingivitis**
      1. **Inflammation of the Gingiva.** Signs of inflammation in the gingiva include swollen, glazed, and spongy tissues that are red to deep purple in appearance (Fig. 15-5). Gingival bleeding is also a common sign. Areas of spontaneous bleeding usually are characterized by intermittent oozing of blood.
         a. In a study of 1,093 adult inpatients undergoing chemotherapy treatment for leukemia, 14.9% of patients manifested gross bleeding from the mouth during the course of chemotherapy (41). The most common oral bleeding sites were the lips, tongue, and gingiva.
         b. In children, the prevalence of gingival inflammation is highest in the maintenance phase of chemotherapy followed by the induction phase with radiotherapy (36).
      2. **Gingival Enlargement.** Gingival enlargement is a common characteristic, initially beginning at the interdental papilla followed by marginal and attached gingiva.

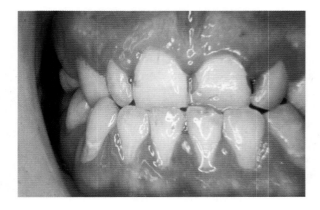

Figure 15-5. Leukemia-Associated Gingivitis. Note the swollen, red gingival tissues in this patient with leukemia. (Courtesy of Dr. Ralph Arnold, San Antonio, TX.)

B. Oral Mucositis

1. **Oral mucositis** is an inflammation of the oral mucous membranes caused when chemotherapy attacks and kills the rapidly dividing cells of the mucous membranes. Cells of the oral mucosa have a lifespan of only 10 to 14 days. Therefore, during chemotherapy, mucosal cells are dying at a faster rate than new cells can be produced.

2. Sloughing of mucosal surfaces can be localized or generalized involving the buccal mucosa, palate, floor of the mouth, gingiva, lips, and/or tongue. Ulcerations of the oral cavity also are a common complication of chemotherapy.

C. Xerostomia

1. Xerostomia may occur due to damage of the salivary glands during radiation therapy. A reduction in salivary flow alters the self-cleaning mechanisms of the oral cavity resulting in rapid biofilm accumulation and the development of dental caries.

2. Lack of saliva also can result in diminished taste perception and/or difficulty in swallowing and talking.

3. Reduced salivary flow and xerostomia can encourage the growth of *C. albicans* and the development of oral candidiasis (42).

3. **Leukemia: Implications for the Dental Hygienist**

A. The dental team can act as an important point of contact for early screening and diagnosis of undiagnosed leukemia. In some individuals, the first signs of leukemia show up in the oral cavity (35,43).

1. When a dental patient has spontaneous gingival bleeding and/or gingival enlargement for no apparent reason—combined with symptoms such as facial swelling, tiredness, poor appetite, lethargy, musculoskeletal pain—the individual should be referred to a medical specialist (35,43).

2. The fact that leukemia frequently presents with early oral manifestations emphasizes the need for dental professionals who are aware of the early oral signs of leukemia and can provide a timely referral.

B. Frequent unfavorable oral conditions of individuals undergoing anticancer therapy for leukemia highlight the responsibility of the otolaryngologist to refer these patients to the dental office (36,44). The planning of anticancer therapy for leukemia should include dental professionals in the multidisciplinary oncology team.

1. Immune suppression during chemotherapy may cause serious oral infections. Therefore, professional diagnosis and elimination of oral infection foci must be carried out as early as possible before chemotherapy. Aggressive chemotherapy causes xerostomia and as a consequence an increased risk for oral diseases.

2. Adequate oral care before, during, and after chemotherapy is necessary to prevent oral diseases and systemic complications of oral origin. Frequent dental care is essential for improvement in oral conditions that may diminish patient suffering and prevent the spread of serious infections from the oral cavity to other parts of the body (36).

3. Chemotherapy can cause a sore and sensitive mouth that bleeds easily. Soft toothbrushes with gentle brushing should be recommended. If the mouth is too sensitive to tolerate toothbrushing, soft dental sponges (available from a pharmacy) can be recommended.

C. Pain from oral mucositis afflicts from 40% to 70% of patients receiving chemotherapy or radiation therapy. Current methods of clinical pain management (e.g., topical anesthetics, systemic analgesics) have limited success (45).

1. Oral mucositis is common in children undergoing chemotherapy. In 2011, a study by Soares et al. (40) suggest that the prophylactic use of 0.12% chlorhexidine gluconate reduces the frequency of oral mucositis and oral pathogens in children with leukemia.

2. In a pilot study, Berger examined the ability of oral capsaicin to provide temporary relief of oral mucositis pain.
   a. Capsaicin (cap-SAY-sin) is the active ingredient in chili peppers. Along with being very spicy, capsaicin also helps to relieve pain. It has anti-inflammatory effects, much like aspirin or ibuprofen.
   b. The oral capsaicin taffy recipe in Box 15-1, developed by nurses, uses just enough of the cayenne pepper to get the anti-inflammatory effects and produces temporary pain reduction (45). Clinicians should monitor patients with care, however, since this sugar containing candy may increase the risk of developing dental caries.
D. Good nutrition can become challenging due to mouth sores and/or xerostomia during anticancer treatment for leukemia. Table 15-1 summarizes recommendations for good nutrition.
E. Care should be coordinated with other health professionals. Interprofessional collaboration among professionals such as physicians, dental professionals, dieticians, and case managers is an essential component of patient-centered care (46).

Box 15-1. Oral Capsaicin Taffy Recipe

You may wonder why you would want to put something spicy into your mouth if it is sore from cancer treatment. *You should never put regular cayenne pepper into your sore mouth.* This would be very painful. The following recipe, however, was developed by nurses and uses just enough of the cayenne pepper to get the anti-inflammatory pain relief, without the spicy-hot burning.

Total Time: 35 minutes
Ingredients:
1 cup sugar
¾ cup light corn syrup
⅔ cup water
1 tablespoon cornstarch
2 tablespoons butter or margarine
1 teaspoon salt
2 teaspoons vanilla
½ to 1½ teaspoons powdered cayenne pepper (red pepper)[a]

Preparation:
- Combine all ingredients except vanilla and cayenne pepper in a stove-top pot.
- Cook over medium heat, stirring constantly, until the mixture reaches 256°F (use a candy thermometer).
- Remove from heat, and stir in vanilla and cayenne pepper.
- When cool enough to handle, pull taffy until firm. Lay out in a thin layer and let cool on waxed paper.
- When taffy is stiff, cut into strips, then small pieces. Wrap taffy in waxed paper and store in a cool place.

[a]Start by using only ½ teaspoon of cayenne pepper in the first batch. You can add more cayenne pepper to the next batch if this gives you better pain relief and does not cause any burning sensation. You can add up to 1½ teaspoons of cayenne pepper per batch of taffy.

TABLE 15-1. WHAT TO EAT WHEN YOU HAVE MOUTH SORES

What to Eat	What to Avoid
Soft food and foods that contain liquids; soften food with items such as milk; soy, almond, or rice milk; juice, broth, or yogurt	Avoid caffeinated drinks and foods, such as coffee, tea, soda, colas, and chocolate
Add a little olive oil to food to make it slippery and easier to swallow	Avoid alcohol, including hard liquor, mixed drinks, beer, and wine
Use a blender to mash fruits or vegetables	Avoid tobacco including cigarettes, chewing tobacco, and pipes
For dry mouth, use saliva substitutes and moisturizers	Avoid mouthwashes that contain alcohol
Examples of soft foods and foods containing liquids: smoothies, shakes, nutritional supplement drinks, warm (not hot) soups, cooked cereals (such as oatmeal thinned with extra water or milk, yogurt, pudding, mashed potatoes	Examples of foods to avoid: acidic foods such as citrus fruits and juices (orange, grapefruit, tomato, lemon, lime), spicy foods, salty foods, raw vegetables, rice, chips, breads, and cakes

HIV INFECTION

1. **Characteristics of Human Immunodeficiency Virus (HIV) Infection**
   A. Acquired immunodeficiency syndrome (AIDS) is a communicable disease caused by HIV. People with AIDS are at an increased risk for developing certain cancers and for infections that usually occur only in individuals with a weak immune system.
   B. In most developed countries, the death rate from AIDS among adults has declined largely because of newer antiretroviral therapies and improved access to these therapies (47,48). Nevertheless, because of the large numbers of existing plus new cases of HIV infection, dental and medical practitioners will still be required to treat oral and periodontal conditions in HIV-infected adults and children (49).
   C. Periodontal diseases strongly associated with HIV infection are classified as linear gingival erythema and necrotizing periodontal diseases (47,50). Necrotizing periodontal diseases are discussed in Chapters 9 and 28.

2. **Linear Gingival Erythema**
   A. **Characteristics**
      1. Gingival manifestations of HIV infection were formerly known as HIV-associated gingivitis but currently are designated as linear gingival erythema. **Linear gingival erythema** (LGE) is characterized by a 2- to 3-mm marginal band of intense erythema (redness) in the free gingiva (Fig. 15-6) (51).
      2. The band of gingival erythema may extend into the attached gingiva and/or extend beyond the mucogingival line into the alveolar mucosa (51). Linear gingival erythema may be localized to one or two teeth but is more commonly a generalized gingival condition.
      3. The lack of response of linear gingival erythema to conventional self-care and periodontal therapy is an important criterion in its diagnosis (52).

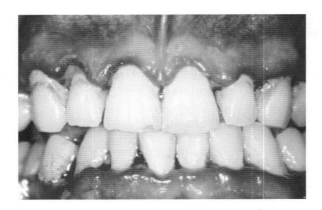

Figure 15-6. Linear Gingival Erythema. Gingival changes associated with linear gingival erythema. Note the marginal band of intense erythema in the free gingiva.

4. The etiology of linear gingival erythema is not well understood. Research suggests that organisms not generally associated with gingivitis, such as *Candida* species, are associated with linear gingival erythema (51,53).

5. With the advent of antiretroviral therapy for HIV-positive patients, the prevalence of HIV-specific lesions has been dramatically reduced (3,54,55).

3. **HIV-Infected Individuals: Implications for the Dental Hygienist**

A. HIV-infected individuals should be monitored to prevent irreversible periodontal damage. The need for early periodontal therapy and more frequent maintenance visits should be stressed. Continuity of dental care remains important for HIV-positive patients even when they are being treated with antiretroviral therapies (55–58). Dental healthcare providers should emphasize the importance of careful self-care at home and frequent professional care visits (56).

B. The initial treatment for linear gingival erythema should be standard periodontal therapy plus the use of 0.12% chlorhexidine gluconate as a mouth rinse. Consideration may be given to the use of antibiotics (52).

C. Care should be coordinated with other health professionals. Interprofessional collaboration among professionals such as physicians, dental professionals, social workers, dieticians, and case managers is an essential component of patient-centered care (46,59).

D. Despite the beneficial effects of antiretroviral therapies, drug interactions with other medications have been observed. For instance, fluconazole, ketoconazole, itraconazole, metronidazole, ciprofloxacin, midazolam, and triazolam can interact with some antiretroviral medications, such as zidovudine, nevirapine, and ritonavir. Dental professionals need to understand drug interaction in HIV infection in order to establish a better control during periodontal treatment (47).

HORMONAL FLUCTUATIONS DURING PUBERTY, PREGNANCY, AND MENOPAUSE

Hormonal fluctuations during puberty, pregnancy, and menopause impact the periodontal tissues.

1. **Puberty**

A. **Impact of Puberty on the Periodontium**

1. During puberty there are increased levels of estradiol in females and testosterone in males. Increased levels of sex hormones during puberty cause increased blood circulation to the gingival tissues and may cause an increased sensitivity to local irritants, such as plaque biofilms, resulting in **pubertal gingivitis.**

2. Pubertal gingivitis occurs equally in girls and boys. The tendency for plaque-induced gingivitis usually decreases as the young person progresses through puberty.
3. Clinical features of pubertal gingivitis include
   a. Accumulation of plaque biofilm
   b. Red, inflamed, swollen gingival tissue; bleeding upon probing
   c. Reversible with meticulous daily self-care; reversible following puberty
B. Implications for the Dental Hygienist
   1. Dental hygienists should stress that daily attention to biofilm control (self-care) and frequent professional care are very important for gingival health during puberty (60).
   2. The American Dental Association (ADA) recommends the use of antimicrobial mouth rinses, antibiotic therapy, and aggressive periodontal therapy for any severe cases of puberty gingivitis.

2. Pregnancy
   A. Impact of Pregnancy on the Periodontium
      1. Inflammation of the gingiva increases in pregnant women in the presence of even small amounts of plaque biofilm.
         a. The likelihood of gingival inflammation increases in the second and third trimesters when enhanced estrogen levels in the blood increase sensitivity to plaque biofilm and other local irritants (61). Pregnant women, near or at term, produce large quantities of estradiol, estriol, and progesterone.
         b. Elevated progesterone levels in pregnancy enhance capillary permeability and dilation resulting in increased gingival exudate and edema (62).
         c. During pregnancy profound changes in immune response impact the periodontal tissues (63). High levels of progesterone and estrogen associated with pregnancy have been shown to suppress the immune response to dental plaque biofilm. PMN chemotaxis and phagocytosis have been reported to be depressed in response to high levels of gestational hormones (64).
      2. Gingival inflammation initiated by plaque biofilms, and exacerbated by hormonal changes in the second and third trimesters of pregnancy, is referred to as **pregnancy gingivitis**.
         a. The gingival tissue may be edematous and dark red, with bulbous interdental papillae (Figs. 15-7 and 15-8).
         b. In some cases, a gingival papilla can react so strongly to plaque biofilm that a large, localized overgrowth of gingival tissue called a **pregnancy-associated pyogenic granuloma** (pregnancy tumor), may form on the interdental gingiva or on the gingival margin (Fig. 15-9).
            1. These growths are benign and are generally not painful.
            2. If the growth persists after delivery, it can be surgically removed.
         c. Probing depths, bleeding on probing, and crevicular fluid flow are increased in pregnancy gingivitis.
   B. Expectant Patient: Implications for the Dental Hygienist
      1. Dental professionals and gynecologists should educate pregnant patients about the importance of oral health. The perinatal period is an ideal time to educate and perform dental treatment on expectant mothers (65,66). Pregnancy provides an opportunity to educate women regarding oral health with self-care and future child care (67).

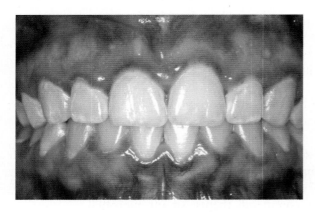

Figure 15-7. Pregnancy Gingivitis. Clinical appearance of reddened, swollen tissues of pregnancy gingivitis. (Courtesy of Dr. Richard Foster, Guilford Technical Community College, Jamestown, NC.)

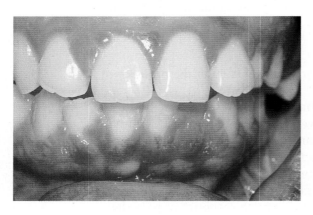

Figure 15-8. Hormonal Gingivitis. Hormonal gingivitis is evident 3 weeks postpartum (after giving birth) in this female patient. (Used with permission from Langlais RP. *Color Atlas of Common Oral Diseases.* Philadelphia, PA: Wolters Kluwer; 2003.)

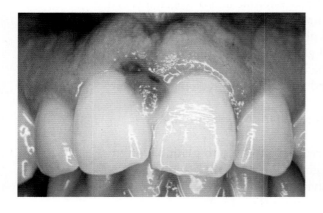

Figure 15-9. Pregnancy-Associated Pyogenic granuloma. The clinical appearance of a pyogenic granuloma (pregnancy tumor).

a. The effects of pregnancy on the gingival tissues and the importance of thorough daily self-care for plaque control in combination with regular professional care should be stressed.

b. The dental hygienist should ask the expectant woman if she has any concerns about getting dental care while pregnant and be ready to address her concerns.

c. Expectant women should be advised that prevention, diagnosis, and treatment of oral diseases—including needed dental x-ray and use of local anesthesia—is safe, beneficial, and can be undertaken any time during pregnancy (68). Also, acute/emergency care may be provided at any time during pregnancy.

d. Hygienists should encourage behaviors that support good oral health.
   1. Meticulous daily self-care for biofilm control.

2. Prenatal vitamins, including folic acid to reduce the risk of birth defects such as cleft lip and palate.

3. Chewing xylitol-containing gum to decrease caries risk.

2. Expectant women experiencing frequent nausea and vomiting should be advised that erosion of tooth surfaces might be reduced by

   a. Eating more frequent, smaller meals consisting of nutritious foods.

   b. Using a rinse comprised of one-teaspoon baking soda in a cup of water should be used to rinse and spit out after vomiting. Avoiding toothbrushing directly after vomiting as the effect of erosion can be exacerbated.

3. A comprehensive periodontal treatment plan should be developed for preventive, treatment, and maintenance care throughout pregnancy. In addition, the importance of regular dental care during the postpartum period and thereafter should be emphasized.

4. Dental care should be coordinated with the expectant woman's medical care professional to ascertain whether other risk factors—such as gestation diabetes—are present and to advise the medical professional of the periodontal status of the patient and any proposed treatment.

3. Menopause and Postmenopause

   A. Impact of Menopause on the Periodontium

   1. After menopause, some women become more susceptible to periodontal disease. Dental healthcare providers often are the first professionals to notice changes that occur during menopause. The periodontium is extremely susceptible to hormonal changes that take place just before menopause. A literature review by Dutt, Chaudhary, and Kumar compiled data on the major orodental complications observed during menopause. This review observed that the health of the periodontium is most severely affected, followed by dry mouth and burning mouth; which, in turn, may increase the occurrence of oral mucosal and dental diseases, such as candidiasis (69).

   2. If menopause does affect the gingiva, it is called **menopausal gingivostomatitis**. Menopausal gingivostomatitis is characterized by gingivae that bleed readily, with an abnormally pale, dry, shiny erythematous appearance (70).

   3. During menopause there is a decline in hormonal levels, most notably, a rapid decline in estrogen levels. Lack of estrogen during and after menopause may cause the loss of bone. The rapid decline in estrogen can lead to systemic bone loss. **Osteoporosis** is a reduction in bone mass that causes an increased susceptibility to fractures (Fig. 15-10). **Osteopenia** is a condition in which there is a lower than average bone density but not necessarily an increase in the risk or incidence of fracture.

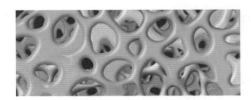

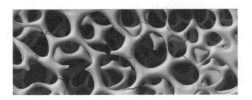

Figure 15-10. Healthy Bone Versus Bone with Osteoporosis. The upper illustration depicts the structure of healthy bone. The lower illustration depicts the reduction in bone mass commonly seen in osteoporosis.

4. Bisphosphonates are the most commonly prescribed medications to inhibit the bone resorption of systemic osteoporosis. In dentistry, there is concern about bisphosphonate-associated osteonecrosis of the jaw (71). Osteonecrosis of the jaw is a rare disorder characterized by painful areas of exposed bone in the mouth that fail to heal after an extraction or oral surgery procedure. Bisphosphonates and osteonecrosis are discussed in Chapter 26, Host Modulation.

5. The same processes that lead to loss of bone in the spine and hips can also lead to loss of alveolar bone.
   a. There may be a link between skeletal osteoporosis, alveolar bone loss in the jaw, and tooth loss (72–74). Preliminary studies report significant correlations between mandibular bone mineral density and hipbone mineral density (74,75). Some studies suggest that females with osteoporosis are at an increased risk of periodontal attachment loss and tooth loss (72,75,76).
   b. The American Academy of Periodontology considers osteoporosis to be a risk factor for periodontal disease (77). The relationship between alveolar bone loss and systemic bone loss, however, is not yet fully understood (78).
   c. In and of itself, however, osteoporosis does not initiate periodontitis. Loss of density of the alveolar bone, however, may exacerbate the bone resorption seen in pre-existing periodontitis.
   d. Estrogen replacement therapy improves bone density in postmenopausal women. In a 3-year study, hormone/estrogen replacement therapy significantly increased alveolar bone mass compared with placebo and tended to improve alveolar crest (79).

6. Genco and Grossi (80) have proposed a model for estrogen deficiency as a risk factor for periodontal disease (Fig. 15-11).

B. **Menopause: Implications for the Dental Hygienist**
   1. Dental hygienists and gynecologists should educate postmenopausal women about osteoporosis and interventions such as calcium supplements and weight-bearing exercise.
   2. Meticulous daily self-care, combined with regular professional care, decreases the likelihood of periodontal problems during menopause.

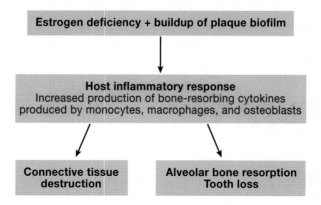

Figure 15-11. Postulated Effects of Estrogen Deficiency on the Periodontium.

Section 2
Genetic Risk Factors for Periodontitis

Periodontitis is widely recognized as a complex disease. For many years, clinical observations that severe periodontitis can occur in successive generations of some families led to speculation about the potential role of genetic factors in periodontitis. Research has begun to clarify the true role of genetics as a risk factor in this complex disease.

1. Rare Genetic Syndromes Associated with Periodontitis
   A. It is common knowledge today that genes within cell nuclei have a huge influence on most of our characteristics. Mutations or variations within these genes can lead to specific diseases, and sometimes these diseases can even affect the periodontium.
   B. There are several rare genetic disorders that in addition to creating multiple medical problems for patients can also lead to very unusual forms of periodontitis.
      1. Examples of some of these rare disorders include conditions such as Chédiak–Higashi syndrome, leukocyte adhesion deficiency syndrome, Job syndrome, Papillon–Lefèvre syndrome, Crohn disease, acute monocytic leukemia, as well as cyclic and chronic neutropenia.
      2. Many of these rare disorders are accompanied by a PMN malfunction that makes patients more susceptible to infections such as periodontitis (Fig. 15-12). Abnormalities in PMN function can lead to overwhelming systemic bacterial infections and are often associated with increased susceptibility to severe periodontal destruction.
      3. *Dental hygienists are unlikely to encounter patients with most of these severe genetic disorders outside a hospital dentistry setting.*

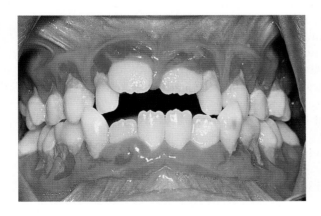

Figure 15-12. Cyclic Neutropenia. This individual with cyclic neutropenia exhibits pronounced gingival erythema. (Used with permission from Langlais RP. *Color Atlas of Common Oral Diseases.* Philadelphia, PA: Wolters Kluwer; 2003.)

2. Down Syndrome and Periodontitis. Though most of these rare genetic syndromes are unlikely to be encountered by the dental hygienist outside a hospital setting, *persons with Down syndrome are frequently treated by members of the dental team in general and periodontal dental offices.* Down syndrome is one of the most common birth defects.
   A. Genetic Changes in Down Syndrome
      1. Normally, the nucleus of each cell contains 46 chromosomes. In Down syndrome, however, the nucleus contains 47 chromosomes. Most cases of Down syndrome occur because there are three copies of the 21st chromosome. For this reason, Down syndrome is also referred to as trisomy 21.

2. Due to advances in medical treatment, individuals with Down syndrome are living longer. As the mortality rate associated with Down syndrome decreases, the prevalence of adults with Down syndrome in our society will increase. More and more dental healthcare providers will interact with individuals with this condition, increasing the need for education and acceptance.

B. **Orofacial Features Characteristic of People with Down Syndrome.** Among the most common orofacial traits of individuals with Down syndrome are:
1. An underdeveloped midfacial region, affecting the appearance of the lips, tongue, and palate.
   a. The maxilla, the bridge of the nose, and the bones of the midface region are smaller than in the general population, creating a prognathic occlusal relationship. Mouth breathing may occur because of smaller nasal passages, and the tongue may protrude because of a smaller midface region. People with Down syndrome often have a strong gag reflex due to placement of the tongue, as well as anxiety associated with any oral stimulation.
   b. The palate, although normal sized, may appear highly vaulted and narrow. This deceiving appearance is due to the unusual thickness of the sides of the hard palate. This thickness restricts the amount of space the tongue can occupy in the mouth and affects the ability to speak and chew.
   c. The lips may grow large and thick. Fissured lips may result from chronic mouth breathing. In addition, decreased muscle tone may cause the mouth to droop and the lower lip to protrude. Increased drooling, compounded by a chronically open mouth, contributes to angular cheilitis.
   d. The tongue also develops cracks and fissures with age; this condition can contribute to halitosis.
2. Malocclusion is found in most people with Down syndrome because of the delayed eruption of permanent teeth and underdevelopment of the maxilla. A smaller maxilla contributes to an open bite, leading to poor positioning of teeth and increasing the likelihood of periodontal disease and dental caries.

C. **Medical and Developmental Problems of Patients with Down Syndrome**
1. Children are at increased risk for congenital heart defects, susceptibility to infection, respiratory problems, gastrointestinal abnormalities, and childhood leukemia.
2. Abnormal PMN function is seen in about half of all patients with Down syndrome.
3. Most individuals with Down syndrome have IQs in the mild to moderate range of mental retardation. Those who receive good medical care and experience a supportive social environment can attend school, hold jobs, and participate in decisions that affect them (Fig. 15-13).

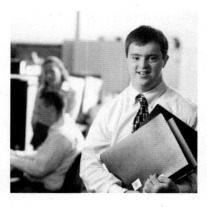

Figure 15-13. Individuals with Down Syndrome in the Workforce. With appropriate training and support people with Down Syndrome can and do make a huge contribution to their workplace. (Courtesy of Getty Images.)

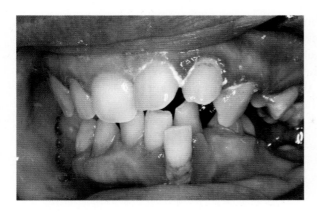

Figure 15-14. Periodontitis and Down Syndrome. A 25-year-old patient with Down syndrome exhibits severe periodontal destruction. (Courtesy of Dr. Richard Foster, Guilford Technical Community College, Jamestown, NC.)

D. Implications of Down Syndrome for the Periodontium
   1. It is widely known that individuals with Down syndrome often develop severe, aggressive periodontitis.
      a. The prevalence of periodontal disease ranges from 58% to 96% in young adults under 35 years of age with Down syndrome (81).
      b. Substantial plaque biofilm formation, deep periodontal pockets, and extensive gingival inflammation characterize periodontal disease in Down syndrome (Figs. 15-14 and 15-15A–C) (82).
   2. Children experience rapid, destructive periodontal disease. Consequently, large numbers of them lose their permanent anterior teeth in their early teens.
      a. At least some children with Down syndrome are congenitally missing at least one salivary gland (83).
      b. Studies indicate that various periodontal pathogens colonize the gingival tissues in the very early childhood years of children with Down syndrome (84).
   3. The etiology of periodontal disease in persons with Down syndrome is complex. The prevalence of periodontal disease cannot simply be attributed to poor daily self-care. In recent years, much focus has been placed on the altered immune response resulting from the underlying genetic disorder (81,85).
      a. Impaired PMN chemotaxis and phagocytosis most likely explain the high prevalence and increased severity of periodontitis associated with Down syndrome.
      b. Impaired cellular motility of gingival fibroblasts that prevents wound healing and regeneration of periodontal tissues may be involved in the etiology of Down syndrome periodontitis (86).
E. Down Syndrome: Implications for the Dental Hygienist
   1. Early and frequent professional treatment and meticulous daily care at home can mitigate the severity of periodontal disease in individuals with Down syndrome.
      a. Some people with Down syndrome can brush and floss independently, but many need help from caregivers.
      b. Encourage independence in daily self-care in those individuals who are capable on their own. Involve patients in hands-on demonstrations of brushing and interdental cleaning aids.
      c. Hygienists should educate caregivers about daily self-care. Dental healthcare providers should not assume that all caregivers know the basics; demonstrate proper brushing and flossing techniques. A power toothbrush or a floss holder can simplify oral care.

1. The hygienist can demonstrate techniques to caregivers on techniques to access the oral cavity, such as having the person close slightly for improved access to the posterior teeth and where to sit or stand to gain easier access to different areas of the dentition.

2. The hygienist should emphasize to the caregiver the importance of establishing a daily routine for oral care.

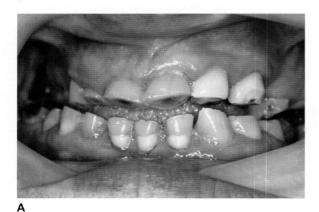

A

Figure 15-15. Periodontitis and Down Syndrome. Photos **A** to **C** show an individual with Down syndrome. **A:** This patient exhibits pronounced attrition and localized loss of attachment. (Courtesy of Dr. Richard Foster, Guilford Technical Community College, Jamestown, NC).

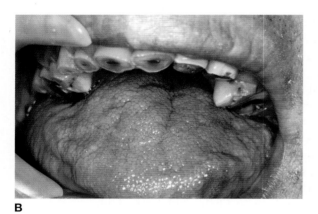

B

B: Pronounced attrition of the maxillary teeth in an individual with Down syndrome. (Courtesy of Dr. Richard Foster, Guilford Technical Community College, Jamestown, NC).

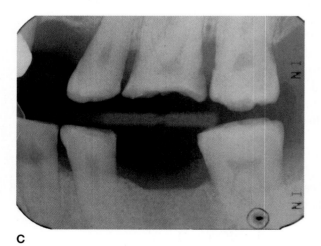

C

C: This bitewing radiograph shows attrition and localized loss of attachment on the left side of the mouth in an individual with Down syndrome. (Courtesy of Dr. Richard Foster, Guilford Technical Community College, Jamestown, NC.)

Section 3
Systemic Medications with Periodontal Side Effects

Many medications used to treat systemic diseases can cause oral complications. Effects of medications can modify oral hygiene habits, plaque biofilm composition, size of gingival tissues, level of bone, and salivary flow. Educating patients about potential oral side effects is critical to reducing the medication-related risks of periodontal disease. Commonly prescribed medications that can affect the periodontium are summarized in Table 15-2.

TABLE 15-2. HARMFUL EFFECTS OF COMMONLY PRESCRIBED MEDICATIONS ON PERIODONTIUM		
Medication Class	**Generic Name (Brand Name)**	**Effect on Periodontium**
Anticonvulsant	Phenytoin (Dilantin)	Gingival overgrowth
Antianxiety agents	Alprazolam (Zoloft)	Decreased biofilm formation
Antihypertensive	Enalapril (Vasotec)	Increased gingival inflammation
Calcium blocker	Nifedipine (Procardia)	Gingival overgrowth
Immunosuppressive	Cyclosporine (Sandimmune)	Gingival overgrowth

1. Medications that Alter Plaque Biofilm Composition, pH, or Salivary Flow
   A. Plaque Biofilm Composition or pH
      1. Many oral medications alter plaque biofilm composition and pH in ways that are harmful to the periodontium.
      2. Sugar is a major component of some cough drops, liquid medications, cough syrups, tonics, chewable vitamins, antacid tablets, and other medications. Medications that contain sugar add significantly to the alteration of pH and composition of the biofilm.
      3. Sugar is metabolized by bacteria to form acid, causing enamel to demineralize. The demineralized areas are rough and act as attachment sites for bacteria, keeping bacterial plaque biofilm against tissues and eventually resulting in inflammation of the gingiva.
      4. Some over-the-counter (OTC) preparations contain sugar and vitamin C. This combination delivers sugar and the vitamins cause an acid pH.
      5. Products that alter the plaque biofilm pH significantly can cause root-surface caries in older adults and have an effect on the metabolism of periodontal pathogens (87,88).
   B. Salivary Flow and pH
      1. Adequate saliva flow is necessary for the maintenance of healthy oral tissues. The ability of saliva to limit the growth of pathogens is a major determinant of systemic and oral health.
         a. The physical flow of the saliva helps to dislodge microbes from the teeth and mucosa surfaces. Saliva can also cause bacteria to clump together, so that they can be swallowed before they become firmly attached.

    b. Saliva is rich in antimicrobial components. Certain molecules in saliva can directly kill or inhibit a variety of microbes.

2. Patients with xerostomia suffer from an increase in the incidence of oral candidiasis, coronal and root-surface caries, as well as excess plaque biofilm formation. Xerostomia is discussed more fully in Chapter 33, Oral Malodor and Xerostomia.

3. More than 400 OTC and prescription drugs have xerostomia as a possible side effect (89).

4. Some of the more common groups of medications that cause xerostomia are cardiovascular medications (blood pressure, diuretics, calcium channel blockers); antidepressants; sedatives; anti-parkinsonism medications; allergy medications; and antacids (90).

2. Drug-Influenced Gingival Enlargement

A. Introduction

1. **Drug-influenced gingival enlargement** is an esthetically disfiguring overgrowth of the gingiva that is a side effect associated with certain medications.

2. *Drugs associated with gingival enlargement can be broadly divided into three categories: anticonvulsants, calcium channel blockers, and immunosuppressants* (Table 15-2). These three classes of medications influence gingival fibroblasts to overproduce collagen matrix when stimulated by gingival inflammation (91).

    a. More than 20 medications have been shown to have the potential to induce gingival enlargement.

    b. Among longstanding and relatively newer pharmacologic agents involved in gingival enlargement, overall, the anticonvulsant phenytoin still has the highest prevalence rate with calcium channel blockers and immunosuppressant-associated enlargements about half as prevalent (92).

3. The clinical characteristics of drug-influenced gingival enlargement include enlargement of the gingiva, tendency to occur more often in the anterior gingiva, prevalence in younger age groups, and onset within 3 months of use (93).

B. Anticonvulsants

1. **Phenytoin** (FEN-i-toyn) is one of the most commonly used anticonvulsant medications used to control convulsions or seizures in the treatment of epilepsy. Phenytoin is marketed under various trade names including Dilantin 4, Dilantin Kapseals 4, and Phenytoin. Phenytoin is among the 20 most prescribed drugs in the world.

2. Overgrowth of the gingiva is one of the most common side effects of phenytoin. It has been estimated that 40% to 50% of the millions of individuals who take phenytoin will develop gingival overgrowth to some extent (92). Overgrowths appear to be more common in children and young adults.

3. Gingival overgrowth begins with enlargement of the interdental papillae.

    a. The interdental papillae overgrow, forming firm triangular tissue masses that protrude from the interdental area.

    b. Gradually the enlarged papillae may fuse mesially and distally and partially cover the anatomical crown with marginal gingiva (Fig. 15-16). Overgrowths are most commonly seen on the facial aspect of the anterior teeth.

    c. In the presence of good biofilm control, the enlarged tissue is pink in color and firm and rubbery in consistency. In the presence of poor biofilm control, the tissue appears red, edematous, and spongy.

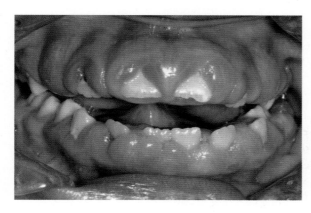

Figure 15-16. Phenytoin-Influenced Gingival Overgrowth. Severe enlargement of the gingiva associated with phenytoin (Dilantin) medication in an individual with epilepsy. (Courtesy of Dr. Ralph Arnold, San Antonio, TX.)

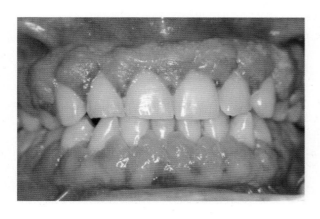

Figure 15-17. Cyclosporine-Influenced Gingival Overgrowth. The clinical appearance of cyclosporine-associated gingival overgrowth resembles that of phenytoin-associated gingival enlargement. (Courtesy of Dr. Ralph Arnold, San Antonio, TX.)

C. **Immunosuppressants**
   1. **Cyclosporine** (SIGH-kloe-spor-een) belongs to the group of medicines known as immunosuppressive agents used for prevention of transplant rejection as well as for management of a number of autoimmune conditions such as rheumatoid arthritis.
   2. The incidence of cyclosporine-associated gingival overgrowth affects approximately 25% of patients taking the medication.
   3. The clinical appearance of cyclosporine-associated gingival overgrowth resembles that of phenytoin-associated gingival enlargement (Fig. 15-17).
D. **Calcium Channel Blockers**
   1. Antihypertensive drugs in the calcium channel blocker group are used extensively in elderly patients who have angina or peripheral vascular disease.
   2. The use of calcium channel blockers is associated with an increased risk of gingival hyperplasia (94,95).
      a. **Nifedipine** (nye-FED-I-peen), one type of calcium channel blocker, is used as a coronary vasodilator in the treatment of hypertension, angina, and cardiac arrhythmias. Calcium channel blockers are a class of drugs that block the influx of calcium ions through cardiac and vascular smooth muscle cell membranes. This results in the dilation of the main coronary and systemic arteries.
      b. Various other calcium channel blocking medications, such as diltiazem, felodipine, nitrendipine, and verapamil also may induce gingival enlargement.
   3. The clinical appearance of gingival overgrowth associated with calcium channel blockers resembles that of phenytoin-associated gingival enlargement (Figs. 15-18 and 15-19).

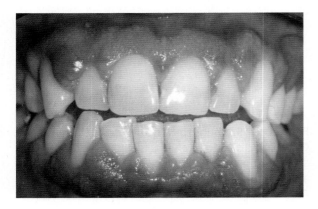

Figure 15-18. Gingival Overgrowth Associated with Nifedipine. Gingival overgrowth in a patient who takes nifedipine for the treatment of cardiac arrhythmia. (Courtesy of Dr. Ralph Arnold, San Antonio, TX.)

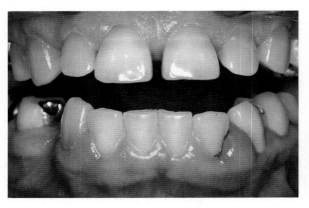
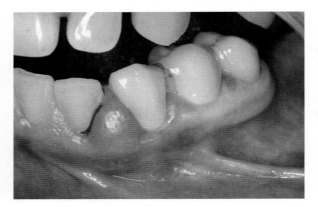

Figure 15-19. Gingival Enlargement Associated with Calcium Channel Blocking Drugs. Gingival enlargement of the papilla between the lateral incisor and canine induced by the calcium channel blocking medication Norvasc. (Courtesy of Dr. Richard Foster, Guilford Technical Community College, Jamestown, NC.)

  E. **Systemic Medications: Implications for the Dental Hygienist**
    1. Dental hygienists should be alert for patient medications that can alter biofilm composition, pH, or salivary flow.
      a. Sugar-containing liquid or chewable medications are sometimes used in the treatment of children with chronic medical problems. Parents should be made aware of the oral health consequences of such medications. Giving the medications at mealtimes instead of between meals is helpful.
      b. Some OTC preparations contain sugar and vitamin C. This combination delivers sugar and the vitamins cause an acid pH. Examples of products containing sugar and vitamin C include chewable vitamin C tablets, certain cough drops, and certain liquid cough preparations.
    2. Closer collaboration between medical and dental clinical teams is necessary for the joint management of individuals being treated with anticonvulsants, calcium channel blockers, or immunosuppressants (46). Patients receiving cyclosporine are usually medically compromised, requiring close consultation with the patient's physician to assure safe management of the patient's periodontal condition. In addition to professional and at-home plaque biofilm control, it has been shown that azithromycin induced a striking reduction in cyclosporine-induced gingival hyperplasia (96).
    3. Treatment of gingival enlargement should include consultation with the physician, substitution of the current medication for another whenever possible,

nonsurgical periodontal therapy, frequent periodontal maintenance, and surgical therapy, if needed (96).

a. The hygienist should emphasize the importance of meticulous daily self-care and involve patients in hands-on demonstrations of brushing and interdental cleaning aids.

b. Surgical elimination of the tissue overgrowth is often required. Unfortunately, the gingival overgrowth is likely to recur within 1 to 2 years even in the presence of good plaque biofilm control, especially if the patient is younger than 25 years. If plaque biofilm control is inadequate, the regrowth will occur rapidly. The patient should be advised of the likelihood of the recurrence of the gingival overgrowth following surgery.

Chapter Summary Statement

The presence of dental plaque biofilm does not necessarily mean that an individual will experience periodontitis. Additional factors play a role in determining why some individuals are more susceptible to periodontitis than others. Significant systemic contributing factors include diabetes mellitus, leukemia, AIDS, hormonal fluctuations, genetic risk factors, and systemic medications. Contributing risk factors must be evaluated to develop the best treatment plan for each individual. Dental professionals should provide health promotion education that contributes to overall systemic and periodontal health and collaborate with medical team members for joint patient management.

Section 4
Focus on Patients

Clinical Patient Care

CASE 1

A patient, who has been previously treated for chronic periodontitis and has been followed by your dental team for several years, calls your dental office with a concern. She is scheduled to undergo a liver transplant and has been warned by her physician that the medications she will need will make her more susceptible to infections. She asks if these medications might have an effect on her continuing treatment for periodontitis. How might you respond to her concern?

CASE 2

The parents of a young patient currently being treated by your dental team inform you that following a lengthy illness, their daughter has recently been diagnosed by her physician with a neutrophil defect. Neutrophils are also known as polymorphonuclear leukocytes. They inquire about any dental implications of this diagnosis. How might you respond to this inquiry?

Evidence in Action

CASE 1

A new patient in your office reports that she has recently been diagnosed with diabetes mellitus and that her physician suggested that she should have a dental checkup. The patient confides in you that she feels like this disease is really changing her lifestyle. She laughingly says "I have always had such good reports from my previous dentist, and I just don't really see why I need to be worried about my teeth now." Based upon what is known about the relationship between diabetes and periodontal disease, how might you explain the need for the recommended dental exam to the patient?

Ethical Dilemma

You have just recently married and moved across the country to the city where your husband was raised. His parents helped you secure a full-time dental hygiene position with their family dentist, Dr. Ramos. You are quite happy working with the office staff, as well as meeting and getting to know many of your in-law's family and friends, who are patients of the practice as well.

Today your mother-in-law, June, is scheduled for her 6-month recall appointment. This is the first time you will be treating her. You review her medical history, and she states that lately she's been feeling tired, lethargic, and has a poor appetite. She assumed she was just overtired from all the wedding planning and festivities. She hasn't been able to workout regularly, as she has musculoskeletal aches and pains.

Your clinical examination reveals gingival enlargement and spontaneous gingival bleeding, despite excellent self-care. Her tissues are swollen, glazed, and spongy, red to deep purple in appearance, and ooze blood intermittently. She also appears to have facial swelling. You review the notes from her last appointment, which was 6 months ago, and see that her tissues were classified as normal and healthy.

You become very concerned that June may have a serious medical condition, and you are not sure what to do. You feel that you need to discuss this with your husband before saying anything to June.

1. What systemic condition do you think could be causing June's signs/symptoms?
2. What ethical principles are in conflict in this dilemma?
3. What is the best way for you to handle this ethical dilemma?

References

1. Wild S, Roglic G, Green A, et al. Global prevalence of diabetes: estimates for the year 2000 and projections for 2030. *Diabetes Care.* 2004;27(5):1047–1053.
2. Christgau M, Palitzsch KD, Schmalz G, et al. Healing response to non-surgical periodontal therapy in patients with diabetes mellitus: clinical, microbiological, and immunologic results. *J Clin Periodontol.* 1998;25(2):112–124.
3. Deshpande K, Jain A, Sharma R, et al. Diabetes and periodontitis. *J Indian Soc Periodontol.* 2010;14(4):207–212.
4. Preshaw PM, Alba AL, Herrera D, et al. Periodontitis and diabetes: a two-way relationship. *Diabetologia.* 2012;55(1):21–31.
5. Botero JE, Yepes FL, Roldan N, et al. Tooth and periodontal clinical attachment loss are associated with hyperglycemia in patients with diabetes. *J Periodontol.* 2012;83(10):1245–1250.
6. Demmer RT, Holtfreter B, Desvarieux M, et al. The influence of type 1 and type 2 diabetes on periodontal disease progression: prospective results from the Study of Health in Pomerania (SHIP). *Diabetes Care.* 2012;35(10):2036–2042.
7. Haseeb M, Khawaja KI, Ataullah K, et al. Periodontal disease in type 2 diabetes mellitus. *J Coll Physicians Surg Pak.* 2012;22(8):514–518.

8. Diabetes and periodontal diseases. Committee on Research, Science and Therapy. American Academy of Periodontology. *J Periodontol.* 2000;71(4):664–678.

9. Mealey BL, Oates TW, American Academy of Periodontology. Diabetes mellitus and periodontal diseases. *J Periodontol.* 2006;77(8):1289–1303.

10. Preshaw PM, Bissett SM. Periodontitis: oral complication of diabetes. *Endocrinol Metab Clin North Am.* 2013;42(4): 849–867.

11. Salvi GE, Yalda B, Collins JG, et al. Inflammatory mediator response as a potential risk marker for periodontal diseases in insulin-dependent diabetes mellitus patients. *J Periodontol.* 1997;68(2):127–135.

12. Taylor JJ, Preshaw PM, Lalla E. A review of the evidence for pathogenic mechanisms that may link periodontitis and diabetes. *J Periodontol.* 2013;84(4 suppl):S113–S134.

13. Apoorva SM, Sridhar N, Suchetha A. Prevalence and severity of periodontal disease in type 2 diabetes mellitus (non-insulin-dependent diabetes mellitus) patients in Bangalore city: an epidemiological study. *J Indian Soc Periodontol.* 2013;17(1): 25–29.

14. Daniel R, Gokulanathan S, Shanmugasundaram N, et al. Diabetes and periodontal disease. *J Pharm Bioallied Sci.* 2012;4(suppl 2):S280–S282.

15. Monea A, Mezei T, Monea M. The influence of diabetes mellitus on periodontal tissues: a histological study. *Rom J Morphol Embryol.* 2012;53(3):491–495.

16. Tervonen T, Karjalainen K. Periodontal disease related to diabetic status. A pilot study of the response to periodontal therapy in type 1 diabetes. *J Clin Periodontol.* 1997;24(7):505–510.

17. Westfelt E, Rylander H, Blohme G, et al. The effect of periodontal therapy in diabetics. Results after 5 years. *J Clin Periodontol.* 1996;23(2):92–100.

18. Gugliucci A. Glycation as the glucose link to diabetic complications. *J Am Osteopath Assoc.* 2000;100(10):621–634.

19. Busato IM, Ignacio SA, Brancher JA, et al. Impact of xerostomia on the quality of life of adolescents with type 1 diabetes mellitus. *Oral Surg Oral Med Oral Pathol Oral Radiol Endod.* 2009;108(3):376–382.

20. Lin CC, Sun SS, Kao A, et al. Impaired salivary function in patients with noninsulin-dependent diabetes mellitus with xerostomia. *J Diabetes Complications.* 2002;16(2):176–179.

21. Moore PA, Guggenheimer J, Etzel KR, et al. Type 1 diabetes mellitus, xerostomia, and salivary flow rates. *Oral Surg Oral Med Oral Pathol Oral Radiol Endod.* 2001;92(3):281–291.

22. Ueta E, Osaki T, Yoneda K, et al. Prevalence of diabetes mellitus in odontogenic infections and oral candidiasis: an analysis of neutrophil suppression. *J Oral Pathol Med.* 1993;22(4):168–174.

23. Dye BA, Genco RJ. Tooth loss, pocket depth, and HbA1 c information collected in a dental care setting may improve the identification of undiagnosed diabetes. *Evid Based Dent Pract.* 2012;12(3 suppl):12–14.

24. Genco RJ. Periodontal disease and association with diabetes mellitus and diabetes: clinical implications. *J Dent Hyg.* 2009;83(4):186–187.

25. Al-Khabbaz AK, Al-Shammari KF, Al-Saleh NA. Knowledge about the association between periodontal diseases and diabetes mellitus: contrasting dentists and physicians. *J Periodontol.* 2011;82(3):360–366.

26. Lalla E, Kunzel C, Burkett S, et al. Identification of unrecognized diabetes and pre-diabetes in a dental setting. *J Dent Res.* 2011;90(7):855–860.

27. Kanjirath PP, Kim SE, Rohr Inglehart M. Diabetes and oral health: the importance of oral health-related behavior. *J Dent Hyg.* 2011;85(4):264–272.

28. Strauss SM, Singh G, Tuthill J, et al. Diabetes-related knowledge and sources of information among periodontal patients: is there a role for dental hygienists? *J Dent Hyg.* 2013;87(2):82–89.

29. Valerio MA, Kanjirath PP, Klausner CP, et al. A qualitative examination of patient awareness and understanding of type 2 diabetes and oral health care needs. *Diabetes Res Clin Pract.* 2011;93(2):159–165.

30. Yuen HK, Marlow NM, Mahoney S, et al. Oral health content in diabetes self-management education programs. *Diabetes Res Clin Pract.* 2010;90(3):e82–e84.

31. Yuen HK, Wolf BJ, Bandyopadhyay D, et al. Oral health knowledge and behavior among adults with diabetes. *Diabetes Res Clin Pract.* 2009;86(3):239–246.

32. Chapple IL, Genco R; working group 2 of the joint EFPAAPw. Diabetes and periodontal diseases: consensus report of the Joint EFP/AAP Workshop on Periodontitis and Systemic Diseases. *J Periodontol.* 2013;84(4 suppl):S106–S112.

33. Lopes MH, Southerland JH, Buse JB, et al. Diabetes educators' knowledge, opinions and behaviors regarding periodontal disease and diabetes. *J Dent Hyg.* 2012;86(2):82–90.

34. Lalla E, Cheng B, Lal S, et al. Diabetes mellitus promotes periodontal destruction in children. *J Clin Periodontol.* 2007;34(4):294–298.

35. Sepulveda E, Brethauer U, Fernandez E, et al. Oral manifestations as first clinical sign of acute myeloid leukemia: report of a case. *Pediatr Dent.* 2012;34(5):418–421.

36. Azher U, Shiggaon N. Oral health status of children with acute lymphoblastic leukemia undergoing chemotherapy. *Indian J Dent Res.* 2013;24(4):523.

37. Bektas-Kayhan K, Kucukhuseyin O, Karagoz G, et al. Is the MDR1 C3435T polymorphism responsible for oral mucositis in children with acute lymphoblastic leukemia? *Asian Pac J Cancer Prev.* 2012;13(10):5251–5255.

38. Javed F, Utreja A, Bello Correa FO, et al. Oral health status in children with acute lymphoblastic leukemia. *Crit Rev Oncol Hematol.* 2012;83(3):303–309.

39. Mathur VP, Dhillon JK, Kalra G. Oral health in children with leukemia. *Indian J Palliat Care.* 2012;18(1):12–18.

40. Soares AF, Aquino AR, Carvalho CH, et al. Frequency of oral mucositis and microbiological analysis in children with acute lymphoblastic leukemia treated with 0.12% chlorhexidine gluconate. *Braz Dent J.* 2011;22(4):312–316.

41. Dreizen S, McCredie KB, Keating MJ. Chemotherapy-associated oral hemorrhages in adults with acute leukemia. *Oral Surg Oral Med Oral Pathol.* 1984;57(5):494–498.

42. Mikulska M, Calandra T, Sanguinetti M, et al.; Third European Conference on Infections in Leukemia Group. The use of mannan antigen and anti-mannan antibodies in the diagnosis of invasive candidiasis: recommendations from the Third European Conference on Infections in Leukemia. *Crit Care.* 2010;14(6):R222.

43. Silva BA, Siqueira CR, Castro PH, et al. Oral manifestations leading to the diagnosis of acute lymphoblastic leukemia in a young girl. *J Indian Soc Pedod Prev Dent.* 2012;30(2):166–168.

44. Thomaz EB, Mouchrek JC Jr., Silva AQ, et al. Longitudinal assessment of immunological and oral clinical conditions in patients undergoing anticancer treatment for leukemia. *Int J Pediatr Otorhinolaryngol.* 2013;77(7):1088–1093.
45. Berger A, Henderson M, Nadoolman W, et al. Oral capsaicin provides temporary relief for oral mucositis pain secondary to chemotherapy/radiation therapy. *J Pain Symptom Manage.* 1995;10(3):243–248.
46. Bridges DR, Davidson RA, Odegard PS, et al. Interprofessional collaboration: three best practice models of interprofessional education. *Med Educ Online.* 2011;16.
47. Goncalves LS, Goncalves BM, de Andrade MA, et al. Drug interactions during periodontal therapy in HIV-infected subjects. *Mini Rev Med Chem.* 2010;10(8):766–772.
48. Ryder MI, Nittayananta W, Coogan M, et al. Periodontal disease in HIV/AIDS. *Periodontol 2000.* 2012;60(1):78–97.
49. Hirnschall G, Harries AD, Easterbrook PJ, et al. The next generation of the World Health Organization's global antiretroviral guidance. *J Int AIDS Soc.* 2013;16:18757.
50. Mataftsi M, Skoura L, Sakellari D. HIV infection and periodontal diseases: an overview of the post-HAART era. *Oral Dis.* 2011;17(1):13–25.
51. Armitage GC. Development of a classification system for periodontal diseases and conditions. *Ann Periodontol.* 1999; 4(1):1–6.
52. Yin MT, Dobkin JF, Grbic JT. Epidemiology, pathogenesis, and management of human immunodeficiency virus infection in patients with periodontal disease. *Periodontol 2000.* 2007;44:55–81.
53. Velegraki A, Nicolatou O, Theodoridou M, et al. Paediatric AIDS–related linear gingival erythema: a form of erythematous candidiasis? *J Oral Pathol Med.* 1999;28(4):178–182.
54. Kroidl A, Schaeben A, Oette M, et al. Prevalence of oral lesions and periodontal diseases in HIV-infected patients on antiretroviral therapy. *Eur J Med Res.* 2005;10(10):448–453.
55. Fricke U, Geurtsen W, Staufenbiel I, et al. Periodontal status of HIV-infected patients undergoing antiretroviral therapy compared to HIV-therapy naive patients: a case control study. *Eur J Med Res.* 2012;17:2.
56. Lemos SS, Oliveira FA, Vencio EF. Periodontal disease and oral hygiene benefits in HIV seropositive and AIDS patients. *Med Oral Patol Oral Cir Bucal.* 2010;15(2):e417–e421.
57. Stojkovic A, Boras VV, Planbak D, et al. Evaluation of periodontal status in HIV infected persons in Croatia. *Coll Antropol.* 2011;35(1):67–71.
58. Vernon LT, Demko CA, Whalen CC, et al. Characterizing traditionally defined periodontal disease in HIV+ adults. *Community Dent Oral Epidemiol.* 2009;37(5):427–437.
59. Hein C. Translating evidence of oral-systemic relationships into models of interprofessional collaboration. *J Dent Hyg.* 2009;83(4):188–189.
60. Kara C, Demir T, Tezel A. Effectiveness of periodontal therapies on the treatment of different aetiological factors induced gingival overgrowth in puberty. *Int J Dent Hyg.* 2007;5(4):211–217.
61. Gursoy M, Gursoy UK, Sorsa T, et al. High salivary estrogen and risk of developing pregnancy gingivitis. *J Periodontol.* 2013;84(9):1281–1289.
62. Straka M. Pregnancy and periodontal tissues. *Neuro Endocrinol Lett.* 2011;32(1):34–38.
63. Armitage GC. Bi-directional relationship between pregnancy and periodontal disease. *Periodontol 2000.* 2013;61(1):160–176.
64. Lundgren D, Magnusson B, Lindhe J. Connective tissue alterations in gingivae of rats treated with estrogen and progesterone. A histologic and autoradiographic study. *Odontol Revy.* 1973;24(1):49–58.
65. Boggess KA, Society for Maternal-Fetal Medicine Publications C. Maternal oral health in pregnancy. *Obstet Gynecol.* 2008;111(4):976–986.
66. Silk H, Douglass AB, Douglass JM, et al. Oral health during pregnancy. *Am Fam Physician.* 2008;77(8):1139–1144.
67. Boggess KA, Edelstein BL. Oral health in women during preconception and pregnancy: implications for birth outcomes and infant oral health. *Matern Child Health J.* 2006;10(5 suppl):S169–S174.
68. American College of Obstetricians and Gynecologists Women's Health Care Physicians, Committee on Health Care for Underserved Women. Committee Opinion No. 569: oral health care during pregnancy and through the lifespan. *Obstet Gynecol.* 2013;122(2 Pt 1):417–422.
69. Dutt P, Chaudhary S, Kumar P. Oral health and menopause: a comprehensive review on current knowledge and associated dental management. *Ann Med Health Sci Res.* 2013;3(3):320–323.
70. Friedlander AH. The physiology, medical management and oral implications of menopause. *J Am Dent Assoc.* 2002;133(1):73–81.
71. Carey JJ, Palomo L. Bisphosphonates and osteonecrosis of the jaw: innocent association or significant risk? *Cleve Clin J Med.* 2008;75(12):871–879.
72. Al Habashneh R, Alchalabi H, Khader YS, et al. Association between periodontal disease and osteoporosis in postmenopausal women in Jordan. *J Periodontol.* 2010;81(11):1613–1621.
73. Bertulucci Lde A, Pereira FM, de Oliveira AE, et al. [Periodontal disease in women in post-menopause and its relationship with osteoporosis]. *Rev Bras Ginecol Obstet.* 2012;34(12):563–567.
74. Vishwanath SB, Kumar V, Kumar S, et al. Correlation of periodontal status and bone mineral density in postmenopausal women: a digital radiographic and quantitative ultrasound study. *Indian J Dent Res.* 2011;22(2):270–276.
75. Jeffcoat M. The association between osteoporosis and oral bone loss. *J Periodontol.* 2005;76(11 suppl):2125–2132.
76. Chang WP, Chang WC, Wu MS, et al. Population-based 5-year follow-up study in Taiwan of osteoporosis and risk of periodontitis. *J Periodontol.* 2014;85(3):e24–e30.
77. American Dental Association. Council on Access, Prevention, and Interprofessional Relations. Women's Oral Health Issues. Chicago, IL: American Dental Association, 2006, pp. 46 (Oral health care series).
78. Pilgram TK, Hildebolt CF, Yokoyama-Crothers N, et al. Relationships between longitudinal changes in radiographic alveolar bone height and probing depth measurements: data from postmenopausal women. *J Periodontol.* 1999;70(8):829–833.
79. Civitelli R, Pilgram TK, Dotson M, et al. Alveolar and postcranial bone density in postmenopausal women receiving hormone/estrogen replacement therapy: a randomized, double-blind, placebo-controlled trial. *Arch Intern Med.* 2002;162(12):1409–1415.
80. Genco RJ, Grossi SG. Is estrogen deficiency a risk factor for periodontal disease? *Compend Contin Educ Dent Suppl.* 1998(22):S23–S29.
81. Morgan J. Why is periodontal disease more prevalent and more severe in people with Down syndrome? *Spec Care Dentist.* 2007;27(5):196–201.

82. Barr-Agholme M, Dahllof G, Modeer T, et al. Periodontal conditions and salivary immunoglobulins in individuals with Down syndrome. *J Periodontol.* 1998;69(10):1119–1123.

83. Odeh M, Hershkovits M, Bornstein J, et al. Congenital absence of salivary glands in Down syndrome. *Arch Dis Child.* 2013;98(10):781–783.

84. Amano A, Kishima T, Kimura S, et al. Periodontopathic bacteria in children with Down syndrome. *J Periodontol.* 2000;71(2):249–255.

85. Cavalcante LB, Tanaka MH, Pires JR, et al. Expression of the interleukin-10 signaling pathway genes in individuals with Down syndrome and periodontitis. *J Periodontol.* 2012;83(7):926–935.

86. Murakami J, Kato T, Kawai S, et al. Cellular motility of Down syndrome gingival fibroblasts is susceptible to impairment by Porphyromonas gingivalis invasion. *J Periodontol.* 2008;79(4):721–727.

87. Steele JG, Sheiham A, Marcenes W, et al. Clinical and behavioural risk indicators for root caries in older people. *Gerodontology.* 2001;18(2):95–101.

88. Touger-Decker R, van Loveren C. Sugars and dental caries. *Am J Clin Nutr.* 2003;78(4):881S–892S.

89. Ciancio SG. Medications' impact on oral health. *J Am Dent Assoc.* 2004;135(10):1440–1448; quiz 68–69.

90. Guggenheimer J, Moore PA. Xerostomia: etiology, recognition and treatment. *J Am Dent Assoc.* 2003;134(1):61–69; quiz 118–119.

91. Dongari-Bagtzoglou A; Research, Science and Therapy Committee, American Academy of Periodontology. Drug-associated gingival enlargement. *J Periodontol.* 2004;75(10):1424–1431.

92. Mohan RP, Rastogi K, Bhushan R, et al. Phenytoin-induced gingival enlargement: a dental awakening for patients with epilepsy. *BMJ Case Reports.* 2013;2013. doi:10.1136/bcr-2013–008679.

93. Drug-induced gingival hyperplasia. *Prescrire Int.* 2011;20(122):293–294.

94. Sanz M. Current use of calcium channel blockers (CCBs) is associated with an increased risk of gingival hyperplasia. *J Evid Based Dent Pract.* 2012;12(3 suppl):147–148.

95. Parwani RN, Parwani SR. Management of phenytoin-induced gingival enlargement: a case report. *Gen Dent.* 2013;61(6): 61–67.

96. Ramalho VL, Ramalho HJ, Cipullo JP, et al. Comparison of azithromycin and oral hygiene program in the treatment of cyclosporine-induced gingival hyperplasia. *Ren Fail.* 2007;29(3):265–270.

 STUDENT ANCILLARY RESOURCES

A wide variety of resources to enhance your learning and understanding of this chapter are available on thePoint®.

- Visit thePoint to access:
  - Audio Glossary
  - Animations
  - Suggested Readings
  - Answers to Review Questions
  - Case Studies

16

Local Factors Contributing to Periodontal Disease

Clinical Application.
As discussed in other chapters of this book, periodontal diseases are infections. Many individuals, however, have local contributing factors that can (1) make it more likely that they will develop periodontal disease or (2) affect the progress of existing periodontal disease. Members of the dental team must identify these local factors when they exist and minimize the impact of these factors for periodontal therapy to be truly successful. This chapter outlines these local contributing factors and explains how these factors can alter periodontal disease in patients.

Learning Objectives

- Define the terms pathogenicity and local contributing factors.

- Describe local etiologic factors that contribute to the retention and accumulation of microbial plaque biofilm.

- Explain the meaning of the phrase "pathogenicity of plaque biofilm."

- Identify and differentiate the location, composition, modes of attachment, mechanisms of mineralization, and pathologic potential of supra- and subgingival calculus deposits.

- Describe local contributing factors that can lead to direct damage to the periodontium.

- Explain the role of trauma from occlusion as a possible contributing factor in periodontal disease.

Key Terms

Local contributing factors
Disease site
Dental calculus
Pellicle
Morphology
Overhanging restoration
Palatogingival groove
Pathogenicity
Plaque biofilm pathogenicity

Food impaction
Tongue thrusting
Mouth breathing
Biologic width
Embrasure space
Encroaching on the
    embrasure space
Prosthesis
Removable prosthesis

Trauma from occlusion
Primary trauma from occlusion
Secondary trauma from
    occlusion
Functional occlusal forces
Parafunctional occlusal forces
Clenching
Bruxism
Occlusal adjustment

Section 1
Introduction to Local Contributing Factors

As will be discussed in subsequent chapters, it is clear that both gingivitis and periodontitis have bacterial plaque biofilm as their primary etiology. There are, however, certain local contributing factors that can increase the risk of developing gingivitis and periodontitis or that can increase the risk of developing more severe disease when gingivitis and periodontitis are already established (1–3). **Local contributing factors** for periodontal disease are oral conditions or habits that increase an individual's susceptibility to periodontal infection or that can damage the periodontium in specific sites within the dentition. Local contributing factors do not actually initiate either gingivitis or periodontitis, but these factors can contribute to the disease process previously initiated by bacterial plaque biofilm.

It is critical for the dental team to recognize local contributing factors for periodontal disease during a periodontal assessment. The dental team should always eliminate or at least minimize the impact of existing local contributing factors during the nonsurgical periodontal treatment.

The conditions discussed in this chapter refer to circumstances that favor periodontal breakdown and can contribute to gingivitis or periodontitis in individual sites in the mouth. In the context of this discussion, a **disease site** is an individual tooth or specific surface of a tooth. For instance, a local contributing factor might increase the susceptibility to periodontal infection on the distal surface of a maxillary premolar tooth. Examples of potential local contributing factors can include dental calculus, faulty dental restorations, developmental defects in teeth, dental decay, certain patient habits, and trauma from occlusion.

MECHANISMS FOR INCREASED DISEASE RISK

Local contributing factors can increase the risk of developing gingivitis or periodontitis through several mechanisms or through combinations of these mechanisms. Table 16-1 summarizes mechanisms for increasing disease risk in local sites, and each of these mechanisms is discussed in detail in the following sections of this chapter. There are three primary mechanisms by which local factors can increase the risk of developing periodontal disease or increase the severity of existing periodontal disease.
1. A local factor can increase plaque biofilm retention.
2. A local factor can increase plaque biofilm pathogenicity (disease-causing potential).
3. A local factor can cause direct damage to the periodontium.

TABLE 16-1. MECHANISMS FOR INCREASING DISEASE RISK IN LOCAL SITES	
Mechanism	**Clinical Example**
Local factor that increases plaque biofilm retention	Rough edge on a restoration harbors plaque biofilm and makes it difficult to remove plaque biofilm with a brush and floss
Local factor that increases plaque biofilm pathogenicity (disease-causing potential)	Calculus which harbors plaque biofilm, allowing it to grow uninhibited for an extended period of time
Local factor that can inflict damage to the periodontium	Ill-fitting dental appliance that puts excessive pressure on the gingiva

Section 2
Local Factors That Can Increase Biofilm Retention

This section discusses local factors that can increase plaque biofilm retention. Most often these local contributing factors include rough or irregular surfaces that decrease the effectiveness of a patient's self-care and lead to the increased plaque biofilm retention.

1. **Dental Calculus.** Dental calculus is the most obvious example of a local contributing factor that can lead to increased plaque biofilm retention. **Dental calculus** is mineralized bacterial plaque biofilm, covered on its external surface by nonmineralized, living bacterial plaque biofilm. Mineralization of plaque biofilm can begin from 48 hours up to 2 weeks after plaque biofilm formation.

   A. **Effects of Calculus on the Periodontium**
      1. The surface of a calculus deposit at the microscopic level is quite irregular in contour and is always covered with disease-causing bacteria. Thus, even calculus that has not built up enough to result in a ledge or grossly altered tooth contour can lead to plaque biofilm retention at the site simply because of the rough nature of the calculus surface and its tendency to harbor bacteria.
      2. As dental calculus deposits build up, they can lead to even more irregular surfaces, ledges on the teeth, and other alterations of the contours of the teeth (Fig. 16-1). As calculus deposits accumulate, they create more and more areas of plaque biofilm retention that are difficult or impossible for a patient to clean.

   B. **Pathologic Potential**
      1. Since a layer of living bacterial plaque biofilm always covers a calculus deposit, dental calculus plays a significant role as a local contributing factor in periodontal disease.
      2. It is difficult to bring either gingivitis or periodontitis under control in the presence of dental calculus on affected teeth, and the importance of removing these deposits in patients with gingivitis and periodontitis cannot be overemphasized. The removal of dental calculus is discussed in Chapter 22.

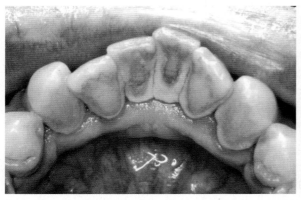
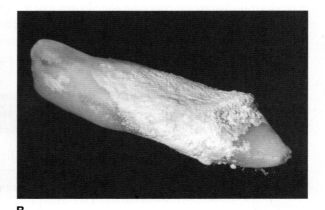

A   **B**

Figure 16-1. Irregular Surface of Calculus Deposits. A: Heavy calculus deposits on the lingual surfaces of the mandibular anterior teeth. These deposits are so large that they interfere with the patient's self-care efforts. In addition, calculus deposits harbor living bacteria that can be in constant contact with the gingival tissue.
B: Calculus deposit on the crown and root surfaces of an extracted mandibular canine. (Photograph **B** courtesy of Dr. Don Rolfs, Periodontal Foundations, Wenatchee, WA.)

C. **Composition of Dental Calculus.** Calculus comprises an inorganic (or mineralized) component and an organic component.
   1. Inorganic Portion of Calculus
      a. The inorganic part of calculus makes up 70% to 90% of the overall composition of calculus.
      b. This inorganic part of dental calculus is primarily calcium phosphate, but the dental calculus also contains some calcium carbonate and magnesium phosphate.
      c. The inorganic part of calculus is similar to the inorganic components of bone.
   2. Organic Portion of Calculus
      a. The organic part of calculus makes up 10% to 30% of the overall composition of calculus.
      b. Components of the organic part include materials derived from plaque biofilm, derived from dead epithelial cells, and derived from dead white blood cells. It can also include living bacteria within the deposits of calculus.
D. **Types of Dental Calculus**
   1. Crystalline Forms of Dental Calculus. As calculus ages on a tooth surface, the inorganic component changes through several different crystalline forms. It is interesting to note that some of these crystalline forms of calculus are quite similar to the crystal forms in the tooth itself.
      a. Newly formed calculus deposits appear as a crystalline form called brushite.
      b. In calculus deposits that are a bit more mature, but less than 6 months old, the crystalline form is primarily octacalcium phosphate.
      c. In mature deposits that are more than 6 months old, the crystalline form is primarily hydroxyapatite.
   2. Location of Calculus Deposits
      a. Supragingival calculus deposits are calculus deposits located coronal to (above) the gingival margin. Other terms that have been used to refer to deposits coronal to the gingival margin are supramarginal calculus and salivary calculus.
         1. Though supragingival calculus deposits can be found on any tooth surface, they usually are found in localized areas of the dentition, such as lingual surfaces of mandibular anterior teeth, facial surfaces of maxillary molars, and on teeth that are crowded or in malocclusion. It is interesting to note that supragingival calculus is frequently found in areas adjacent to large salivary ducts (such as the lingual surfaces of mandibular anterior teeth and the facial surfaces of maxillary posterior teeth).
         2. Though supragingival calculus can form in any shape, these deposits most often are irregular, large deposits.
      b. Subgingival deposits are calculus deposits located apical to (below) the gingival margin. Other terms that have been used for deposits apical to the gingival margin are submarginal calculus or serumal calculus.
         1. The distribution of subgingival deposits may be localized in certain areas or generalized throughout the mouth.
         2. The shape of subgingival deposits is most often flattened. It is thought that the shape of the deposit may be guided by pressure of the pocket wall against the deposit.
E. **Modes of Attachment to Tooth Surfaces.** Dental calculus attaches to tooth surfaces through several different modes, and different attachment mechanisms can even exist in the same calculus deposit.

1. **Attachment by Means of Pellicle**
   a. Calculus can attach to the tooth surface by attaching to **pellicle** on the surface. The pellicle is a thin, bacteria-free membrane that forms on the surface of the tooth during the late stages of eruption.
   b. This mode of attachment occurs most commonly on enamel surfaces.
   c. Calculus deposits attached via the pellicle are usually removed easily because this attachment is on the surface of the pellicle (and not actually locked into the tooth surface).
2. **Attachment to Irregularities in the Tooth Surface**
   a. Calculus can also attach to irregularities in tooth surfaces. These irregularities include cracks in the teeth, tiny openings left where periodontal ligament fibers are detached, and grooves in cemental surfaces created as the result of faulty instrumentation during previous calculus removal procedures.
   b. Complete calculus removal in areas of irregularities in tooth surfaces is usually difficult since the deposits can be sheltered in these tooth defects.
3. **Attachment by Direct Contact of the Calcified Component and the Tooth Surface**
   a. Calculus can also attach to tooth surfaces by attaching directly to the calcified component of the tooth. In this mode of attachment, the matrix of the calculus deposit is interlocked with the inorganic crystals of the tooth.
   b. Deposits, firmly interlocked in the tooth surface, are usually difficult to remove.

2. **Tooth Morphology. Morphology** is the study of the anatomic surface features of the teeth. There are a variety of local contributing factors that relate to tooth morphology. Some of these variations in tooth morphology can occur when a tooth requires a restoration, and some of them occur simply because of variations in the way teeth form.
   A. **Poorly Contoured Restorations**
      1. When a dentist places a restoration, it is not always possible to contour the restoration perfectly smoothly with the existing tooth structure. When a restoration is not smoothly contoured with the tooth surfaces, this condition is referred to as an **overhanging restoration** or overhang (Fig. 16-2).
      2. Because of difficulty of access to tooth surfaces protected by an overhanging restoration, it is often impossible for a patient to remove plaque biofilm effectively from the tooth surface. This leads to plaque biofilm retention at the site and can subsequently lead to increased severity of either gingivitis or periodontitis at the site.
   B. **Dental Caries.** Untreated tooth decay is another example of a local contributing factor that can increase plaque biofilm retention. Since tooth decay can result in defects in tooth structure (dental cavities), these defects (cavities) can also act as protected environments for bacteria that cause gingivitis and periodontitis to live and grow undisturbed (Fig. 16-3).

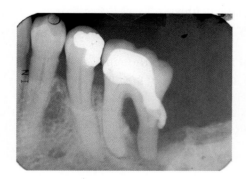

Figure 16-2. Radiographic Evidence of Poorly Contoured Restorations. Note that the restoration margins on the distal surfaces of the second premolar and first molar are not smoothly contoured with the actual tooth surfaces. This leads to increased biofilm retention of these areas. (Courtesy of Dr. Richard Foster, Guilford Technical Community College, Jamestown, NC.)

C. Tooth Grooves or Concavities

1. Naturally occurring developmental grooves and concavities in tooth surfaces frequently lead to difficulty in self-care at the site and can also be a local contributing factor for gingivitis and periodontitis because of the increase in plaque biofilm retention at the site.

2. During the natural development of some incisor teeth, a groove forms on the palatal surface of the tooth. This groove is a developmental defect called a **palatogingival groove** and is most frequently seen on maxillary lateral incisors. Plaque biofilm retention is a common problem associated with a palatogingival groove since the groove is often difficult or impossible to clean effectively (Fig. 16-4).

3. Some tooth root surfaces have naturally occurring concavities or depressions that can lead to plaque biofilm retention (Fig. 16-5). The mesial surface of maxillary first premolar teeth often has a pronounced concavity in the surface. This concavity is a natural contour for that tooth, but if exposed in the oral cavity, can make it extremely difficult for a patient to maintain effective self-care at the site. Figure 16-6 illustrates how a tooth concavity can prevent thorough self-care even for a patient skilled in use of dental floss.

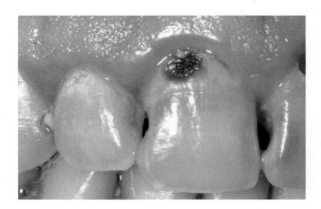

Figure 16-3. Untreated Decay. Note that this untreated tooth decay leaves an actual hole (cavity) in the tooth surface that can then harbor periodontal pathogens and can allow them to grow undisturbed by self-care efforts. (Courtesy of Dr. Ralph Arnold.)

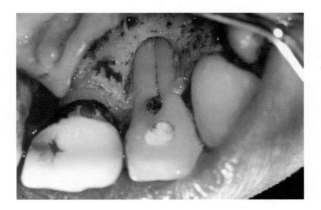

Figure 16-4. Palatogingival Groove. A palatogingival groove on the lingual surface of this maxillary lateral incisor is revealed during a periodontal surgical procedure. The gingiva has been lifted off the bone and tooth root. The palatal side of the root and the alveolar bone level is clearly visible. The palatogingival groove allowed plaque biofilm to mature undisturbed in the depth of the groove and has contributed to the extensive alveolar bone loss. (Courtesy of Dr. Ralph Arnold.)

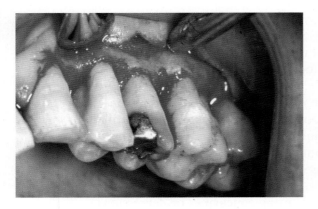

Figure 16-5. Root Concavity. The mesial root concavity on a maxillary first premolar. This photograph was taken during a periodontal surgical procedure designed to allow better visualization and treatment of the root concavity. (Courtesy of Dr. Ralph Arnold.)

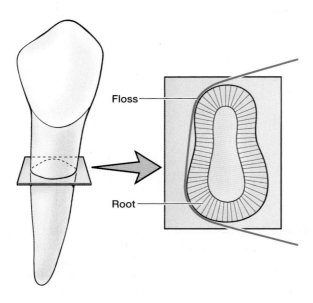

Floss

Root

Figure 16-6. Flossing a Tooth Surface with a Concavity. Note that even if floss is closely adapted to the tooth surfaces, the floss will not dislodge the plaque biofilm in the base of the concavity.

Section 3
Local Factors That Can Increase Biofilm Pathogenicity

Pathogenicity can be described as the ability of a disease-causing agent to actually produce the disease. In the dental context, pathogenicity can be thought of as the ability of the dental plaque biofilm to cause periodontal disease. Plaque biofilm pathogenicity relates to the character of the plaque biofilm rather than simply an increase in the amount of plaque biofilm.

1. **Undisturbed Plaque Biofilm Growth**
   A. **Plaque Biofilm Maturation**
      1. Plaque biofilm allowed to grow undisturbed is said to "mature." As plaque biofilm matures, it becomes colonized with larger and larger numbers of bacteria.
      2. Starting with a perfectly clean tooth surface, plaque biofilm bacteria accumulate in a predictable pattern on any tooth surface not being cleaned by the patient.
         a. Immediately after cleaning, salivary proteins attach to the tooth surface and form the pellicle.
         b. Within the first 2 days, the pellicle becomes colonized with gram-positive aerobic cocci and rods. These bacteria can cause gingivitis but do not cause periodontitis.
         c. Over the next week, other bacteria enter the plaque biofilm. These new bacteria include those that can cause periodontitis.
            1. The bacteria in this stage of plaque biofilm development include some gram-negative anaerobic cocci and gram-negative rods.
            2. In addition, at this stage specific periodontal pathogens can colonize the plaque biofilm including Fusobacterium species and *Prevotella intermedia*.
         d. Later, other bacteria including *Porphyromonas gingivalis* colonize the plaque biofilm. Some of these other bacteria are also associated with periodontitis.
   B. **Increased Plaque Biofilm Pathogenicity**
      1. The concept of **plaque biofilm pathogenicity** refers to the ability of the bacteria in the dental plaque biofilm to produce periodontal disease.
         a. It is important to understand that all plaque biofilm that is left undisturbed and allowed to mature (i.e., age) on a tooth surface is eventually colonized by bacteria known to cause periodontitis.
         b. As plaque biofilm matures into a true plaque biofilm it becomes more pathogenic than the plaque biofilm that first developed on the tooth surface since it includes more of the bacteria that are the causative agents in periodontitis (Fig. 16-7).
      2. Increased plaque biofilm pathogenicity is closely related to some plaque biofilm retention factors. Plaque biofilm retention factors not only allow an increase in the amount of plaque biofilm at the site but can also allow plaque biofilm to mature and increase in its pathogenicity.

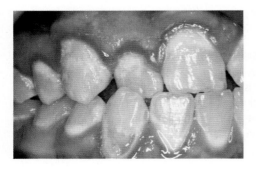

Figure 16-7. Mature Dental Plaque Biofilm. Note the thick dental plaque biofilm at the gingival margin of the teeth in this photograph. This plaque biofilm has been present for several weeks and is more pathogenic than a less mature plaque biofilm because it now harbors periodontal pathogens. (Courtesy of Dr. Richard Foster, Guilford Technical Community College, Jamestown, NC.)

Section 4
Local Factors That Cause Direct Damage

This section discusses a few of the local contributing factors that may actually cause direct damage to the periodontium. These factors also may alter the progress of periodontitis at individual sites. Some local contributing factors that can directly damage the periodontium include food impaction, patient habits, and faulty restorations or appliances.

1. Direct Damage Due to Food Impaction
   A. **Definition.** Food impaction refers to forcing food (such as pieces of tough meat) between teeth during chewing, trapping the food in the interdental area.
   B. **Effect of Food Impaction**
      1. Food forced into a tooth sulcus can strip the gingival tissues away from the tooth surface and contribute to periodontal breakdown in addition to the more obvious danger of serving as nutrients for tooth decay–causing bacteria.
      2. Food impaction not only damages the gingival tissues directly but can also lead to alterations in gingival contour that result in interdental areas that are difficult for patients to clean (Fig. 16-8).
2. Direct Damage from Patient Habits. In some patients, habits such as tongue thrusting, mouth breathing, or the improper use of toothbrushes, toothpicks, and other dental cleaning aids can also cause direct damage to the periodontium.
   A. **Improper Use of Plaque Biofilm Control Aids.** Improper use of plaque biofilm control aids can result in direct damage to the gingival tissues causing alteration of the natural contours of the tissues (Fig. 16-9).

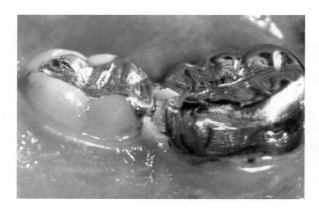

Figure 16-8. Food Impaction. Note the food impaction between the two molar teeth. As this patient chews food, the food is forced between these teeth and produces direct damage to the periodontium. (Courtesy of Dr. Don Rolfs, Periodontal Foundations, Wenatchee, WA.)

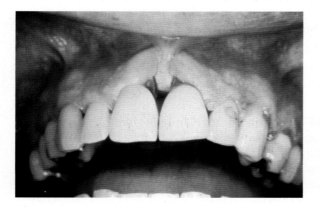

Figure 16-9. Misuse of Toothpick. The interdental papilla between the two central incisors has been destroyed by the patient's habit of repeatedly forcing a toothpick between the teeth. This damage to the papillae is an example of direct damage to the periodontium.

B. **Tongue Thrusting. Tongue thrusting** is the application of forceful pressure against the anterior teeth with the tongue.
1. Tongue thrusting is often the result of an abnormal tongue positioning during the initial stage of swallowing.
2. This oral habit exerts excessive lateral pressure against the teeth and may be traumatic to the periodontium (Fig. 16-10).
C. **Mouth Breathing. Mouth breathing** is the process of inhaling and exhaling air primarily through the mouth rather than the nose, and often occurs while the patient is sleeping. Mouth breathing has a tendency to dry out the gingival tissues in the anterior region of the mouth.

3. **Direct Damage Due to Faulty Restorations and Appliances**
A. **Inappropriate Crown Placement.** A crown is a metal, ceramic, or ceramic-bonded-to-metal covering for a badly damaged tooth. Placing a crown on a damaged tooth is a common mechanism used to preserve a badly damaged tooth.
1. Crowns can sometimes be placed inappropriately when tooth structure is minimal. There can be direct damage to the periodontium when the edges of a crown (called margins) are placed below the gingival margin and too near the alveolar bone.
2. A crown margin that is closer than 2 mm to the crest of the alveolar bone can result in resorption of alveolar bone (Fig. 16-11).

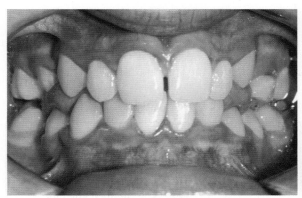
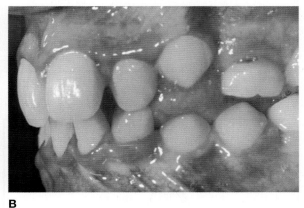

A   **B**

Figure 16-10. Tongue Thrust. A: Facial view of a patient with a tongue thrust. As this patient swallows, the patient applies lateral pressure with her tongue against the teeth. **B:** Side view of the tongue thrust. The tongue is visible in the canine region of the mouth as the patient presses her tongue forward when swallowing. (Courtesy of Dr. Don Rolfs, Periodontal Foundations, Wenatchee, WA.)

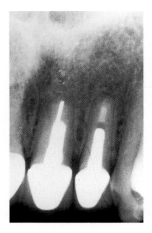

Figure 16-11. Direct Damage to the Periodontium. This radiograph reveals a crown with a margin that is approximately 1 mm from the alveolar bone. This distance is too close to bone to allow for normal soft tissue attachment to the tooth.

3. **Biologic width** refers to the space on the tooth surface occupied by the junctional epithelium and the connective tissue attachment fibers immediately apical to (below) the junctional epithelium (Fig. 16-12). This biologic width can be "violated" or damaged by restoration margins. The drawings in Figure 16-13 show the biologic width and its relationship to a properly placed margin and a restoration margin that violates or damages the biologic width.

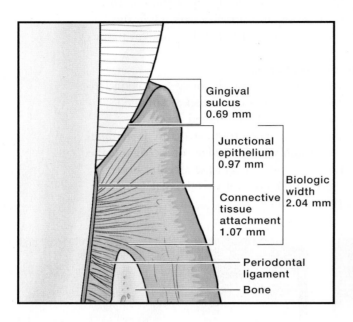

Figure 16-12. Biologic Width in Health. Illustration showing the biologic width in health with average dimensions that have been reported in the literature.

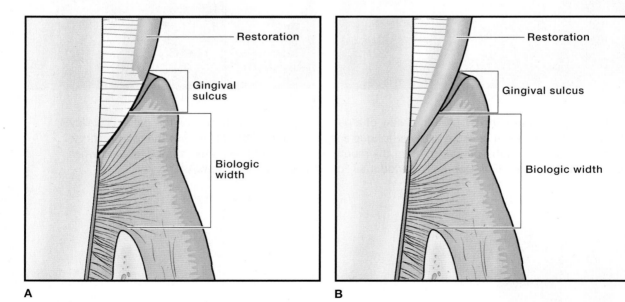

A   B

Figure 16-13. Margins of a Restoration. A: Illustration showing the placement of a restoration margin in a position that leaves the biologic width undamaged by the restoration. **B:** Illustration showing the placement of a restoration margin in a position that violates or damages the biologic width.

B. **Improperly Contoured Restorations**
1. Bulky or overcontoured crowns or restorations can result in inadequate space between the teeth to accommodate the natural form of the interdental papilla.
2. The open space apical to the contact area of two adjacent teeth is referred to as an **embrasure space**. In health, the embrasure space is filled by an interdental papilla.
3. Bulky crowns reduce the size of the embrasure space, so that inadequate space exists between the teeth to accommodate the interdental papilla. In this situation, the bulky crowns are described as **encroaching on the embrasure space** (Fig. 16-14).

C. **Faulty Removable Prosthesis**
1. A **prosthesis** is an appliance used to replace missing teeth.
   a. A **removable prosthesis** is one that the patient can remove for cleaning and before going to bed. A removable prosthesis that replaces a few teeth is commonly called a removable partial denture.
   b. A removable prosthesis should be differentiated from a fixed prosthesis. A fixed prosthesis is a prosthesis that is cemented to the teeth (also known as a fixed bridge).
2. A damaged or poorly fitting removable prosthesis can impinge on gingival tissue and favor plaque biofilm accumulation and thus hasten the progress of periodontitis (Fig. 16-15).

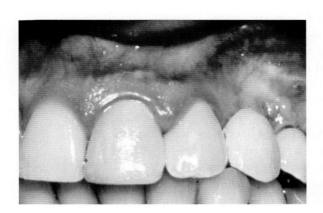

Figure 16-14. Bulky Crown Encroaching on Interdental Space. The crowns shown here are so bulky in contour on their proximal surfaces that they fill the embrasure space leaving no room for the natural form of the papilla. Note the papilla between the central and lateral incisor appears enlarged because it is being pushed from between the teeth.

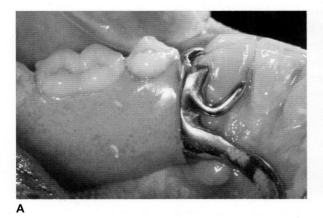

A

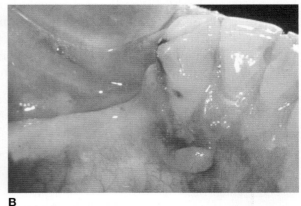

B

Figure 16-15. Tissue Damage by a Poorly Fitting Removable Prosthesis. A: Clinical photograph showing a removable prosthesis (lower partial denture) that replaces extracted posterior teeth. **B:** With the prosthesis removed, the tissue damage to the mandibular canine is revealed. Gingival recession on the canine is due in part to the clasp of the faulty prosthesis impinging upon the gingival tissue. (Courtesy of Dr. Don Rolfs, Wenatchee, WA.)

4. **Direct Damage From Occlusal Forces**
   A. **Trauma from Occlusion**
      1. Direct damage to the periodontium can result from excessive occlusal (or biting) forces on the teeth.
      2. When excessive occlusal forces cause damage to the periodontium, this is referred to as **trauma from occlusion.**
         a. When trauma from occlusion occurs, some alveolar bone resorption can result simply because of increased pressure placed on the surrounding alveolar bone.
         b. When there is loss of some alveolar bone due to pressures from trauma from occlusion, there can be a more rapid destruction by any existing periodontitis.
      3. A thorough clinical exam and a thorough radiographic exam can frequently reveal signs of trauma from occlusion.
         a. Some of the clinical signs of trauma from occlusion that have been reported include the following:
            1. Tooth mobility
            2. Sensitivity to pressure
            3. Migration of teeth
         b. Some of the radiographic signs of trauma from occlusion that have been reported include the following:
            1. Enlarged, funnel-shaped periodontal ligament space.
            2. Alveolar bone resorption. Figure 16-16 shows a radiograph of a tooth that has been subjected to excessive occlusal forces (trauma from occlusion).
      4. Trauma from occlusion has been classified in the dental literature for many years as either primary trauma from occlusion or secondary trauma from occlusion.
         a. **Primary trauma from occlusion** is defined as excessive occlusal forces on a sound periodontium.
            1. Examples of causes of primary trauma from occlusion include accidental placement of a high restoration or insertion of a fixed bridge or partial denture that places excessive force on the supporting teeth.
            2. The changes seen in primary occlusal trauma include a wider periodontal ligament space, tooth mobility, and even tooth and jaw pain. These changes are reversible if the trauma is removed.
         b. **Secondary trauma from occlusion** is defined as normal occlusal forces on an unhealthy periodontium previously weakened by periodontitis.
            1. Secondary trauma from occlusion occurs to a tooth in which the surrounding periodontium has experienced apical migration of the junctional epithelium, loss of connective tissue attachment, and loss of alveolar bone. In this type of trauma, the periodontium was unhealthy

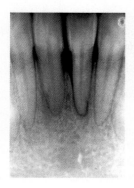

Figure 16-16. Radiographic Evidence of Trauma from Occlusion. Note the dramatic widening of the periodontal ligament space along the lateral root surfaces on the mandibular right central incisor (center tooth on radiograph). The alveolar bone has been destroyed because of the pressures resulting from trauma from occlusion.

before experiencing excessive occlusal forces. Table 16-2 summarizes definitions of some terms used to describe trauma from occlusion.

2. A tooth with an unhealthy, inflamed periodontium that is subjected to excessive occlusal forces is thought to be subject to more rapid bone loss and pocket formation.

3. Teeth can be tipped laterally easily when subjected to lateral occlusal forces. These tipping forces frequently accompany trauma from occlusion and can create areas of pressure and tension within the periodontal ligament (PDL) that are transmitted to the bone. Figure 16-17 illustrates how this tipping can occur. As alveolar bone loss progresses, this lateral tipping becomes even more likely because of the longer lever arm created by the part of the tooth out of the bone compared to the part of the tooth encased in bone.

4. Teeth with reduced alveolar bone support can have additional damage to the periodontium because of the tipping action of lateral forces placed on the teeth. Figure 16-18 shows a series of drawings that illustrate this concept.

B. Parafunctional Occlusal Forces

1. A series of other terms has been used to describe excessive occlusal forces. Two of these terms are functional and parafunctional occlusal forces.

   a. **Functional occlusal forces** are the normal forces produced during the act of chewing food.

   b. **Parafunctional occlusal forces** result from tooth-to-tooth contact made when not in the act of eating.

      1. Examples of these parafunctional habits are clenching of the teeth together as a release of nervous tension or grinding the teeth together for the same release.

         a. **Clenching** is the continuous or intermittent forceful closure of the maxillary teeth against the mandibular teeth.

         b. **Bruxism** is forceful grinding of the teeth.

         c. These parafunctional habits can occur without the person having conscious knowledge of the habit. Some individuals exhibit these habits while asleep.

      2. Parafunctional habits can exert excessive force on the teeth and to the periodontium.

2. There are several clinical therapies that can be used by a dentist to help control the damage from trauma from occlusion.

   a. When the trauma is a result of a faulty bite (referred to as a faulty occlusion), the dentist can make minor adjustments in the bite to minimize the damaging forces. This procedure is called an **occlusal adjustment**.

   b. When the trauma is a result of bruxism, the dentist can fabricate an acrylic appliance known sometimes referred to as a night guard appliance that can protect the teeth during part of each day.

TABLE 16-2. TERMS ASSOCIATED WITH TRAUMA FROM OCCLUSION

Term	Definition
Trauma from occlusion	Injury to the periodontium resulting from excessive occlusal forces
Primary trauma from occlusion	Injury to a healthy periodontium resulting from excessive occlusal forces
Secondary trauma from occlusion	Injury from normal occlusal forces applied to a periodontium previously damaged by periodontitis

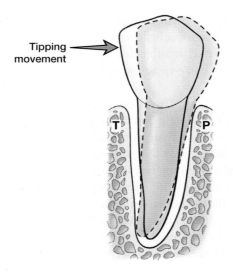

Figure 16-17. Tipping Movement from Lateral Occlusal Forces. Tipping of a tooth within the socket due to lateral occlusal forces often accompanies trauma from occlusion. This tipping can result in areas of pressure and tension within the PDL. In the illustration, "P" indicates an area of pressure in the PDL and alveolar bone. The letter "T" indicates an area of tension. Bone under pressure tends to undergo resorption.

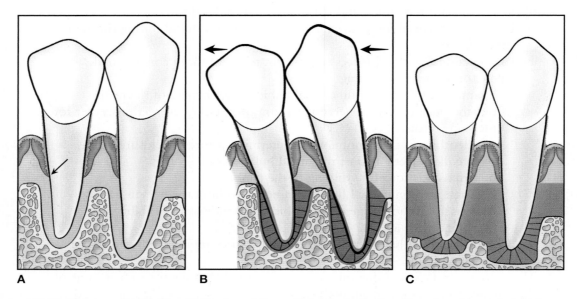

Figure 16-18. Damage to Teeth with Reduced Bone Height. A: Teeth with reduced bone height from existing periodontitis. **B:** Teeth being subjected to lateral forces and being moved laterally by those forces. **C:** Additional bone loss to the periodontium as a result of pressure on bone from the lateral tooth movement. This additional bone loss can be additive to the bone loss already occurring in a periodontitis patient.

Chapter Summary Statement

Local contributing factors can increase the risk of developing gingivitis or periodontitis or increase the risk of developing more severe disease when gingivitis or periodontitis is already established. The three mechanisms in which local factors can increase the risk of periodontal disease are by (1) increasing plaque biofilm retention, (2) increasing plaque biofilm pathogenicity, and (3) causing direct damage to the periodontium. As will be discussed in Chapter 19, the dental team must identify these local contributing factors during a clinical assessment, so that any local contributing factors can be eliminated or minimized during the nonsurgical periodontal treatment.

Section 5
Focus on Patients

Clinical Patient Care

CASE 1

Examination of a patient reveals gingivitis. In addition, the patient has generalized calculus deposits and numerous restorations with overhangs. What steps might be necessary to bring the gingivitis under control in this patient?

CASE 2

Examination of a patient reveals periodontitis. The patient also has a severe tooth-clenching habit. Explain how the tooth-clenching habit could be related to the progress of the periodontitis.

Evidence in Action

CASE 1

In a dental hygiene journal you find an article that refers to mature dental plaque biofilm. Explain what the author means by this term mature dental plaque biofilm.

References

1. Genco RJ. Current view of risk factors for periodontal diseases. *Journal of periodontology.* 1996;67(10 Suppl):1041-9. doi: 10.1902/jop.1996.67.10.1041. PubMed PMID: 8910821.
2. Leknes KN. The influence of anatomic and iatrogenic root surface characteristics on bacterial colonization and periodontal destruction: a review. *Journal of periodontology.* 1997;68(6):507-16. doi: 10.1902/jop.1997.68.6.507. PubMed PMID: 9203093.
3. Pihlstrom B. Treatment of periodontitis: key principles include removing subgingival bacterial deposits; providing a local environment and education to support good home care; providing regular professional maintenance. *Journal of periodontology.* 2014;85(5):655-6. doi: 10.1902/jop.2014.140046. PubMed PMID: 24773135.

 STUDENT ANCILLARY RESOURCES

A wide variety of resources to enhance your learning and understanding of this chapter are available on thePoint®.

- Visit thePoint to access:
  - Audio Glossary
  - Animations
  - Suggested Readings
  - Answers to Review Questions
  - Case Studies

CHAPTER

17

Nutrition, Inflammation, and Periodontal Disease

Clinical Application. Though the precise relationship between nutrition and periodontal disease is not fully understood, all members of the dental team must be aware of what is known about this relationship and understand how to apply this information to guide patients with nutritional issues that may have an impact upon periodontal health. This chapter outlines emerging understanding related to the association between nutrition and periodontal disease and provides some practice in applying this information to a clinical setting.

Learning Objectives

- Discuss the link between obesity and periodontal disease.
- Discuss the role of polymorphonuclear leukocytes in the production of reactive oxygen species in response to plaque biofilm.
- Discuss how antioxidants may influence periodontal disease onset and progression.
- Describe the proposed roles of micronutrients and macronutrients in periodontal disease.
- List some oral symptoms associated with ascorbic acid–deficiency gingivitis.
- Explain the role of dental healthcare providers in addressing obesity and nutrition in the management of periodontal disease.

Key Terms

Body mass index (BMI)
Reactive oxygen species (ROS)
Micronutrients

Antioxidants
Macronutrients
Ascorbic acid–deficiency gingivitis

Historically, periodontal disease has been seen as an inflammatory disease with limited associations to nutrition. Many early studies into the relationship between nutrition and periodontal disease failed to show associations between nutritional status and periodontal disease. These studies, however, used poor methodologies, tended to study nutrients in isolation, and failed to control for confounding variables (such as smoking). Improved understanding of periodontal disease at the cellular level and more stringent nutritional methodologies have created a renewed interest in the relationship between nutrition and periodontal disease. *Recent research is focused on (1) the association between obesity and periodontal inflammation and (2) the role of antioxidants in the prevention and treatment of periodontal disease.*

Section 1
Association Between Obesity and Periodontal Disease

1. Obesity Overview
   A. Obesity is an excess amount of body fat in proportion to lean body mass, to the extent that health is impaired (1).
      1. The most commonly used measure of body fat is the body mass index (BMI), which is defined as a person's weight in kilograms divided by the square of his/her height in meters. The World Health Organization and the National Heart, Lung, and Blood Institute define overweight as a body mass index of 25 to 29.9 and obesity as a BMI of equal to or greater than 30 (2).
      2. More than 65% of the United States adult population has a body mass index of greater than or equal to 25 kg/m2 and 15.8% of children aged 6 to 11 years, and 16.1% of adolescents aged 12 to 19 years, are overweight (3).
      3. More than a third of adults (35%) and 17% of youth (age 2 to 19) were obese in 2011 to 2012, with no significant change for either group since 2003 to 2004, Ogden et al. reported in the *Journal of the American Medical Association*. However, more women over 60 became obese with the prevalence rising to 38% from 31.5% in that group during that time. The CDC data comes from an analysis of the National Health and Nutrition Examination Survey (NHANES) 2011 to 2012 involving 9,120 people in the United States (4). International trends are similar to those in the United States. The International Obesity Task Force estimates that over 1 billion adults are overweight (5).
   B. Adipose tissue is a complex and metabolically active endocrine organ that secretes numerous immunomodulatory factors and plays a major role in regulating metabolic and vascular biology (6). Obese individuals are reported to have elevated levels of circulating TNF-α and IL-6 compared to normal weight controls (7,8).
2. The Obesity–Periodontal Disease Link
   A. Recent research indicates a link between obesity and periodontal disease (9–19).
      1. An analysis of data from The Third National Health and Nutrition Examination Survey (NHANES III) involving over 13,000 individuals having one or more sites with clinical attachment loss found a positive correlation between BMI and the severity of periodontal attachment loss (20).
      2. Al-Zahrani et al. conducted a study of a representative sample of participants in the NHANES III survey who were 18 years or younger and had undergone a periodontal examination.

    a. The purpose of the study was to examine the relation between body weight and periodontal disease in a representative United States sample. Body mass index and waist circumference were used as measures of overall and abdominal fat content, respectively.

    b. Study results indicate that even in a younger population, overall and abdominal obesity are associated with increased prevalence of periodontal disease while underweight (BMI < 18.5) is associated with decreased prevalence (9).

3. In another analysis of the NHANES III data, Al-Zahrani et al. found that individuals who maintained normal weight, exercised regularly, and followed a diet utilizing the U.S. Department of Agriculture Center for Nutrition Policy and Promotions' dietary guidelines were 40% less likely to have periodontitis (21).

4. In the United States, the Forsyth Institute conducted an ongoing case control study. The study reported that obesity is related to a marked increase in plaque biofilm accumulation, attachment loss, deep pockets, and bleeding on probing and an increase in the proportion of *Tannerella forsythia (Bacteroides forsythus)* (22).

B. Among lifestyle-related risk factors, smoking displays the greatest impact on periodontitis. Both smoking and obesity are independent risk indicators for periodontitis. Nishida et al. (23) suggested that obesity is second only to smoking as the strongest lifestyle-related factor for inflammatory periodontal disease destruction.

3. **Biological Mechanisms Linking Obesity with Periodontal Disease.** The mechanism of how obesity modifies the pathogenesis of periodontal disease at the molecular level currently is poorly understood, but what is known is that obesity has several harmful biological effects that might be related to the pathogenesis of periodontitis (16).

A. **Release of Proinflammatory Cytokines from Adipose Tissue.** Further studies are needed to determine if obesity is a true risk factor for periodontal disease. Several researchers have suggested that the association most likely lies in the commonality of their inflammatory pathways. According to Genco (24), the relentless release of proinflammatory cytokines into the systemic circulation from adipose tissue in obese individuals provides a "systemic inflammatory overload." The relentless release of cytokines provides a possible explanation of how obesity intensifies infections, including periodontal disease.

1. Adipose tissue secretes several cytokines and hormones that are involved in inflammatory processes, suggesting that similar pathways are involved in the pathogenesis of obesity and periodontitis. The adverse effect of obesity on the periodontium may be mediated through proinflammatory cytokines like interleukins (IL-1, IL-6, and TNF-α), adipokines (leptin and adiponectin), and reactive oxygen species (ROS), which may affect the periodontal tissues directly (25).

2. Adiponectin is a circulating hormone secreted by the adipose tissue involved in glucose and lipid metabolism.
    a. Adiponectin production is ***decreased*** in obese individuals.
    b. Low levels of adiponectin are associated with increased systemic inflammation (26).

3. Leptin is secreted from adipose tissue and plays an important role in regulating appetite and metabolism.
    a. Leptin acts to suppress appetite and increase energy expenditure.
    b. Most obese individuals have elevated leptin levels ***that do not suppress appetite.*** Many researchers consider leptin resistance to be one of the features contributing to obesity's pathology (27). It has been demonstrated

that human leptin is present within healthy gingival tissue and decreases in concentration with increased probing depths (28).

4. Obesity-associated tumor necrosis factor-α (TNF-α) is primarily secreted from macrophages accumulated in abdominal adipose tissue. It is thought that increased circulating TNF-α from adipose tissue contributes to general systemic inflammation (29).

5. Interleukin-6 (IL-6) is secreted by adipose tissue and is produced in greater amounts by abdominal fat.

B. **Increased Levels of Reactive Oxygen Species**

1. Reactive oxygen species (ROS) are chemically reactive molecules containing oxygen. ROS are products of normal cellular metabolism, but excessive production induces damage by oxidizing DNA, lipids, and proteins (30). ROS clearly can be toxic to cells. One of the best-known toxic effects of oxygen radicals is damage to cellular membranes.

2. Emerging scientific evidence indicates that obesity appears to play a role in the multifactorial etiology of periodontitis through the increased production of ROS and an increase in inflammatory cytokines (9–19). Figure 17-1 shows a suggested model for the link between obesity and periodontal disease.

3. Normally, cells defend themselves against ROS damage with enzymes and small molecule antioxidants such as ascorbic acid (vitamin C), tocopherol (vitamin E), uric acid, and glutathione.

4. **The Role of the Dental Team in Managing Obesity and Periodontal Disease.** Periodontists and dental hygienists must be aware of the increasing numbers of obese persons and of the significance of obesity as a multiple risk factor for oral health. Addressing obesity in the management of periodontal disease is clearly important in patients who have both conditions. This necessitates the cooperation and collaboration of all healthcare professionals to educate patients regarding the implications of obesity and periodontitis and to encourage counseling, weight reduction, and treatment.

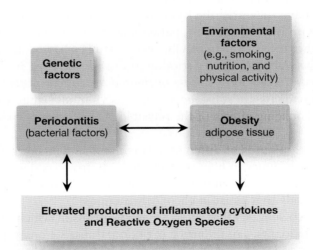

Figure 17-1. Hypothesis Linking Obesity and Periodontal Disease. One hypothesis linking obesity and periodontal disease is that both conditions are associated with an elevated production of both inflammatory cytokines and reactive oxygen species. Of course, both conditions are also affected by other background factors such as genetic factors and environmental factors, which make identifying a precise link between them difficult.

Section 2
Micronutrients, Antioxidants, and Periodontal Disease

Nutrients are divided into six categories: vitamins, minerals, proteins, lipids, carbohydrates, and water. **Micronutrients** are nutrients that are needed in tiny quantities each day. Vitamins and calcium are two examples of micronutrients. Proteins, lipids, and carbohydrates are **macronutrients**, which provide energy or calories.

1. Micronutrients and Oxidation
   A. **Oxidation.** As oxygen interacts with cells of any type—a ripening banana or a cell in the body—oxidation occurs. Oxidation produces some type of change in the cell. The banana may rot or in time, dead body cells are replaced with new cells.
      1. Oxidative stress occurs with the production of harmful molecules called free radicals.
      2. Free radicals containing oxygen, known as **reactive oxygen species (ROS)**, are the most biologically significant free radicals.
      3. It is impossible for the cells of the body to avoid damage by free radicals. Free radicals arise from sources both inside and outside the body. Oxidants develop from processes within the body as the result of normal metabolism and inflammation. Outside the body free radicals form from environmental factors such as pollution, sunlight, smoking, and radiation.
      4. In response to plaque biofilm, polymorphonuclear leukocytes (PMNs) produce reactive oxygen species during phagocytosis as part of the host response to infection.
         a. Individuals with periodontal disease display increased PMN number and activity.
         b. It has been suggested that this proliferation results in a high degree of ROS release, culminating in heightened damage to gingival tissue, periodontal ligaments, and alveolar bone (31–34).
         c. Studies also have suggested the ROS stimulate osteoclast activation (35). Compared with healthy controls, patients with chronic periodontitis generate higher levels of many ROS. Several studies have demonstrated a correlation between ROS and periodontal disease activity (36,37).
      5. *The damage mediated by ROS can be mitigated by antioxidants* (38).
   B. **Antioxidants.** Antioxidants are substances—such as vitamins—that are capable of counteracting the damaging effects of the physiological process of oxidation in a living organism.
      1. Nature provides thousands of different antioxidants in fruits, vegetables, nuts, whole grains, and legumes to help protect the body from oxidation.
      2. Dietary antioxidants include vitamins and minerals as well as enzymes (proteins in the body that assist in chemical reactions).
      3. Data from research suggests that there are mechanisms in which nutrition, particularly antioxidants, can influence periodontal disease onset, progression, and wound healing (31). Antioxidants are thought to be important in the downregulation of proinflammatory responses. While additional information is needed, nutrients can act as antioxidants that may modulate gingival inflammation (31,38).

2. Vitamins and Minerals
   A. **Vitamins.** Vitamins are organic antioxidants that are not synthesized by the body and are necessary for normal metabolism. Vitamin C is the most common water-soluble antioxidant while vitamin E is one of the most common fat-soluble antioxidants.

1. Vitamin C
   a. Vitamin C has effective antioxidant properties that are important for maintaining the integrity of cell membranes and protection against the ROS generated during inflammatory responses (39).
   b. In addition, vitamin C has the ability to enhance neutrophil, monocyte, and natural killer cell functions (40,41).
   c. An epidemiologic study of vitamin C intake demonstrated an association between low vitamin C intake and periodontal disease, especially among smokers (42).
   d. Vitamin C is a water-soluble vitamin that cannot be stored by the body except in insignificant amounts.
      1. Since the human body lacks the ability to synthesize and make vitamin C, it depends on dietary sources to meet vitamin C needs.
      2. Vitamin C is found in fresh fruits and vegetables such as oranges, berries, tomatoes, leafy greens, and kiwi fruit. Consumption of fruits and vegetables or fortifying diets with vitamin C supplements is essential to avoid ascorbic acid deficiency.
   e. Ascorbic acid–deficiency gingivitis is an inflammatory response of the gingiva caused by plaque biofilm that is aggravated by chronically low vitamin C (ascorbic acid) levels.
      1. Ascorbic acid–deficiency gingivitis manifests clinically as bright red, swollen, ulcerated gingival tissue that bleeds with the slightest provocation (43,44).
      2. An example of infantile vitamin C deficiency is shown in Figures 17-2 and 17-3.

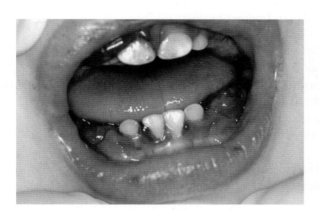

Figure 17-2. Ascorbic Acid–Deficiency Gingivitis. This 15-month-old boy had a history of unexplained gingival bleeding for several weeks and fever for 2 days. He had been fed only cow's milk and oatmeal since age 4 months. Laboratory blood tests revealed that his vitamin C levels were low. (Used with permission from Riepe FG, Eichmann D, Oppermann HC, et al. Special feature: picture of the month. *Arch Pediatr Adolesc Med.* 2001;155:607; copyright 2001 American Medical Association. All rights reserved.)

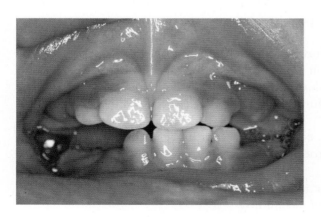

Figure 17-3. After Treatment with Vitamin C. The same boy shown in Figure 17-2 after 3 days treatment with vitamin C. (Courtesy of Dr. Felix G. Riepe, MD, Christian Albrechts University, Kiel, Germany.)

2. Vitamin A
   a. Vitamin A appears to be essential for epithelial cell differentiation, cell-mediated immunity, and supporting a T-helper anti-inflammatory response (45).
   b. Vitamin A has a key role in epithelial maintenance. Severe vitamin A deficiency, however, is rare in industrialized nations. The NHANES III study found no significant relationship between serum vitamin A and risk for periodontitis (46).
   c. Foods high in vitamin A include milk, eggs, liver, carrots, pumpkin, and mangoes.
3. Vitamin D
   a. Vitamin D promotes the differentiation of monocytes to macrophages (47,48).
   b. Vitamin D may reduce susceptibility to gingival inflammation through its anti-inflammatory effects (49). Studies of gingival tissue suggest a mitigating effect of vitamin E on periodontal inflammation and collagen breakdown. Lower gingival levels of vitamin E are associated with periodontal disease (34,50,51).
   c. Vitamin D is found in some foods but is mostly produced within the skin in response to sunlight; good sources of dietary vitamin D include egg yolk, liver, and oily fish.
4. Vitamin E
   a. Vitamin E is considered the most important fat-soluble antioxidant that protects cell membranes from oxidative damage and reduces the production of prostaglandin E2 in macrophages (52).
   b. Recent in vitro studies show vitamin E to have mitigating effects on indicators of gingival inflammation (34,51).
   c. Several clinical studies have shown positive effects of supplementation of vitamin E on the immune response, particularly in aged populations (53).
   d. Good dietary sources include nuts, seeds, and wheat germ.
5. Folic Acid
   a. Folic acid is a water-soluble vitamin belonging to the B-complex group of vitamins. With the exception of folic acid, there is little evidence that B vitamins are vital to periodontal health.
   b. Folic acid is involved with DNA synthesis. Cells with rapid turnover, such as those in the gingival epithelium, have high folic acid requirements.
   c. A deficiency of folic acid may reduce the ability of the gingival tissue to act as a barrier to bacteria.
   d. Recently published data from the NHANES survey showed that low serum foliate was independently associated with periodontal disease in older adults (54).
   e. In Canada and the United States, grains marketed as enriched have been fortified with folic acid since 1998. Other good dietary sources include broccoli, asparagus, Brussels sprouts, peas, and brown rice.
B. Minerals: Calcium
   1. The micronutrient calcium is intricately involved in the calcification process and, therefore, has a role in the formation and maintenance of alveolar bone. Nishida et al. found a 54% increased risk of periodontal disease in females who ingested less than 499 mg/d of calcium and a 27% increased risk in those with intakes below 800 mg/d (42,55).
   2. In another interesting longitudinal study, elderly adults with higher daily calcium intake had a decreased risk for tooth loss than adults who consumed lower calcium levels (56).
   3. Consumption of milk, yogurt, and cheese (preferably lower-fat varieties) is important in ensuring adequate intakes of calcium.

Section 3
Macronutrients and Periodontal Disease

Proteins, lipids, and carbohydrates are macronutrients, which provide energy or calories. Many of the pathways to inflammation are related to high caloric intake from refined carbohydrates and oxidative stress, which is stimulated by changes in the metabolism of adipose tissue (57).

1. Proteins
   A. Protein deficiency can have an effect on the host defenses that could modulate the progress of periodontitis. Cell-mediated immunity, the complement system, phagocyte activity, and production of cytokines are all impaired by protein deficiency (58).
   B. The effect of protein–energy malnutrition on periodontal disease risk was extensively reviewed by Enwonwu (32), who observed that aggressive periodontal disease was more prevalent and severe in undernourished individuals than in well-nourished ones. The immune depression that occurs in protein–energy malnutrition promotes vulnerability of the periodontium to inflammatory stimuli from the plaque biofilm.

2. **Refined Carbohydrates and Lipids.** Diets rich in refined carbohydrates and saturated fats may play a role in increasing the risk for periodontal disease. Excessive energy intake causes obesity, which has been shown to be associated with increased risk of periodontitis.
   A. Excess consumption of refined carbohydrates can affect the immune response and may lead to continued destruction of the periodontium in patients with existing periodontitis through mechanisms such as the action of enzymes (i.e., collagenase) and proinflammatory mediators (i.e., interleukin-1 and interleukin-6) (57). These destructive mechanisms have been discussed in other chapters of this book.
   B. Diets high in refined carbohydrates and saturated fats cause rapid release of glucose into the bloodstream (Table 17-1). High blood glucose levels increase triglyceride levels and stimulate the release of insulin, which decreases the ability of the body to break down fat stored in adipose depots (57).
   C. As discussed earlier in this chapter, obesity increases the circulation of ROS, which, in turn, causes oxidative damage, and progression of periodontal disease (10,17,38,59–61).

3. **The Role of the Dental Team in Promoting Good Nutrition**
   A. Making an appropriate connection between diet, nutrients, and periodontal disease can allow clinicians to make specific suggestions to improve a patient's diet. When indicated clinically, nutritional counseling, with an emphasis on periodontal health and root caries prevention, should be offered to periodontal patients. Teaching patients good dietary habits can be accomplished using standard diet forms, counseling techniques, and analysis procedures (62).
   B. Table 17-1 contains a summary of potential ways that diet and nutrition may modify periodontal disease.

TABLE 17-1. SUMMARY OF THE ASSOCIATION BETWEEN NUTRITION OF PERIODONTAL DISEASE

Dietary Component	Association with Periodontal Disease
Dietary antioxidants	Antioxidant status is compromised in periodontal disease (38,63)
Vitamin C	An epidemiologic study demonstrated a positive association between low vitamin C intake and periodontal disease, especially among smokers (42)
Vitamin E	In vitro studies show that vitamin E can dampen gingival inflammation (37,53)
Folic acid	Supplementation with folic acid reduces gingival inflammation (39,64,65)
Calcium	Lower intake of calcium has been shown to be independently associated with increased risk of periodontitis (42,55)
Protein	Protein malnutrition increases risk and enhances progression of aggressive periodontal disease (32)
Refined carbohydrates and lipids	Excessive energy intake causes obesity, which has been shown to be associated with increased risk of periodontitis Obesity increases the circulation of ROS which, in turn, causes oxidative damage and progression of periodontal disease (10,38,61)

Chapter Summary Statement

Though periodontal disease cannot be caused by nutritional deficiencies, some nutritional deficiencies do indeed appear to modify the severity and extent of the periodontal disease.

- Research links specific nutrient deficiencies and foods high in refined carbohydrates to increased inflammation—the very kind that triggers the host-mediated inflammatory response seen in periodontal disease.
- Reports of the relationship between obesity and periodontal disease are increasing. At this time, it is not possible to determine whether obesity predisposes an individual to periodontal disease or periodontal disease affects lipid metabolism, or both. Future longitudinal studies with more precise measures of adiposity on large populations are needed to clarify whether obesity is one of the risk factors for periodontal disease or simply a risk indicator.
- Data from research suggests that there are mechanisms in which nutrition, particularly antioxidants, can influence periodontal disease onset, progression, and wound healing.
- It is wise to counsel patients with periodontal disease to be thoughtful food shoppers and to prepare meals and snacks that are rich in specific nutrients.

Section 4
Focus on Patients

Clinical Patient Care

Directions for Clinical Patient Cases: Analyze the information and 24-Hour Diet Recall (Tables 17-2 and 17-3) on the two fictitious periodontal patients, to answer the following questions:

1. Can you identify any eating patterns (healthy or unhealthy)? If so, what are they?
2. List diet practices that have the potential to be most detrimental to the individual's periodontal health.
3. List two diet behaviors that the individual could modify to benefit his/her periodontal health.

CASE 1

Fictitious Periodontal Patient—Mr. Phillip Burgess

Mr. Phillip Burgess is a 39-year-old male. Mr. Burgess is 5'8" in height and weighs 280 lb (173 cm and 127 kg). His periodontal diagnosis is generalized mild chronic periodontitis.

TABLE 17-2. MR. BURGESS: 24-HOUR DIET RECALL

Time	Food/Beverage	Amount	Reason
6:00 AM	Two cups of coffee with nondairy creamer and two packets of sugar	Two medium cups	Breakfast
	Honey Nut Cheerios cereal and milk	Medium-sized bowl	
10:00 AM	Apple Danish pastry with icing		Snack
12:00 PM	Double hamburger with cheese, lettuce, tomato, onion	Supersize	Lunch
	French fries	Large	
	Regular Coke	Large	
2:00 PM	Regular Coke	One can	Snack
	Bag of potato chips	Small bag	
7:00 PM	Steak	Large	Dinner
	French fries	Large serving	
	Tossed salad with Italian dressing	Small bowl	
	Garlic toast	Two pieces	
	Water		
9:00 PM	Ice cream	Medium bowl	Snack while watching TV

CASE 2

Fictitious Periodontal Patient—Mrs. Glenda Bissada

Mrs. Bissada is a 70-year-old female. Mrs. Bissada is 5'1" in height and weighs 160 lb (155 cm and 73 kg). Her periodontal diagnosis is generalized severe chronic periodontitis.

TABLE 17-3. MRS. BISSADA: 24-HOUR DIET RECALL

Time	Food/Beverage	Amount	Reason
7:00 AM	Coffee with organic nondairy cream Whole grain English muffin Peanut butter and jelly	One large mug One	Breakfast
10:30 AM	Green grapes	25	Hungry
11:00 AM	M&M's	Three handfuls	Stressed (arguing with daughter on the phone)
12:30 PM	Philly cheese steak (fried shaved beef, onions, and green peppers, covered with cheese sauce in a large white "hoagie" bun) Potato chips Iced tea sweetened with sugar	 One bag One glass	Lunch
2:00 PM	Caramel-coated popcorn mix	Two handfuls	Stressed/hungry
6:00 PM	Fried hamburger patty with brown gravy Baked potato with sour cream and real bacon bits Peas Coffee with sugar		Dinner
7:00 PM	Glass of water		Thirsty
8:00 PM	Popcorn with butter	Medium bowl	Watching a movie

Ethical Dilemma

Stuart Fisher, your next patient, is new to the practice. He is a 48-year-old male, who is married with three young children. He owns a successful restaurant, where he works as the head chef. As he is self-employed, he doesn't carry dental insurance.

You review Stuart's medical history, and he states that he is scheduled for lap band surgery next month. Stuart admits that he has neglected his general and oral health for many years, due to his busy lifestyle. He also notes that although he knows better, his diet is poor. After cooking in the restaurant all day and night, the last thing he wants to do is prepare food for himself. So, both before and after work, he stops for "fast food."

Your radiographs and examination reveal that Stuart presents with generalized chronic periodontitis and moderate bone loss throughout his mouth, as well as localized furcation involvement.

You review the treatment plan with Stuart, which includes periodontal instrumentation with anesthesia, nutritional counseling, and referral to a periodontist. Stuart refuses to agree with your suggestions, as he states that he doesn't carry dental insurance. He only scheduled this appointment, as his surgeon required it prior to his surgery. He wants to receive the minimal dental treatment, and will not "go for" anything more.

1. What is the best way for you to handle this ethical dilemma?
2. What is the best way to address/discuss Stuart's treatment plan with him?
3. What ethical principles are in conflict in this dilemma?

References

1. Aronne LJ, Segal KR. Adiposity and fat distribution outcome measures: assessment and clinical implications. *Obes Res.* 2002;10(Suppl 1):14S–21S.
2. Executive summary of the clinical guidelines on the identification, evaluation, and treatment of overweight and obesity in adults. *Arch Intern Med.* 1998;158(17):1855–1867.
3. National Center for Health Statistics (U.S.). *Health, United States, 2005: with Chartbook on Trends in the Health of Americans.* Hyattsville, MD: Dept. of Health and Human Services, Centers for Disease Control and Prevention, National Center for Health Statistics; 2005:xix, 535.
4. Ogden CL, Carroll MD, Kit BK, et al. Prevalence of childhood and adult obesity in the U.S., 2011–2012. *JAMA.* 2014;311(8):806–814.
5. James PT, Rigby N, Leach R; International Obesity Task Force. The obesity epidemic, metabolic syndrome and future prevention strategies. *Eur J Cardiovasc Prev Rehabil.* 2004;11(1):3–8.
6. Trayhurn P, Wood IS. Adipokines: inflammation and the pleiotropic role of white adipose tissue. *Br J Nutr.* 2004;92(3):347–355.
7. Kern PA, Ranganathan S, Li C, et al. Adipose tissue tumor necrosis factor and interleukin-6 expression in human obesity and insulin resistance. *Am J Physiol Endocrinol Metab.* 2001;280(5):E745–E751.
8. Ziccardi P, Nappo F, Giugliano G, et al. Reduction of inflammatory cytokine concentrations and improvement of endothelial functions in obese women after weight loss over one year. *Circulation.* 2002;105(7):804–809.
9. Al-Zahrani MS, Bissada NF, Borawskit EA. Obesity and periodontal disease in young, middle-aged, and older adults. *J Periodontol.* 2003;74(5):610–615.
10. Dahiya P, Kamal R, Gupta R. Obesity, periodontal and general health: relationship and management. *Indian J Endocrinol Metab.* 2012;16(1):88–93.
11. Gorman A, Kaye EK, Nunn M, et al. Changes in body weight and adiposity predict periodontitis progression in men. *J Dent Res.* 2012;91(10):921–926.
12. Krejci CB, Bissada NF. Obesity and periodontitis: a link. *Gen Dent.* 2013;61(1):60–63.
13. Kumar PM, Kumar PA, Rao A, et al. Periodontal disease and obesity. *J Stomat Occ Med.* 2013;6:1–5.
14. Lawande S. Obesity and periodontal disease: a multidirectional relationship? *J Pharm Biomed Sci.* 2012;25(25):252–256.
15. Morita I, Okamoto Y, Yoshii S, et al. Five-year incidence of periodontal disease is related to body mass index. *J Dent Res.* 2011;90(2):199–202.
16. Ritchie CS. Obesity and periodontal disease. *Periodontol 2000.* 2007;44:154–163.
17. Saito T, Shimazaki Y, Koga T, et al. Relationship between upper body obesity and periodontitis. *J Dent Res.* 2001;80(7):1631–1636.
18. Shimazaki Y, Shirota T, Uchida K, et al. Intake of dairy products and periodontal disease: the Hisayama Study. *J Periodontol.* 2008;79(1):131–137.
19. Wood N, Johnson RB, Streckfus CF. Comparison of body composition and periodontal disease using nutritional assessment techniques: Third National Health and Nutrition Examination Survey (NHANES III). *J Clin Periodontol.* 2003;30(4):321–327.

20. Genco RJ, Grossi SG, Ho A, et al. A proposed model linking inflammation to obesity, diabetes, and periodontal infections. *J Periodontol.* 2005;76(11 Suppl):2075–2084.

21. Al-Zahrani MS, Borawski EA, Bissada NF. Periodontitis and three health-enhancing behaviors: maintaining normal weight, engaging in recommended level of exercise, and consuming a high-quality diet. *J Periodontol.* 2005;76(8):1362–1366.

22. Socransky SS, Haffajee AD. Periodontal microbial ecology. *Periodontol 2000.* 2005;38:135–187.

23. Nishida N, Tanaka M, Hayashi N, et al. Determination of smoking and obesity as periodontitis risks using the classification and regression tree method. *J Periodontol.* 2005;76(6):923–928.

24. Genco R. The three-way street. In: *Oral and Whole Body Health.* New York, NY: Scientific American, Inc.; 2006.

25. Ylostalo P, Suominen-Taipale L, Reunanen A, et al. Association between body weight and periodontal infection. *J Clin Periodontol.* 2008;35(4):297–304.

26. Nisoli E, Carruba MO. Emerging aspects of pharmacotherapy for obesity and metabolic syndrome. *Pharmacol Res.* 2004;50(5):453–469.

27. Correia ML, Haynes WG. Obesity-related hypertension: is there a role for selective leptin resistance? *Curr Hypertens Rep.* 2004;6(3):230–235.

28. Johnson RB, Serio FG. Leptin within healthy and diseased human gingiva. *J Periodontol.* 2001;72(9):1254–1257.

29. Berg AH, Scherer PE. Adipose tissue, inflammation, and cardiovascular disease. *Circ Res.* 2005;96(9):939–949.

30. Ahsan H, Ali A, Ali R. Oxygen free radicals and systemic autoimmunity. *Clin Exp Immunol.* 2003;131(3):398–404.

31. Chapple IL. Role of free radicals and antioxidants in the pathogenesis of the inflammatory periodontal diseases. *Clin Mol Pathol.* 1996;49(5):M247–M255.

32. Enwonwu CO. Cellular and molecular effects of malnutrition and their relevance to periodontal diseases. *J Clin Periodontol.* 1994;21(10):643–657.

33. Enwonwu CO, Phillips RS, Falkler WA Jr. Nutrition and oral infectious diseases: state of the science. *Compend Contin Educ Dent.* 2002;23(5):431–434, 436, 438 passim; quiz 448.

34. Offenbacher S, Odle BM, Green MD, et al. Inhibition of human periodontal prostaglandin E2 synthesis with selected agents. *Agents Actions.* 1990;29(3–4):232–238.

35. Hall TJ, Schaeublin M, Jeker H, et al. The role of reactive oxygen intermediates in osteoclastic bone resorption. *Biochem Biophys Res Commun.* 1995;207(1):280–287.

36. Cao CF, Smith QT. Crevicular fluid myeloperoxidase at healthy, gingivitis and periodontitis sites. *J Clin Periodontol.* 1989;16(1):17–20.

37. Marton IJ, Balla G, Hegedus C, et al. The role of reactive oxygen intermediates in the pathogenesis of chronic apical periodontitis. *Oral Microbiol Immunol.* 1993;8(4):254–257.

38. Ritchie CS, Kinane DF. Nutrition, inflammation, and periodontal disease. *Nutrition.* 2003;19(5):475–476.

39. Vojdani A, Bazargan M, Vojdani E, et al. New evidence for antioxidant properties of vitamin C. *Cancer Detect Prev.* 2000;24(6):508–523.

40. Heuser G, Vojdani A. Enhancement of natural killer cell activity and T and B cell function by buffered vitamin C in patients exposed to toxic chemicals: the role of protein kinase-C. *Immunopharmacol Immunotoxicol.* 1997;19(3):291–312.

41. Siegel BV, Morton JI. Vitamin C and immunity: natural killer (NK) cell factor. *Int J Vitam Nutr Res.* 1983;53(2):179–183.

42. Nishida M, Grossi SG, Dunford RG, et al. Dietary vitamin C and the risk for periodontal disease. *J Periodontol.* 2000;71(8):1215–1223.

43. Moran JR, Greene HL. The B vitamins and vitamin C in human nutrition. II. 'Conditional' B vitamins and vitamin C. *Am J Dis Child.* 1979;133(3):308–314.

44. Riepe FG, Eichmann D, Oppermann HC, et al. Special feature: picture of the month. *Arch Pediatr Adolesc Med.* 2001;155(5):607–608.

45. Stephensen CB. Vitamin A, infection, and immune function. *Annu Rev Nutr.* 2001;21:167–192.

46. Chapple IL, Milward MR, Dietrich T. The prevalence of inflammatory periodontitis is negatively associated with serum antioxidant concentrations. *J Nutr.* 2007;137(3):657–664.

47. Bikle DD. Vitamin D and the immune system: role in protection against bacterial infection. *Curr Opin Nephrol Hypertens.* 2008;17(4):348–352.

48. Kreutz M, Andreesen R, Krause SW, et al. 1,25-dihydroxyvitamin D3 production and vitamin D3 receptor expression are developmentally regulated during differentiation of human monocytes into macrophages. *Blood.* 1993;82(4):1300–1307.

49. Dietrich T, Nunn M, Dawson-Hughes B, et al. Association between serum concentrations of 25-hydroxyvitamin D and gingival inflammation. *Am J Clin Nutr.* 2005;82(3):575–580.

50. Asman B, Wijkander P, Hjerpe A. Reduction of collagen degradation in experimental granulation tissue by vitamin E and selenium. *J Clin Periodontol.* 1994;21(1):45–47.

51. Cohen ME, Meyer DM. Effect of dietary vitamin E supplementation and rotational stress on alveolar bone loss in rice rats. *Arch Oral Biol.* 1993;38(7):601–606.

52. Meydani SN, Beharka AA. Vitamin E and immune response in the aged. *Bibl Nutr Dieta.* 2001;(55):148–158.

53. Han SN, Meydani SN. Impact of vitamin E on immune function and its clinical implications. *Expert Rev Clin Immunol.* 2006;2(4):561–567.

54. Yu YH, Kuo HK, Lai YL. The association between serum folate levels and periodontal disease in older adults: data from the National Health and Nutrition Examination Survey 2001/02. *J Am Geriatr Soc.* 2007;55(1):108–113.

55. Nishida M, Grossi SG, Dunford RG, et al. Calcium and the risk for periodontal disease. *J Periodontol.* 2000;71(7):1057–1066.

56. Krall EA, Wehler C, Garcia RI, et al. Calcium and vitamin D supplements reduce tooth loss in the elderly. *Am J Med.* 2001;111(6):452–456.

57. Chapple IL. Potential mechanisms underpinning the nutritional modulation of periodontal inflammation. *J Am Dent Assoc.* 2009;140(2):178–184.

58. Woodward B. Protein, calories, and immune defenses. *Nutr Rev.* 1998;56(1 Pt 2):S84–S92.

59. Boesing F, Patino JS, da Silva VR, et al. The interface between obesity and periodontitis with emphasis on oxidative stress and inflammatory response. *Obes Rev.* 2009;10(3):290–297.

60. Saito T, Shimazaki Y, Kiyohara Y, et al. Relationship between obesity, glucose tolerance, and periodontal disease in Japanese women: the Hisayama study. *J Periodontal Res.* 2005;40(4):346–353.

61. Tomofuji T, Yamamoto T, Tamaki N, et al. Effects of obesity on gingival oxidative stress in a rat model. *J Periodontol.* 2009;80(8):1324–1329.
62. Sroda R. *Nutrition for a Healthy Mouth.* 2nd ed. Philadelphia, PA: Lippincott Williams & Wilkins; 2010:xviii, 350.
63. Brock GR, Butterworth CJ, Matthews JB, et al. Local and systemic total antioxidant capacity in periodontitis and health. *J Clin Periodontol.* 2004;31(7):515–521.
64. Pack AR, Thomson ME. Effects of topical and systemic folic acid supplementation on gingivitis in pregnancy. *J Clin Periodontol.* 1980;7(5):402–414.
65. Vogel RI, Fink RA, Frank O, et al. The effect of topical application of folic acid on gingival health. *J Oral Med.* 1978;33(1):22–32.

 STUDENT ANCILLARY RESOURCES

A wide variety of resources to enhance your learning and understanding of this chapter are available on thePoint®.

- Visit thePoint to access:
  - Audio Glossary
  - Animations
  - Suggested Readings
  - Answers to Review Questions
  - Case Studies

18

Tobacco, Smoking, and Periodontal Disease

Clinical Application. Smoking may be one of the most significant risk factors in the development and progression of periodontal disease. Dental hygienists have a professional responsibility to provide tobacco cessation services as a routine component of dental hygiene practice. Smoking cessation guidelines recommend that dental team members should check the smoking status of their patients at least once a year and should advise all smokers to stop smoking. This chapter summarizes what is known about tobacco as a risk for periodontitis and provides suggestions for brief, effective tobacco cessation counseling in the dental setting.

Learning Objectives

- Discuss the implications of smoking/the use of tobacco products on periodontal health status.
- Discuss the implications of smoking on the host response to periodontal disease.
- Discuss the effects of smoking on periodontal treatment outcomes.
- Discuss current theories as to why smokers have more periodontal disease than nonsmokers.
- Explain why tobacco cessation counseling is a valuable part of patient care in the dental setting.
- Value the importance of providing tobacco cessation counseling as a routine part of periodontal treatment.

Key Terms

Dental implant
Peri-implant mucositis

Peri-implantitis
Environmental tobacco smoke

Tobacco cessation counseling

Section 1
Tobacco as a Risk Factor for Periodontal Disease

Inflammation is a critical component of normal tissue repair, as well as being fundamental to the body's defense against infection. Environmental factors, such as smoking, have been reported to modify the host response and hence modify the progression, severity, and outcome of the inflammatory response. Therefore, a comprehensive understanding of how smoking affects inflammation is vital for preventive and therapeutic strategies on a clinical level.

EPIDEMIOLOGY OF TOBACCO IN PERIODONTAL PATIENTS

- Evidence accumulated over the past three decades indicates that cigarette smoking is considered to be a very strong risk factor for periodontal disease (1–4). Cigarette smoking increases the risk for periodontal disease by at least 2 to 3 times (1).
- Tooth loss is the ultimate outcome of untreated periodontitis. Smokers are at higher risk for tooth loss due to periodontal disease (3,5–7).
- Cigar and pipe smoking are also significant risk factors for attachment loss (7–9).
- Smokeless tobacco use is associated with severe recession and loss of attachment to buccal surfaces of teeth, where the smokeless tobacco was placed (10).

SMOKING AND PERIODONTITIS

- There is a wealth of literature outlining the role that cigarette smoking has on periodontal disease and treatment, and a number of reviews cover this topic in detail (4,11,12).
- Results from the first National Health and Nutrition Examination Survey (NHANES) demonstrated that smokers have greater periodontal destruction than former and never smokers (8).
- More recently the NHANES III study concluded that approximately half of periodontitis cases could be attributed to either current (42.9%) smoking or former smoking (10.9%) (8,13). Current estimates indicate smoking also increases the prevalence of periodontitis in excess of 20% in younger segments of the adult population (7).
- The effect of smoking and periodontal destruction are said to be dose dependent with total exposure to cigarette smoking being a widely used measure of dose (7). Heavy smokers (more than 10 cigarettes/day) have greater odds for more severe attachment loss compared to nonsmokers (Fig. 18-1) (14).

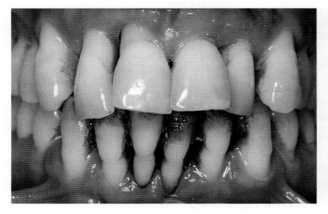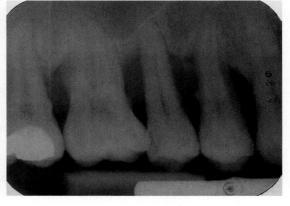

Figure 18-1. Attachment Loss Associated with Smoking. Clinical and radiographic evidence shows advanced periodontitis with horizontal and vertical bone loss in this 37-year-old male, cigarette smoker, with 20 pack-years of smoking.

Section 2
Mechanisms of Smoking-Mediated Periodontal Disease

More than 4,000 toxins are present in cigarette smoke including poisons such as carbon monoxide, oxidizing radicals, carcinogens (e.g., nitrosamines) and addictive psychoactive substances such as nicotine (3,7). Oral problems associated with smoking include halitosis, dry mouth, dental staining (Fig. 18-2), periodontal disease, and cancer (3,12,13). Smoking affects the periodontium in several ways. Some of the possible mechanisms are highlighted in Figure 18-3.

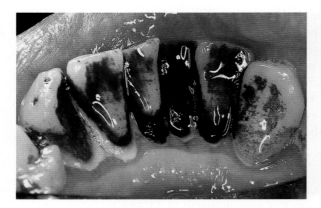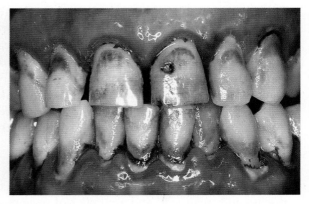

Figure 18-2. Oral Problems Associated With Smoking. Heavy tobacco staining and plaque biofilm accumulation are evident in a smoker along with accompanying signs of periodontitis.

EFFECTS OF SMOKING ON THE PERIODONTIUM

Smoking affects the periodontium in several ways. Some of the possible mechanisms are highlighted in Figure 18-3.

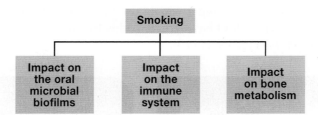

Figure 18-3. Mechanisms of Smoking-Mediated Destruction.

1. Impact of Smoking on the Oral Microbial Biofilms
    A. There are conflicting reports on how smoking affects the oral microflora. A few studies indicate that there are no differences in the subgingival bacteria between smokers and nonsmokers (15–17).
        1. Other investigations, however, show that the subgingival microbial profile associated with periodontitis in smokers is diverse and distinct from that of nonsmokers (16,18–20).
        2. Multiple studies have shown that plaque biofilm in smokers is more likely to be colonized by *Porphyromonas gingivalis* and other potential periodontal pathogens (21–25).

   B. Cigarette smoking is associated with a lower oxygen tension in the periodontal pocket and thus is favorable for the growth of anaerobic bacteria (13).
   C. A recent study by Kumar et al. (18) examined the impact of smoking on composition and proinflammatory characteristics of the biofilm during formation. The authors reported that smoking favors early acquisition and colonization of periodontal pathogens in oral biofilms.
2. Impact of Smoking on the Immune system
   A. From both a biological and epidemiological viewpoint, numerous studies suggest that smoking enhances the risk of periodontal disease (3,12,26). Smoking affects both the human immune system and cellular and humoral inflammatory response systems (3,27,28).
   B. Smokers have decreased signs of inflammation and a decreased gingival crevicular blood flow that is indicative of impaired gingival blood flow in smokers. This is due to the vasoconstrictor properties of nicotine.
   C. Although smokers have a higher number of neutrophils, neutrophil function in the peripheral circulation is impaired. Neutrophils have shown decreased adherence, chemotaxis, and phagocytosis in smokers (29).
   D. Antibody production is another protective mechanism impacted by smoking (29). Smoking generally decreased IgG2 antibody production that, in turn, leads to decreased serum immunoglobulin G (IgG) concentrations. IgG2 antibody production is also reported to occur in patients with aggressive periodontitis (23,29,30).
3. Smoking and Bone Metabolism
   A. Bone is one of the tissues most affected by smoking (31). Smoking is associated with a greater amount of alveolar bone destruction in comparison to nonsmokers (29,31–33). In a 10-year longitudinal study, reduction in bone height was 2.7 times greater in adult smokers compared to nonsmokers (31).
      1. At least one longitudinal cohort study has reported the bone mineral content among smokers was 10% to 30% lower compared to nonsmokers (2).
      2. Bone loss in smokers also appears to be dose dependent with odds ratios ranging from 3.25 for light smokers to 7.28 for heavy smokers (34).
   B. Although the mechanisms of how nicotine contributes to alveolar bone damage are not fully understood, several pathways have been proposed.
      1. In vitro studies have shown that nicotine suppresses osteoblasts while stimulating alkaline phosphatase activity (35,36).
      2. Nicotine also increases the secretion of interleukin-6 (IL-6) and tumor necrosis factor alpha (TNF-α) in osteoblasts (37).
      3. Lastly, nicotine is also known to alter normal bone remodeling by increasing the release of matrix metalloproteinases (33).
4. Impact of Environmental Tobacco Smoke
   A. Nonsmokers exposed to **environmental tobacco smoke**—"secondhand smoke" or "passive smoking"—are at increased risk for periodontitis. An analysis of NHANES III data concluded that the odds of having periodontitis are 1.6 times higher for nonsmoking adults who are exposed to environmental tobacco smoke than adults who are not exposed to passive smoke (38).
      1. Sanders et al. (39) conclude that exposure to environmental tobacco smoke and presence of severe periodontitis among nonsmokers had a dose-dependent relationship. Their research findings show that individuals exposed to environmental tobacco smoke for 1 to 25 hours per week have a 29% increased risk of severe periodontitis. For those exposed to environmental

tobacco smoke for 26 hours or more per week, the odds were twice as high for severe periodontitis as individuals not exposed.

    2. A more recent investigation of 3,137 subjects evaluated the association between environmental tobacco smoke and periodontitis in nonsmokers. This study concluded that adults with high environmental tobacco smoke exposure had two times the odds of periodontitis in comparison with subjects with negligible exposure (40).

  B. Nishida et al. (26) determined that passive smoke exposure was correlated to an elevation of interleukin-1β, albumin, and aspartate aminotransferase (AST) levels in the saliva.

5. **Electronic Cigarettes (E-cigarettes)**
  A. The electronic cigarette was introduced to the United States market in 2007. "E-cigarettes" don't contain tobacco. Instead, there's a mechanism that heats up liquid nicotine, which turns into a vapor that smokers inhale and exhale.
    1. Laboratory analysis of electronic cigarette conducted by the U.S. Food and Drug Administration shows quite clearly that the fluid and aerosol in e-cigarettes contains known toxins, including propylene glycol, heavy metals, volatile organic compounds, and tobacco-specific nitrosamines. (http://www.fda.gov/NewsEvents/PublicHealthFocus/ucm173146.htm. Accessed February 12, 2014.)
    2. At this time, the possible side effects of inhaling nicotine vapor, as well as other health risks e-cigarettes may pose—both to users and to the public—are unknown.
  B. The environmental tobacco smoke generated from a single cigarette is 32 $\mu g/m^3$ compared to 3.3 $\mu g/m^3$ from a single e-cigarette. Thus, it may be that e-cigarettes have proportionally less impact (factor of 10 times) on the periodontium than would exposure to environmental tobacco smoke from a cigarette (41).

EFFECTS OF SMOKING ON PERIODONTAL THERAPY

1. **Impact of Chemical Products and Toxins in Cigarette Smoke on Periodontal Therapy**
  A. Chemical products and toxins in tobacco smoke may delay wound healing by impairing the biologic progression of healing and by inhibiting the basic cellular functions necessary for the initiation of wound healing (29).
  B. Volatile components of cigarette smoke—namely acrolein and acetaldehyde—may inhibit gingival fibroblast attachment and proliferation. Fibroblasts exposed to nicotine produce less extracellular matrix, less collagen, and more collagenase. These negative effects on fibroblast functions influence wound healing and progression of periodontitis (3,12).

2. **Smoking and Response to Periodontal Treatment.** Smoking not only increases the risk for developing periodontal disease, but it also impacts the response to periodontal treatment. Smokers show a poorer response to periodontal therapy compared to nonsmokers (42–44).
  A. Smokers exhibit less reduction in probing depth and less gain in clinical attachment after treatment compared to ex-smokers or nonsmokers (45).
  B. In a 6-year longitudinal study, nonsmokers had approximately a 50% higher rate of improvement in probing depth and clinical attachment levels after periodontal therapy than did active smokers (34).
  C. Periodontal treatment in smokers, both surgical and nonsurgical therapies, has been associated with improvements in periodontal outcomes. Comparison of the outcomes, however, showed significantly less improvement in smokers compared with nonsmokers (45–52).

Section 3
Smoking and Peri-Implant Disease

A **dental implant** is a nonbiologic (artificial) device surgically inserted into the jawbone to (1) replace a missing tooth or (2) provide support for a prosthetic denture. The **peri-implant tissues** are the tissues that surround the dental implant. In many ways, the peri-implant tissues are similar to the periodontium of a natural tooth. Dental implants are discussed in detail in Chapter 31, Maintenance of the Dental Implant.

- Peri-implant mucositis (also called peri-implant gingivitis) is plaque-induced gingivitis (with no loss of supporting bone) that is localized in the gingival tissues surrounding a dental implant and is characterized by edema, change in color (red or red-blue), bleeding and/or purulence on probing, with probing depts of equal to or greater than 4 mm, and no evidence of radiographic peri-implant bone loss (53).
- Peri-implantitis is a more advanced inflammatory disease—essentially chronic periodontitis—that exhibits deep probing depths (5 mm or greater), bleeding on probing (BOP) and/or purulence, and radiographic evidence of loss of alveolar bone (54).

THE IMPACT OF SMOKING ON DENTAL IMPLANTS

- Heat produced by smoking, as well as, the toxic by-products of cigarette smoking, such as nicotine, carbon monoxide, and hydrogen cyanide, have been implicated as risk factors for impaired healing after implant surgery (55).
- Smokers experience almost twice as many implant failures compared with nonsmokers and are more prone to show peri-implant bone loss in the maxilla (56–63).
- Risk indicators associated with increased peri-implant mucositis and peri-implantitis include poor plaque biofilm control, a history of periodontitis, diabetes, and smoking (55,59,61–63).
- The combination of smoking and a history of periodontitis (treated or untreated) increases the risk of peri-implant bone loss (Figs. 18-4 and 18-5) (56,62).

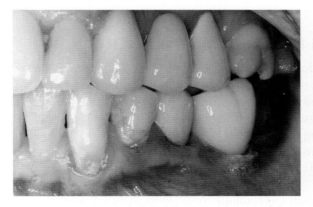

Figure 18-4. Peri-implant Mucositis. Clinical signs of peri-implant mucositis of the mandibular first molar.

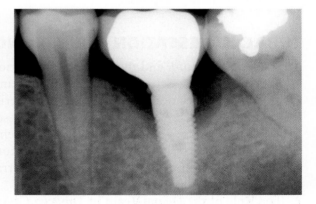

Figure 18-5. Peri-implantitis. Radiographic evidence of peri-implantitis featuring circumferential angular bone loss.

Section 4
Tobacco Cessation for the Periodontal Patient

EFFECTS OF TOBACCO CESSATION ON THE PERIODONTIUM

There have been few publications in the periodontal literature to specifically address the impact of smoking cessation on the periodontium, most probably because of the common challenges in motivating patients to quit smoking. Fiorini et al. conducted a systematic review of the literature to evaluate the effect of smoking cessation on periodontitis progression and response to periodontal therapy. Based on the limited available evidence, Fiorini et al. (1) concluded that smoking cessation seems to have a positive influence on periodontitis occurrence and periodontal healing.

1. The Effect of Smoking Cessation on Periodontal Status
   A. Current smokers usually have significantly worse periodontal conditions (greater probing depths, more attachment loss, and alveolar bone loss) than either never smokers or former smokers. The NHANES III study concluded that approximately half of periodontitis cases could be attributed to either current (42.9%) smoking or former smoking (10.9%) (8,13).
   B. In general, the periodontal health status of former smokers is not as good as that of never smokers but is better than that of current smokers (64). These findings suggest that while the past effects of smoking on the periodontium cannot be reversed, smoking cessation is beneficial to periodontal health (65).
   C. The American Academy of Periodontology strongly recommends that inclusion of tobacco cessation counseling is an integral part of periodontal therapy (66).
2. The Effect of Smoking Cessation on Periodontal Treatment Outcomes
   A. Studies have confirmed that treatment outcomes in former smokers are generally similar to those that can be expected in never smokers but are usually better than those that can be expected in current smokers (65).
   B. The benefits of smoking cessation on the periodontium likely result from (1) a reduction in pathogenic bacteria in the subgingival plaque biofilm, (2) improved circulation in the gingiva, and (3) improvements in the host's immune-inflammatory response.

TOBACCO CESSATION COUNSELING IN PERIODONTAL THERAPY

1. Smoking Cessation and the Prevention of Periodontal Disease
   A. The knowledge that smoking is a significant risk factor suggests that in smokers, smoking cessation might prevent more periodontal disease than daily plaque control self-care. All patients should be assessed for smoking status and smokers should be given smoking cessation counseling (67).
   B. Tobacco cessation counseling includes information on smoking cessation and prevention of tobacco use, as well as referrals to other health professionals for tobacco cessation programs.
2. The Role of the Dental Team in Tobacco Cessation Counseling
   A. The World Health Organization (WHO) advocates that all health providers must be involved in tobacco cessation efforts, including oral health professionals who reach a large proportion of the healthy population (68).

B. Dental team members have regular contact with patients, are the first to see the effects of tobacco in the mouth, and are the only health professionals who frequently see "medically healthy" patients. Dental hygienists, thus, are in an ideal position to reinforce the antitobacco message, as well as being able to motivate and support smokers willing to quit.

C. Dental hygienists have a professional responsibility to provide tobacco cessation services as a routine component of dental hygiene practice. Smoking cessation guidelines recommend that all health professionals, including dental team members, should check the smoking status of their patients at least once a year, and should advise all smokers to stop smoking (1,68,69).

A USER-FRIENDLY MODEL FOR COUNSELING THE PERIODONTAL PATIENT

1. Counseling Time Commitment. *In the vast majority of cases, dental teams will only be involved in delivering brief advice to smokers. This should take less than 5 minutes of their time.*

2. Key Elements in Providing Brief Advice
   A. All patients should have their smoking/tobacco use status (current, ex-, never smoked) established and checked at regular intervals. This information should be recorded in the patient's chart.
   B. Smokers should then be asked some simple questions, in order to assess their degree of interest in stopping smoking/tobacco use.
   C. All smokers and chewers of tobacco should be advised both of the value of stopping, and of the health risks of continuing. The advice should be clear, firm, and personalized.
   D. Although most people know of the risks of tobacco use in relation to cancers and heart disease, fewer are aware of the detrimental effects on the mouth. Dental teams, thus, have a unique opportunity to highlight the dangers of tobacco use. The early signs of tobacco use—such as tooth staining, changes to the soft tissues and halitosis—are easily identified and are reversible, and these provide a useful means of motivating smokers to stop.
   E. All smokers and chewers of tobacco should be advised of the value of the support offered by quitlines. **Quitlines** are toll-free telephone centers staffed by trained tobacco cessation experts. It takes as little as 30 seconds to refer a patient to a quitline. Smokers who are interested and motivated to stop should be referred to these services. The U.S. Department of Health & Human Services has a national quitline number: **1–800-QUIT-NOW** (1–800–784–8669).

3. A Pathway and Sample Dialogs for Cessation Counseling. A tobacco cessation care pathway for dental practice is summarized in Figure 18-6 (70). Boxes 18-1 to 18-3 provide sample dialogs for cessation counseling.

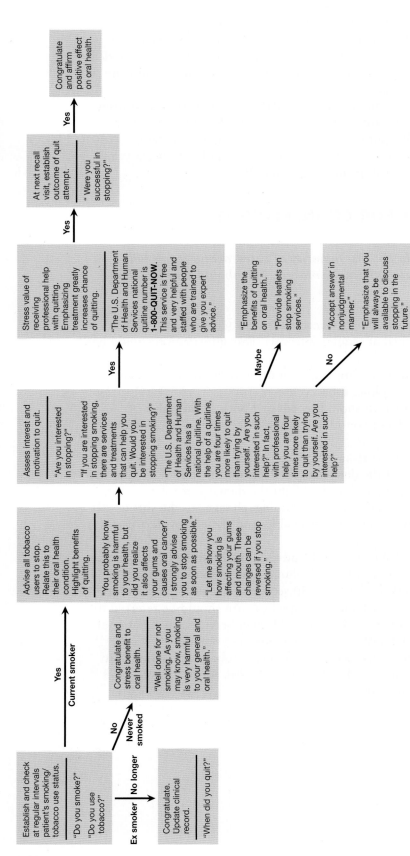

Figure 18-6. A Pathway for Tobacco Cessation Counseling.

Box 18-1. Sample Cessation Counseling Dialog #1

Ms. W is a 22-year-old radiology technician who has come to the dental office for her biannual exam. Ms. W has no significant health history. She has periodontitis on exam. Ms. W began smoking at age 12 and has smoked ¾ to 1 pack a day for almost 10 years. She is very excited because she has just become engaged but admits that her fiancé will not set a wedding date until she has quit smoking.

Clinician: Your oral exam shows evidence of damage from smoking. How do you feel about quitting?

Ms. W: I want to quit. My fiancé hates that I am smoking. Every day I tell myself not to smoke but I just cannot seem to quit.

Clinician: What is the most difficult part about quitting? What is your biggest barrier?

Ms. W: I feel like cigarettes are my best friends! The only time I relax is when I smoke—or when I am out drinking and smoking with my friends. Almost all my friends smoke.

Clinician: Have you ever tried to quit?

Ms. W: Every day!! But nothing works! And then my fiancé yells at me, so I feel worse and end up smoking more. I feel so guilty and so embarrassed!

Clinician: It sounds like you are in a vicious circle that is probably making it harder to quit. Let's put this in perspective. Of all addictions, it is harder to take control over the nicotine addiction than any other. It is also harder for women to quit than for men. But the good news is that there are more things available to help smokers quit than ever before. And quitting at your young age will be so beneficial in every way—including your oral health! The longer we do anything, the harder it is to stop. So stopping now would be the best thing you will ever do for yourself and while it will be very difficult, it will definitely be easier than if you continue to smoke for another 20 years.

Ms. W: What is the best way to quit?

Clinician: Probably the most important thing for you to do is make the decision to quit. That is even more important than wanting to quit. Rather than telling yourself, "today I am not going to smoke," set a firm quit date within 1 to 2 weeks of this appointment and make plans on how not to smoke. Think of quitting as taking on a new job. With all the other responsibilities you have, quitting has to be your priority for about 3 months. And get help—the more support you have the better.

Ms. W: What kind of help? My fiancé tells me to just stop—that if I really wanted to quit I could.

Clinician: A lot of people think smokers should just stop. But that is like telling an alcoholic to just stop drinking and we wouldn't do that. We tell other addicts to get quit therapy and that's what smokers should do! It is about learning how to quit. We rarely get what we want in life unless we work at it.

Ms. W: I never thought of it that way. I thought I couldn't stop because I am weak or just don't have any will power.

Clinician: Not at all. I would suggest calling 1 800 QUIT NOW. This is a free service that provides counseling on how to quit. This quitline can also tell you about programs near you if you are interested in more intensive treatment. And as your provider I will assist you in any way I can—including educate you about the medications that help people quit.

Ms. W: Thank you. I will call the quitline and let you know what I decide to do.

Clinician: Good for you. You will miss your "best friend" but your life will be so much better once you have made the break!

Box 18-2. Sample Cessation Counseling Dialog #2

Ms. G is a 50-year-old grant writer who has come to the dental office for follow-up care. Ms. G has type 2 diabetes, COPD (chronic bronchitis), and severe enough periodontal disease that most of her teeth have been extracted in the past few years. Ms. G began smoking at age 13 and has smoked a pack a day for most of her life. About a year ago she decreased her daily consumption to half a pack.

Clinician: Congratulations on being able to cut down on your smoking! Have you thought about quitting completely? We might be able to save your remaining teeth if you are able to quit.

Ms. G: I know I should quit but I really love my cigarettes.

Clinician: Has it been hard for you to cut down?

Ms. G: Actually it's been horrible.

Clinician: What has been the most difficult part for you?

Ms. G: I can't stop thinking about my next cigarette. I find myself thinking about when I can get the next cigarette in as soon as I put one out!

Clinician: It almost sounds like the cigarettes have become even more important to you since you cut down! While quitting is the most difficult thing you might ever do, it might in fact make your life easier to not have to worry about when you can get in your next cigarette.

Ms. G: That's true—it would be so nice to not to have to think about them anymore.

Clinician: So you still love your cigarettes but don't love that you are smoking!

Ms. G: Yes that is exactly it. I hate that I am still smoking. I know it is so bad for my health. I feel that I must quit but I have tried to quit before and the longest I have ever gone without a cigarette has only been 4 hours! Cigarettes are the only things that calm me down.

Clinician: How soon do you smoke when you first get up in the morning and do you ever smoke if you wake during the night?

Ms. G: I smoke before my feet hit the ground every morning and I often take a couple of drags if I wake up during the night.

Clinician: It sounds like you have a strong physical addiction as well as a significant psychological addiction. Have you considered using medication to help you quit? You would be a good candidate for pharmacotherapy.

Ms. G: No. I take insulin for my diabetes and I don't want to take anything that would interfere with that.

Clinician: Actually, smoking interferes with controlling your diabetes much more than a quit-smoking medication. And were you aware that with every cigarette your blood sugar goes up? So your diabetes would be much easier to control if you quit.

Ms. G: I had no idea that was the case.

Clinician: One suggestion would be to look at quitting the same way you look at having diabetes. A nicotine addiction is a chronic condition just as diabetes is. You do whatever you can to control your blood sugar with diet, exercise, and medication in order to enhance your quality of life and decrease risks—even though you may not want to do all those things. Try to look at quitting that way. Even though you love cigarettes, you will benefit by taking control! Look at quitting as something you are doing for yourself rather than to yourself. That approach may make it easier to let go of smoking.

Ms. G: I like that. It puts me in control of the situation—rather than letting the cigarettes control me! Maybe I will consider trying a medication to help me.

Box 18-3. Sample Smoking Cessation Counseling Dialog #3

Mr. R is a 48-year-old attorney who has come to the dental office for his care. Mr. R has hypertension and high cholesterol. He has periodontal disease on exam. Mr. R. began smoking at age 17 and has smoked 2 packs a day for 30 years.

Clinician: As you know, your oral exam shows significant damage from smoking and your blood pressure is elevated today. Have you tried to quit since our last visit?

Mr. R: Not really. And I don't want to talk about it. Everyone is on me. My doctors, my wife, my kids, and now I suppose you are going to give me a hard time too.

Clinician: I don't want to give you a hard time. But I do want to encourage you to at least try and quit. The more times you try, the more chance you have of success. I am not going to tell you how dangerous it is to smoke. But I am going to remind you that by quitting you can reverse so much of the damage cigarettes have caused in you.

Mr. R: Look I really don't want to quit. I exercise and I watch what I eat. I'll keep coming to you for my teeth and take medicine for my heart problems and hope for the best.

Clinician: You are such a "take charge" person in every other aspect of your life. How about taking control over this addiction rather than hoping for the best?

Mr. R: I will quit when I am ready. I know myself. When I decide to do something, it gets done.

Clinician: Take advantage of that! Consider what is available to help you quit now. It is possible to quit even if you don't want to quit or don't feel ready.

Mr. R: It would get people off my back anyway. My kids nag me every day.

Clinician: People in your life are concerned about you. But you cannot quit for them. You can use the fact that you will have a longer, better quality life with your kids as a motivation, though the decision to quit is yours. No one, nothing, can make you quit but there are plenty of us who can help you quit.

Mr. R: If I do this, I am doing it on my own.

Clinician: I understand your wanting to take that approach. However, it would be so much easier if you use a medication. You have been smoking for a long time and a medication would increase your chance of permanent success.

Mr. R: Is it ok to take something with all my heart problems?

Clinician: Absolutely. In fact the medication, Chantix, has the highest success rates. It should be started 1 to 2 weeks before quitting and once there is a therapeutic dose in your system, you should notice a significant decrease in your desire to smoke. I can provide you with more information and arrange for a prescription.

Mr. R: I have heard that makes you feel depressed.

Clinician: That is been reported but only in a tiny minority. Feeling depressed is very common with quitting! I will show you a list of the most common withdrawal symptoms, so you will be aware of what to expect. And also give you information on the other six FDA-approved medications, so you will have all the options. Think about setting a quit date within a couple of weeks and let me know how I can best assist you through the process. I will keep working with you until you are able to quit.

Mr. R: OK I will try but this is just between you and me.

Clinician: I understand and will respect that. At some point people in your life will be aware that you are trying to quit and it might help you to let them know what they can do to help you—including NOT nag you! I am very proud of you for making the attempt. You will not regret it!

Chapter Summary Statement

Tobacco use is a major risk factor for the onset and progression of periodontal disease. Smoking affects the periodontium in several ways by impacting oral biofilms, host immune response, and bone metabolism. There is sufficient evidence for the benefits of tobacco cessation on a wide variety of oral health outcomes, including periodontal treatment. Advice and assistance on tobacco cessation is therefore an integral part in the management of all patients seeking periodontal care.

Section 5
Focus on Patients

Clinical Patient Care

CASE 1

A new patient with severe chronic periodontitis has a history of smoking one to two packs of cigarettes each day. The patient informs you that he will do "anything" to save his teeth, but that he cannot quit smoking. What counsel would you provide this patient about the effect of the smoking habit on the likelihood of long-term control of his periodontitis?

References

1. Fiorini T, Musskopf ML, Oppermann RV, et al. Is there a positive effect of smoking cessation on periodontal health? A systematic review. *J Periodontol.* 2014;85(1):83–91.
2. Gelskey SC. Cigarette smoking and periodontitis: methodology to assess the strength of evidence in support of a causal association. *Community Dent Oral Epidemiol.* 1999;27(1):16–24.
3. Johannsen A, Susin C, Gustafsson A. Smoking and inflammation: evidence for a synergistic role in chronic disease. *Periodontol 2000.* 2014;64(1):111–126.
4. Johnson GK, Guthmiller JM. The impact of cigarette smoking on periodontal disease and treatment. *Periodontol 2000.* 2007;44:178–194.
5. Ahlqwist M, Bengtsson C, Hollender L, et al. Smoking habits and tooth loss in Swedish women. *Community Dent Oral Epidemiol.* 1989;17(3):144–147.
6. Holm G. Smoking as an additional risk for tooth loss. *J Periodontol.* 1994;65(11):996–1001.
7. Tonetti MS. Cigarette smoking and periodontal diseases: etiology and management of disease. *Ann Periodontol.* 1998;3(1):88–101.
8. Albandar JM, Streckfus CF, Adesanya MR, et al. Cigar, pipe, and cigarette smoking as risk factors for periodontal disease and tooth loss. *J Periodontol.* 2000;71(12):1874–1881.
9. Tomar SL, Asma S. Smoking-attributable periodontitis in the United States: findings from NHANES III. National Health and Nutrition Examination Survey. *J Periodontol.* 2000;71(5):743–751.
10. Anand PS, Kamath KP, Bansal A, et al. Comparison of periodontal destruction patterns among patients with and without the habit of smokeless tobacco use–a retrospective study. *J Periodontal Res.* 2013;48(5):623–631.
11. Heasman L, Stacey F, Preshaw PM, et al. The effect of smoking on periodontal treatment response: a review of clinical evidence. *J Clin Periodontol.* 2006;33(4):241–253.
12. Johnson GK, Hill M. Cigarette smoking and the periodontal patient. *J Periodontol.* 2004;75(2):196–209.
13. Johnson GK, Slach NA. Impact of tobacco use on periodontal status. *J Dent Educ.* 2001;65(4):313–321.
14. Grossi SG, Genco RJ, Machtei EE, et al. Assessment of risk for periodontal disease. II. Risk indicators for alveolar bone loss. *J Periodontol.* 1995;66(1):23–29.
15. Bostrom L, Bergstrom J, Dahlen G, et al. Smoking and subgingival microflora in periodontal disease. *J Clin Periodontol.* 2001;28(3):212–219.
16. Preber H, Bergstrom J. Occurrence of gingival bleeding in smoker and non-smoker patients. *Acta Odontol Scand.* 1985;43(5):315–320.
17. Stoltenberg JL, Osborn JB, Pihlstrom BL, et al. Association between cigarette smoking, bacterial pathogens, and periodontal status. *J Periodontol.* 1993;64(12):1225–1230.
18. Kumar PS, Matthews CR, Joshi V, et al. Tobacco smoking affects bacterial acquisition and colonization in oral biofilms. *Infect Immun.* 2011;79(11):4730–4738.

19. Shchipkova AY, Nagaraja HN, Kumar PS. Subgingival microbial profiles of smokers with periodontitis. *J Dent Res.* 2010;89(11):1247–1253.

20. van Winkelhoff AJ, Bosch-Tijhof CJ, Winkel EG, et al. Smoking affects the subgingival microflora in periodontitis. *J Periodontol.* 2001;72(5):666–671.

21. Bagaitkar J, Daep CA, Patel CK, et al. Tobacco smoke augments Porphyromonas gingivalis-Streptococcus gordonii biofilm formation. *PLoS One.* 2011;6(11):e27386.

22. Eggert FM, McLeod MH, Flowerdew G. Effects of smoking and treatment status on periodontal bacteria: evidence that smoking influences control of periodontal bacteria at the mucosal surface of the gingival crevice. *J Periodontol.* 2001;72(9):1210–1220.

23. Haffajee AD, Socransky SS. Relationship of cigarette smoking to attachment level profiles. *J Clin Periodontol.* 2001;28(4):283–295.

24. Kamma JJ, Nakou M, Baehni PC. Clinical and microbiological characteristics of smokers with early onset periodontitis. *J Periodontal Res.* 1999;34(1):25–33.

25. Zambon JJ, Grossi SG, Machtei EE, et al. Cigarette smoking increases the risk for subgingival infection with periodontal pathogens. *J Periodontol.* 1996;67(10 suppl):1050–1054.

26. Nishida N, Yamamoto Y, Tanaka M, et al. Association between passive smoking and salivary markers related to periodontitis. *J Clin Periodontol.* 2006;33(10):717–723.

27. Kinane DF, Chestnutt IG. Smoking and periodontal disease. *Crit Rev Oral Biol Med.* 2000;11(3):356–365.

28. Palmer RM, Wilson RF, Hasan AS, et al. Mechanisms of action of environmental factors–tobacco smoking. *J Clin Periodontol.* 2005;32(suppl 6):180–195.

29. Jacob V, Vellappally S, Smejkalova J. The influence of cigarette smoking on various aspects of periodontal health. *Acta Medica.* 2007;50(1):3–5.

30. Mooney J, Hodge PJ, Kinane DF. Humoral immune response in early-onset periodontitis: influence of smoking. *J Periodontal Res.* 2001;36(4):227–232.

31. Bergstrom J, Eliasson S. Cigarette smoking and alveolar bone height in subjects with a high standard of oral hygiene. *J Clin Periodontol.* 1987;14(8):466–469.

32. Kerdvongbundit V, Wikesjo UM. Effect of smoking on periodontal health in molar teeth. *J Periodontol.* 2000;71(3):433–437.

33. Razali M, Palmer RM, Coward P, et al. A retrospective study of periodontal disease severity in smokers and non-smokers. *Br Dent J.* 2005;198(8):495–498.

34. Grossi SG, Zambon JJ, Ho AW, et al. Assessment of risk for periodontal disease. I. Risk indicators for attachment loss. *J Periodontol.* 1994;65(3):260–267.

35. Fang MA, Frost PJ, Iida-Klein A, et al. Effects of nicotine on cellular function in UMR 106–01 osteoblast-like cells. *Bone.* 1991;12(4):283–286.

36. Rosa GM, Lucas GQ, Lucas ON. Cigarette smoking and alveolar bone in young adults: a study using digitized radiographs. *J Periodontol.* 2008;79(2):232–244.

37. Kamer AR, El-Ghorab N, Marzec N, et al. Nicotine induced proliferation and cytokine release in osteoblastic cells. *Int J Mol Med.* 2006;17(1):121–127.

38. Yamamoto Y, Nishida N, Tanaka M, et al. Association between passive and active smoking evaluated by salivary cotinine and periodontitis. *J Clin Periodontol.* 2005;32(10):1041–1046.

39. Sanders AE, Slade GD, Beck JD, et al. Secondhand smoke and periodontal disease: atherosclerosis risk in communities study. *Am J Public Health.* 2011;101(suppl 1):S339–S346.

40. Sutton JD, Ranney LM, Wilder RS, et al. Environmental tobacco smoke and periodontitis in U.S. non-smokers. *J Dent Hyg.* 2012;86(3):185–194.

41. Goniewicz ML, Kuma T, Gawron M, et al. Nicotine levels in electronic cigarettes. *Nicotine Tob Res.* 2013;15(1):158–166.

42. James JA, Sayers NM, Drucker DB, et al. Effects of tobacco products on the attachment and growth of periodontal ligament fibroblasts. *J Periodontol.* 1999;70(5):518–525.

43. Machuca G, Rosales I, Lacalle JR, et al. Effect of cigarette smoking on periodontal status of healthy young adults. *J Periodontol.* 2000;71(1):73–78.

44. Preber H, Bergstrom J. The effect of non-surgical treatment on periodontal pockets in smokers and non-smokers. *J Clin Periodontol.* 1986;13(4):319–323.

45. Kaldahl WB, Johnson GK, Patil KD, et al. Levels of cigarette consumption and response to periodontal therapy. *J Periodontol.* 1996;67(7):675–681.

46. Ah MK, Johnson GK, Kaldahl WB, et al. The effect of smoking on the response to periodontal therapy. *J Clin Periodontol.* 1994;21(2):91–97.

47. Grossi SG, Skrepcinski FB, DeCaro T, et al. Response to periodontal therapy in diabetics and smokers. *J Periodontol.* 1996;67(10 suppl):1094–1102.

48. Kinane DF, Radvar M. The effect of smoking on mechanical and antimicrobial periodontal therapy. *J Periodontol.* 1997;68(5):467–472.

49. Miller PD Jr. Root coverage with the free gingival graft. Factors associated with incomplete coverage. *J Periodontol.* 1987;58(10):674–681.

50. Preber H, Bergstrom J. Effect of cigarette smoking on periodontal healing following surgical therapy. *J Clin Periodontol.* 1990;17(5):324–328.

51. Rosen PS, Marks MH, Reynolds MA. Influence of smoking on long-term clinical results of intrabony defects treated with regenerative therapy. *J Periodontol.* 1996;67(11):1159–1163.

52. Tonetti MS, Pini-Prato G, Cortellini P. Effect of cigarette smoking on periodontal healing following GTR in infrabony defects. A preliminary retrospective study. *J Clin Periodontol.* 1995;22(3):229–234.

53. Sanz M, Chapple IL; Working Group 4 of the VEWoP. Clinical research on peri-implant diseases: consensus report of Working Group 4. *J Clin Periodontol.* 2012;39(suppl 12):202–206.

54. Tomasi C, Derks J. Clinical research of peri-implant diseases–quality of reporting, case definitions and methods to study incidence, prevalence and risk factors of peri-implant diseases. *J Clin Periodontol.* 2012;39(suppl 12):207–223.

55. Levin L, Schwartz-Arad D. The effect of cigarette smoking on dental implants and related surgery. *Implant Dent.* 2005;14(4):357–361.

56. Anner R, Grossmann Y, Anner Y, et al. Smoking, diabetes mellitus, periodontitis, and supportive periodontal treatment as factors associated with dental implant survival: a long-term retrospective evaluation of patients followed for up to 10 years. *Implant Dent.* 2010;19(1):57–64.

57. Cavalcanti R, Oreglia F, Manfredonia MF, et al. The influence of smoking on the survival of dental implants: a 5-year pragmatic multicentre retrospective cohort study of 1727 patients. *Eur J Oral Implantol.* 2011;4(1):39–45.

58. Charalampakis G, Rabe P, Leonhardt A, et al. A follow-up study of peri-implantitis cases after treatment. *J Clin Periodontol.* 2011;38(9):864–871.

59. Heitz-Mayfield LJ. Peri-implant diseases: diagnosis and risk indicators. *J Clin Periodontol.* 2008;35(8 suppl):292–304.

60. Heitz-Mayfield LJ, Huynh-Ba G. History of treated periodontitis and smoking as risks for implant therapy. *Int J Oral Maxillofac Implants.* 2009;24(suppl):39–68.

61. Klokkevold PR, Han TJ. How do smoking, diabetes, and periodontitis affect outcomes of implant treatment? *Int J Oral Maxillofac Implants.* 2007;22(suppl):173–202.

62. Koldsland OC, Scheie AA, Aass AM. Prevalence of implant loss and the influence of associated factors. *J Periodontol.* 2009;80(7):1069–1075.

63. Rodriguez-Argueta OF, Figueiredo R, Valmaseda-Castellon E, et al. Postoperative complications in smoking patients treated with implants: a retrospective study. *J Oral Maxillofac Surg.* 2011;69(8):2152–2157.

64. Bolin A, Eklund G, Frithiof L, et al. The effect of changed smoking habits on marginal alveolar bone loss. A longitudinal study. *Swed Dent J.* 1993;17(5):211–216.

65. Preshaw PM, Heasman L, Stacey F, et al. The effect of quitting smoking on chronic periodontitis. *J Clin Periodontol.* 2005;32(8):869–879.

66. Position paper. tobacco use and the periodontal patient. Research, Science and Therapy Committee of the American Academy of Periodontology. *J Periodontol.* 1999;70(11):1419–1427.

67. Binnie VI. Addressing the topic of smoking cessation in a dental setting. *Periodontol 2000.* 2008;48:170–178.

68. The world health report: report of the Director-General / 2003. *Shaping the Future.* Geneva: WHO; 2003. XV, 193.

69. West R, McNeill A, Raw M. Smoking cessation guidelines for health professionals: an update. Health Education Authority. *Thorax.* 2000;55(12):987–999.

70. Needleman I, Warnakulasuriya S, Sutherland G, et al. Evaluation of tobacco use cessation (TUC) counselling in the dental office. *Oral Health Prev Dent.* 2006;4(1):27–47.

 ## STUDENT ANCILLARY RESOURCES

A wide variety of resources to enhance your learning and understanding of this chapter are available on thePoint®.

- Visit thePoint to access:
  - Audio Glossary
  - Animations
  - Suggested Readings
  - Answers to Review Questions
  - Case Studies

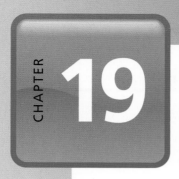
Clinical Periodontal Assessment

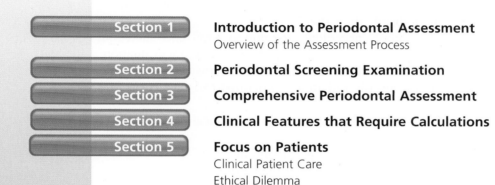
Clinical Application. Clinical periodontal assessment is a critical step in the care of all patients with periodontal diseases. This step serves as the foundation for assigning a periodontal diagnosis, the foundation for developing plans for treating patients, and the foundation for monitoring the success or failure of periodontal treatment performed. The rigorous standards for care in effect today require every clinician participating in patient care to be familiar with the details of performing and documenting a clinical periodontal assessment. This chapter describes how to perform a clinical periodontal assessment, how to document the findings of the assessment, and how to perform calculations needed during the assessment.

Learning Objectives

- Compare and contrast a periodontal screening examination and a comprehensive periodontal assessment.

- Describe how to perform one type of periodontal screening examination.

- List the components of a comprehensive periodontal assessment.

- Describe how to evaluate each component of a comprehensive periodontal assessment.

- Explain how to calculate the width of attached gingiva.

- Explain how to calculate clinical attachment level given several different clinical scenarios.

- Given a clinical scenario, calculate and document the clinical attachment levels for a patient with periodontitis.

Key Terms

Clinical periodontal
   assessment
Baseline data
Periodontal screening
   examination
Periodontal Screening and
   Recording (PSR)

World Health Organization
   (WHO) probe
PSR Code
Comprehensive periodontal
   assessment
Exudate
Horizontal tooth mobility

Vertical tooth mobility
Fremitus
Furcation probes
Gingival crevicular fluid
Attached gingiva
Clinical attachment level
   (CAL)

Section 1
Introduction to Periodontal Assessment

OVERVIEW OF THE ASSESSMENT PROCESS

1. **Clinical periodontal assessment** is a fact-gathering process designed to provide a comprehensive picture of the patient's periodontal health status.
   A. Importance of Periodontal Assessment
      1. This assessment is one of the most important duties performed by any dental team.
         a. The dental team is obligated to perform and document findings of a periodontal assessment for every patient when the patient first enters the dental practice and periodically thereafter (1).
         b. Periodontal assessment requires meticulous attention to detail since successful patient care is dependent on a thorough and accurate periodontal evaluation.
      2. The information gathered during the clinical periodontal assessment forms the basis of both a periodontal diagnosis and an individualized treatment plan for the patient.
   B. Objectives of Periodontal Assessment. The objectives of the clinical periodontal assessment process include the following:
      1. Detect clinical signs of inflammation in the periodontium.
      2. Identify damage to the periodontium already caused by disease or trauma.
      3. Provide the dental team with data used to assign a periodontal diagnosis.
      4. Document features of the periodontium to serve as baseline data for long-term patient monitoring.
   C. Two Types of Periodontal Assessment. Two commonly used types of periodontal assessment are periodontal screening examinations and comprehensive periodontal assessments.
      1. Periodontal Screening Examination. Periodontal screening examination is a rapid information-gathering process that may be used to determine if a periodontium appears healthy, displays signs of gingivitis, or displays signs of periodontitis.
      2. Comprehensive Periodontal Assessment. Comprehensive periodontal assessment is an intensive information-gathering process used to gather the detailed data needed to document the complete periodontal health status of a patient.
2. Standard of Care
   A. *The standard of care is for dentists and dental hygienists to complete an accurate and thorough periodontal assessment on every patient.*
   B. Without a thorough clinical periodontal assessment, periodontal diseases are often not diagnosed or are misdiagnosed, inevitably leading to either undertreatment or overtreatment of the patient.
3. Documentation of Assessment Findings
   A. The clinical periodontal assessment is not complete until all of the information gathered during the assessment has been accurately recorded in the patient's dental chart.
   B. The importance of the accuracy of the documentation cannot be overstated.
      1. Findings documented during the clinical periodontal assessment serve as baseline data used to evaluate the success or failure of an episode of periodontal therapy. Baseline data refers to clinical information gathered prior to periodontal therapy that can be used for comparison to clinical information gathered at a subsequent appointment.
      2. Documented findings also provide the baseline data used in the long-term monitoring of the patient's periodontal health status. An example of when patient monitoring may occur is at periodontal maintenance visits following successful treatment.

Section 2
Periodontal Screening Examination

In some dental offices a periodontal screening examination is used as one of the first steps in evaluating the periodontal status of a patient. A periodontal screening examination is a rapid information-gathering process that may be used to determine if a periodontium appears healthy, displays signs of gingivitis, or displays signs of periodontitis. The Periodontal Screening and Recording (PSR) is one example of an easy-to-use screening system that can aid in the detection of periodontal disease.

1. Periodontal Screening and Recording (PSR)
    A. Characteristics of Periodontal Screening and Recording (PSR)
        1. The PSR can help separate patients into broad categories: those who seem to have periodontal health, gingivitis, or periodontitis.
        2. When the PSR screening examination indicates the presence of periodontal health or gingivitis, in a very few instances no further clinical periodontal assessment may be needed beyond the PSR. It is important to note that individual states have different rules related to the use of this screening examination.
    B. Techniques for Performing the PSR Screening Examination
        1. Special Probe. A World Health Organization (WHO) probe is used for this examination. The WHO probe has a colored band (called the reference mark) located 3.5 to 5.5 mm from the probe tip. This color-coded reference mark is used when performing the PSR screening examination.
        2. One Code Per Sextant. Each sextant of the mouth is examined and assigned an individual PSR code. The unique aspects of the PSR screening system are the manner in which the probe is read and the minimal amount of information that needs to be recorded.
            a. Instead of reading and recording six precise measurements per tooth, the clinician only needs to observe the position of the color-coded reference mark in relation to the gingival margin and a few other clinical features such as the presence of bleeding on probing, the presence of calculus, or the presence of an overhang on a restoration.
            b. Each of the sextants is examined as a separate unit during the PSR screening (i.e., only one PSR code number will be assigned to the entire sextant).
            c. *Only one PSR code is recorded for each sextant in the mouth.* Each sextant is assigned a single PSR code; the highest code obtained for the sextant is recorded.
            d. An "X" is recorded instead of a PSR code if the sextant is edentulous.
        3. Probing Technique
            a. The probe is "walked" circumferentially around each tooth in the sextant being examined. Walking a periodontal probe refers to moving the probe in small increments circumferentially around a tooth.
            b. The color-coded reference mark is monitored continuously as the probe is walked around each tooth. At each site probed, the color-coded reference mark will be (a) completely visible, (b) partially visible, or (c) not visible at all.
2. The PSR Codes
    A. Use of PSR Codes
        1. A PSR code is assigned to each sextant according to the criteria shown in Table 19-1. *The code assigned to a sextant should represent the most advanced periodontal finding on any tooth in that sextant.*
        2. The PSR codes are used to guide further clinical documentation.

a. For some patients with low PSR codes in all sextants (codes 0, 1, or 2), the PSR screening may be adequate documentation of the patient's periodontal health status. Note, however, that the dentist may request a comprehensive periodontal assessment even when low PSR codes are found, since many periodontal conditions must be monitored in more detail than that included in the PSR.

b. For patients with higher PSR codes in one or more sextants (codes 3 or 4), a comprehensive periodontal examination should be performed as outlined in Section 3 of this chapter.

B. **Cautions for Interpreting PSR Codes.** The PSR codes can mislead a clinician in certain patients. As already pointed out, lower codes usually mean periodontal health or gingivitis, and higher codes usually mean periodontitis. *When interpreting the results of the PSR, the clinician must be alert for teeth with gingival enlargement or with gingival recession. In the presence of either of these conditions the PSR can give misleading results.*

TABLE 19-1. CRITERIA FOR ASSIGNING PSR CODES	
CODE 0:	• Color-coded reference mark is *completely visible* in deepest sulcus or pocket of the sextant • No calculus or defective margins on restorations are present • Gingival tissues are healthy with no bleeding evident on gentle probing
CODE 1:	• Color-coded reference mark is *completely visible* in deepest sulcus or pocket of the sextant • No calculus or defective margins on restorations are present • Bleeding *is evident* on probing
CODE 2:	• Color-coded reference mark is *completely visible* in deepest sulcus or pocket of the sextant • Supragingival or subgingival calculus and/or defective margins are detected
CODE 3:	• Color-coded reference mark is *only partially visible* in the deepest sulcus or pocket of the sextant • Code 3 indicates a probing depth between 3.5 and 5.5 mm
CODE 4:	• Color-coded reference mark is *not visible* in the deepest sulcus or pocket of the sextant • Code 4 indicates a probing depth of greater than 5.5 mm
CODE *:	• The * (star) symbol is added to the code of any sextant that exhibits any of the following: 1. Furcation involvement 2. Mobility 3. Mucogingival problems 4. Recession extending into the colored area of the probe • The * (star) symbol is recorded next to the sextant code. For example, "4*"

Section 3
Comprehensive Periodontal Assessment

A comprehensive periodontal assessment is an intensive clinical periodontal evaluation used to gather information about the periodontium. This section of the chapter outlines the clinical features that should be noted and documented during a comprehensive periodontal assessment. It is important to note that special precautions are necessary when examining dental implants. These examination techniques are presented in Chapter 31.

The comprehensive periodontal assessment normally includes clinical features such as probing depth measurements, bleeding on probing, presence of exudate, level of the free gingival margin, level of the mucogingival junction, tooth mobility, furcation involvement, presence of calculus, presence of plaque biofilms, gingival inflammation, radiographic evidence of alveolar bone loss, and presence of local contributing factors.

It should be noted that there are a number of excellent electronic tools that can be used during parts of a comprehensive periodontal assessment; for example, periodontal probes are available that can record probing depths directly in computer software. The discussion in this chapter focuses only on the basic concepts underlying each of the clinical factors being assessed with the knowledge that a clinician who understands the basic concepts can easily apply any of the available electronic tools appropriately.

1. Components of the Comprehensive Periodontal Assessment
   A. **Probing Depth Measurements.** Probing depth measurements are made from the free gingival margin to the base of the pocket (or base of the sulcus).
      1. Probing depths are recorded to the nearest full millimeter. Measurements are normally rounded up to the next higher whole number (e.g., a reading of 3.5 mm is recorded as 4 mm, and a 5.5 mm reading is recorded as 6 mm).
      2. Probing depth measurements are recorded for six specific sites on each tooth: (i) distofacial, (ii) middle facial, (iii) mesiofacial, (iv) distolingual, (v) middle lingual, and (vi) mesiolingual.
   B. **Bleeding on Probing**
      1. Bleeding on gentle probing represents bleeding from the soft tissue wall of a periodontal pocket where the wall of the pocket is ulcerated (i.e., where portions of the epithelium have been destroyed) (Fig. 19-1).
      2. Bleeding can occur immediately after the site is probed or can be slightly delayed in occurrence. An alert clinician will observe each site for a few seconds before moving on to the next site.

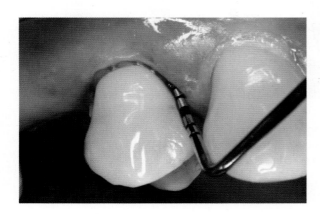

Figure 19-1. A Bleeding Site. Bleeding from the soft tissue wall is a sign of disease. This bleeding was evident upon gentle probing. (Courtesy of Dr. Richard Foster, Guilford Technical Community College, Jamestown, NC.)

C. Presence of Exudate

1. **Exudate** (sometimes referred to as suppuration) is pus that can be expressed from a periodontal pocket. Pus is composed mainly of dead white blood cells and can occur in response to any infection, including periodontal disease.

2. Exudate can be recognized as a pale yellow material oozing from the orifice of a pocket. It is usually easiest to detect when the gingiva is manipulated in some manner. For example, light finger pressure on the gingiva can reveal exudate when it is present (Fig. 19-2). Figure 19-3 illustrates the clinical appearance of exudate in a patient with periodontitis.

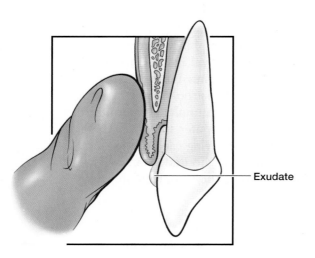

Exudate

Figure 19-2. Using Finger Pressure to Detect Exudate. Exudate can be detected in a periodontal pocket by placing an index finger on the soft tissue in the area of the pocket and exerting slight pressure. This slight pressure can force the exudate out of the pocket, making it readily visible to the clinician.

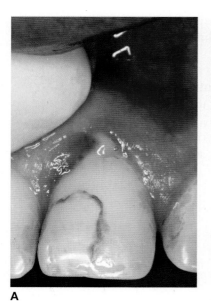
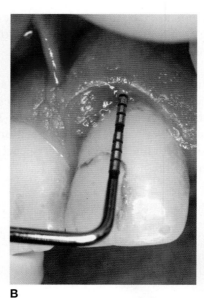
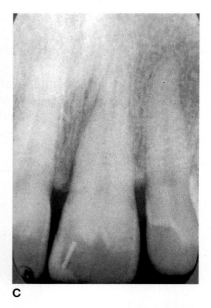

A   B   C

Figure 19-3. Exudate. A: Pressure with the clinician's finger on the gingiva reveals exudate from the gingival tissue adjacent to the central incisor. **B:** Exudate also is visible during probing. **C:** Radiograph of the incisor shown in A and B. (Courtesy of Dr. Richard Foster, Guilford Technical Community College, Jamestown, NC.)

D. Level of the Free Gingival Margin
   1. The level of the free gingival margin in relationship to the cementoenamel junction (CEJ) should be recorded on the dental chart. This level can simply be drawn on the facial and lingual surfaces of the dental chart.
   2. Several possible relationships exist between the free gingival margin and the CEJ:
      a. **Free gingival margin can be slightly coronal to (above) the CEJ.** This is the natural level of the gingival margin and represents the expected position of the gingival margin in the absence of disease or trauma.
      b. **Free gingival margin can be significantly coronal to the CEJ.** The gingival margin can be significantly coronal to the CEJ due to (1) swelling (edema), (2) overgrowth (as seen in patients taking certain medications), or (3) increase in fibrous connective tissue (as seen in long-standing inflammation of tissue).
      c. **Free gingival margin can be apical to the CEJ.** This relationship, known as gingival recession, results in exposure of a portion of the root surface.
   3. Box 19-1 outlines the technique for determining the free gingival margin level.
   4. When the gingival margin is apical to the CEJ (i.e., gingival recession is present), the severity of gingival recession can be classified using the Miller classification system for gingival recession. This system is outlined in Figure 19-4A–D.

Box 19-1. Technique for Determining the Level of the Gingival Margin

When tissue swelling or recession is present, a periodontal probe is used to measure the distance the gingival margin is apical or coronal to the CEJ. Keep in mind that the natural or expected level of the gingival margin in the absence of disease or trauma is slightly coronal to the CEJ.

1. **For gingival recession.** If gingival recession is present, the distance between the CEJ and the gingival margin is measured using a calibrated periodontal probe. This distance is recorded as the gingival margin level.
2. **For gingival enlargement.** If gingival enlargement is present, the distance between the CEJ and the gingival margin is also measured using a calibrated periodontal probe. This distance is estimated using the following technique:
   a. Position the tip of the probe at a 45-degree angle to the tooth surface.
   b. Slowly move the probe tip beneath the gingival margin until the junction between the enamel and cementum is detected as a slight discrepancy in the smoothness of the tooth surface.
   c. Measure the distance between the gingival margin and the CEJ. This distance is recorded as the gingival margin level.

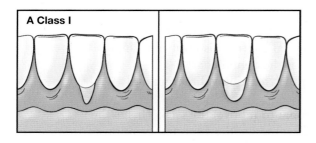

Figure 19-4A: Miller Class I Defect. In a Miller Class I gingival defect the recession is isolated to the facial surface and the interdental papillae fill the adjacent interdental spaces. Class I recession does not extend to the mucogingival line. These Class I defects can be further subdivided into narrow or wide.

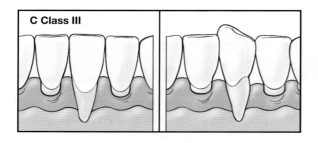

Figure 19-4B: Miller Class II Defect. In a Miller Class II gingival defect the recession is isolated to the facial surface and the papillae remain intact and fill the interdental spaces. Class II recession does extend beyond the mucogingival line into the mucosa.

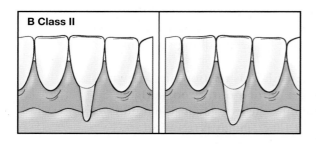

Figure 19-4C: Miller Class III Defect. In a Miller Class III gingival defect the recession is quite broad with the interdental papillae missing due to damage from disease. The Class III defect extends beyond the mucogingival line into the mucosa.

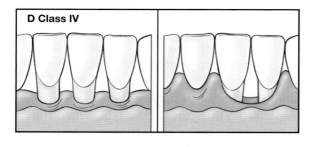

Figure 19-4D: Miller Class IV Defect. In a Miller Class IV gingival defect the recession extends to or beyond the mucogingival junction with loss of alveolar bone resulting in open interdental areas.

E. **Level of Mucogingival Junction**
1. The level of the mucogingival junction represents the junction between the keratinized gingiva and the nonkeratinized mucosa. The level of the mucogingival junction is used in calculation of the width of the attached gingiva as will be described in Section 4 of this chapter.
2. The mucogingival junction is usually readily visible since the keratinized gingiva is normally pale pink and opaque while the surface of the mucosa consists of thin, translucent tissue (Fig. 19-5).
3. Occasionally, the mucogingival junction can be difficult to detect visually. In this case, the tissue can be manipulated by pulling on the patient's lip or pushing on the tissue with a blunt instrument to distinguish the movable mucosa from the more firmly attached gingiva.

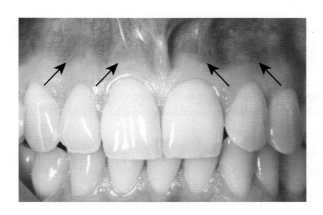

Figure 19-5. Mucogingival Junction. The mucogingival junction represents the junction between the keratinized gingiva and nonkeratinized mucosa and is usually readily visible.

F. **Tooth Mobility and Fremitus**
1. **Horizontal tooth mobility,** movement of a tooth in a facial to lingual direction, is assessed by trapping the tooth between two dental instrument handles.
   a. Alternating moderate pressure is applied in the facial–lingual direction against the tooth first with one, then the other instrument handle.
   b. Mobility can be observed by using an adjacent tooth as a stationary point of visual reference during attempts to move the tooth being examined.
2. **Vertical tooth mobility,** the ability to depress the tooth in its socket, can be assessed using the end of an instrument handle to exert pressure against the occlusal or incisal surface of the tooth (Fig. 19-6).
3. Even though the periodontal ligament allows some slight movement of the tooth in its socket, the amount of this natural tooth movement is so slight that it cannot normally be seen with the naked eye. Thus, when visually assessing mobility, the clinician should expect to find no visible movement in a periodontally healthy tooth.
4. There are many rating scales for recording clinically visible tooth mobility. One useful scale is indicated in Table 19-2.
5. In some dental offices, the dentist may also wish to assess fremitus.
   a. **Fremitus** is a palpable or visible movement of a tooth when in function.
   b. Fremitus can be assessed by gently placing a gloved index finger against the facial aspect of the tooth as the patient either taps the teeth together or simulates chewing movements. Fremitus is easy to detect if the finger pressure is gentle.

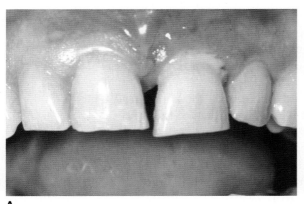
A

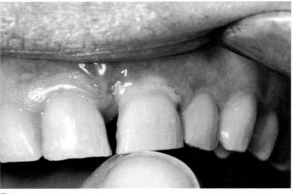
B

Figure 19-6. Vertical Tooth Mobility. A: The patient came to the dental office complaining of a loose tooth. Note the position of the maxillary left central incisor. **B:** The patient then demonstrated how he could push this tooth upward by applying pressure with his index finger against the incisal edge. This central incisor has vertical mobility. (Courtesy of Dr. Don Rolfs, Wenatchee, WA.)

TABLE 19-2. SCALE FOR RATING VISIBLE TOOTH MOBILITY

Classification	Description
Class I	Slight mobility, up to 1 mm of horizontal displacement in a facial–lingual direction
Class II	Moderate mobility, greater than 1 mm but less than 2 mm of horizontal displacement in a facial–lingual direction
Class III	Severe mobility, greater than 2 mm of displacement in a facial–lingual direction or vertical displacement (tooth depressible in the socket)

G. Furcation Involvement
1. A furcation probe is used to assess furcation involvement on multirooted teeth. Most molar teeth are multirooted, but some maxillary premolar teeth also develop with two roots creating the potential for a furcation involvement on some premolars also.
2. **Furcation probes** are curved, blunt-tipped instruments that allow easy access to the furcation areas; straight periodontal probes cannot be relied upon to detect furcation involvements accurately.
3. Furcation involvement occurs on a multirooted tooth when periodontal infection invades the area between and around the roots, resulting in a loss of attachment and loss of alveolar bone between the roots of the tooth.
   a. Mandibular molars are usually bifurcated (with mesial and distal roots), with potential furcation involvement on both the facial and lingual aspects of the tooth (Fig. 19-7A,B).
   b. Maxillary molar teeth are usually trifurcated (with mesiobuccal, distobuccal, and palatal roots) with potential furcation involvement on the facial, mesial, and distal aspects of the tooth.
   c. Maxillary first premolars that have bifurcated roots (buccal and palatal roots) have the potential for furcation involvement on the mesial and distal aspects of the tooth.

4. Furcation involvement frequently signals a need for periodontal surgery after completion of nonsurgical therapy, so detection and documentation of furcation involvement is a critical component of the comprehensive periodontal assessment.

5. Furcation involvement should be recorded using a scale that quantifies the severity (or extent) of the furcation invasion. Table 19-3 shows a commonly used scale for rating furcation invasions of multirooted teeth.

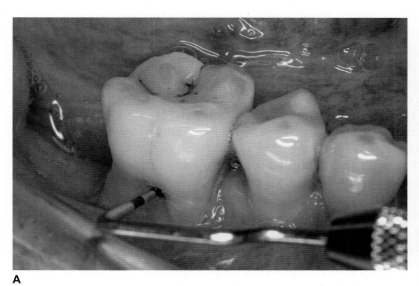
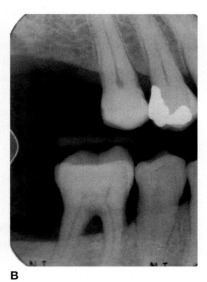

A   B

Figure 19-7. Furcation Involvement. A: Furcation involvement as viewed from the facial aspect of a mandibular first molar. **B:** The radiograph of the same molar shows bone loss between the roots of this molar.

TABLE 19-3. SCALE FOR RATING FURCATION INVOLVEMENT

Classification	Description
Class I	Curvature of the concavity leading to the furcation can be felt with the probe tip; however, the probe penetrates the furcation no more than 1 mm
Class II	The probe penetrates into the furcation greater than 1 mm but does not pass completely through the furcation
Class III	The probe passes completely through the furcation. In mandibular molars, the probe passes completely through the furcation between the mesial and distal roots. In maxillary molars, the probe passes between the mesiobuccal and distobuccal roots and will touch the palatal root.
Class IV	Same as Class III furcation, except that the entrance to the furca is clinically visible because of the presence of advanced gingival recession.

H. Presence of Calculus Deposits on the Teeth
1. The presence of dental calculus on the teeth should be noted since these deposits must later be identified and removed as part of the nonsurgical therapy.
2. Calculus is a local contributing factor in both gingivitis and periodontitis; thus, the identification and removal of these deposits is a critical component of successful patient treatment.
3. Calculus deposits can be located through several techniques that include the following:
   a. Direct visual examination using a mouth mirror to locate supragingival deposits.
   b. Visual examination while using compressed air to dry the teeth to aid in locating supragingival deposits.
   c. Tactile examination using an explorer to locate subgingival calculus deposits.

I. Presence of Plaque Biofilm on the Teeth
1. The presence of plaque biofilm on the teeth should be noted during a comprehensive periodontal assessment since these deposits contain living periodontal pathogens that can lead to both gingivitis and periodontitis.
2. Plaque biofilm can be identified using disclosing dyes or by moving the tip of an explorer or a periodontal probe along the tooth surface adjacent to the gingival margin.
3. There are many ways to record the presence of plaque biofilms, but most dental offices record the results of the plaque assessment in terms of the percentage of tooth surfaces with plaque biofilm evident at the gingival margin. A useful formula for recording plaque percentages is shown in Box 19-2.
   a. Note that in using the calculation shown in Box 19-2, a plaque score of 90% indicates that 90% of the total available tooth surfaces have plaque biofilm at the gingival margin.
   b. One goal of therapy would be for the patient to learn and perform plaque biofilm control measures that would bring the plaque score as close to 0% as possible (or at least to bring the percentage of tooth surfaces with plaque biofilm as low as possible).
4. As discussed previously in this book, plaque biofilm is the primary etiologic factor for both gingivitis and periodontitis. Identification of the presence and distribution of plaque biofilm on the teeth is a critical piece of information needed when planning appropriate therapy and patient education.

Box 19-2. Formula for Calculating Plaque Percentages

$$\frac{\text{Number of tooth surfaces with plaque}}{\text{Total number of tooth surfaces}} \times 100 = \text{percentage score}$$

J. Gingival Inflammation
1. A thorough periodontal assessment includes recording the overt signs of inflammation. The overt signs of inflammation of the gingiva include erythema (redness) and edema (swelling) of the gingival margins resulting in readily identifiable changes in gingival color and contour.
2. It is always important to be aware that inflammation can be present in the deeper structures of the periodontium without necessarily involving any obvious clinical signs of inflammation of the gingival margin.

a. When assessing the presence of inflammation, it is important to remember that bleeding on probing also can be a sign of inflammation.

b. Thus, when a clinician is identifying gingival inflammation for purposes of planning treatment, the visible signs such as color, contour, and consistency changes in the gingiva must be correlated with the other signs such as bleeding on probing or the presence of exudate.

K. **Radiographic Evidence of Alveolar Bone Loss.** Radiographic interpretation is discussed in Chapter 20.

1. It is important for the clinician to remember, however, that radiographs play an important role in arriving at the periodontal diagnosis and in developing an appropriate plan for nonsurgical periodontal therapy.

2. Radiographic evidence of alveolar bone loss is always an important part of a clinical periodontal assessment.

L. **Presence of Local Contributing Factors**

1. A thorough periodontal assessment will always include identification of local contributing factors.

2. These factors are discussed in Chapter 16. The plan for treatment for any periodontal patient will always include measures to eliminate or to minimize the impact of these local factors.

2. **Supplemental Diagnostic Tests**

A. **Overview of Supplemental Diagnostic Tests**

1. Clinical periodontal assessment using the parameters discussed in Section 3 will result in an accurate periodontal diagnosis and can serve as a sound basis for designing an appropriate plan for therapy for the patient with gingival or periodontal disease. There are, however, a number of supplemental diagnostic tests that can be used for certain patients.

2. Clinicians might consider using some of these supplemental tests for patients who have periodontitis that is failing to respond to conventional periodontal therapy or periodontitis that shows other unusual signs of disease progression.

3. There are a number of supplemental tests that have been suggested for use, and much research is continuing related to these types of tests. Most of these tests fall into three general types:

a. Tests related to bacteria

b. Tests that analyze gingival crevicular fluid content

c. Tests for genetic susceptibility to periodontal disease.

4. It is critical for the clinician to realize that based upon current research, none of these supplemental diagnostic tests should be ordered routinely on all patients with periodontal disease.

B. **Tests Related to Bacteria.** Table 19-4 presents an overview of the tests related to bacteria. It is important to keep in mind that conventional periodontal therapy brings periodontal pathogens to low enough levels that disease progression can be halted without the need for identifying specific periodontal pathogens in most patients.

C. **Tests that Analyze Gingival Crevicular Fluid Content**

1. Gingival Crevicular Fluid

a. **Gingival crevicular fluid** is the fluid that flows into the sulcus from the adjacent gingival connective tissue; the flow is slight in health and increases in the presence of inflammatory disease.

b. Gingival crevicular fluid originates in connective tissue and flows into periodontal pockets. It has long been believed that this gingival crevicular fluid can contain markers for periodontal disease progression, and quite a bit of research time has been devoted to the study of this fluid.

2. Examples of Gingival Crevicular Contents That Have Been Studied

   a. Collagenase (an enzyme that breaks down collagen) is an example of one of the gingival crevicular fluid contents that has been studied, though no test for this is currently in widespread use.

   b. Prostaglandin E2 is another such gingival crevicular fluid ingredient that has been studied. Prostaglandin E2 is associated with arachidonic acid that is involved with inflammatory reactions such as those seen in periodontal disease.

D. **Tests for Genetic Susceptibility to Periodontal Disease**

1. Genetic Susceptibility

   a. It is obvious that a patient's genetic makeup affects susceptibility to many diseases including periodontal disease.

   b. This genetic makeup is inherited and cannot normally be altered.

2. Tests for Interleukin-1

   a. One test for genetic susceptibility to periodontal disease has been studied extensively and has resulted in a test that has been marketed to clinicians. The first version of this test was the PST Genetic Susceptibility Test from Interleukin Genetics Incorporated, Waltham, MA. A new version of this genetic susceptibility test, called PerioPredict is scheduled to be released.

   b. Both of these tests identify patients with genetic programming to produce high levels of interleukin-1 (an inflammatory mediator produced in response to the presence of periodontal pathogens).

      1. Higher levels of interleukin-1 in patients tend to predispose the patients to more inflammation in the periodontium and have been associated with increased risk for severe and progressive periodontal disease.

      2. It has been reported that 30% of the people in the United States have the genetic makeup to produce high levels of interleukin-1 in response to periodontal pathogens.

E. **The Future.** It would be extremely helpful if clinicians had access to a diagnostic test that could indicate which patients are undergoing or are likely to undergo attachment loss. It is safe to assume that as more research is completed additional useful clinical tests will be developed in this area.

TABLE 19-4. TESTS RELATED TO BACTERIA

Test Name	Purpose of Test	Special Considerations
Phase contrast microscopic study of plaque sample	Used for patient education and motivation	Test cannot identify specific bacterial species
Culture and sensitivity	Used to determine the sensitivity of bacteria to specific antibiotics	Sampling techniques for this test and the transport of bacterial samples to the laboratory are difficult
DNA (deoxyribonucleic acid) probe analysis	Used to identify specific periodontal pathogens in a patient's mouth	Only a few bacterial species can be identified by this test

Section 4
Clinical Features that Require Calculations

Some judgments that are made as part of the clinical periodontal assessment may require some calculations. The most common features that may require some calculations are the width of the attached gingiva and clinical attachment level.

1. **Calculating the Width of Attached Gingiva**
   A. **Description.** The **attached gingiva** is the part of the gingiva that is firm, dense, and tightly connected to the cementum on the cervical-third of the root or to the periosteum (connective tissue cover) of the alveolar bone. The attached gingiva lies between the free gingiva and the alveolar mucosa, extending from the base of the sulcus (or pocket) to the mucogingival junction.
      1. The functions of the attached gingiva are to keep the free gingiva from being pulled away from the tooth and to protect the gingiva from trauma.
      2. The width of the attached gingiva is not measured on the palate since it is not possible to determine where the attached gingiva ends and the palatal mucosa begins.
      3. *The attached gingiva does not include any portion of the gingiva that is separated from the tooth by a crevice, sulcus, or periodontal pocket.*
   B. **Significance.** The width of the attached gingiva on a tooth surface is an important clinical feature for the dentist to keep in mind when planning many types of restorative procedures. If there is no attached gingiva on a tooth surface, the dentist is limited in the types of restorations that can be placed. Therefore, it is important to use the information collected during the comprehensive periodontal assessment to calculate this clinical feature.
   C. **Method of Calculation.** The method of calculation of the width of attached gingiva is shown in Box 19-3. Note that the information needed to calculate the width of the attached gingiva already would have been recorded during the periodontal assessment.

Box 19-3. Calculating the Width of Attached Gingiva

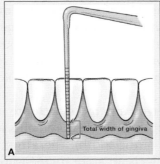
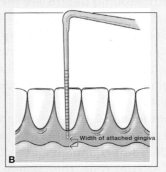

Formula: To calculate the width of attached gingiva at a specific site, measure the width of the gingiva and subtract the probing depth from the total width using the steps below:

Step 1: Measure the total width of the gingiva from the gingival margin to the mucogingival junction.

Step 2: Measure the probing depth (from the gingival margin to the base of the pocket).

Step 3: Calculate the width of the attached gingiva by subtracting the probing depth from the total width of the gingiva.

2. **Calculating the Clinical Attachment Level (CAL)**
   A. **Definition.** The clinical attachment level (CAL) is a clinical measurement of the true periodontal support around the tooth as measured with a periodontal probe. Box 19-4 outlines a comparison of probing depths and clinical attachment levels.
   B. **Significance of Clinical Attachment Levels**
      1. An attachment level measurement is a more accurate indicator of the periodontal support around a tooth than is a probing depth measurement.
         a. Probing depths are measured from the free gingival margin to the base of the sulcus or pocket. The position of the gingival margin may change with tissue swelling, overgrowth of tissue, or recession of tissue. Since the position of the gingival margin can change (move coronally or apically), probing depths do not provide an accurate means to monitor changes in periodontal support over time in a patient.
         b. CAL provides an accurate means to monitor changes in periodontal support over time. The CAL is calculated from measurements made from a fixed point on the tooth that does not change (i.e., the CEJ of the tooth).
      2. The presence of loss of attachment is a critical factor in distinguishing between gingivitis and periodontitis.
         a. Inflammation with no attachment loss is characteristic of gingivitis.
         b. Inflammation with attachment loss is characteristic of periodontitis.

Box 19-4. Comparison of Probing Depths and Clinical Attachment Levels

Monitoring the periodontal support of teeth over time is a vital component of long-term care of patients with periodontal disease. There are two measurements used to describe the amount of periodontal support for teeth: (1) probing depths and (2) clinical attachment levels (CALs). Probing depths are frequently used, whereas clinical attachment levels are less commonly used. Clinicians should be aware that the use of probing depths alone may not be in some patients' best interests.

- **Probing depths** alone are not the most reliable indicators of the amount of periodontal support for a tooth. Probing depths are measured from the gingival margin; the position of the gingival margin often changes over time. Changes in the level of the gingival margin occur with gingival swelling, overgrowth of gingiva, or gingival recession. So, a change in probing depth over time may indicate a change in the amount of periodontal support for a tooth, but it may also only indicate that there has been some change in the level of the gingival margin (which may well be unrelated to the actual periodontal support of the tooth).
- **Clinical attachment levels (CALs)** are the preferred and more accurate indicator of the actual amount of periodontal support for a tooth. CAL measurements are made from a fixed point that does not change (i.e., the CEJ of the tooth). Therefore, when there is a change in the CAL over time, this change reflects an accurate measurement of a true change in the periodontal support of a tooth.

C. Calculating the Clinical Attachment Level
   1. **When the gingival margin is near the CEJ.** When the gingival margin is at its natural location (i.e., near the CEJ of the tooth), the probing depth and the clinical attachment level readings are the same for all practical purposes.
   2. **When the gingival margin is apical to the CEJ (i.e., there is gingival recession).** When gingival recession is present, a straight calibrated periodontal probe is used to measure the distance the gingival margin is apical to the CEJ (Fig. 19-8A–C), and the same probe is used to measure the probing depth at the site. Both of these measurements will have been made and recorded as part of the comprehensive periodontal assessment. To calculate the CAL, simply add these two measurements (i.e., the amount of gingival recession plus the amount of the probing depth at the site).
   3. **When the gingival margin is significantly coronal to the CEJ (i.e., there is gingival enlargement).** When gingival enlargement is present, a straight calibrated periodontal probe is used to measure the distance the gingival margin is coronal to the cementoenamel junction (Fig. 19-8A–C). Remember that the natural position for the gingival margin is either at or slightly coronal to the CEJ, but there are many instances when the gingival margin will be found to be significantly (several millimeters) coronal to the CEJ. If the gingival margin is significantly coronal to the CEJ, the distance between the margin and the CEJ is estimated using the following technique:
      a. Position the tip of the straight calibrated probe at a 45-degree angle to the tooth surface.
      b. With light force, slowly move the probe beneath the gingival margin until the junction between the enamel and cementum is detected.
      c. Measure the distance between the gingival margin and the cementoenamel junction, and measure the probing depth at this site.
      d. Subtract the distance from the gingival margin to the CEJ from the probing depth to determine the CAL at the site.
D. **Recording the Gingival Margin on a Periodontal Chart.** Customarily, the notations 0, −, or + are used to indicate the position of the gingival margin on a periodontal chart (Box 19-5).

Box 19-5. Notations that Indicate the Position of the Free Gingival Margin

- A zero **(0)** indicates the free gingival margin is slightly coronal to the CEJ.
- A negative number **(−)** indicates the free gingival margin significantly covers the CEJ.
- A positive number **(+)** indicates the free gingival margin is apical to the CEJ (recession).

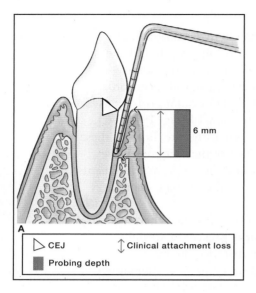

Figure 19-8A: Calculating Clinical Attachment Level when the Gingival Margin is Slightly Coronal to the Cementoenamel Junction. When the gingival margin is slightly coronal to the CEJ, no calculations are needed since the probing depth and the clinical attachment level are equal.

For example:
Probing depth measurement: 6 mm
Gingival margin level: 0 mm
Clinical attachment loss: 6 mm

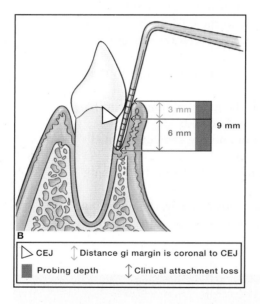

Figure 19-8B: Calculating Clinical Attachment Level when the Gingival Margin is Significantly Coronal to the Cementoenamel Junction. When the gingival margin is significantly coronal to the CEJ, the CAL is calculated by SUBTRACTING the gingival margin level from the probing depth.

For example:
Probing depth measurement: 9 mm
Gingival margin level: −3 mm
Clinical attachment loss: 6 mm

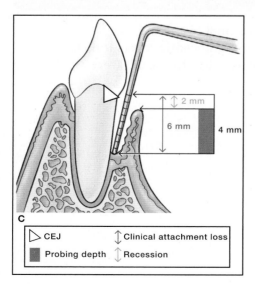

Figure 19-8C: Calculating Clinical Attachment Level in the Presence of Gingival Recession. When recession is present, the CAL is calculated by ADDING the probing depth to the gingival margin level.

For example:
Probing depth measurement: 4 mm
Gingival margin level: +2 mm
Clinical attachment loss: 6 mm

Chapter Summary Statement

The information gathered by the members of the dental team during the clinical periodontal assessment forms the basis for an individualized treatment plan for the patient. This chapter discusses two types of clinical periodontal assessment: a periodontal screening examination and the comprehensive periodontal assessment. The Periodontal Screening and Recording (PSR) is an example of an efficient periodontal screening system for the detection of periodontal disease.

The comprehensive periodontal assessment is a complete clinical periodontal assessment used to gather information about the periodontium. The information collected in a comprehensive periodontal assessment includes probing depth measurements, bleeding on probing, presence of exudate, level of the free gingival margin, level of the mucogingival junction, tooth mobility, furcation involvement, presence of calculus, presence of plaque biofilm, gingival inflammation, radiographic evidence of alveolar bone loss, and presence of local contributing factors. Supplemental diagnostic tests are indicated for certain patients. Some judgments made during a clinical periodontal assessment require calculation. These include the width of attached gingiva and clinical attachment levels. Detection of clinical attachment level is important in determining whether gingivitis or periodontitis is present at a site of inflammation.

Section 5
Focus on Patients

Clinical Patient Care

CASE 1

While visiting a dental office, you observe a member of the dental team performing a periodontal assessment. You note that while searching for furcation invasion, the clinician is using a straight calibrated periodontal probe. What critical information might be lost because of instrument selection for this step in a periodontal assessment?

CASE 2

During a comprehensive periodontal assessment you note severe inflammation of the gingiva over the facial surface of a lower right molar tooth. On the dental chart you are using there is no obvious mechanism to record this important piece of periodontal information. How should you proceed?

CASE 3

During a periodontal assessment of a periodontitis patient, you are trying to determine the clinical attachment level on the facial surface of a canine tooth. On the facial surface of the canine tooth you have measured 3 mm of gingival recession and a probing depth of 6 mm. How much attachment has been lost on the facial surface of this canine tooth?

Ethical Dilemma

Your next patient is Marlene Perkins, who is a new patient to your practice. She is a 37-year-old married mother of two small daughters, who works part-time as a lawyer. Her chief complaint is "bleeding gums." She left her last dental practice because she questioned if she was receiving quality dental services.

The radiographs, you have taken today, show that there is very slight horizontal bone loss on her anterior teeth. Marlene's pocket readings range from 1 to 4 mm throughout her mouth, and there is generalized bleeding on probing. She presents with heavy plaque biofilm and moderate supragingival and subgingival calculus, although states that she had her teeth cleaned 4 months ago. She states that she "isn't a very good flosser, and was always reprimanded by the hygienist at her former dental practice, to do a better job."

She notes that she has a history of periodontal disease in her family, as both her mother and father have had "extensive gum surgeries." She asked the dentist and hygienist in her last practice if periodontal disease was hereditary and if there was a way to predict if she also would have periodontal disease. She was told that each person is an individual, and that if she "took care of her teeth and gums," she would be just fine.

1. What is the best way for you to handle this ethical dilemma?
2. What is the best way to address/discuss Marlene's treatment plan?
3. What ethical principles are in conflict in this dilemma?

Reference

1. American Academy of Periodontology. Comprehensive periodontal therapy: a statement by the American Academy of Periodontology. *J Periodontol.* 2011;82(7):943–949.

 STUDENT ANCILLARY RESOURCES

A wide variety of resources to enhance your learning and understanding of this chapter are available on thePoint®.

- Visit thePoint to access:
  - Audio Glossary
  - Animations
  - Suggested Readings
  - Answers to Review Questions
  - Case Studies

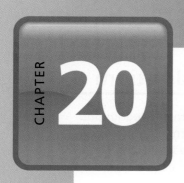

Radiographic Analysis of the Periodontium

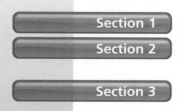
Clinical Application. Interpretation of radiographic images is an integral part of the diagnosis for patients with most types of periodontal diseases. Members of the dental team will need to rely on their skills in radiographic interpretation on a daily basis. This chapter outlines some information about radiographic image interpretation that all members of the dental team will find helpful.

Learning Objectives

- Recognize the radiographic characteristics of normal and abnormal alveolar bone.
- Recognize and describe early radiographic evidence of periodontal disease.
- Distinguish between vertical and horizontal alveolar bone loss.
- Recognize potential etiologic agents for periodontal disease radiographically.
- Gain practical experience in radiographic assessment by applying information from this chapter in the clinical setting.

Key Terms

Radiolucent
Radiopaque

Cortical bone
Lamina dura

Crestal irregularities
Triangulation

Section 1
Radiographic Appearance of the Periodontium

Dental radiographs are an important adjunct to the clinical assessment of the periodontium. To recognize disease, the dental hygienist must be able to recognize the normal radiographic appearance of the periodontium. Periodontal anatomy visible on radiographic images includes the alveolar bone, periodontal ligament space, and cementum. The gingiva is a noncalcified soft tissue that cannot usually be seen on a radiograph.

1. Radiolucent and Radiopaque Structures and Materials
   A. Radiolucent materials and structures are easily penetrated by x-rays.
      1. Most of the x-rays will be able to pass through these objects and structures to expose the radiograph. Radiolucent areas appear as dark gray to black on the radiograph.
      2. Examples of radiolucent structures are the tooth pulp, periodontal ligament space, a periapical abscess, marrow spaces in the bone, and bone loss defects.
   B. Radiopaque materials and structures absorb or resist the passage of x-rays.
      1. Radiopaque areas appear light gray to white on the radiograph. These structures absorb most of the x-rays, so that very few x-rays reach the radiograph.
      2. Examples of radiopaque structures and materials are metallic silver (amalgam restorations) and newer composite restorations, enamel, dentin, pulp stones, and compact or cortical bone.
2. Identification of the Periodontium on Radiographic images. The components of the periodontium that can be identified on radiographic images include the alveolar bone, periodontal ligament space, and cementum (Fig. 20-1).
   A. Cortical Bone
      1. Cortical bone is the outer surface of the bone and is composed of layers of bone closely packed together.
         a. On the maxilla, the cortical bone is a thin shell.
         b. On the mandible, the cortical bone is a dense layer.
      2. Radiographic Appearance of Cortical Bone
         a. Inferior border of the mandible appears on the radiograph as a thick white border.
         b. Interdental alveolar crests between the teeth of both jaws appear on the radiograph as a thin white line on the outside of crestal bone.
         c. The lattice-like pattern of the cancellous bone that fills the interior portion of the alveolar process appears on the radiograph as a pattern of delicate white tracings within the bone.

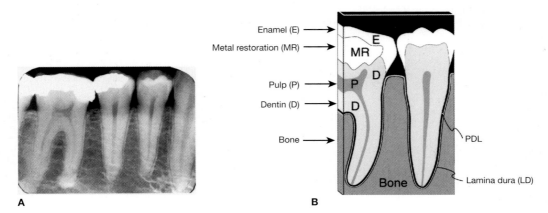

Figure 20-1. Radiographic Structures of the Periodontium.

B. **Alveolar Crest.** *The normal level of the alveolar bone is located approximately 2 mm apical to (below) the cementoenamel junction (CEJ).*
   1. If the coronal bone level is within 3 mm of the CEJ, the bone level is considered normal.
   2. It is unlikely that bone loss less than 3 mm can be detected on a radiograph.
C. **Crestal Contour of the Interdental Bone**
   1. The contour of the crest of the interproximal bone is a good indicator of periodontal health. *The contour of the interproximal crest is parallel to an imaginary line drawn between the CEJs of adjacent teeth.*
   2. In posterior sextants, the contour of the interproximal crest is parallel to an imaginary line drawn between the CEJs of the adjacent teeth.
      a. Horizontal crest contour. The crest of the interproximal bone will have a horizontal contour when the CEJs of the adjacent teeth are at the same level (Fig. 20-2).
      b. Angular crest contour. The crest of the interproximal bone will have a vertical contour when one of the adjacent teeth is tilted or erupted to a different height (Fig. 20-3).

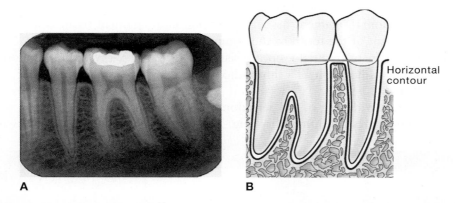

A   B

Figure 20-2. A: Normal Alveolar Bone Height. This radiograph shows a normal alveolar bone height that is 1.5 to 2 mm below and parallel to the cementoenamel junction. In this example, alveolar crest is a dense radiopaque line similar in density to the lamina dura surrounding the root of the tooth. **B: Horizontal Crest Contour.** The crest of the interproximal bone will have a horizontal contour when the CEJs of the adjacent teeth are at the same level.

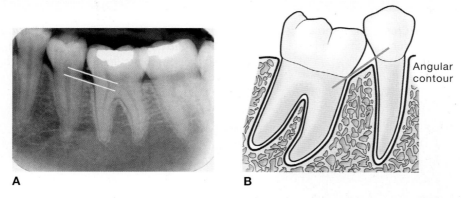

A   B

Figure 20-3. Angular Crest Contour. The crest of the interproximal bone will have a vertical contour when one of the adjacent teeth is tilted or erupted to a different height.

D. Alveolar Crestal Bone
1. Alveolar bone is the part of the jawbone that supports the teeth.
2. The surfaces of the bony crests are smooth and covered with a thin layer of cortical (dense, hard) bone that may be seen as a thin, white line on a radiograph.
3. *The most important radiographic feature of the alveolar crest is that it forms a smooth intact surface between adjacent teeth with only the width of the periodontal ligament space separating it from the adjacent root surface.*
   a. The crest of the interdental septa between incisors is thin and pointed.
   b. The crest of the interdental septa between the posterior teeth is rounded or flat (Fig. 20-4).

E. Lamina Dura
1. The alveolar bone proper is the thin layer of dense bone that lines a normal tooth socket. In radiographic images, the alveolar bone proper is identified as the lamina dura. On a radiograph, the lamina dura appears as a continuous white (radiopaque) line around the tooth root (Fig. 20-5).
2. On a radiograph, the lamina dura is continuous with the cortical bone layer of the crest of the interdental septa.

F. Periodontal Ligament Space
1. The space between the tooth root and the lamina dura of the socket is filled with the periodontal ligament tissue. The periodontal ligament tissue functions as the attachment of the tooth to the lamina dura of the socket.
2. Periodontal ligament tissue does not resist penetration of x-rays and, therefore, appears on the radiograph as a thin radiolucent black line surrounding the tooth root (Fig. 20-5).
3. In most cases, a widening of the periodontal ligament space (PDLS) on the radiograph indicates tooth mobility (Fig. 20-6).

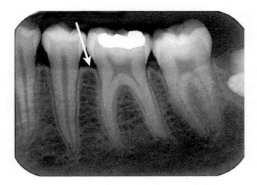

Figure 20-4. Alveolar Crest. The alveolar crest (indicated by an *arrow*) forms a smooth intact surface between adjacent teeth.

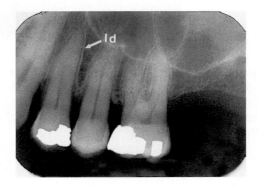

Figure 20-5. Lamina Dura and Periodontal Ligament Space. The lamina dura (ld) appears as a continuous white line around the tooth root.

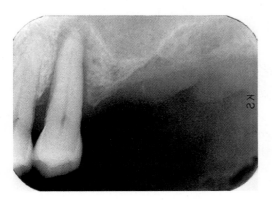

Figure 20-6. Widening of the PDL Space. This maxillary second premolar has a uniformly widened periodontal ligament space (PDL) that is characteristic of tooth mobility.

Section 2
Use of Radiographic Images for Periodontal Evaluation

1. Techniques for Good Radiographic Quality
   A. **Long-Cone Paralleling Technique.** The long-cone paralleling technique provides a radiograph that is more anatomically accurate when compared with other intraoral techniques such as bisecting angle.
   B. **Long Gray Scale Low Contrast Images.** Long-scale contrast radiographic images have many visible shades of gray that make it easier to see subtle changes such as bone loss in periodontal disease. These images can be obtained using high kVp exposures (70 to 100 kVp) or using digital imaging software adjustments to maximize the gray scale of normally exposed images. Many software programs now provide presets to optimize for detection of periodontal disease.
2. **Limitations of Radiographs for Periodontal Evaluation.** There are limitations in the use of the radiograph in the diagnosis of periodontal disease.
   A. **A Two-Dimensional Image.** A radiograph provides a two-dimensional image of a complex three-dimensional structure. The fact that the radiograph is a two-dimensional image can be misleading to the viewer. For example, the buccal alveolar bone can hide bone loss on the lingual aspect of a tooth, and the palatal root makes it difficult to detect furcation involvement of a maxillary molar.
   B. **Information Limited to Noncalcified Structures.** In addition, radiographic images do not provide any information about the noncalcified components of the periodontium.
   C. **Limited Information on Periodontium.** Radiographic images *do not reveal* the following: the presence or absence of periodontal pockets, early bone loss, exact morphology of bone destruction, tooth mobility, early furcation involvement, condition of the alveolar bone on the buccal and lingual surfaces, or the level of the epithelial attachment.
      1. Periodontal Pockets
         a. *The only reliable method of locating a periodontal pocket and evaluating its extent is by careful periodontal probing.*
         b. The periodontal pocket is composed of soft tissue, so it will not be visible on the radiograph.
      2. Early Bone Loss
         a. *The very earliest signs of periodontitis must be detected clinically, not radiographically.* By the time periodontal bone loss becomes detectable on the radiograph, it usually has progressed beyond the earliest stages of the disease.
            1. Interseptal bony defects smaller than 3 mm usually cannot be seen on radiographic images.
            2. Bone height on the facial and lingual aspects is difficult to evaluate radiographically because the teeth are superimposed over the bone.
         b. *A radiograph cannot accurately display the shape of bone deformities because it is not three dimensional.*
         c. A radiograph with poor technique and excessive vertical angulation can obscure bone loss. Periapical radiographs may over- or underestimate the actual outline of the alveolar bone (Fig. 20-7) (1).
            1. For this reason the bitewing radiograph should be the primary radiograph used to evaluate crestal bone height rather than the periapical radiograph.
            2. Proper long-cone paralleling technique can prevent distortion of crestal bone height on periapical radiographic images and improve their usefulness.

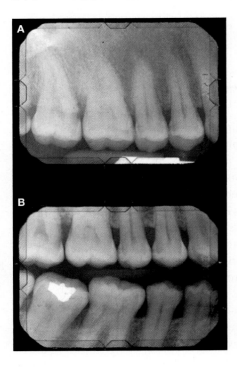

Figure 20-7A: Excessive Vertical Angulation. Note how the crestal bone height is exaggerated in the periapical radiograph shown here as opposed to the bitewing radiograph shown below.

Figure 20-7B: Bitewing Radiograph. The bitewing shown here reveals the true bone height of the teeth shown in Figure 20-7A.

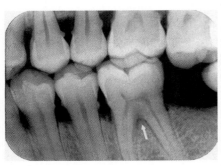

Figure 20-8. Furcation Involvement. The radiolucency on the mandibular first molar should be evaluated using a furcation probe.

3. Early Furcation Involvement
    a. Radiographic images usually ***show more interradicular bone***—bone between the roots of the teeth—than is actually present. The facial and lingual aspects of the alveolar bone will often be superimposed over the furcation and hide bone loss from view.
    b. ***Variations in alignment of the x-ray beam may conceal the presence or extent of furcation involvement.***
    c. Furcation involvement (bone loss between the roots) is detected by clinical examination with a furcation probe. The furcation area of a tooth should be examined with a furcation probe even if the radiograph shows a very small radiolucency or an area of diminished radiodensity at the furcation (Fig. 20-8).
4. Extensive Bone Loss
    a. ***Crestal bone loss of 5 mm or greater may cause the coronal bone to be poorly visualized or not seen at all on normal bitewing radiographic images.***
    b. Vertically oriented bitewings may be used in these situations.
    c. An adaptor is available for most film holders to accomplish this.
    d. The long axis of the film is rotated 90 degrees to be perpendicular to the occlusal plane instead of the short axis (Fig. 20-9).

e. Vertical bitewing radiographic images show more of the coronal bone than regular bitewings especially when the teeth are widely separated by the film holder (Fig. 20-10).

5. Disease Activity
   a. Just as clinical attachment levels only indicate past disease destruction, *radiographic images do not show **disease activity**, but only the **effects of the disease**.*
   b. *Because of these limitations, the radiographic examination is never a satisfactory substitute for a clinical periodontal assessment.*

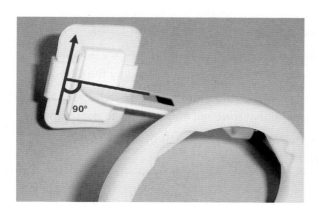

Figure 20-9. Film Placement for Vertical Bitewing. A #2 periapical film positioned for taking a vertical bitewing radiograph. Note how the film is rotated 90 degrees from the usual orientation.

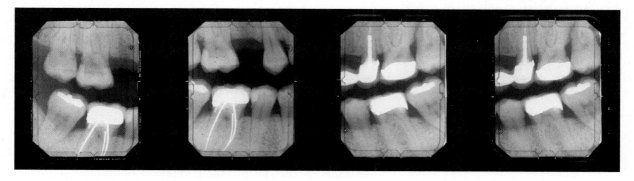

Figure 20-10. Four Film Vertical Bitewing Series. Note how much coronal bone is visible on these vertical bitewings despite the separation of the teeth by the positioning device.

3. **Benefits of Radiographs for Periodontal Evaluation.** Despite the radiograph's limitations, the periodontal examination is incomplete without accurate radiographic images. Radiographs will demonstrate the following: most of the bony changes associated with periodontitis, the tooth root morphology, relationship of the maxillary sinus to the periodontal deformity, widening of periodontal ligament space, advanced furcation involvement, periodontal abscesses, and local factors such as overhanging restorations, marginal ridge height discrepancies, open contacts, and calculus (Table 20-1) (1).

A. **Assessment of Bony Changes.** Early radiographic signs of periodontitis are (1) fuzziness at the crest of the alveolar bone, (2) a widened periodontal ligament space (PDLS), and (3) radiolucent areas in the interseptal bone (Fig. 20-11).

   1. **Crestal Irregularities.** **Crestal irregularities** are the appearance of breaks or fuzziness instead of a nice clean line at the crest of the interdental alveolar bone.

TABLE 20-1. BENEFITS OF RADIOGRAPHS IN THE DETECTION OF PERIODONTAL DISEASE

Condition	Radiographic Sign(s)
Early bony changes	Break or fuzziness at the crest of the interdental alveolar bone Widening of the periodontal ligament space at crestal margin Presence of finger-like radiolucent projections into the interdental alveolar bone
Horizontal bone loss	Can be measured from a plane that is parallel to a tooth-to-tooth line drawn from the CEJs of adjacent teeth
Vertical bone loss	Seen as more bone loss on the interproximal aspect of one tooth than on the adjacent tooth; bone level is at an angle to a line joining the CEJs
Bone defects	Are radiolucent due to bone loss and, therefore, visible on radiographic images, although three-dimensional structure may be hard to determine
Furcation involvement	Loss of bone in furcation area may be detectable as triangular radiolucency especially on mandibular molars

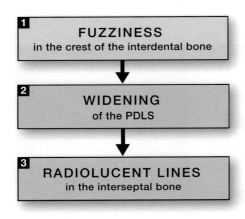

Figure 20-11. Early Radiographic Signs. Sequence of radiographic changes that occur in periodontitis.

2. Triangulation (Funneling). Triangulation is the widening of the PDLS caused by the resorption of bone along either the mesial or distal aspect of the interdental (interseptal) crestal bone (Fig. 20-12).
3. Interseptal Bone Changes
   a. Another radiographic sign of periodontitis is the existence of finger-like radiolucent projections extending from the crestal bone into the interdental alveolar bone (Fig. 20-13).
   b. These finger-like radiolucent lines represent a reduction of mineralized tissue (bone) adjacent to blood vessel channels within the alveolar bone.

   c. If chronic periodontitis goes untreated and much of the alveolar bone around the tooth is destroyed, the tooth will seem to "float in space" on the radiograph. This represents the "terminal stage" of the disease process.

B. Extent or Direction of Bone Loss. The extent or direction of bone loss is determined using the cementoenamel junction (CEJ) of adjacent teeth as the points of reference.

   1. Horizontal Bone Loss. Horizontal bone loss is bone destruction that is parallel to an imaginary line drawn between the CEJs of adjacent teeth (Fig. 20-14).

   2. Vertical Bone Loss. Vertical (or angular) bone loss occurs when there is greater bone destruction on the interproximal aspect of one tooth than on the adjacent tooth, so that the bone meets the tooth at an acute angle (Fig. 20-15).

C. Assessment of Bone Loss

   1. The radiograph is an indirect method of detecting bone loss. *Periodontitis is a disease process with active and inactive periods, so the radiograph is only a snapshot of an instant in time in the disease process.*

   2. The radiograph reveals the bone remaining rather than the amount of bone actually lost. Bone loss occurs on all surfaces; however, the tooth root tends to mask (or hide) bone loss on the facial and lingual surfaces of the tooth.

   3. Mesial or distal bone loss is evaluated primarily by examining the interproximal septal bone on the radiograph. The amount of bone loss is estimated as the difference between the level of the remaining bone and the normal bone height.

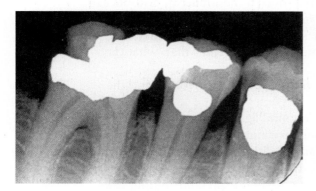

Figure 20-12. Triangulation. The crestal bone between these mandibular teeth demonstrates triangulation, a pointed, triangular appearance.

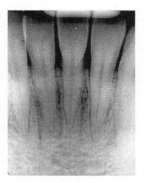

Figure 20-13. Finger-Like Radiolucent Projections. The nutrient canals within the bone are seen as finger-like projections extending between and beyond the roots of the mandibular incisors on this radiograph.

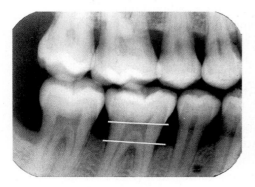

Figure 20-14. Horizontal Bone Loss. Horizontal bone loss is parallel to an imaginary line drawn between the CEJs of adjacent teeth.

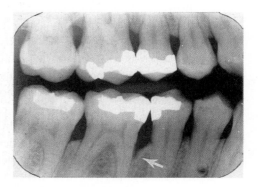

Figure 20-15. Vertical Bone Loss. The *arrow* points to vertical bone loss on the mesial surface of the mandibular first molar.

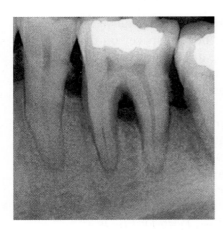

Figure 20-16. Furcation Involvement. The furcation involvement is easily visible on the mandibular first molar in this radiograph.

D. **Assessment of Furcation Involvement**
   1. Furcation involvement will not be seen on the radiograph until the bone resorption extends past the furcation area.
      a. Furcation involvement of mandibular molars is easier to detect on a radiograph than is furcation involvement of maxillary molars. This is because mandibular molars have only two roots, a mesial root and a distal root (Fig. 20-16).
      b. Furcation involvement on maxillary molars is more difficult to detect on a radiograph. Maxillary molars have three roots, a mesiobuccal, distobuccal, and palatal root. The palatal root is often superimposed over the furcation of the tooth on the radiograph and masks (hides) any radiolucency there.
   2. It is a general rule that furcation involvement is often *greater* than what the radiograph reveals.
   3. If using the radiograph to aid in the detection of furcation involvement, the following rules should be kept in mind:
      a. If there is a slight thickening of the periodontal ligament space in the furcation area, the area should be examined clinically with a furcation probe.
      b. If severe bone loss is evident on the mesial or distal surface of a multirooted tooth (especially maxillary molars), furcation involvement should be suspected.
E. **Recognition of Local Contributing Risk Factors.** Several local contributing risk factors that may be revealed by the radiograph are calculus deposits, faulty restorations, and food packing areas.
   1. Calculus Deposits
      a. *The only accurate way **to detect calculus deposits** is with an explorer,* however, large calculus deposits *may be visible* on a radiograph.
         1. The radiograph may show large, heavy interproximal calculus deposits.
         2. Calculus deposits may be visible on the facial and lingual surfaces of the anterior teeth (smooth surface calculus or calcified plaque)
         3. Calculus deposits may be visible on the facial and lingual surfaces of teeth when there is severe bone loss on these surfaces.
      b. The ability to visualize calculus radiographically depends on the degree of mineralization within the calculus and the angulation factors of the x-ray beam.
   2. Faulty Restorations. Inadequate dental restorations and prostheses are common causes of gingival inflammation, periodontitis, and alveolar bone resorption. In many cases, faulty restorations can be detected on a radiograph (Fig. 20-17).
   3. Trauma from Occlusion
      a. The radiograph is used only as a supplemental aid in recognizing trauma from occlusion.

b. Radiographic signs of trauma from occlusion include the following:
   1. Increased width of the periodontal ligament spaces on the mesial and distal sides of the tooth due to resorption of the lamina dura.
   2. Vertical or angular bone destruction often times wider at the crestal margins where maximum force is directed during trauma.

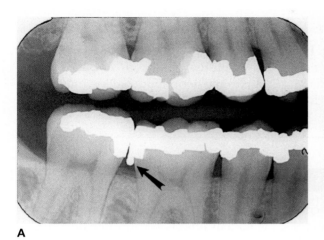
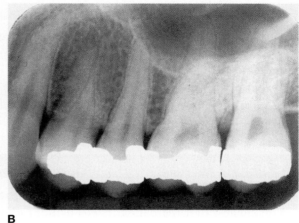

A   B

Figure 20-17. Faulty Restorations. A: The distal surface of the mandibular first molar, indicated by the arrow, has a faulty restoration that creates a food trap and harbors plaque biofilm. **B:** The distal proximal tooth surface of the maxillary first molar and the mesial tooth surface of the second molar have not been restored to their original shape and contour. These faulty contours create an open contact that can allow food impaction.

Chapter Summary Statement

When the limitations of radiographic images are recognized, they can be an important diagnostic aid in the examination and diagnosis of patients with periodontitis. Radiographic images are extremely useful tools in the detection of bony changes due to periodontitis such as crestal irregularities, triangulation, interseptal bone loss, assessment of bone defects, and furcation involvement.

Section 3
Focus on Patients

Clinical Patient Care

CASE 1

Mr. Jones is a new patient in your dental office. He brings with him some recent full-mouth radiographs that reveal no evidence of alveolar bone loss. While studying a copy of the patient's dental chart, you note that there is a diagnosis of chronic periodontitis. How might you explain the apparent discrepancy between the lack of radiographic evidence of bone loss and the diagnosis of periodontitis?

CASE 2

During a periodontal assessment for a new patient, you detect clinical attachment loss. When you suggest that the patient needs dental radiographs, the patient objects because she does not want to be exposed to "unnecessary x-rays." How should you respond?

CASE 3

While reviewing a new set of dental radiographs for a patient, you note numerous sites of obvious bone loss. The bone loss appears to be vertical (or angular), where there is much more bone loss on one tooth surface compared with the immediately adjacent tooth surface. How might the dental team use this vertical pattern of bone loss when developing the periodontal diagnosis?

Ethical Dilemma

Philomena C is your first patient of the morning. She was born in Italy, and moved to the United States with her family when she was 10. She is a 60-year-old homemaker, who appears slightly overweight, and admits to high blood pressure and high cholesterol, both controlled by medication. She has been a patient in the practice of your dentist's sister, Dr. Lynne, who has an office across town, for the last 30 years. She recently decided to change dental practices as our office is near her residence.

Philomena has been faithful with her recall visits and has followed all the treatments that Dr. Lynne and the various hygienists have suggested during her years as a patient in that practice, including routine radiographs.

You begin probing and Philomena questions what you are doing. She states that "no one has ever done that to her teeth and gums," and quite frankly finds it very uncomfortable. Philomena says that she thought her oral health could be evaluated by the "full set of x-rays" that she received every few years.

Your clinical exam reveals that Philomena presents with generalized tooth mobility and early furcation involvement, especially on the maxillary molars. Her probe readings are generalized 4 to 6 mm in the posterior sextants. She assumed that her mouth was in good health and is shocked to find out otherwise.

1. What ethical principles are in conflict in this dilemma?
2. What is the best way for you to handle this ethical dilemma?
3. What is the best way to address/discuss Philomena's treatment plan?

Reference

1. Bragger U. Radiographic parameters: biological significance and clinical use. *Periodontol 2000.* 2005;39:73–90.

 STUDENT ANCILLARY RESOURCES

A wide variety of resources to enhance your learning and understanding of this chapter are available on thePoint®.

- Visit thePoint to access:
  - Audio Glossary
  - Animations
  - Suggested Readings
  - Answers to Review Questions
  - Case Studies

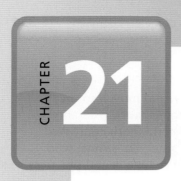

Best Practices for Periodontal Care

Clinical Application. All clinicians face the daunting problem of making sure that they are providing the best possible care for their patients. Dental hygienists must continuously update their knowledge about periodontal diseases and about the care patients with these diseases require. Faced with the fact that there is continuous publication of scientific information about these topics, keeping up-to-date can be difficult. This chapter outlines strategies that any dental hygienist (or any member of the dental team) can employ to ensure that he or she is indeed able to provide patient care based upon the latest scientific information available.

Learning Objectives

- Summarize how the explosion of knowledge is impacting practitioners and patients.
- Identify the three components of evidence-based decision making.
- Discuss the benefits and limitations of experience.
- Describe the role of the patient in the evidence-based model.
- List locations for accessing systematic reviews.
- Explain the difference between a peer-reviewed journal and trade magazine.
- State three desired outcomes from attending continuing education courses.
- Formulate a question using the PICO process.

Key Terms

Best practice
Best evidence
Databases
Association
Levels of evidence

Cochrane Collaboration
Causal factor
Systematic review
MEDLINE (PubMed)
Evidence-based practice

PICO process
Peer-reviewed journals
Confirmation bias

Section 1
What is Best Practice?

Providing the best possible care to patients is the foremost goal of all dental healthcare providers. Yet it is generally acknowledged that periodontal care may vary from office to office and even by regions of the country. *As new procedures and techniques become available, hygienists committed to excellence must regularly update and adapt their strategies for providing patient care.* The approach known as "best practice" is an important tool in helping hygienists provide high quality care to their patients.

1. Overview of the Concept of Best Practice
   A. Definition. Best practice refers to practices/treatments/therapies that are based on the best available evidence (1).
   B. Goals and Considerations
      1. The goal of best practice is consistent, superior patient outcomes.
         a. The outcomes should be measurable such as a reduction in probing depths.
         b. The outcome should be reproducible. For example, if a technique produces a certain result on one patient, it is reasonable to expect a similar outcome when the technique is used with other patients.
      2. Best practice is derived from evidence-based care. It is the process of using the best available evidence in patient interventions (1).
2. Circumstances That Prompted the Best Practice Approach to Patient Care
   A. Direct Access to Rapidly Emerging Clinical Research Information
      1. Explosion of Information
         a. Information about new techniques, tests, procedures, and products for periodontal care is emerging at an astonishing rate. Hundreds of articles are published in dental journals each year.
         b. In addition to the information in dental journals, relevant articles are published each year in medical and specialty journals. An example of articles in other disciplines that are relevant to periodontal health are those on the topic of the oral/systemic link. Important research on this topic can be found in journals such as the *New England Journal of Medicine* or *Diabetes Care*.
      2. Direct Access to Information
         a. In the past, dental healthcare providers relied on what they learned in school and the advice of recognized experts to determine how to provide care. Patients had little or no input into this process. Knowledge of new or cutting edge research was limited to a few practitioners with access to an educational or healthcare institution.
         b. Today, with the Internet, clinicians and patients have instant access to the results of federally funded clinical trials on treatment methods, equipment, and materials. PubMed, a gateway to more than 23 million research citations, can be accessed by anyone for free.
         c. *Practicing dental hygienists are expected to remain current with new techniques, devices, and materials that will result in improvements in periodontal care.* Dental hygienists in private practice cannot continue to use the same treatments and techniques learned in dental hygiene school year after year. The best practice 2 years ago may not represent the highest standard of care today.

B. **Active Patient Role in Decision Making**
1. Today's patient expects to be a partner in the decision-making process about his or her own periodontal care. Patients may arrive at the dental office with information downloaded from the Internet.
2. Before the widespread use of information technology, patients depended on the expertise of a healthcare provider for advice, and in most cases accepted that advice without question.
3. Patients who are more engaged in their healthcare experience report a better experience and 3 to 5 times greater satisfaction with their providers (2).

3. **Ability to Interpret the Literature**
A. **Not All Studies are Significant to Clinical Care.** Even though hundreds of studies are published yearly, very few are significant enough on their own to merit a change in clinical care.
1. The merit or weight of study is influenced by its design. For example, a randomized clinical trial is considered a higher level of evidence than a case series.
2. No study is completely free of bias. Reputable journals require investigators to declare a conflict of interest and disclose corporate financial support for studies.
3. Many studies either are not designed to provide an answer to the needs of the clinician or provide results that are too weak to merit implementation.

B. **New Does Not Necessarily Mean Better**
1. New treatments and products need to demonstrate consistent superiority to established methods.
2. Some new products and therapies are also significantly more costly to implement, and these costs are ultimately passed down to patients.

C. **Associations Are Not the Same as Cause and Effect**
1. An **association** is a relationship between an exposure and a disease that implies the exposure *might* cause the disease (3).
2. A **causal factor** (causality) is an event or condition that plays a role in producing an occurrence of a disease. An example of a causal factor is exposure to the bacterium called *Mycobacterium tuberculosis*. Exposure to this bacterium may cause an individual to develop the infectious disease tuberculosis (TB).
   a. Investigations/studies are undertaken to demonstrate a link—relationship or association—between an agent and a disease. On a population basis:
      1. An increase in the level of a causal factor will be accompanied by an increase in the incidence of disease (all other things being equal). So, if a population—such as, a large group of people in the confined area of refugee camp—is exposed to many persons in the camp who are infected with the bacterium *M. tuberculosis,* then it is likely that there will be an increase in the number of new cases of tuberculosis.
      2. If the causal factor is eliminated or reduced, the frequency of tuberculosis will decline.
3. Finding an association between an event and a disease does not make it causal.
   a. Over the past several years, many studies have looked at the relationship between periodontal disease and a host of systemic conditions.
   b. For instance, while many studies do show that periodontal disease is *associated* with cardiovascular disease, at the time of this writing, periodontal disease cannot be said to be a causal factor for cardiovascular disease (4).

Section 2
Role of Evidence-Based Decision Making in Best Practice

1. **Introduction to Evidence-Based Decision Making.** Knowledge of the most recent and relevant evidence is the foundation for best practice. The ADHA advocates evidence-based, patient-/client-centered *dental hygiene* practice.
   A. **Definition.** The ADHA defines **evidence-based practice** as the conscientious, explicit, and judicious use of current best evidence in making decisions about the care of individual patients. The practice of evidence-based dental hygiene requires the integration of individual clinical expertise and patient preferences with the best available external clinical evidence from systematic research (5).
   B. **Why is there a need for evidence-based decision making?**
      1. The Journal of Evidence-Based Dental Practice states "Care that is important is often not delivered; care that is delivered is often not important." Whether this stems from lack of knowledge on the part of the provider or lack of support for implementation within the dental practice, the ultimate result is that the patient does not receive the highest level of care (6).
      2. Studies of appropriateness of dental and dental hygiene care confirm that there is a lag time between the discovery of new scientific findings and implementation into private practice (7). Studies on dental hygienists' knowledge and practices relating to oral cancer detection and caries prevention showed variation in knowledge and practices (8–10).
      3. A recent study identified several key barriers for dental hygienists in the implementation of evidence-based care. These included a lack of support by the dentist employer, nonclinical personnel dictating care, a monetary preoccupation, and level of comfort in continuing to do procedures the same way (7).
      4. Dental hygienists were more likely to utilize evidence-based decision making when there was an aligned practice philosophy that included supportive leadership and common goals. A commitment to continuing education also is important (7).
   C. **About Evidence-Based Decision Making**
      1. Evidence-based decision making emerged from the work of Dr. David Sackett and others at McMaster University in Ontario, Canada. In 1981, this group began publishing articles to help clinicians critically appraise the literature, so the best evidence could be identified to help solve patient problems (11).
      2. Evidence-based decision making includes three foundational elements: (1) incorporation of the best scientific evidence with (2) the healthcare provider's clinical expertise and judgment, and (3) patient's preferences and values. Figure 21-1 illustrates these three foundational elements of evidence-based health care. Box 21-1 provides an example of evidence-based practice.
      3. Evidence is not meant to replace experience or clinical skills. The addition of evidence to decision making brings balance to the process. It helps close the gap between "what we do" and science. It has the ability to enhance patient care and outcomes (12).

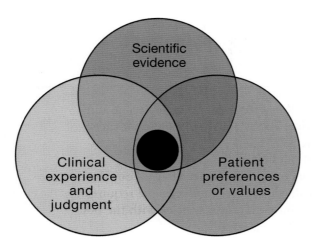

Figure 21-1. The Three Foundational Elements of Evidence-Based Health Care. Evidence-based care has three equal components: scientific evidence, clinical experience, and patient preferences or values.

Box 21-1. Evidence-Based Practice: An Example

Evidence-based practice is built on information obtained from research.

For example, perhaps a dental hygienist was taught in school that ultrasonic instrumentation should be used sparingly and only for the removal of large supragingival calculus deposits. In addition, the hygienist learned in school that hand instruments produce the best results for periodontal instrumentation.

- After reading current research on ultrasonic instrumentation, the hygienist learns that modern slim-tipped ultrasonic instruments can be used subgingivally and that a combination of ultrasonic and hand instrumentation leads to excellent results.
- This evidence motivates the dental hygienist to attend a continuing education course on ultrasonic instrumentation and to incorporate ultrasonic instrumentation in treating patients with periodontitis.

D. Foundational Elements of Evidence-Based Decision Making
  1. Evidence-based care recognizes that essential skills are needed in order to engage in evidence-based decision making and obtain the best health outcomes (12).
     a. Over time, healthcare providers gain clinical expertise by engaging in clinical experiences (i.e., treating patients and observing the results).
     b. Patients' preferences may be the result of many factors including past dental experiences, current medical and dental status, perceived needs, health values, and economic considerations.
     c. The most challenging essential skill for a healthcare professional to develop is the ability to assess "evidence."
  2. Clinical experience is both valuable and limiting. It signifies the ability of a clinician to grow in skill and knowledge through experience.
     a. Experience helps the practitioner make thoughtful clinical judgments about the applicability of research findings to individual patient situations. Yet all patients are different, they may present with complicated or complex medical and dental histories.
     b. Experience is valuable when it is used as a learning rather than reinforcement tool. Ideally, a clinician uses his or her clinical experiences in making better treatment decisions.

    c. Experience can be limiting. The limitation is that not all individuals are able to learn and grow from experience. To acquire "practical wisdom" the clinician needs to learn how to be reflective and analyze his or her own performance.

      1. There is a human tendency to look for or interpret information that confirms our beliefs. This tendency is called **confirmation bias.**

      2. Confirmation bias can lead practitioners to misinterpret information based on beliefs, positive or negative, about a treatment or device.

  3. Patient preference or values is an important consideration in treatment selection. If due consideration is not given to the individual patient's preferences, values, and concerns as well as their unique clinical circumstances, the likelihood of the patient fully accepting the clinician's recommendation is diminished.

    a. It is the dental hygienist's responsibility to understand the evidence and its implications for periodontal treatment and communicate it effectively to a patient. Ultimately, it will be the patient who chooses which therapy he or she prefers.

    b. In helping a patient decide which periodontal treatment is right for him or her, there are several elements that should be discussed, including:

      1. The evidence about a particular treatment option.

      2. The treatment of choice based on the evidence.

      3. All possible treatment alternatives.

      4. The risks of no treatment at all.

    c. In addition to the efficacy of a proposed treatment, a patient may place equal weight on other aspects of treatment such as:

      1. Cost. Patients usually are concerned about what a treatment will cost. In addition, patients decide if the treatment has benefits that they perceive as being worth the cost.

      2. Pain. Assurances about pain control and management help lessen these concerns.

      3. Time lost from work. Different jobs and work environments have varying levels of flexibility in allowing employees time off for health-related matters.

      4. Impact on family. Caregivers of young children or elderly family members may feel that they do not have the time to devote to periodontal treatment. Individuals with chronic health problems may believe that periodontal care is no longer a priority.

      5. Insurance benefits. A practice reality is that patients will sometimes choose care based on what insurance will pay for versus the full treatment recommendation.

2. **Evaluation of Scientific Evidence. All scientific evidences are not created equal.**

  A. **Levels of Evidence. Best evidence** is the highest level of evidence available for a specific clinical question.

    1. **Levels of evidence** is a ranking system used in evidence-based care to describe the strength of the results measured in a clinical trial or research study. In simple terms, one way of looking at levels of evidence is as follows (the higher the level, the better the quality; the lower, the greater the bias). Figure 21-2 illustrates the levels of evidence.

    2. Based on a hierarchy of levels of evidence, systematic reviews of randomized controlled trials constitute the highest level of current best evidence, and expert opinion is lower-level evidence.

    3. The highest level of evidence available represents the current best evidence for a specific clinical question.

B. **Systematic Reviews: The Highest Ranked Source of Evidence**
1. A **systematic review** is a concise summary of individual research studies on a treatment or device to determine the overall validity and clinical applicability of that treatment or device.
   a. The systematic review process strives to identify and track down all the literature on a given topic. Once the literature is complied, the review process strives to summarize, appraise, and communicate the results and implications in a concise form for healthcare professionals who need this information to keep up-to-date.
   b. Internationally, the stimulus for systematic reviews has come from the Cochrane Collaboration, a worldwide group of subject and methodological specialists who aim to identify and synthesize the research in all aspects of health care.
2. Systematic reviews are, by their very nature, efficient. As an information management tool, they provide a way of coping with large volumes of data in a concise and manageable form.
   a. With more than two million articles published in medical and dental journals annually, it is impossible for any one healthcare provider to read and utilize all the new information.
   b. Systematic reviews of randomized clinical trials represent one of the highest levels of evidence (13).
   c. Systematic reviews also facilitate the development of clinical practice guidelines by bringing together all that is known about a given topic in a nonbiased manner. This provides useful mechanisms for bringing research to practice (13).
3. Because of the emphasis on evidence-based care, there are more systematic reviews conducted in dentistry than ever before.
4. The systematic review makes incorporating evidence-based care easier. In the past, practitioners were encouraged to do their own searching for research. Since most busy practitioners do not have the time or expertise to do this, the systematic review fills this gap.

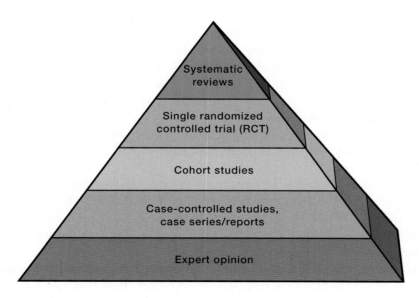

Figure 21-2. Levels of Evidence. The importance or merit of a research study usually is evaluated through its design. Systematic reviews and randomized controlled trials represent the best levels of evidence. Case reports and expert opinion are the lowest levels of evidence.

Section 3
Finding Clinically Relevant Information

Today, all that is required to have access to research information is a computer with Internet access. Determining which studies are of the highest evidence and the most clinically relevant for a particular need is much more challenging. The most comprehensive process for finding and critically evaluating clinical evidence involves a five-step process. This five-step process is summarized in Box 21-2. Steps 1 to 3 of this five-step process are discussed below.

Box 21-2. Five-Step Process for Finding and Evaluating Clinical Evidence

1. Develop an answerable clinical question from a patient problem or need
2. Conduct a computerized search to locate the best available evidence
3. Critically appraise the evidence for clinical applicability
4. Apply the results to your particular clinical situation
5. Evaluate the process and the results

Adapted from Forrest JL. Evidence-based decision making: Introduction and formulating good clinical questions. 2012. Available online at: http://www.dentalcare.com/en-US/dental-education/continuing-education/ce311/ce311.aspx?ModuleName=introduction&PartID=−1&SectionID=−1. Accessed April 30, 2014.

---

1. **Developing an Answerable Question.** A clinical question may develop from questions that arise relative to patient care or from an area in which the hygienist wants updated knowledge. In order to find the best information to help patients, it is fundamental to learn how to ask the "right questions." This is more challenging than it seems. It involves converting problems into answerable questions.
   A. **Use Four Components to Structure the Question.** The structure for asking a clear and focused question entails four critical components, known as the **PICO Process** (12). The PICO process involves the combination of four separate components to form an answerable question: "Patient, Intervention, Comparison, and Outcome."
      1. P (Patient or Problem). An example of the P component might be "*A periodontal maintenance patient with bleeding and gingivitis.*"
      2. I (Intervention)
         a. An intervention is a specific diagnostic test, treatment, adjunctive therapy, medication, product, or clinical procedure.
         b. An example of an intervention being questioned is "*brushing and daily home irrigation.*"
      3. C (Comparison)
         a. Identifies the specific alternative therapy or device that you wish to compare to the main intervention.
         b. An example of the "C" segment of the question is "*compared to brushing and flossing.*"
      4. O (Outcome)
         a. Identifies the measurable outcome you plan to accomplish, improve, or influence.
         b. An example of the "O" segment of the question is "*reduce gingivitis and bleeding within 4 weeks.*"

B. **Formulate the Question.** Once each of the PICO components has been determined, the clinician combines them into an answerable question. Using the above examples, the question would read *"For a periodontal maintenance patient with bleeding and gingivitis, will brushing and daily home irrigation OR brushing and flossing provide a better reduction in bleeding and gingivitis within 4 weeks?"*

2. **Conduct a computerized search to find the best evidence**

A. **Databases**

1. The most efficient way to go about finding relevant research is to use an online index of published articles, such as PubMed, MEDLINE, or CINAHL (Cumulative Index of Nursing and Allied Health Literature).

2. These indexes—known as **databases**—list all articles published in a given period of time by journals in a particular profession or group of professions.

3. **MEDLINE** is the U.S. National Library of Medicine's (NLM) premier database that contains over 19 million references to journal articles in life sciences with a concentration on biomedicine. MEDLINE enables quick access to locate relevant clinical evidence in the published dental/periodontal literature (Fig. 21-3).

   a. A distinctive feature of MEDLINE is that the records are indexed with NLM *Medical Subject Headings* (MeSH).

   b. Anyone can access MEDLINE for free using **PubMed**—a gateway hosted by the National Library of Medicine.

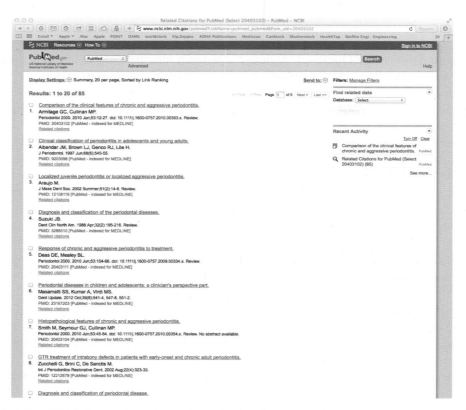

Figure 21-3. PubMed Website. PubMed search results for the topic "chronic periodontitis." (Courtesy of the U.S. National Library of Medicine, Bethesda, MD.)

B. **Systematic Reviews.** Many healthcare providers do not have the time or expertise needed to do their own systematic reviews of a question. Fortunately, there are numerous trustworthy resources for busy practitioners who want to implement high-quality science into patient care.

1. **The Cochrane Collaboration Database of Systematic Reviews**
   a. The **Cochrane Collaboration** was established in 1993 by a British epidemiologist, who recognized that ready access to systematic reviews of available evidence would facilitate better-informed decisions by healthcare providers.
   b. *The Cochrane Database of Systematic Reviews* includes systematic reviews of healthcare interventions that are produced and disseminated by The Cochrane Collaboration, a global not-for-profit organization.
      1. The Cochrane Library is published online. Abstracts of reviews are free.
      2. Also, many health science libraries subscribe to the Cochrane databases, so that faculty and students have online access.
   c. The Cochrane review group relevant to periodontics is the "Oral Health Review Group." An example of a systematic review conducted by the Oral Health Group is on the topic of psychological interventions to improve adherence to oral hygiene instructions in adults with periodontal diseases.
   d. A complete listing of topics and abstracts can be accessed at http://www.cochrane.org/reviews/index.htm

2. **The PubMed Clinical Query: The National Library of Medicine**
   a. One feature of the MEDLINE database is the PubMed Clinical Query, which provides specialized searches using an evidence-based filter.
   b. An online tutorial for the PubMed Clinical Query tool can be accessed online at http://www.nlm.nih.gov/bsd/disted/pubmedtutorial/020_570.html

3. **Systematic Reviews by Professional Organizations.** Many professional organizations are developing systematic reviews. The American Dental Association recently developed a web-based Center for Evidence-Based Dentistry (http://ebd.ada.org).

4. **Systematic Reviews in Evidence-Based Journals**
   a. Evidence-based journals publish summaries of valid research studies to simplify the evidence-based process for dental healthcare providers.
   b. For example, The Journal of Evidence-Based Dental Practice scans the top dental journals and a panel reviews the selected articles for clinical relevance to practice.
   c. Other examples of evidence-based journals include Evidence-Based Dentistry, Evidence-Based Medicine, Evidence-Based Healthcare, and Evidence-Based Nursing.

5. **Appraisal of the Evidence for Clinical Applicability.** In medicine, the use of point-of-care electronic databases and algorithms are emerging to help practitioners evaluate and implement evidence-based decision making (11).
   a. The use of electronic records is integral to this process as it allows individual patient characteristics to be automatically linked to the best evidence (1).
   b. Table 21-1 outlines preappraised evidence resources including interactive drug databases that are a key part of clinical care decision support systems (11).

3. **Using the PICO Process to Find Clinically Relevant Information.** Figure 21-4 shows how the PICO process can be incorporated in a three-step approach to finding clinically relevant information.

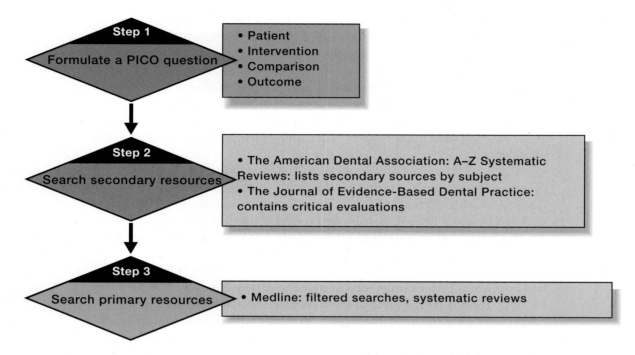

Figure 21-4. Strategy for Finding Clinically Relevant Evidence. The Center for Evidence-Based Medicine recommends a straightforward approach based on (1) formulating a PICO question, (2) searching evaluated (secondary) resources, and (3) then examining primary text documents.

CLINICAL CASE EXAMPLE

A dental hygienist used the following steps to find evidence-based clinically relevant information.

1. Step 1: Formulate a PICO Question
   - Patient: *adult female patient with chronic periodontitis; new patient in the dental office*
   - Intervention: *periodontal instrumentation*
   - Comparison: *full-mouth disinfection versus quadrant instrumentation*
   - Outcome: *resolution of inflammation*
   - Question: *For a patient with chronic periodontitis, will full-mouth disinfection OR quadrant instrumentation provide a better reduction in inflammation?*
2. Step 2: Search Online Evidence-Based Sources
   a. ADA Center for Evidence-Based Dentistry at http://ebd.ada.org
   b. PubMed at http://pubmed.gov
3. The results of the search suggest that both the traditional quadrant approach and the newer the full-mouth debridement could be equally effective (Box 21-3).
4. In this instance, the dental hygienist presented both options to the patient, explaining that both treatment options are equally effective.
5. The patient chose full-mouth debridement because it would be less disruptive for her to be away from work for 1 day rather than four shorter appointments over a period of several weeks.

Box 21-3. Search Results

Main Results

The search identified 216 abstracts. Review of these abstracts resulted in 12 publications for detailed review. Finally, seven randomized controlled trials (RCTs) which met the criteria for eligibility were independently selected by two review authors. None of the studies included reported on tooth loss. All treatment modalities led to significant improvements in clinical parameters after a follow-up of at least 3 months. For the secondary outcome, reduction in probing depth, the mean difference between full-mouth disinfection and control was 0.53 mm (95% confidence interval (CI) 0.28 to 0.77) in moderately deep pockets of single-rooted teeth and for gain in probing attachment 0.33 mm (95% CI 0.04 to 0.63) in moderately deep single- and multirooted teeth. Comparing FMD and FMS, the mean difference in one study for gain in probing attachment amounted to 0.74 mm in favor of FMS (95% CI 0.17 to 1.31) for deep pockets in multirooted teeth, while another study reported a mean difference for reduction in bleeding on probing of 18% in favor of FMD (95% CI −34.30 to −1.70) for deep pockets of single-rooted teeth. No significant differences were observed for any of the outcome measures, when comparing full-mouth disinfection and control.

Authors' Conclusions

In patients with chronic periodontitis in moderately deep pockets slightly more favorable outcomes for pocket reduction and gain in probing attachment were found following full-mouth disinfection compared to control. However, these additional improvements were only modest and there were only a very limited number of studies available for comparison, thus limiting general conclusions about the clinical benefit of full-mouth disinfection.

TABLE 21-1. PREAPPRAISED EVIDENCE RESOURCES

Level 6 Clinical Decision Support Systems: Interactive Drug Databases

Clinical Key	http://www.clinicalkey.com
Comprehensive Drug Database; Interactions	http://www.lexi.com
Integrative Medicine with Evidence-Based Grading System	http://www.naturalstandard.com
UpToDate	http://www.uptodate.com

Level 5 Summaries: Clinical Practice Guidelines

American Academy of Pediatric Dentistry	http://www.aapd.org/policies/
American Academy of Periodontology	http://www.perio.org/resources-products/posppr2.html
ADA Clinical Recommendations	http://ebd.ada.org/ClinicalRecommendations.aspx
ADHA Position Papers and Consensus Statements	http://www.adha.org/profissues/index.html
American Heart Association	http://my.americanheart.org/professional/Statements-Guidelines/Statements-Guidelines_UCM_316885_Sub-HomePage.jsp
Centers for Disease Control and Prevention	http://www.cdc.gov/OralHealth/guidelines.htm
PubMed (article type limited to "Practice Guideline")	http://pubmed.gov
Scottish Intercollegiate Guidelines Network	http://www.sign.ac.uk/guidelines/index.html
The Evidence-Based Dental Library	http://www.ebdlibrary.com

Level 4 Synopses of Systemic Reviews: Critically Appraised Systemic Reviews

ADA Center for Evidence-Based Dentistry (Critical Summary)	http://ebd.ada.org/en/evidence/
Database of Abstracts of Reviews of Effects (DARE)	http://www.crd.york.ac.uk/crdweb/SearchPage.asp
PubMed (look for comments on systemic reviews)	http://pubmed.gov
Evidence-Based Dentistry	http://www.nature.com/ebd/index.html
Journal of Evidence-Based Dental Practice	http://www.jebdp.com

Level 3 Systemic Reviews

ADA Center for Evidence-Based Dentistry	http://ebd.ada.org/en/evidence/
Cochrane Database of Systemic Reviews	http://www.thecochranelibrary.com
PubMed (article filter limit to "systemic review")	http://pubmed.gov
Evidence-Based Dentistry	http://www.nature.com/ebd/index.html
Journal of Evidence-Based Dental Practice	http://www.jebdp.com

Level 2 Synopses of Individual Studies: Critically Appraised Randomized Controlled Trials (RCTs)

Database of Abstracts of Reviews of Effects (DARE)	http://www.crd.york.ac.uk/crdweb/SearchPage.asp
PubMed (limit to "RCT" or "clinical trial"; look for comments)	http://pubmed.gov
Evidence-Based Dentistry	http://www.nature.com/ebd/index.html
Journal of Evidence-Based Dental Practice	http://www.jebdp.com

Level 1 Original Studies: Individual Research Studies (Original studies and not preappraised)

PubMed (limit to "RCT" or "clinical trial")	http://pubmed.gov
Journal publications, that is, Journal of Dental Hygiene, International Journal of Dental Hygiene, Dental Specialty Groups, etc.	http://www.adha.org/publications/index.html jada.ada.org http://www.ifdh.org/publications.html

Courtesy of Miller SA and Forrest JL, National Center for Dental Hygiene Practice & Research ©2012 (Forrest JL, Overman P. Keeping current: a commitment to patient care excellence through evidence based practice. *J Dent Hyg.* 2013;87(Suppl 1):33–40).

Section 4
Lifelong Learning Skills for Best Practice

One of the most challenging but important aspects of getting to best practices involves self-evaluation. Practitioners continually need to think about whether the care they are providing is still the best level care. There are several questions a dental hygienist should think about on a regular basis.

1. How sure am I that what I do is right?
    A. Do I know where to access systematic reviews? Do I keep up with journal reading?
        1. Peer-Reviewed Journals. Peer-reviewed journals (also called refereed journals) use a panel of experts to review research articles for study design, statistics, and conclusions. Peer-reviewed journals:
            a. Are good sources for randomized clinical trials, and learning about new research findings. Sometimes will publish systematic reviews.
            b. May be expensive to purchase a subscription; some highly ranked peer-reviewed journals from professional associations have begun to allow free access to full studies 6 months after publication.
            c. Are a good source of higher levels of evidence—systematic reviews and randomized clinical trials.
        2. Practice or Trade Magazines
            a. Can be commercial in nature
            b. May or may not be peer reviewed; generally provide more of the "expert" opinion
            c. May or may not be supported with references
            d. Vary widely in quality
            e. Provide the lowest quality of evidence
        3. Textbooks
            a. Provide a broad overview of a subject
            b. May not provide specifics on the research
            c. May be dated because of the amount of time involved in writing and publishing a textbook; always check the publication date
    B. Do I attend continuing education courses? How do I decide which courses to attend?
        1. Content: Is the subject matter something you like or something that you need? It is important to take the time to evaluate learning/practice needs. Conferring with coworkers or your employer can facilitate more objective choices.
        2. Speaker: Is he or she an expert, a facilitator, or both? A well-rounded speaker will provide information on the latest research findings along with providing some practical advice based on experience.
        3. Outcomes: A well-rounded continuing education course will do three things (14):
            a. Reaffirm: The course information provides support for your current ways of providing treatment.
            b. Reenergize: The course supports changes in areas that you have previously identified and provides the motivation and impetus to begin making those changes.
            c. Reexamine: The course addresses new research findings that merit further study and investigation as to the appropriateness of incorporation into practice.
    C. Am I active in my professional association?
        1. Networking with colleagues exposes dental hygienists to other practicing professionals who can provide guidance and mentoring to younger members.

2. Membership in a professional organization can provide free access to peer-reviewed journals.
3. Active membership provides the opportunity to help shape evidence-based policies and guidelines for the organization.
4. Provides immediate access to any Clinical Practice Guidelines the association may develop.

D. How well developed is my clinical judgment? Am I able to combine evidence and clinical experience to make a good decision?

E. Do I take into consideration what my patient wants?
   1. Do I listen to my patients?
   2. Do I provide them with enough information and direction to make a good decision?
   3. Do I respect their autonomy and choices?

F. Are there things that I should stop doing?
   1. Am I holding on to what I do because "that's what I learned in school" even though it was several years ago?
   2. Is what I am doing making the best use of office and patient resources, both financial and human?

G. Are there things I need to change?
   1. Are there better, more efficient, or cost-effective tools available such as specific diagnostic tests, treatments, adjunctive therapies, medications, products, or procedures than what I am currently using?
   2. Do I have the appropriate amount of time scheduled or equipment provided for the highest level of patient care?

Chapter Summary Statement

Best practice is a process of care with the goal of achieving consistent, superior patient outcomes. Best practice is founded on evidence-based data. The highest ranked level of evidence today is the systematic review, an evaluation of a body of research on a treatment or device through rigorous scientific methods to determine the overall validity and clinical applicability of that treatment or device. In addition to scientific data, best practice incorporates sound clinical judgment and patient values into the process. Achieving best practice requires that dental hygienists question and think about what they are doing and be open to learning new techniques. By using this approach to periodontal care, hygienists can meet the challenges of continuing to provide quality care in a rapidly changing field of dental health care.

Section 5
Focus on Patients

Clinical Patient Care

CASE 1

You have just started working in a new office and find that the other dental hygienist in the practice, Debbie, "doesn't believe" in using the ultrasonic equipment. Debbie states she has been practicing for 20 years, that is what she learned in school and she knows what she sees, good results with hand scaling. It is a little intimidating since you have less experience (only 5 years) but have routinely used ultrasonic instruments and mention to her "that is what you learned in school." For a while you pass it off as no big deal, a difference of opinions, but because Debbie didn't use the ultrasonic equipment, the equipment in the office is old and doesn't function at the level it should. You speak to your employer about getting a new machine, but he said, "Debbie doesn't use it, why do you?"

1. How would you answer your employer?
2. What types of evidence would you try to locate to justify your position?
3. Where would you search?
4. What types of key words would you use?
5. How would you manage your conflict with Debbie?

CASE 2

Your patient, Ms. Karen Jones, is a healthy, nonsmoking 30-year-old. Her only medication is birth control pills of 5 years duration, and a daily multivitamin. She has been coming in for regular maintenance every 6 months. She brushes two times per day and flosses when she remembers, perhaps once a week and she states she finds the procedure difficult. The exam shows some 4-mm probing depths and significant bleeding. As you have done several times in the past, you show the patient how to use the manual brush and floss and really "lay it on the line" about improving oral health and warn her she will need to come in more frequently if her habits do not improve. The patient states that "she tries" and is visibly upset when she leaves office. While you hate to see her upset, you hope she finally got the message.

About a month after her visit, you get a message that Karen Jones would like you call her. When you reach Karen, she tells you she has been "researching" her gum problem, and she has found out she has several alternatives to a manual toothbrush and floss. Karen reports she has looked on the Internet and talked to a relative who is also a dental hygienist. She has learned about automatic toothbrushes, automatic flossing devices, and oral irrigators, and how they could help her. In fact, she has purchased one of everything and feels her mouth is improving. Not only that, the power-flossing device makes the task so much easier. "Why didn't you tell me about this!" she demands. "I am unhappy, and going to have my records transferred elsewhere!"

1. What are some of the reasons the dental hygienist may have for not telling Karen about these products?
2. Ethically, is not telling a patient about all self-care products that have evidence to support their use the same as not telling a patient about all available professional treatment options? Why or why not?
3. What steps could the dental hygienist take to improve her knowledge on self-care products?

Ethical Dilemma

You have been working as a hygienist in the same periodontal practice for the last 10 years and are quite happy there. There are four dentists in the group, so you have a very full schedule, which allows you to work 4 10-hour days. The practice is very flexible and generous with their resources and benefits. They pay for continuing education courses for all staff members. Unfortunately, you haven't taken any courses since you have worked there, even though you know you are in violation of your state practice act. You have been very busy in your personal life over the last number of years, as you got engaged, married, had two children within the span of 2 years, and are now caring for your aging parents. You just can't squeeze anything else into your life.

Your next patient Richie G, is a 63-year-old real estate agent, who was referred to your practice for a periodontal evaluation 3 months ago. Richie comes armed with questions, articles, and information that he has downloaded from the Internet. Although Dr. Willis, the periodontist, suggested periodontal surgery for Richie's treatment, Richie is inquiring about laser procedures as well as bone and tissue regeneration. He asks for your opinion on the articles and studies he has in hand, and if you think there are superior options to "gum surgery."

While you want Richie to be a partner in the decision about his periodontal care, you feel very uncomfortable discussing this with him. You know you are not current in your dental knowledge, and do not know how to accurately interpret the literature Richie presents to you. Unfortunately, you have not updated or adapted your own treatment strategies, and still rely on what you learned in school over 10 years ago.

1. What ethical principles are in conflict in this dilemma?
2. What is the best way for you to handle this ethical dilemma?

References

1. Hartford Center for Geriatric Nursing Excellence. Best practices for healthcare professionals. Available online at: http://www.nursing.uiowa.edu/hartford/best-practices-for-healthcare-professionals.
2. Alston C, Paget L, Halvorson G, et al. *Communicating with Patients on Health Care Evidence*. Washington, DC: Institute of Medicine; 2012. Available online at: http://www.iom.edu/evidence.
3. Bhopal R. Causes in epidemiology: the jewels in the public health crown. *J Public Health (Oxf)*. 2008;30(3):224–225; discussion 32–33.
4. Brunette DM. Causation, association and oral health–systemic disease connections. In: Glick M, ed. *The Oral-Systemic Health Connection: A Guide to Patient Care*. Chicago, IL: Quintessence Publishing Co.; 2014:312.
5. American Dental Hygienists' Association. *ADHA Policy Manual*. 2013. Available online at: http://www.adha.org/resources-docs/7614_Policy_Manual.pdf.
6. Building a business case for evidence-based medicine. *J Evid Based Dent Pract*. 2013;13(2):74–76.
7. Asadoorian J, Hearson B, Satyanarayana S, et al. Evidence-based practice in healthcare: an exploratory cross-discipline comparison of enhancers and barriers. *J Healthc Qual*. 2010;32(3):15–22.
8. Forrest JL, Drury TE, Horowitz AM. U.S. dental hygienists' knowledge and opinions related to providing oral cancer examinations. *J Cancer Educ*. 2001;16(3):150–156.
9. Forrest JL, Horowitz AM, Shmuely Y. Caries preventive knowledge and practices among dental hygienists. *J Dent Hyg*. 2000;74(3):183–195.
10. Forrest JL, Horowitz AM, Shmuely Y. Dental hygienists' knowledge, opinions, and practices related to oral and pharyngeal cancer risk assessment. *J Dent Hyg*. 2001;75(4):271–281.
11. Forrest JL, Overman P. Keeping current: a commitment to patient care excellence through evidence based practice. *J Dent Hyg*. 2013;87(Suppl 1):33–40.
12. Forrest JL. Evidence-based decision making: Introduction and formulating good clinical questions. 2012. Available online at: http://www.dentalcare.com/en-US/dental-education/continuing-education/ce311/ce311.aspx?ModuleName=introduction&PartID=-1&SectionID=-1. Accessed April 30, 2014.
13. Prato GP, Pagliaro U, Buti J, et al. Evaluation of the literature: evidence assessment tools for clinicians. *J Evid Based Dent Pract*. 2013;13(4):130–141.
14. Jahn CA. Product focus: continuing education. *Access*. 2008;22:30–32.

 STUDENT ANCILLARY RESOURCES

A wide variety of resources to enhance your learning and understanding of this chapter are available on thePoint®.

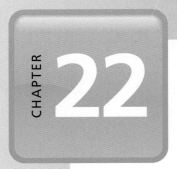

22

Nonsurgical Periodontal Therapy

Clinical Application. Treating patients with periodontal diseases is a dynamic process that requires constant monitoring and reorientation of ongoing therapy. Periodontal therapy is often divided into phases and one of the first phases of therapy following comprehensive periodontal assessment is the nonsurgical therapy phase. Members of the dental team need to have a clear understanding of the importance of nonsurgical periodontal therapy and the decisions that are required following this therapy. This chapter provides an overview of nonsurgical periodontal therapy, discusses some of the problems that can arise during this therapy and outlines the decisions needed following reevaluation of the nonsurgical therapy.

Learning Objectives

- Explain the term and name four goals for nonsurgical periodontal therapy.
- Write a typical plan for nonsurgical therapy for (1) a patient with plaque-induced gingivitis and (2) a patient with slight chronic periodontitis.
- Describe the type of healing to be expected following instrumentation of root surfaces.

- Explain strategies for managing dental hypersensitivity during nonsurgical therapy.
- Explain why reevaluation is an important step during nonsurgical therapy.
- List steps in an appointment for reevaluation of the results of nonsurgical therapy.

Key Terms

Nonsurgical periodontal
   therapy
Periodontal instrumentation
Long junctional epithelium

Dentinal hypersensitivity
Dentinal tubules
Odontoblastic process
Smear layer

Reevaluation
Nonresponsive disease sites

Section 1
Overview of Nonsurgical Periodontal Therapy

UNDERSTANDING NONSURGICAL PERIODONTAL THERAPY

1. Nonsurgical Periodontal Therapy Defined
   A. Nonsurgical periodontal therapy is a term used to describe the many nonsurgical steps used to eliminate inflammation in the periodontium of a patient with periodontal disease in an attempt to return the periodontium to a healthy state that can then be maintained by a combination of both professional care and patient self-care.
      1. Many terms have been used to describe nonsurgical periodontal therapy, and this fact may create some confusion. Some of the other terms that have been used to describe this same phase of treatment include initial periodontal therapy, initial therapy, hygienic phase, anti-infective phase, cause-related therapy, phase I treatment, and soft tissue management.
      2. Nonsurgical periodontal therapy, however, is one of the most frequently used terms for this phase of periodontal care.
      3. It is convenient to view nonsurgical periodontal procedures as the initial step in the periodontal treatment for a patient, but for many patients this initial step is all that is needed to bring periodontal disease under control.
   B. Philosophy for Nonsurgical Periodontal Therapy
      1. The basic philosophy for developing a sensible plan for nonsurgical periodontal therapy should be to plan treatment that will provide for the control, elimination, or minimization of (1) primary etiologic factors for periodontal disease, (2) local risk factors for periodontal disease, and (3) systemic risk factors for periodontal disease.
      2. Procedures included in a plan for nonsurgical periodontal therapy should be selected to meet the needs of each individual patient; therefore, nonsurgical therapy plans can vary from patient to patient.

NONSURGICAL THERAPY RELATED TO THE PERIODONTAL DIAGNOSIS

Nonsurgical periodontal therapy is indicated for many patients but not all patients. It may be helpful to view some common periodontal diagnoses and to see how nonsurgical periodontal therapy normally relates to these diagnoses.
1. A Diagnosis of Plaque-Induced Gingivitis
   A. Nonsurgical periodontal therapy is the primary type of care provided for most patients with plaque-induced gingivitis.
   B. Thorough nonsurgical therapy can normally bring plaque-induced gingivitis under control and bring it to a point that periodontal health can be maintained by a combination of both professional care and patient self-care.
   C. This general relationship between nonsurgical therapy and a diagnosis of plaque-induced gingivitis should not be interpreted to mean that patients with this diagnosis never need periodontal surgery, since periodontal surgery is sometimes needed to correct other existing problems (i.e., gingival recession or gingival overgrowth) in gingivitis patients.

2. A Diagnosis of Slight to Moderate Chronic Periodontitis
   A. Thorough nonsurgical therapy can also bring many cases of slight to moderate chronic periodontitis under control and bring it to a point that periodontal health can be maintained by a combination of both professional care and patient self-care (1–4).
   B. It should be noted that some patients with a diagnosis of moderate chronic periodontitis will require periodontal surgery to correct damage done by the disease (i.e., furcation involvement or attachment loss) (5).
   C. It should also be noted that periodontal surgery is sometimes used to correct other problems (i.e., gingival recession) and may indeed be indicated in any patient.
3. A Diagnosis of Severe Chronic Periodontitis
   A. For most patients with more advanced periodontal disease, such as severe chronic periodontitis, control of the periodontitis will not only require thorough nonsurgical periodontal therapy, but it will also require more advanced periodontal procedures such as periodontal surgery.
   B. Although periodontal surgery is frequently indicated for patients with more advanced periodontitis, it should be understood that *most patients with chronic periodontitis can benefit from undergoing nonsurgical therapy prior to periodontal surgical intervention.*
   C. Nonsurgical periodontal therapy is frequently successful in minimizing the extent of any surgery subsequently needed and may be needed to improve the outcomes of that periodontal surgery.
4. A Diagnosis of One of the Other Forms of Periodontitis
   A. Members of the dental team should be aware that nonsurgical periodontal therapy may not be the treatment of choice for all patients with other types of periodontitis.
   B. For example, nonsurgical periodontal therapy is not necessarily the best therapy for patients with other types of periodontitis, such as aggressive periodontitis.

GOALS OF NONSURGICAL PERIODONTAL THERAPY

The goals of nonsurgical periodontal therapy are discussed below and summarized in Box 22-1.

1. Goal 1: To minimize the bacterial challenge to the patient
   A. Control of the bacterial challenge usually involves intensive training of the patient in appropriate techniques for self-care in combination with frequent professional care for the removal of calculus deposits and bacterial products from tooth surfaces (6).
   B. Removal of calculus deposits and bacterial products contaminating the tooth surfaces is an important step in achieving control of the bacterial challenge. Calculus deposits are always covered with living bacterial biofilms that are associated with continuing inflammation if not removed (7).
2. Goal 2: To eliminate or control local contributing factors for periodontal disease
   A. Local contributing factors can increase the risk of developing periodontitis in localized sites. For example, defective restorations with overhangs can lead to plaque biofilm retention in a localized area. Local contributing factors are discussed in Chapter 16.
   B. Biofilm retention at a site over time allows periodontal pathogens to live, multiply, and lead to damage of the periodontium.
   C. A thorough plan for nonsurgical periodontal therapy will always include minimizing the impact of local environmental contributing factors.

3. Goal 3: To minimize the impact of systemic factors for periodontal disease
   A. It is apparent that there are certain systemic diseases or conditions that can increase the risk of developing periodontitis or can increase the risk of developing more severe periodontitis where periodontitis already exists. Two examples of systemic factors are uncontrolled diabetes mellitus and smoking. Systemic factors are discussed in Chapter 15 of this book.
   B. A thorough plan for nonsurgical therapy always includes measures to minimize the impact of systemic risk factors. For example, a periodontitis patient with a family history of diabetes mellitus should be evaluated to rule out undiagnosed diabetes as a contributing systemic factor to the periodontitis. This medical evaluation should occur as part of the nonsurgical periodontal therapy. Another example would be that a patient who smokes should receive smoking cessation counseling.
4. Goal 4: To stabilize the attachment level
   A. The ultimate goal of nonsurgical periodontal therapy in chronic periodontitis patients is to stabilize the level of attachment by eliminating inflammation in the periodontium.
   B. Stabilization of the attachment level by eliminating inflammation involves control of all of the factors listed in the other goals of nonsurgical periodontal therapy.

Box 22-1. Goals of Nonsurgical Periodontal Therapy

Goal 1: To minimize the bacterial challenge to the patient
Goal 2: To eliminate or control local environmental risk factors for periodontal disease
Goal 3: To minimize the impact of systemic risk factors for periodontal disease
Goal 4: To stabilize the attachment level by eliminating inflammation

---

TYPES OF PROCEDURES INCLUDED IN NONSURGICAL THERAPY

Box 22-2 lists of some of the nonsurgical therapy procedures that the dental team may utilize for patients. The list of procedures that may be included in nonsurgical therapy is lengthy, but it should be evident that while some of the procedures are included in the treatment of all patients, other procedures are utilized only rarely. Since each patient presents unique treatment challenges, members of the dental team will need to customize the selection of the nonsurgical procedures included for each individual.

1. **Customized Self-Care Instructions.** One important aspect of nonsurgical periodontal therapy is effective daily self-care by the patient. Thus, patients need to be taught self-care skills and also be motivated to use those skills. These important topics are discussed in Chapters 23, 24, and 25.
2. **Instrumentation of Tooth Surfaces.** Periodontal instrumentation is always an important component of nonsurgical periodontal therapy. The thoroughness of the performance of this step can determine the overall success of nonsurgical periodontal therapy in most patients.
3. **Use of antimicrobial agents.** A variety of antimicrobial agents are available in the form of irrigation solutions and gel applications. Antimicrobial agents are discussed in Chapter 25.
4. **Correction of Local Contributing Factors.** Correction of local contributing factors such as overhanging margins on restorations or control of food impaction is a critical component of nonsurgical periodontal therapy in many patients. Local contributing factors are discussed in Chapter 16.

5. **Correction of Systemic Risk Factors.** Correction of systemic risk factors such as undiagnosed diabetes is also a critical component of nonsurgical periodontal therapy in some patients. This component often demands careful coordination of care with other healthcare providers such as physicians. Systemic risk factors are discussed in Chapter 15.

6. **Modulation of Host Defenses.** When indicated, modulation of host defenses can also be a component of nonsurgical periodontal therapy. Modulation of host defenses is discussed in Chapter 26.

Box 22-2. Procedures that May be Included in Nonsurgical Periodontal Therapy

1. Customized self-care instructions including
   a. Mechanical plaque biofilm control
   b. Chemical plaque biofilm control
2. Periodontal instrumentation of tooth surfaces
3. Use of antimicrobial agents
4. Correction of local contributing factors
5. Correction of systemic risk factors
6. Modulation of host defenses

TYPICAL TREATMENT PLANS FOR NONSURGICAL PERIODONTAL THERAPY

A treatment plan for nonsurgical therapy is a list of nonsurgical procedures or interventions that addresses a patient's periodontal health needs as identified during the periodontal assessment. Although it is critical for a treatment plan for nonsurgical therapy to meet the needs of each individual patient, beginning clinicians often find it helpful to view examples of typical treatment plans. A properly designed treatment plan for nonsurgical periodontal therapy could include procedures to be carried out *by the dental hygienist, by the dentist, or by the patient.*

1. **Examples of Typical Treatment Plans**
   A. **Plaque-Induced Gingivitis.** A typical plan for nonsurgical therapy for a patient with moderate plaque-induced gingivitis might include the following:
      1. Customized self-care instructions including patient education and motivation.
      2. Periodontal instrumentation (typically a dental prophylaxis in American Dental Association terminology).
      3. Elimination of plaque-retentive factors such as overhanging restorations, caries, or ill-fitting dental prostheses.
      4. Reevaluation of the patient's periodontal status.
         a. Response to nonsurgical therapy is normally delayed, since it takes some time for the body's defense mechanisms to respond to individual treatment steps.
         b. Because of this delay time in healing, the dental team is obligated to reevaluate the results of nonsurgical periodontal therapy after a period of healing to ensure that all appropriate measures have been included and to identify any other measures that might be needed.

c. It is wise for the dental team to include this reevaluation step in the plan for nonsurgical therapy, so that the patient has a clear understanding from the outset how future treatment decisions will be made.

B. **Slight to Moderate Chronic Periodontitis.** As already discussed, it is always important to customize the nonsurgical therapy for the needs of each patient, but again it may be helpful to look at a typical nonsurgical plan for a patient with slight to moderate chronic periodontitis. This typical plan might include the following:

1. Customized self-care instructions including patient education and motivation.
2. Periodontal instrumentation (typically scaling and root planing in American Dental Association terminology).
3. Control of local risk factors to include steps such as removal of overhanging restorations, restoration of caries, or minimizing excessive occlusal forces.
4. Correction of systemic risk factors to include steps such as smoking cessation counseling or referral for control of diabetes.
5. Reevaluation of patient's periodontal status.

C. **Severe Chronic Periodontitis.** Most patients with severe chronic periodontitis can include complicating factors such as advanced attachment loss, deep probing depths, advanced alveolar bone loss, furcation involvements, or mucogingival problems that require some more advanced treatment procedures later in therapy.

1. A typical treatment plan for nonsurgical therapy for a patient with severe chronic periodontitis would look much like a treatment plan for a patient with moderate periodontitis.
2. Periodontal surgery would not normally be part of a plan for the nonsurgical periodontal therapy, but the dental team would be wise to document the possible need for this more advanced treatment and inform the patient when the need for such treatment appears likely. This can avoid confusion on the part of the patient later in the therapy.
   a. The members of the dental team should be aware of the possible need for periodontal surgical intervention in patients with more advanced periodontitis.
   b. As the severity of periodontitis increases, it becomes more likely that some periodontal surgery will be needed to bring the disease under control.
   c. The need for periodontal surgical therapy should be reevaluated after the completion of nonsurgical periodontal therapy. Surgical periodontal therapy is discussed in Chapter 27.

Section 2
Instrumentation During Nonsurgical Therapy

OVERVIEW OF INSTRUMENTATION IN NONSURGICAL THERAPY

1. Objective of Periodontal Instrumentation During Nonsurgical Therapy
   A. The objective of the mechanical removal of calculus and plaque biofilm is the physical removal of microorganisms and their products to prevent and treat periodontal infections.
      1. Because of the structure of biofilms, physical removal of plaque biofilm is the most effective mechanism of control, though chemical agents are sometimes used to improve the patient response to these procedures.
      2. Most subgingival biofilm within pockets *cannot* be reached by brushes, floss, or antibacterial rinses.
         a. For this reason, frequent periodontal instrumentation of subgingival root surfaces to remove or disrupt plaque biofilms mechanically is an essential component of the treatment of most patients with periodontitis.
         b. In fact, periodontal instrumentation is likely to remain an important component of nonsurgical periodontal therapy for the foreseeable future.
   B. Removal of deposits from tooth surfaces is a critical component in any plan for nonsurgical periodontal therapy.
      1. Calculus deposits harbor living bacterial biofilms; thus, if the calculus remains, so do the bacteria, making it impossible to reestablish periodontal health.
      2. Calculus removal is always a fundamental part of nonsurgical periodontal therapy.
2. Evolving Instrumentation Terminology. There has been some evolution in the terminology associated with dental calculus and biofilm removal over the past years. The careful reader will be wise to note the terminology that appears in many dental hygiene journals and textbooks compared to the terminology in dental journals and textbooks. The differences in this terminology are described below.
   A. Traditional Instrumentation Terminology
      1. Scaling is instrumentation of the crown and root surfaces of the teeth to remove plaque biofilm, calculus, etc.
      2. A dental prophylaxis includes scaling and polishing procedures to remove coronal plaque biofilm, calculus, and stains. ***This procedure usually is used for healthy patients and patients with gingivitis.***
      3. Root planing is a treatment procedure designed to remove cementum or surface dentin that is rough, impregnated with calculus, or contaminated with toxins or microorganisms. Root planing is a fundamental treatment procedure for patients with chronic periodontitis.
         a. As traditionally described, root planing involves the routine, intentional removal of cementum and the instrumenting of all root surfaces to a glassy smooth texture.
         b. At one time it was thought that bacterial products were firmly held in cemental surfaces exposed by attachment loss occurring as a result of periodontitis. It was believed that vigorous root planing with intentional removal of most cementum was always needed to ensure the removal of all calculus as well as all bacterial products from the root surfaces.
         c. It is now understood that vigorous root planing is not universally needed to reestablish periodontal health in all sites of periodontitis. Rather than vigorous root planing and removal of most or all of the cementum, it is now known that the bacterial products can be removed from the root surfaces with a minimal amount of deliberate cementum removal.

B. Emerging Instrumentation Terminology
   1. Recently in the dental hygiene literature, increasing numbers of authors are using new terminology that reflects modern therapy better than the traditional terminology. The term "periodontal instrumentation" or "periodontal debridement" is suggested to replace the older terms "dental prophylaxis," "scaling," and "root planning."
   2. **Periodontal instrumentation** (periodontal debridement) is defined as the removal or disruption of plaque biofilm, its by-products, and biofilm-retentive calculus deposits from coronal tooth surfaces and tooth root surfaces to the extent needed to reestablish periodontal health and restore a balance between the bacterial flora and the host's immune responses.
   3. Periodontal instrumentation includes instrumentation of every square millimeter of root surface for removal of plaque biofilm and calculus but does not include the deliberate, aggressive removal of cementum.
      a. Conservation of cementum is one goal of periodontal instrumentation. It is currently believed that conservation of cementum enhances periodontal healing in the form of either repair or regeneration. In periodontal health an important function of cementum is to attach the periodontal ligament fibers to the root surface. During the healing process after disease, cementum is thought to contribute to repair of the periodontium.
      b. During periodontal instrumentation, the extent of instrumentation should be limited to that needed to obtain a favorable tissue response. Root surfaces should be instrumented only to a level that results in resolution of tissue inflammation in the periodontal tissues.
C. Considerations Regarding Emerging Terminology and Insurance Codes
   1. Insurance codes are numeric codes to identify different dental procedures. The most important use of codes is for insurance billing purposes. Insurance codes are entered on insurance forms indicating the dental treatment listed by the appropriate procedure code number. In the United States, insurance codes are published in the *American Dental Association Current Dental Terminology*. These codes are very specific and should be reviewed carefully before specific dental treatment is coded.
   2. The ADA Current Dental Terminology continues to use the traditional terms "prophylaxis" and "scaling and root planing" to describe periodontal instrumentation. This difference in terminology can be confusing to clinicians.
      a. Although the term periodontal instrumentation/debridement as defined in the dental hygiene literature may describe modern periodontal therapy better than older terms, this terminology has not yet replaced the older terms as recognized by the ADA. For this reason, many dentists have been reluctant to embrace the new terminology without changes in ADA codes.
      b. Some authors and clinicians have redefined the term "root planing," so that its meaning is similar to that of periodontal instrumentation/debridement. This approach of redefining the term root planing can be confusing, however, because it is difficult to determine which definition of "root planing" any one person is using.
      c. At this time, *dental team members should use the currently accepted insurance codes when filling out insurance forms and in communications with insurance companies or other third-party payers.*

END POINT FOR INSTRUMENTATION DURING NONSURGICAL THERAPY

The end point of periodontal instrumentation is to return the tissues of the periodontium to a state of health. In this context health means periodontal tissues that are free of inflammation.

1. Healing Following Nonsurgical Instrumentation
   A. After thorough periodontal instrumentation, some healing of the periodontal tissues will normally occur.
      1. The primary type of healing in a site of attachment loss after periodontal instrumentation is through the formation of a long junctional epithelium.
         a. As inflammation in the periodontium resolves, epithelial cells can readapt to the root surface as shown in Figure 22-1.
         b. This adaptation of the epithelial cells to the root surface is referred to as a long junctional epithelium.
      2. It is important to realize that following periodontal instrumentation, there normally is *no formation of new alveolar bone, new cementum, or new periodontal ligament.*

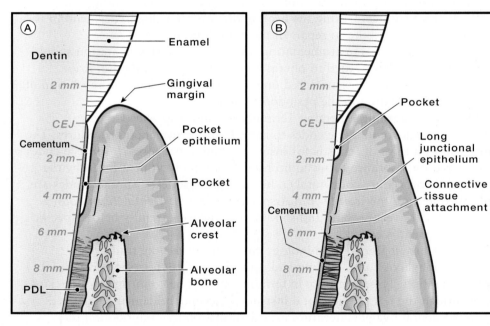

Figure 22-1. Healing after Nonsurgical Periodontal Instrumentation. A: Before therapy, the periodontal pocket has a probing depth of 6 mm. **B:** After periodontal therapy the tissue healing is through the formation of a long junctional epithelium. This results in a probing depth of 3 mm. Note that there is no formation of new bone, cementum, or periodontal ligament during the healing process that occurs after periodontal instrumentation in this example.

   B. Clinically, nonsurgical periodontal therapy, including instrumentation, may certainly result in reduced probing depths. Figure 22-2 shows examples of various soft tissue responses to thorough periodontal instrumentation.
      1. The reduced probing depths result from the formation of a long junctional epithelium combined in many instances with resolution of gingival edema that is usually a part of the inflammatory process. Figure 22-3 shows how some of this reduction in probing depth can occur at the base of a periodontal pocket.

2. Thus, one important clinical feature to monitor following periodontal instrumentation in addition to clinical attachment loss is the probing depths.

3. It should be noted at this point that there are other clinical signs that can correlate with inflammation that can be expected to change following periodontal instrumentation (i.e., bleeding on probing).

2. **Assessing Tissue Healing.** Tissue healing does not occur overnight, and in many patients it is not possible to assess the true tissue response for at least 1 month after the completion of periodontal instrumentation. Assessing tissue healing during and following nonsurgical therapy is discussed in Section 3 of this chapter.

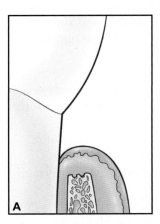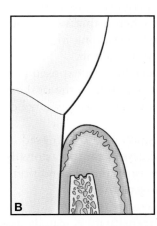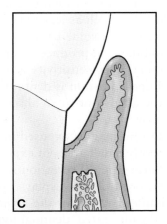

Figure 22-2. Soft Tissue Responses to Thorough Periodontal Instrumentation. This figure shows some of the possible tissue changes that can occur following thorough periodontal debridement of a root surface. **A:** There can be complete resolution of the inflammation resulting in shrinkage of the tissue and a shallow probing depth. **B:** There can be readaptation of the tissues to the root surface forming a long junctional epithelium resulting in shallow probing depths. **C:** There can be very little change in the level of the soft tissues resulting in a residual periodontal pocket.

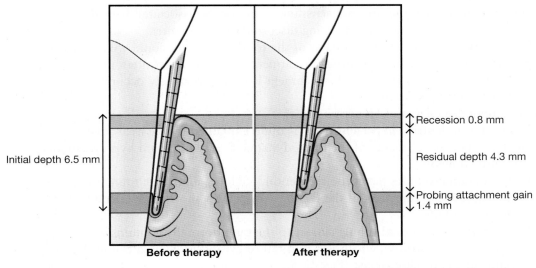

Initial depth 6.5 mm

Recession 0.8 mm

Residual depth 4.3 mm

Probing attachment gain 1.4 mm

Before therapy After therapy

Figure 22-3. Details of Healing at the Base of a Pocket Following Periodontal Instrumentation. Since the tip of a periodontal probe can easily penetrate inflamed soft tissue in the base of periodontal pocket, the probing depth can decrease a small amount following instrumentation because the tissues at the base of the pocket can be much more resistant to accidental penetration by the probe. This figure also depicts slight gingival recession resulting from resolution of inflammation in the tissue.

DENTINAL HYPERSENSITIVITY ASSOCIATED WITH NONSURGICAL THERAPY

Dentinal hypersensitivity as described in this section is not really a periodontal disease or a periodontal condition. However, dentinal hypersensitivity appears so frequently during successful nonsurgical periodontal therapy that clinicians need to be aware of this condition, need to understand its origin and need to understand therapies for the condition.

1. Description of Dental Hypersensitivity
   A. **Dentinal hypersensitivity** is a short, sharp, painful reaction that occurs when areas of exposed dentin are subjected to mechanical, thermal, or chemical stimuli. For example, an individual might experience sensitivity while brushing, when eating cold foods such as ice cream, or when eating sweet, sour, or acidic food such as grapefruit. In some patients simply breathing in cold air while walking outside on a cold day can produce this painful reaction.
   B. Dentinal hypersensitivity is associated with exposed dentin.
      1. Exposed dentin is dentin that is visible in the oral cavity due to the recession of the gingiva or to an absence of some tooth enamel due to damage to the tooth crown.
      2. Dentin may be exposed in a small area or exposed in an extensive area of a tooth; small areas of exposed dentin can occasionally lead to severe pain.
      3. Since gingival recession is a very common condition, it is fortunate that not all exposed dentin displays hypersensitivity.
2. Precipitating Factors for the Hypersensitivity
   A. As already stated, dentinal hypersensitivity is usually associated with gingival recession, though exposure of dentin can also result because of tooth fracture or destruction of enamel.
   B. Resolution of inflammation in the periodontium following successful nonsurgical periodontal therapy in periodontitis patients frequently results in gingival recession that is related to resolution of the inflammatory swelling of the gingiva. This exposure of small areas of the tooth roots can result in dentinal hypersensitivity.
   C. It is common for dentinal hypersensitivity to appear following some types of periodontal surgical therapy, but sensitivity can also be associated with the nonsurgical periodontal therapy being discussed in this chapter.
   D. In the patient's eyes the development of the tooth sensitivity could well appear to be simply a result of the nonsurgical treatment. In reality most often the sensitivity results from areas where clinical attachment loss has previously occurred as a result of existing periodontitis.
3. Theory About the Origin of Hypersensitivity
   A. The origin of dentinal hypersensitivity is often explained by the hydrodynamic theory. Important elements of the hydrodynamic theory of dental hypersensitivity are outlined below.
      1. The **dentinal tubules** penetrate the dentin like long, miniature tunnels extending throughout the thickness of the dentin. Figure 22-4 shows some details of these dentinal tubules.
      2. The part of a dentinal tubule closest to the pulp normally contains an **odontoblastic process**, which is a thin tail of cytoplasm from a cell in the tooth pulp called an odontoblast (Fig. 22-5).
      3. The part of a dentinal tubule not filled by an odontoblastic process is filled by fluids. Stimulation of the root surface may result in fluid flow within the tubules which is theorized to activate the nerve endings near the pulp leading to a painful

sensation experienced by the patient. The stimulation of the surface of the tooth root can arise from mechanical, thermal, or chemical stimuli, as already mentioned.

4. When dentinal tubules are exposed slowly in the oral cavity (as seen in the development of most gingival recession), root surfaces can undergo a natural process of calcification or occlusion (blocking) of the open dentinal tubules; the sealing of the dentinal tubules in this natural process prevents sensitivity from developing. Dentin with calcified tubules has been referred to as sclerosed dentin.

5. In addition, slow exposure of a tooth root can allow for secondary dentin formation within the pulp. Secondary dentin formation can in effect thicken the dentin layer.

6. The occlusion or blocking of dentinal tubules does not always occur, and sometimes the occlusion of the tubules occurs very slowly.

B. Dentinal hypersensitivity may arise following instrumentation during periodontal instrumentation.

1. It should be noted that most dentinal hypersensitivity resulting following periodontal instrumentation is mild and resolves within a few weeks *if the exposed root surfaces are kept biofilm free by thorough self-care.*

2. In its more severe forms, however, dentinal hypersensitivity can result in so much discomfort that it can prevent a patient from performing thorough self-care.

3. It is fortunate that most commonly instrumentation of root surfaces does not result in the development of dentinal hypersensitivity.

4. Sensitivity may not occur in some instances because instrumentation of root surfaces can result in a smear layer of dentin that covers the root surfaces and blocks the tubules.

5. This so-called **smear layer** refers to crystalline debris from the tooth surface that covers or plugs the dentinal tubules during the instrumentation; this smear layer blocks the tubules, inhibits fluid flow, and prevents the development of sensitivity.

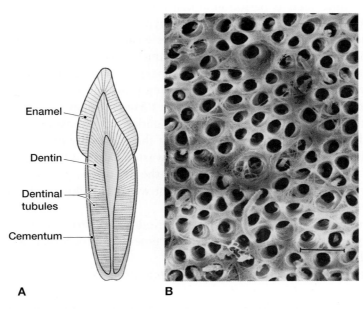

Enamel

Dentin

Dentinal tubules

Cementum

A   **B**

Figure 22-4. Dentinal Tubules. A: Diagram showing the numerous dentinal tubules that penetrate the dentin. **B:** A scanning electron micrograph of the cross section of dentinal tubules adjacent to the pulp chamber of a human tooth. The black line engraved in the lower right is 10 μm long. (Used by permission from Melfi RC. *Permar's Oral Embryology and Microscopic Anatomy.* 10th ed. Philadelphia, PA: Lippincott Williams & Wilkins; 2000:120, Figure 5–8.)

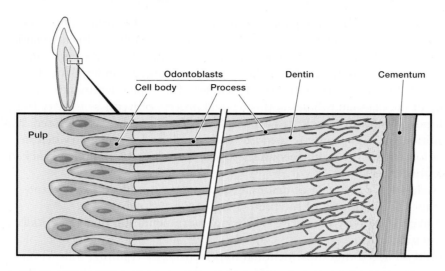

Figure 22-5. Odontoblastic Process. The odontoblastic cell process in the dentinal tubule often fills the part of the dentinal tubule closest to the pulp but can extend farther from the pulp toward the junction of the dentin with the enamel or cementum.

4. **Strategies for Managing Patients with Dentinal Hypersensitivity**
   There are a number of strategies that have been recommended for dealing with dentinal hypersensitivity. These strategies range from simply allowing the open dentinal tubules to seal themselves to performing periodontal surgery. Each of the strategies has proved successful for some patients.
   A. **Periodontal Instrumentation in Patients with Existing Dental Hypersensitivity**
      1. For teeth with existing dentinal hypersensitivity, instrumentation of hypersensitive root surfaces can result in eliciting the sharp pain during a clinical procedure such as periodontal instrumentation.
      2. Since many patients have existing dentinal hypersensitivity, it is critical for dental hygienists to ask patients about hypersensitive teeth before attempting a clinical procedure such as periodontal instrumentation.
      3. For patients with existing hypersensitivity, local anesthesia can be used to control any discomfort that might arise during thorough instrumentation.
   B. **Patient Education—A Critical Element in Patient Management**
      An appropriate strategy for managing patients undergoing nonsurgical periodontal therapy would include educating patients about the possibility of developing hypersensitivity following the procedure. This warning should be given before beginning any treatment and should be part of the discussion preceding informed consent. It may be helpful to provide the patient with the following facts before initiating instrumentation:
      1. Sensitivity to cold can increase following periodontal instrumentation.
      2. If sensitivity resulting from periodontal instrumentation occurs, it will usually gradually disappear over a few weeks.
      3. *Thorough daily plaque biofilm removal during self-care is one of the most important factors in the prevention and control of sensitivity.* It should be noted that without meticulous self-care, treatments for dentinal hypersensitivity are usually not successful.
      4. If dentinal hypersensitivity becomes an ongoing problem, recommendations for in-home therapies can be made that can enhance its resolution, but immediate results should not be expected.

C. **Occluding Patent (Open) Dentinal Tubules with In-Home Therapies**
   1. One important strategy for managing patients with dentinal hypersensitivity involves applying chemicals to the exposed root surface that can help occlude (or block) the dentinal tubules.
   2. The chemicals used to occlude the dentinal tubules often eliminate or minimize associated sensitivity. The mechanism of action of these chemicals has been reported to be precipitating minerals or precipitating proteins within open dentinal tubules resulting in sealing the openings of the tubules.
   3. Many of these chemical agents are available in special formulations of toothpastes, and there are a variety of toothpastes specifically formulated to aid in desensitizing teeth (8–12). Many chemical agents have been reported to help in some patients. Examples of some of the more common chemical agents in toothpaste formulations for dentinal hypersensitivity are potassium nitrate, strontium chloride, sodium citrate, and fluorides. Table 22-1 includes an overview of some of the chemical agents that have been investigated for control of hypersensitivity by blocking dentinal tubules.
   4. The reported efficacy of the chemical agents in controlling dentinal hypersensitivity varies, but this strategy remains the most commonly utilized treatment for this condition.
D. **Occluding Patent Tubules with In-Office Therapies**
   1. There are also professionally applied in-office products that contain chemicals that also have been reported to decrease dentinal hypersensitivity.
   2. A variety of chemical agents have been utilized in in-office remedies for dentinal hypersensitivity. Examples of chemicals that have been reported to decrease hypersensitivity following in-office applications are potassium oxalate, ferric oxalate, and fluorides solutions, or fluoride varnishes.
   3. Note that Table 22-1 includes an overview of some of the chemical agents that have been investigated for control of hypersensitivity by blocking dentinal tubules.
E. **Desensitizing Nerves Associated with the Tubules**
   It has also been reported that applying certain chemicals to the root surface can block the nerve receptors in or near the tooth pulp from activating the painful response.
   1. The chemical agents that can be used to block the nerve receptors from activating a painful response include potassium salts (such as potassium nitrate); potassium nitrate is the active ingredient found in some desensitizing toothpastes and has been shown to be effective in decreasing sensitivity in some patients.
   2. It is thought that potassium depolarizes the nerve fibers associated with the odontoblastic processes, thus preventing pain signals from traveling to the brain.
F. **Treating Exposed Dentin Surfaces with Lasers**
   1. Lasers have been used to treat exposed hypersensitive dentin surfaces with some success.
   2. The mechanism of action of lasers in decreasing dentinal hypersensitivity is not clear at this point.
G. **Blocking Dentinal Tubules with Restorative Materials**
   1. One strategy for blocking some dentinal tubules is to cover the exposed dentin surface with a bonding agent—the same kinds of materials that can sometimes be used to restore caries.
   2. Since the exposure of dentin at some sites can be associated with missing tooth structure resulting from abrasion or erosion of the root surface, bonding a restorative material over that surface can not only block exposed dentinal tubules, it can also restore any missing tooth structure.

3. Examples of restorative materials that have been used to block dentinal tubules include: oxalic acid and resin, glass ionomer cements, composites, and dentin bonding agents.

H. **Blocking Dentinal Tubules with a Periodontal Surgical Procedure**
   1. Another strategy for blocking the open dentinal tubules is to cover the root surface with a gingival grafting material.
   2. This approach can result in rebuilding the gingiva to a more natural level that covers an exposed tooth root, covering the dentinal tubules.

I. **Overview of Dentinal Hypersensitivity**
   1. Figure 22-6 illustrates the wide range of possibilities for dentinal tubules that become exposed in the oral cavity.
   2. Figure 22-7 illustrates the various possibilities for dentinal tubules following therapy.
   3. Table 22-1 provides an overview of chemical agents that have been investigated for the control of dentinal hypersensitivity by occluding dentinal tubules.

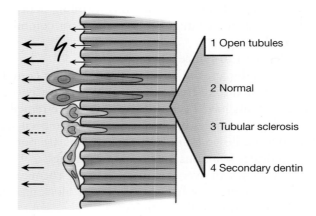

Figure 22-6. The Various Possibilities for Dentinal Tubules Before Therapy and Following Therapy. Dentinal tubules prior to therapy may be open, sclerosed, or insulated from the pulp itself by the formation of secondary dentin.

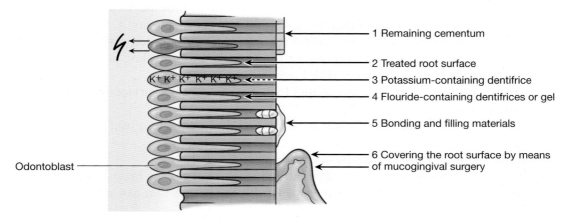

Figure 22-7. The Various Possibilities for Dentinal Tubules Following Therapy. Chemicals can be used to occlude the dentinal tubules and to eliminate or minimize associated dentinal sensitivity.

TABLE 22-1. OVERVIEW OF AGENTS THAT HAVE BEEN INVESTIGATED FOR THE CONTROL OF HYPERSENSITIVITY BY OCCLUDING DENTINAL TUBULES

Agents that can precipitate proteins that can occlude tubules

- Glutaraldehyde
- Silver nitrate
- Zinc chloride
- Strontium chloride

Agents that can precipitate minerals that can occlude dentinal tubules

- Sodium fluoride
- Stannous fluoride
- Strontium chloride
- Potassium oxalate
- Calcium phosphate
- Calcium carbonate
- Arginine
- Bioactive glass

Section 3
Decisions Following Nonsurgical Therapy

THE REEVALUATION APPOINTMENT

Reevaluation refers to a formal step after the completion of nonsurgical therapy. During the reevaluation appointment, the members of the dental team perform another periodontal assessment to gather information about the patient's periodontal status. After comparison with the periodontal status at the time of the initial assessment, the team members make several critical clinical decisions regarding management of the patient's periodontal condition. The reevaluation is described in detail below.

1. Timing of a Reevaluation
    A. Periodontal tissue healing does not occur immediately, and in most cases it is not possible to determine the true tissue response for at least 1 month after the completion of nonsurgical periodontal therapy.
    B. Members of the dental team should usually schedule an appointment for a reevaluation of a chronic periodontitis patient 4 to 6 weeks after completion of nonsurgical therapy.

2. Understanding the Steps in a Reevaluation
    The steps in a typical reevaluation appointment usually include those listed below (Box 22-3).
    A. The first step in the reevaluation appointment is to do a medical status update for the patient. Of course, this is the first step in any patient appointment.
    B. The second step is to perform a thorough periodontal assessment; the nature of a periodontal assessment has already been described in Chapter 19.

C. The third step is to do a comparison of the results of the patient's initial periodontal assessment with the results of the patient's reevaluation assessment.

D. The fourth step is to make appropriate decisions related to the next steps in therapy. Options for treatment following nonsurgical therapy are discussed in the next section.

Box 22-3. Steps in a Typical Reevaluation Appointment

1. Update the medical status of the patient.
2. Perform a periodontal clinical assessment.
3. Compare the initial periodontal assessment with the reevaluation assessment.
4. Make decisions related to the next steps in periodontal therapy.

OPTIONS FOR TREATMENT FOLLOWING REEVALUATION

1. **Managing Nonresponsive Disease Sites.** During the reevaluation, members of the dental team may identify nonresponsive disease sites.
   A. **Nonresponsive disease sites** are areas in the periodontium that show deeper probing depths, continuing loss of attachment, or continuing clinical signs of inflammation in spite of the nonsurgical therapy provided.
   B. Nonresponsive sites should be carefully rechecked for thoroughness of self-care and rechecked for the presence of residual calculus deposits.
   C. If plaque biofilm is discovered at a nonresponsive site, the site should be thoroughly deplaqued with an ultrasonic instrument (unless ultrasonic instrumentation is contraindicated for this patient), and the patient should receive additional self-care motivation and training.
   D. If calculus is found at a nonresponsive site, additional periodontal instrumentation should be performed.
   E. When nonresponsive sites are encountered, the members of the dental team should also consider the possibility that other factors might be contributing to the disease process (such as undiagnosed diabetes or smoking).
   F. In some patients, the nonresponsive disease sites may also require the use of antimicrobial agents.
   G. Some nonresponsive sites represent areas of more advanced destruction from the disease process that will need more advanced care such as periodontal surgery.
2. **Performing Additional Nonsurgical Therapy.** It is common for the reevaluation step to indicate the need for additional nonsurgical periodontal therapy by the dental team, and there are several reasons for this.
   A. Self-care efforts by the patient, though improved, may not be adequate for control of inflammation in the periodontium.
   B. Subgingival calculus deposits are difficult to remove especially in the presence of inflammation resulting in edematous tissue.
   C. An unsuspected systemic condition may be contributing to the disease process.
3. **Establishing a Program for Periodontal Maintenance**
   A. Following appropriate treatment, all patients with periodontitis should be placed on a program of periodontal maintenance.

B. Periodontal maintenance includes all measures used by the dental team and the patient to keep periodontitis under control; periodontal maintenance is discussed in Chapters 30 and 31.

C. The goal of periodontal maintenance is to prevent the recurrence of periodontal diseases.

4. Recognizing the Need for Periodontal Surgery

A. The need for some types of periodontal surgery can often be determined at the time of the initial periodontal assessment.

B. Periodontal surgery to control chronic periodontitis or to regenerate damaged periodontal tissues, however, is frequently best identified at the time of the reevaluation; periodontal surgery and its indications are discussed in Chapter 27.

HOW REEVALUATION OF NONSURGICAL THERAPY RELATES TO OTHER STEPS IN TREATMENT

Figure 22-8 illustrates how reevaluation of nonsurgical periodontal therapy relates to the other steps in the overall management of a periodontal patient.

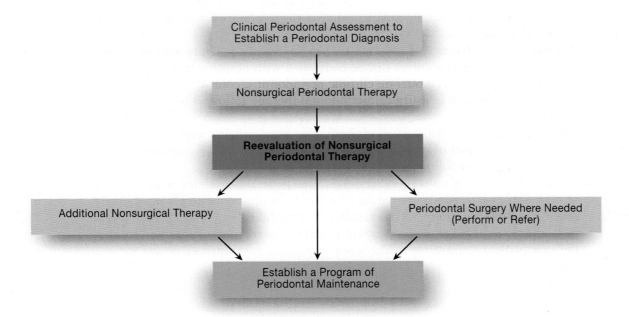

Figure 22-8. Diagram illustrating how reevaluation of nonsurgical periodontal therapy relates to other steps in the overall management of a periodontal patient. Reevaluation of nonsurgical therapy would be performed following the therapy. Decisions made at the reevaluation will primarily involve additional nonsurgical therapy, periodontal surgery, and periodontal maintenance. Periodontal surgery and periodontal maintenance are discussed in Chapters 27, 30, and 31.

THE RELATIONSHIP BETWEEN NONSURGICAL THERAPY AND PERIODONTAL SURGERY

Periodontal surgery can play an important role in therapy for certain patients, and this topic will be discussed in other chapters of this textbook. However, at the time of reevaluation members of the dental team should be aware of the general relationship between nonsurgical periodontal therapy and periodontal surgery and should be able to discuss the possible need for periodontal surgery with patients.

1. **Indications for Surgical Therapy.** As a general rule, periodontal surgery will be needed by patients with more advanced periodontal conditions. Table 22-2 shows an overview of the general relationship of nonsurgical periodontal therapy to surgical periodontal treatment for patients with various periodontal conditions.
   A. **Patients with plaque-induced gingivitis.** For most patients with plaque-induced gingivitis, the gingivitis can be controlled with nonsurgical therapy alone, and only rarely will periodontal surgery be a part of the treatment recommended.
   B. **Patients with slight periodontitis.** For most patients with slight (mild) chronic periodontitis, the periodontitis can be controlled with nonsurgical therapy alone, and only occasionally will periodontal surgery be a part of the treatment recommended.
   C. **Patients with Moderate Chronic Periodontitis.** For some patients with moderate periodontitis, the periodontitis can be controlled with nonsurgical therapy alone. For other patients with moderate chronic periodontitis, control of the periodontitis will require thorough nonsurgical periodontal therapy followed by periodontal surgery.
   D. **Patients with Severe Chronic Periodontitis.** For most patients with severe periodontitis, control of the periodontitis will require thorough nonsurgical periodontal therapy followed by periodontal surgery.
2. **Exceptions.** There will always be exceptions to the general guidelines described above.
   A. One example of an exception would be a patient with moderate plaque-induced gingivitis where the gingivitis has resulted in gingival enlargement. It is common for some types of gingival enlargement to require periodontal surgery to reshape the enlargement to improve aesthetics or to provide for improved access for effective self-care.

TABLE 22-2. INDICATIONS FOR NONSURGICAL AND SURGICAL THERAPY

Disease Status	Nonsurgical Therapy	Surgical Therapy
Plaque-associated gingivitis	Always indicated	Usually not indicated
Slight chronic periodontitis	Always indicated	Usually not indicated
Moderate chronic periodontitis	Always indicated	Sometimes indicated
Severe chronic periodontitis	Always indicated	Usually indicated

B. Another example of an exception to the guidelines would be a patient with slight chronic periodontitis accompanied by severe gingival recession on a tooth. Though surgery is not normally needed in patients with slight chronic periodontitis, periodontal surgery may well be needed to correct the gingival recession.

Chapter Summary Statement

Nonsurgical periodontal therapy refers to all the initial steps used by the dental team to bring gingivitis and periodontitis under control. The goals of nonsurgical periodontal therapy are to control the bacterial challenge to the patient, to minimize the impact of systemic risk factors, to eliminate or control local environmental risk factors, and to stabilize the attachment level. The precise steps included in nonsurgical periodontal therapy should depend on the specific needs of each individual patient.

A vital component of a plan for nonsurgical periodontal therapy is periodontal instrumentation. Biofilms are resistant to topical chemical control; therefore, mechanical periodontal instrumentation of subgingival root surfaces is an essential component of successful nonsurgical periodontal therapy. Dentinal hypersensitivity may occur in some areas of exposed dentin. Thorough daily self-care is the most important factor in the prevention and control of hypersensitivity, but some patients with dentinal hypersensitivity will need additional measures.

Reevaluation is an important step in nonsurgical periodontal therapy. During reevaluation the dental team determines the patient's need for additional nonsurgical therapy or periodontal surgery and establishes a program for periodontal maintenance.

Section 4
Focus on Patients

Clinical Patient Care

CASE 1

A new patient for your dental team has obvious clinical signs of moderate chronic periodontitis with generalized plaque biofilm and dental calculus deposits. Though the patient denies having diabetes, the patient does report having several close family members with this disease. Make a list of steps your dental team might include in an appropriate plan for nonsurgical periodontal therapy for this new patient.

CASE 2

At the time of reevaluation for a patient with a diagnosis of generalized moderate chronic periodontitis, your dental team identifies a few sites of residual subgingival calculus deposits and documents totally ineffective patient self-care. How should the members of your dental team manage the oral health needs of this patient?

CASE 3

One of your patients who has been undergoing nonsurgical periodontal therapy seems a bit upset when he comes in another appointment. After being seated in your treatment room, he states that he gets a sharp pain in his teeth when he tries to eat his favorite desert, ice cream. How should you proceed based upon the patient's complaint?

Ethical Dilemma

You are a retired librarian who just recently lost your husband. You grew up, went to college, married and raised a family all in the same town in which you were born. You are fortunate to be surrounded by many family members and long-time friends.

You are currently a patient in Dr. J. Jay Mack's periodontal practice, and have been for the last 15 or so years. You see Evelyn, the older of the two hygienists in the practice, every 3 months, and have so since you can remember. The only supplemental aids she has suggested that you use, in addition to toothbrushing, are "tufted floss and a tongue scraper."

You are very active in your church and community. At your weekly bridge club gathering, a number of the other participants mention that they also are patients in Dr. Mack's practice. Further discussions revealed that all the patients who saw Evelyn were instructed to use tufted floss and tongue scrapers, for their self-care. However, those patients who saw Anne, the younger hygienist, were instructed to use a variety of self-care aids. It sounds like Anne recommends different aids based on each individual patient's needs. Your bridge partner, Florence who also sees Evelyn, the hygienist, says her teeth are very sensitive to hot, cold, and sweets, yet has only been instructed and educated in the use of tufted floss and a tongue scraper as well.

You wonder why so many patients with differing needs receive the same instructions from the dental hygienist, Evelyn.

1. What ethical principles are in conflict in this dilemma?
2. Should you meet with Dr. Mack to discuss your concerns?
3. How should this ethical dilemma be handled?

References

1. Badersten, A., R. Nilveus, and J. Egelberg, Effect of nonsurgical periodontal therapy. I. Moderately advanced periodontitis. *J Clin Periodontol,* 1981. 8(1): p. 57-72.
2. Cobb, C.M., Clinical significance of non-surgical periodontal therapy: an evidence-based perspective of scaling and root planing. *J Clin Periodontol,* 2002. 29 Suppl 2: p. 6-16.
3. Greenstein, G., Nonsurgical periodontal therapy in 2000: a literature review. *J Am Dent Assoc,* 2000. 131(11): p. 1580-92.
4. Lowenguth, R.A. and G. Greenstein, Clinical and microbiological response to nonsurgical mechanical periodontal therapy. *Periodontol 2000,* 1995. 9: p. 14-22.
5. Stambaugh, R.V., et al., The limits of subgingival scaling. *Int J Periodontics Restorative Dent,* 1981. 1(5): p. 30-41.
6. Drisko, C.H., Nonsurgical periodontal therapy. *Periodontol 2000,* 2001. 25: p. 77-88.
7. Rabbani, G.M., M.M. Ash, Jr., and R.G. Caffesse, The effectiveness of subgingival scaling and root planing in calculus removal. *J Periodontol,* 1981. 52(3): p. 119-23.
8. Kimura, Y., et al., Treatment of dentine hypersensitivity by lasers: a review. *J Clin Periodontol,* 2000. 27(10): p. 715-21.
9. Li, R., et al., Efficacy of a desensitizing toothpaste containing arginine and calcium carbonate on dentin surface pore structure and dentin morphology. *Am J Dent,* 2012. 25(4): p. 210-4.

10. Li, Y., Innovations for combating dentin hypersensitivity: current state of the art. *Compend Contin Educ Dent,* 2012. 33 Spec No 2: p. 10-6.

11. Schwarz, F., et al., Desensitizing effects of an Er:YAG laser on hypersensitive dentine. *J Clin Periodontol,* 2002. 29(3): p. 211-5.

12. Verma, S.K., et al., Laser in dentistry: An innovative tool in modern dental practice. *Natl J Maxillofac Surg,* 2012. 3(2): p. 124-32.

 STUDENT ANCILLARY RESOURCES

A wide variety of resources to enhance your learning and understanding of this chapter are available on thePoint®.

- Visit thePoint to access:
  - Audio Glossary
  - Animations
  - Suggested Readings
  - Answers to Review Questions
  - Case Studies

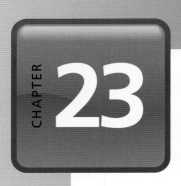

CHAPTER

23

Patient's Role in Nonsurgical Periodontal Therapy

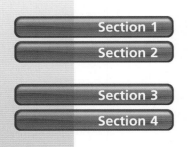
Clinical Application.
For nearly every patient with periodontal disease, the patient plays a major role in nonsurgical periodontal therapy through the patient's own efforts at self-care. Sometimes the self-care techniques required for a patient with periodontitis are far more complicated than the self-care efforts required by a patient with a healthy periodontium. Self-care for a periodontal patient must accommodate changes in the periodontium due to disease—examples of such changes include open embrasure spaces, exposure of root concavities, and attachment loss. This chapter provides guidance for clinicians in both selecting appropriate self-care techniques and training patients with periodontal disease in appropriate self-care.

Learning Objectives

• In a classroom or laboratory setting, explain the criteria for selection and correctly demonstrate the use of the following to an instructor: power toothbrush and interdental aids presented in this chapter.

• Explain why interdental care is of special importance for a patient with periodontitis.

• In a clinical setting, recommend, explain, and demonstrate appropriate interdental aids to a patient with type III embrasure spaces. Assist the patient in selecting an appropriate interdental aid that the patient is willing to use on a daily basis.

• Explain how the presence of exposed root concavities in a dentition would influence your selection of effective self-care aids.

• State the rationale for tongue cleaning and, in the clinical setting, recommend and teach tongue cleaning to an appropriate patient.

Key Terms

Cotherapist
Volatile sulfur compounds

Gingival embrasure space (types I, II, III)
Root concavity

Section 1
Patient Self-Care in Nonsurgical Therapy

Nonsurgical periodontal therapy includes all nonsurgical treatment and educational measures used to help control gingivitis and periodontitis, such as patient self-care, periodontal instrumentation, and chemical plaque control.

1. **Patient as Cotherapist.** Because the primary etiologic factor for periodontitis is plaque biofilm, much of nonsurgical periodontal therapy must be directed toward its daily control by the patient.

   A. Successful nonsurgical periodontal therapy always involves the patient in an intensive training program on self-care techniques.

   B. The patient's efforts at self-care are so critical to the control of periodontitis that some dental teams refer to the patient as having the role of cotherapist in the process of nonsurgical periodontal therapy.

      1. This concept of the patient as cotherapist is used to underscore the vital role the patient plays in establishing control of periodontitis.

      2. The patient should be actively involved in making decisions about his or her own health care and be willing to make a long-term commitment to meticulous self-care and regular professional care.

   C. Mechanical biofilm removal includes self-care efforts by the patient on a daily basis and subgingival periodontal instrumentation by the dental hygienist at regular intervals.

2. **Self-Care**

   A. **What is Self-Care?** There is no single accepted definition of self-care. According to one medical dictionary, it is the personal care performed by the patient usually in collaboration with and after instruction by a healthcare professional (1). This may include activities related to both disease prevention and health maintenance.

      1. Self-care involves instruction on the use and frequency of a product. For example, suggesting the addition of a product such as interdental aid to the daily routine.

      2. Self-care includes collaboration between the dental hygienist and the patient.

         a. The dental hygienist needs to provide input and support while at the same time encouraging patient participation in the final decision on self-care devices.

         b. The optimal device must take patient preference into consideration. Recommending a device that the clinician likes, but that the patient dislikes will not contribute to patient motivation and compliance.

         c. Collaboration hinges on good communication, so the dental hygienist needs to provide education and instruction using words that the patient understands.

   B. **Goals of Self-Care.** The goal of self-care is improved oral health via optimal biofilm removal and the elimination of bleeding and inflammation.

   C. **Self-Care Aids Employed in Biofilm Control**

      1. Toothbrushing is the most frequently used aid for biofilm removal. Unfortunately, it is often the only used device by most patients for daily self-care. *Interdental aids are necessary for most patients and critical for periodontal maintenance patients as the interdental area is generally not accessible to toothbrushing* (2).

      2. Tongue cleaning on a daily basis helps control halitosis and may contribute to a healthy periodontal environment.

Section 2
Self-Care Challenges for Patients with Periodontitis

1. **Anatomical Challenges for the Patient with Periodontitis.** Due to attachment loss, the dentition of an individual with periodontitis often presents anatomical challenges to effective biofilm control, such as recession of the gingival margin, type of embrasure spaces and exposed root concavities.

   A. **Gingival Embrasure Spaces.** The **gingival embrasure space** is the small triangular open space (apical to the contact area) between the curved proximal surfaces of two teeth. The three types of embrasure spaces are shown in Figures 23-1 to 23-3.

      1. In health, the interdental papilla fills the gingival embrasure space. Dental floss is effective in areas of normal gingival contour.

      2. *The tissue destruction characterized by periodontitis usually results in an interdental papilla that is reduced in height or missing, resulting in an open embrasure space. Dental floss is not effective in areas with open embrasure spaces.*

      3. Analysis of the gingival embrasure spaces is critical in determining which interdental aid is likely to be most effective in control of plaque biofilms. Table 23-1 summarizes aids for interdental biofilm removal.

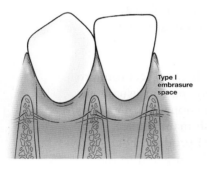

Figure 23-1. Type I Embrasure—Space Filled by the Interdental Papilla. For the patient with excellent self-care compliance and good manual dexterity, dental floss is an effective means of biofilm control.

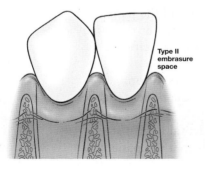

Figure 23-2. Type II Embrasure—Height of Interdental Papilla is Reduced. Interdental brushes and wooden toothpicks are effective means of biofilm control.

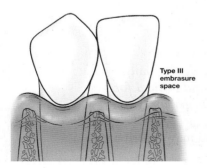

Figure 23-3. Type III Embrasure—the Interdental Papilla is Missing. Interdental brushes and end-tuft brushes are effective means of biofilm control.

B. **Exposed Root Concavities.** A root concavity is a trench-like depression in the root surface. Root concavities commonly occur on the proximal surfaces of anterior and posterior teeth and the facial and lingual surfaces of molar teeth.

1. In health, root concavities are covered with alveolar bone and help to secure the tooth in the bone.
2. Periodontitis results in the apical migration of the junctional epithelium, loss of connective tissue, and destruction of alveolar bone. This tissue destruction results in the exposure of root concavities to the oral environment (either in the presence of tissue recession or, frequently, within a periodontal pocket).
3. Figure 23-4 shows the root surface of a mandibular canine covered in a colored powder; the colored powder represents plaque biofilm. Figures 23-5A,B and 23-6 demonstrate the ineffectiveness of dental floss in cleaning the root concavity of a maxillary premolar.
4. Figures 23-5C,D and 23-6 demonstrate the effectiveness of an interdental brush in cleaning the root concavity of a maxillary premolar. Note that only the interdental brush is effective in reaching the concave surface of the root concavity.

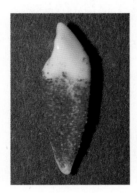

Figure 23-4. Anatomical Challenge: Biofilm Removal from Root Concavity. The proximal surface of this mandibular canine is covered with colored powder representing plaque biofilm. Figures 23-5A,B compare the effectiveness of dental floss and an interdental brush in removing biofilm from an exposed root cavity.

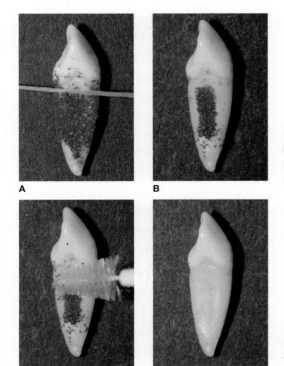

A   B

Figure 23-5A,B: Use of Dental Floss for Biofilm Removal. As seen in figures **(A,B)**, dental floss is not effective in removing the powder (simulated biofilm) from the exposed root concavity.

C   D

Figure 23-5C,D: Use of an Interdental Brush for Biofilm Removal. As seen in figures **(C,D)**, an interdental brush effectively removes the powder (simulated biofilm) from the root concavity.

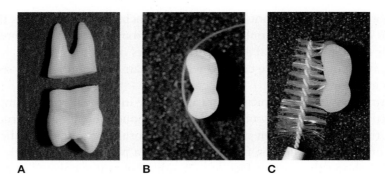

Figure 23-6. Application of Interdental Aids to Root Concavity in Cross Section. A: A maxillary premolar (side view) is cut to expose a cross section of the root. **B:** The root of the same maxillary premolar viewed in cross section; dental floss is unable to clean the root concavity. **C:** The bristles of the interdental brush extend into the root cavity for successful biofilm removal.

TABLE 23-1. AIDS FOR INTERDENTAL PLAQUE BIOFILM REMOVAL

Interdental Aid	Description/Example	Indications for Use
Dental floss	Unwaxed or waxed thread made of silk, nylon, or plastic monofilament fibers	A patient with type I embrasure spaces and excellent compliance to self-care regime
Floss holders	Handheld device to hold the floss or single-use device containing a segment of dental floss (Reach Access Flosser, Glide Floss Picks)	A patient with type I embrasure spaces who is motivated but has dexterity issues
Tufted dental floss	Thickened yarn-like dental floss (J & J Superfloss)	Type II embrasure spaces, fixed bridges, distal surface of last tooth in the arch, proximal surfaces of widely spaced teeth
Interdental brush	Tiny nylon brushes on a handle (Butler Gum Proxabrush), some brands come in varying sizes (TePe Interdental Brushes)	Type II or type III embrasure spaces, distal surface of last tooth in the arch, exposed furcation areas that permit easy insertion of the brush. Embrasure spaces with exposed proximal root concavities
End-tuft brush	Small bristle tuft on a toothbrush-like handle (Butler end-tuft brush)	Type III embrasure spaces, distal surface of the last tooth in arch, lingual surfaces of mandibular teeth, crowded or misaligned teeth, exposed furcation areas
Pipe cleaner	Standard pipe cleaner cut into 3-in lengths	Type III embrasure spaces, exposed furcation areas that permit insertion
Toothpick in holder	A round toothpick in a plastic handle (Marquis Perio-Aid)	Type II or III embrasure spaces, biofilm removal at gingival margin, furcation areas or root concavities
Triangular wooden wedge	A triangular-shaped toothpick generally made of basswood (J & J Stim-U-Dent)	Type II or III embrasure spaces

2. **Selecting Interdental Aids for the Patient with Periodontal Disease**
   A. **Dental Floss**
      1. **Description.** Dental floss is unwaxed or waxed thread made of silk, nylon, or plastic monofilament fibers used to remove dental plaque biofilm from the proximal surfaces of teeth.
      2. **Effectiveness.** While floss tends to be the primary recommendation of most dental hygienists, patient compliance is low. *It has also been shown that a significant number of those that do floss are not able to perform the function effectively* (3).
         a. Evidence indicates that a variety of alternative interdental aids are as effective or more effective than dental floss in removing biofilm and in reducing bleeding and gingivitis (4).
            1. When added to toothbrushing, a study found that dental floss has been shown to significantly reduce bleeding compared to toothbrushing alone (5).
            2. Two systematic reviews of dental floss added to manual toothbrushing found in most cases, the addition of dental floss does not increase biofilm removal or reduce gingivitis (6,7). The authors conclude that practitioners need to determine on an individual basis whether effective flossing is a reasonable and achievable goal (6).
            3. Even though conventional wisdom has long advocated for flossing to reduce decay, the scientific evidence does not bear this out with two systemic reviews finding no studies supporting the effectiveness of flossing in reducing decay in adults (7,8).
            4. It may be easier for some individuals to use floss via a floss holder. Flossing via floss holder has been shown to be as effective as handheld floss and a mechanism for increasing the development of a flossing habit (9). There are many variations of floss holder. Some require manually wrapping the floss onto the holder. Others may be single-use devices with the floss already in place (Fig. 23-7).
         b. *When given a choice, patients often prefer other types of interdental cleaners to dental floss* (4).
         c. Flossing may not be as effective for periodontal patients; recession, attachment loss, and size of the gingival embrasure space are limiting factors (4).
         d. A water flosser has also been shown to be an effective alternative to dental floss, appropriate for patients with many types of oral anatomy and conditions (4). The topic of irrigation is discussed in detail in Chapter 24.
         e. Some mouthrinses have been shown to be an effective alternative to dental floss. Mouthrinses are discussed in detail in Chapter 25.
      3. **Indications for Recommendation of Dental Floss**
         a. Type I embrasures. Dental floss is effective in removing biofilm from tooth crowns and the convex root surfaces in the region of the cementoenamel junction (CEJ). *Dental floss is not effective in removing biofilm from root concavities and grooves.*
         b. Recommended for patients with excellent compliance with self-care. Patient compliance with dental flossing is low with many patients being unable or unwilling to perform daily flossing (3).
         c. Patients who participate in crafting hobbies such as knitting, crocheting, needlepoint, or woodworking may be good candidates for dental floss as they are likely more adept and comfortable at using their hands.

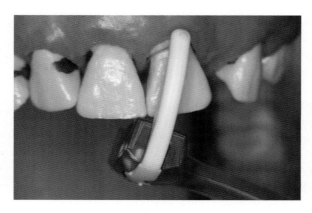

Figure 23-7. Technique for Use of Floss Holder.
Flossing via a floss holder is as effective as handheld flossing provided the patient uses proper technique. The dental floss should be wrapped around the proximal tooth surface in a similar manner to the technique employed with handheld floss.

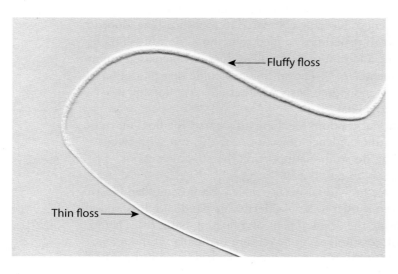

Figure 23-8. Tufted Dental Floss.
This aid is a specialized type of floss consisting of a fluffy segment of yarn-like floss attached to a segment of thin floss.

B. Tufted Dental Floss
1. Description. A specialized type of dental floss that has a segment of ordinary floss attached to a thicker, fluffy, yarn-like segment of floss (Fig. 23-8).
2. Indications
    a. For type II embrasures.
    b. To clean under the pontic of a fixed bridge.
    c. To clean the distal surface of the last tooth in the arch.
    d. To remove plaque biofilm from the proximal surfaces of widely spaced teeth.
3. Technique
    a. For interdental proximal surfaces, the fluffy part of the floss is used interdentally in a C-shape against the tooth, applying pressure with a slight sawing motion against first one proximal surface and then the adjacent proximal tooth surface.
    b. For fixed bridges, the tufted floss is threaded under the pontic and used to clean the undersurface of pontic. Next, the distal surface of the mesial abutment tooth and the mesial surface of the distal abutment tooth are cleaned using the tufted floss.

C. Interdental Brush
1. Description. Tiny conical-shaped or "pine tree"–shaped nylon bristle brush attached to a handle (Fig. 23-9). Brushes are available in different diameters, so that the best size can be selected. The size of the embrasure space determines the correct diameter of the bristle part of the brush. There should be a slight bit of resistance as the brush is moved back and forth between the teeth. Often it is necessary to use different size brushes within one mouth.
2. Indications
   a. A systematic review of interdental brushes found they remove more biofilm than brushing alone (10).
   b. The systematic review also found when compared to dental floss, interdental brushes removed more plaque biofilm. Both flossing and interdental brush use resulted in a similar reduction in inflammation (10).
   c. Excellent for biofilm removal in type II and III embrasure spaces (Fig. 23-10). Interdental brushes should not be used where the interdental papilla fills the interdental space.
   d. *The bristles of an interdental brush are very effective at cleaning root concavities.*
3. Technique. The brush is inserted into the open interdental space and slid in and out of the embrasure space for several strokes. *Always use the interdental brush without toothpaste.* Figure 23-11A–D show techniques for use of interdental brushes.

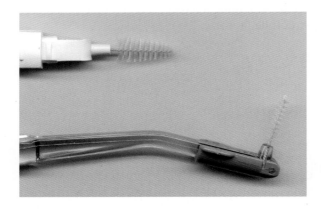

Figure 23-9. Interdental Brushes. Interdental brushes are one of the most useful aids for cleaning root concavities.

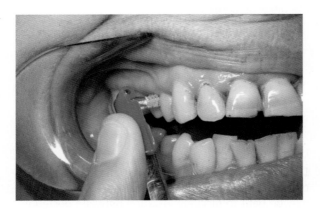

Figure 23-10. Use of Interdental Brush. (Courtesy of Dr. Deborah Milliken, South Florida Community College.)

Figure 23-11. Procedure for Use of an Interdental Brush.

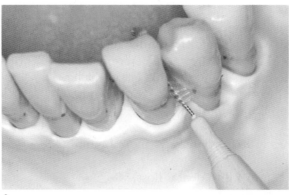

A

A: The brush handle is held between the thumb and index finger and the brush gently pushed between the teeth. The brush should be maintained at a 90-degree angle to the long axis of the tooth.

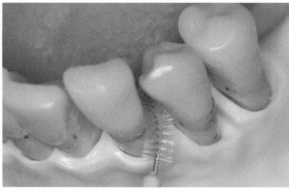

B

B: The bristles can be adapted to tooth surfaces with slight pressure and varying the angle of insertion. For optimal biofilm removal, the brush is slid in and out of the space using the entire length of the bristle part of the brush.

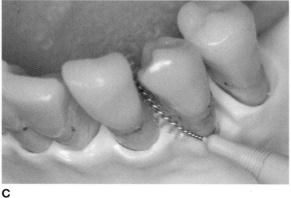

C

C: By changing the angle of insertion, the bristles can be adapted to the mesial surface of the first premolar. Slight pressure with the brush against the gingiva allows the bristles to clean slightly beneath the gingival margin.

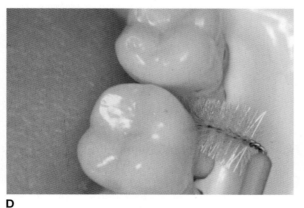

D

D: For posterior areas, advise the patient to close his or her mouth slightly to relax the cheek. The brush may be bent to facilitate insertion between posterior teeth.

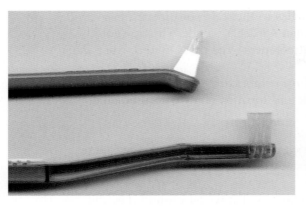

Figure 23-12. End-Tuft Brushes. End-tuft brushes are used to clean areas that are difficult to access with a standard brush.

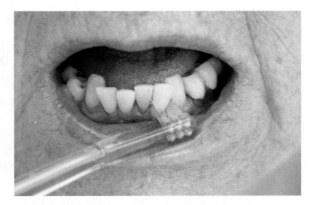

Figure 23-13. Use of End-Tuft Brush. End-tuft brush used around crowded anterior teeth. (Courtesy of Dr. Deborah Milliken, South Florida Community College.)

D. End-Tuft Brush
  1. Description. An end-tuft brush is similar to a standard toothbrush except that the brush head has only a small tuft of bristles (Fig. 23-12). A standard toothbrush easily can be modified to create a customized end-tuft brush by removing some of the bristles.
  2. Indications
     a. Effectively reaches sites around teeth that are difficult for patients to clean, such as the distal surface of the last tooth in the arch, lingual surfaces of mandibular teeth and crowded or misaligned teeth (Fig. 23-13).
     b. Works well to remove biofilm from type III embrasure spaces.
     c. Useful in removing biofilm from an exposed furcation area since the small size of the bristle tufts allows them to partially enter the furcation site.
  3. Technique
     a. The end of the tuft is directed into the embrasure space or furcation area. Gentle circular strokes are used to clean the area.
     b. For difficult-to-reach mandibular lingual tooth surfaces, the brush is used like a standard brush with a sulcular brushing technique.
E. Wooden Toothpick in a Holder
  1. Description. This device consists of a round toothpick in a plastic handle.
  2. Indications
     a. The toothpick in a holder has been shown to reduce biofilm and bleeding as effectively as dental floss (11).
     b. It can be used gently along or slightly below the gingival margin or directed into exposed furcation areas for biofilm removal.
     c. Effective in type II embrasures if the toothpick is easily inserted between the teeth; however, this aid is not effective in cleaning root concavities unless the teeth are widely spaced.
  3. Technique for Use of a Wooden Toothpick in a Holder
     a. A toothpick is secured in the holder and the long end is broken off flush with the holder, so that it will not scratch the inside of the cheek (Fig. 23-14).
     b. The end of toothpick is moistened with saliva.

c. The toothpick tip is applied at right angles to the tooth or directed just beneath the gingival margin at a less than 45-degree angle. The tip should not be directed against the epithelial attachment. The tip is used to trace the gingival margin around each tooth.

d. Where space permits, the tip is angled into embrasure spaces or exposed furcation areas and moved gently back and forth to remove accumulated biofilm.

F. Wooden Wedge

1. Description. This aid is a short wooden stick usually made of softwood. These wedges are triangular, wedge-shaped sticks and should not be confused with round or rectangular toothpicks.

2. Indications. A systematic review of triangular wooden wedges found they did not increase the amount of visible biofilm removal beyond toothbrushing, but they did improve interdental inflammation better than brushing alone (12). To use a wedge, there must be sufficient interdental space available to allow easy placement of the wooden wedge. Long-term use of wooden wedges in type I embrasures may cause a permanent loss of the papillae.

3. Technique for Use of Wooden Wedge

a. The wooden wedge should be moistened thoroughly in the mouth to soften the wood prior to use.

b. The wedge is inserted between the teeth with the *flat side next to the gums* (Fig. 23-15).

c. The wedge is used with gentle in and out motion to clean between the teeth. The wedge should not be forced into tightly spaced teeth. The wedge should be discarded as soon as the first signs of splaying are evident.

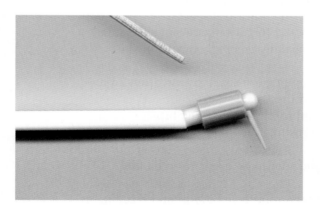

Figure 23-14. Toothpick Holder. To prepare this aid for use, secure a toothpick in the holder and break off the long end, so that it is flush with the plastic holder.

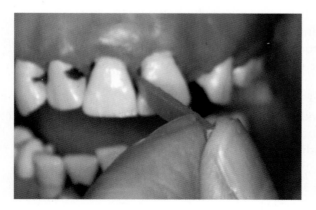

Figure 23-15. Use of Wooden Wedge. The wedge is held between the thumb and index finger with the flat side toward the gingiva. In the upper arch the flat surface faces up, and in the lower arch the flat surface faces down.

Section 3
Tongue Cleaning as an Adjunct

Many patients have coated tongues that make it difficult to maintain fresh breath and cause a lessened sense of taste. *Periodontal patients have been shown to have significantly higher prevalence of tongue coating* (13). Daily tongue cleaning controls halitosis and may help to maintain a healthy periodontal environment.

1. **Tongue Coating and the Role of Volatile Sulfur Compounds in Halitosis**
   The tongue coating is made up of bacteria and other putrefied debris that produces hydrogen sulfide and methyl mercaptan.
   A. **Volatile sulfur compounds (VSCs)** are a family of gases that are responsible for halitosis.
      1. Two members of the VSC family of gases, hydrogen sulfide and methyl mercaptan, are principally responsible for mouth odor. Methyl mercaptan is produced primarily by periodontal pathogens. Some studies have suggested that low concentrations of these gases may be toxic to tissues; however, the research in this area is limited (14).
      2. Most patients are concerned about controlling halitosis and, therefore, are receptive to the introduction of tongue cleaning to their self-care routine.
      3. Tongue coating can contribute to a lessened sense of taste. Tongue cleaning should be recommended to geriatric patients who have a low desire to eat due to depressed taste sensation.
   B. Tongue cleaning is recommended because the bulk of bacteria and debris—especially the periodontal pathogens that produce methyl mercaptan—accumulate mostly within the filiform papillae and on the back of the tongue. The practice of tongue cleaning may not only make a patient feel more confident but may actually help in maintaining a healthy periodontal environment.

2. **Technique for use of Manual Tongue Cleaners.** Manual tongue cleaners come in a variety of styles. The two most common types are specialized toothbrushes and tongue scrapers (Fig. 23-16).
   A. The tongue brush or scraper is positioned as far back on the tongue as possible.
   B. Once the brush or scraper is in position, it is pulled forward gently over the tongue. This procedure is repeated two or three times or until the tongue is clean.
   C. When first learning tongue cleaning, some individuals gag and find the process unpleasant. In the beginning, encourage the patient to place the cleaner wherever it is most comfortable on the tongue. With regular use, most patients become accustomed to the sensation of the tongue brush or scraper and are able to clean further back on the tongue. Over time, most patients become skilled at tongue cleaning.

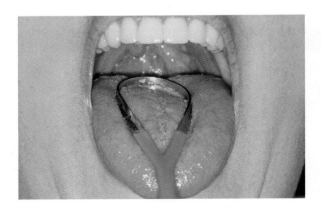

Figure 23-16. Manual Tongue Scraper. Daily tongue cleaning controls halitosis and may help to maintain a healthy periodontal environment.

Chapter Summary Statement

The patient's efforts at self-care are critical to the control of periodontitis. Since the importance of mechanical biofilm control is quite high for the patient with periodontitis, the dental hygienist should be knowledgeable about biofilm control measures and be prepared to recommend appropriate aids based on the individual needs of each patient.

Due to attachment loss, the dentition of an individual with periodontitis often presents anatomical challenges to effective biofilm control, such as recession of the gingival margin, type II or III embrasure spaces, and exposed root concavities. Interdental aids that are especially useful for patients with type II or III embrasure spaces include interdental brushes and end-tuft brushes. Daily tongue cleaning results in reduced amounts of tongue coating and improvements in breath freshness.

Section 4
Focus on Patients

Clinical Patient Care

CASE 1

A patient with slight (or mild) chronic periodontitis has generalized recession of the interdental gingival papillae. What options would you have for training this patient in interdental plaque biofilm control?

CASE 2

You are discussing self-care for biofilm removal with a patient with chronic periodontitis. You point out to the patient how the biofilm control on the facial and lingual surfaces of his teeth is greatly improved and praise him for this success. The patient comments that he likes using his powered toothbrush and has been brushing longer. Unfortunately, you note that there is heavy plaque biofilm on the proximal surfaces of most teeth. The patient tells you that there is "No way that I am going to use that string. It is just too hard to use." The patient has type II embrasure spaces throughout his mouth. What suggestions might you make for interdental biofilm control?

CASE 3

A patient with chronic periodontitis has generalized bone loss and gingival recession, so that the cervical-thirds of the roots are exposed to the oral cavity. What interdental aid would you recommend to clean interproximally (between the roots)?

Evidence in Action

You recently began working as the dental hygienist in an established periodontal practice. The previous hygienist retired after a 20-year career in dental hygiene.

Today is Mrs. J's first maintenance appointment with you. Mrs. J has had periodontal surgery and has type III embrasure spaces throughout her dentition. She also has extensive restorative work in her dentition. According to her patient record, at the past several maintenance visits, Mrs. J has had very little plaque biofilm on the facial and lingual surfaces of her teeth, but moderate biofilm accumulation on the mesial and distal surfaces of her teeth. Today, your assessment reveals a similar pattern of plaque biofilm formation.

You ask Mrs. J about her current self-care program and she explains that she has been instructed to use an electric toothbrush and dental floss daily. She says that she really likes the electric toothbrush but simply cannot use the floss. She complaints that the floss breaks when she tries to get it between her "fillings" and that it is just simply too frustrating to use.

Based on what you know about plaque biofilm control with type III embrasure spaces what suggestions might you offer to Mrs. J as other options for her self-care regimen?

Ethical Dilemma

As a 50-year-old woman who runs a home day care center, you have been referred to Dr. Rogers' periodontal practice by your general dentist Dr. Patel. You now alternate your periodontal maintenance appointments between the two offices, with appointments every 3 months.

Six months ago, the hygienist at Dr. Rogers' office, Khoa, a recent graduate, recommended that you use an interdental brush, due to the recession and large spaces between your teeth. He spent much time educating you in the proper technique, and even watched you use it effectively in your own mouth. However, at home, you find it difficult to use, and due to the osteoarthritis in your fingers, find changing the small nylon brushes on the handle almost impossible. As a result, you have not been using the aid.

You are sitting in front of Khoa again today, and he reviews your medical history and home care regime. You explain that it has been difficult for you to be compliant with the interdental brush, and ask for an alternative periodontal aid. Khoa feels that the interdental brush is the best device for mechanical biofilm control in your situation.

You feel very frustrated and do not think that Khoa is being sensitive to your needs.

1. How should this ethical dilemma be handled?
2. What ethical principles are in conflict in this dilemma?

References

1. O'Toole MT. *Mosby's Medical Dictionary.* 9th ed. St. Louis, MO: Elsevier/Mosby; 2013; xiv: A-43, 1921.

2. Jahn CA. Evidence for self-care products: power brushing and interdental aids. *J Pract Hyg.* 2004;13:24–29.

3. Lang WP, Ronis DL, Farghaly MM. Preventive behaviors as correlates of periodontal health status. *J Public Health Dent.* 1995;55(1):10–17.

4. Asadoorian J. Flossing: Canadian dental hygienists' association position statement. *CJDH.* 2006;40(3):1–10.

5. Graves RC, Disney JA, Stamm JW. Comparative effectiveness of flossing and brushing in reducing interproximal bleeding. *J Periodontol.* 1989;60(5):243–247.

6. Berchier CE, Slot DE, Haps S, et al. The efficacy of dental floss in addition to a toothbrush on plaque and parameters of gingival inflammation: a systematic review. *Int J Dent Hyg.* 2008;6(4):265–279.

7. Sambunjak D, Nickerson JW, Poklepovic T, et al. Flossing for the management of periodontal diseases and dental caries in adults. *Cochrane Database Syst Rev.* 2011;(12):CD008829.

8. Hujoel PP, Cunha-Cruz J, Banting DW, et al. Dental flossing and interproximal caries: a systematic review. *J Dent Res.* 2006;85(4):298–305.

9. Kleber CJ, Putt MS. Formation of flossing habit using a floss-holding device. *J Dent Hyg: JDH/American Dental Hygienists' Association.* 1990;64(3):140–143.

10. Slot DE, Dorfer CE, Van der Weijden GA. The efficacy of interdental brushes on plaque and parameters of periodontal inflammation: a systematic review. *Int J Dent Hyg.* 2008;6(4):253–264.

11. Lewis MW, Holder-Ballard C, Selders RJ Jr., et al. Comparison of the use of a toothpick holder to dental floss in improvement of gingival health in humans. *J Periodontol.* 2004;75(4):551–556.

12. Hoenderdos NL, Slot DE, Paraskevas S, et al. The efficacy of woodsticks on plaque and gingival inflammation: a systematic review. *Int J Dent Hyg.* 2008;6(4):280–289.

13. Yaegaki K, Sanada K. Volatile sulfur compounds in mouth air from clinically healthy subjects and patients with periodontal disease. *J Periodontal Res.* 1992;27(4 Pt 1):233–238.

14. Ratcliff PA, Johnson PW. The relationship between oral malodor, gingivitis, and periodontitis. A review. *J Periodontol.* 1999;70(5):485–489.

 STUDENT ANCILLARY RESOURCES

A wide variety of resources to enhance your learning and understanding of this chapter are available on thePoint®.

- Visit thePoint to access:
  - Audio Glossary
  - Animations
  - Suggested Readings
  - Answers to Review Questions
  - Case Studies

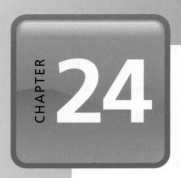

CHAPTER **24**

Supragingival and Subgingival Irrigation

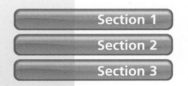
Clinical Application. This chapter addresses the role of supragingival and subgingival irrigation in the treatment of periodontal diseases. The primary objective of *supra*gingival irrigation is to diminish gingival inflammation by disrupting bacterial biofilms. The goal of *sub*gingival irrigation is to reduce the number of bacteria in the periodontal pocket space.

Learning Objectives

- Discuss the oral health benefits of a water flosser for the patient with periodontitis.
- Distinguish the depth of the delivery among the water flosser, a toothbrush, dental floss, and other interdental aids.
- Name the types of agents that can be used in a water flosser.
- In a clinical setting, instruct a patient with periodontitis in the use of a water flosser.
- Summarize research findings that relate to using professional irrigation to deliver chemicals to periodontal pockets.

Key Terms

Water flosser	Flushing zone	Orthodontic irrigation tips
Hydrokinetic activity	Standard irrigation tips	Filament-type irrigation tips
Impact zone	Subgingival irrigation tips	Professional subgingival irrigation

Section 1
Patient-Applied Home Irrigation

1. **What is a Water Flosser?** The water flosser is a generic term for a device that delivers a pulsed irrigation of water or other solution around and between teeth (supragingivally) and into the gingival sulcus or periodontal pocket (subgingivally). This process is commonly referred to as home or oral irrigation. A water flosser jet may also be referred to as a dental water irrigator, home irrigator, or dental water jet.
   A. **Mechanism of Action of a Water Flosser**
      1. A water flosser creates a pulsating fluid stream to flush an area with water or an antimicrobial agent. Figure 24-1 shows examples of devices used for home oral irrigation.
         a. The pulsating fluid delivered by a water flosser incorporates a compression and decompression phase that efficiently displaces biofilm, bacteria, and debris (1,2).
         b. The pulsating fluid creates two zones of fluid movement termed **hydrokinetic activity** (Fig. 24-2).
            1. The area of the mouth of initial fluid contact is called the **impact zone**.
            2. The depth of fluid penetration within a subgingival sulcus or pocket is called the **flushing zone** (3).
      2. Hydrokinetic fluid movement results in subgingival and interdental fluid penetration.
   B. **Fluid Penetration**
      1. A water flosser produces subgingival fluid penetration regardless of the type of tip or attachment used (4,5).
      2. A water flosser has the greatest potential for reaching deeper into a sulcus or pocket over other types of devices including toothbrushes and interdental aids (Table 24-1) (4,5).

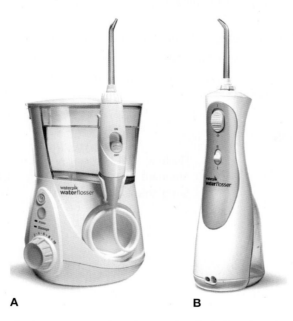

A   **B**

Figure 24-1. Water Flossers. **A:** A countertop dental water jet that plugs into an electrical outlet. **B:** A portable dental water jet that works off of a rechargeable battery. (Courtesy of Water Pik, Inc., Fort Collins, CO.)

2. **Benefits of Home Oral Irrigation.** Studies demonstrate that the water flosser is clinically proven to remove biofilm and reduce bleeding, gingivitis, periodontal pathogens, and inflammatory mediators (6–21).
    A. **Removal of Biofilm.** A water flosser used in combination with manual toothbrushing has been shown to remove 29% more biofilm than traditional brushing and flossing (15).
    B. **Reduction in Bleeding.** Studies consistently show that the water flosser is a valuable tool for helping patients reduce bleeding (6–10,12,13,17,19,20).
        1. Daily irrigation with water significantly reduced bleeding in 14 days (10).
        2. Daily irrigation with water was significantly better than rinsing with 0.12% chlorhexidine at reducing marginal bleeding and bleeding on probing (13).

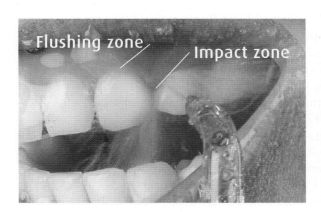

Figure 24-2. The Impact and Flushing Zones. A water flosser creates a pulsating water stream to flush an area with fluid. The area of the mouth where the fluid initially contacts is called the impact zone. The depth of fluid penetration within the subgingival sulcus or pocket is called the flushing zone. (Courtesy of Water Pik, Inc., Fort Collins, CO.)

TABLE 24-1. DEPTH OF DELIVERY OF VARIOUS SELF-CARE PRODUCTS

Oral Hygiene Aid	Penetration	Comments
Toothbrush	1–2 mm	No manual or power toothbrush has clinically proven subgingival access
Rinsing	2 mm	Can reach less accessible areas, but penetrates subgingival areas minimally (4)
Toothpick/wooden wedge	Depends on embrasure size	Effectiveness depends on sufficient interdental space
Interdental brush	Depends on embrasure size	Most effective with an open interdental space
Dental floss	3 mm	Cannot reach into deeper pockets
Waterpik water flosser	6 mm and beyond (4,5)	Clinically proven to remove supra- and subgingival plaque biofilm and bacteria (15,19)

Courtesy of Water Pik, Inc., Fort Collins, CO.

C. **Reduction in Gingival Inflammation.** The water flosser has been shown to reduce the clinical signs of gingivitis (6–8,10,12,13,16,17,21–23).
  1. A water flosser used in combination with manual toothbrushing is more effective in the reduction of gingivitis than manual toothbrushing and flossing (7).
  2. Daily irrigation with water significantly reduces the clinical signs of gingivitis (8).

D. **Reduction of Periodontal Pathogens.** Studies show the dental water jet can reduce subgingival bacteria (3,8,11,18).
  1. The water flosser has demonstrated the ability to reduce periodontal pathogens at up to a 6-mm level within a periodontal pocket (3,11).
  2. Daily irrigation with either water or 0.04% chlorhexidine significantly reduces subgingival bacteria compared to toothbrushing and 0.12% chlorhexidine rinsing (8).

E. **Reduction in Inflammatory Mediators and Destructive Host Response**
  1. Recent studies show that home oral irrigation is effective in significantly reducing inflammatory cytokines Il-1β and PGE2 (8,10). These cytokines have been implicated in attachment loss and alveolar bone loss (24,25).
  2. Irrigation may produce these effects by flushing out loosely adherent plaque and toxins or inflammatory substances, although the exact mechanism of action of irrigation is still speculative (8,17).

3. **Indications for Recommending Home Oral Irrigation**
  A. **Individuals on Periodontal Maintenance.** Studies have shown that daily use of the water flosser may be beneficial for patients with gingivitis or for those in periodontal maintenance (6–10,12,13,17,21). Patients with 5-mm pockets and bleeding who added daily irrigation to traditional home care achieved significant reductions in gingival inflammation and bleeding on probing when compared to patients using only traditional self-care methods (17).

  B. **Individuals Noncompliant with Dental Floss.** While previously considered an adjunctive to brushing and flossing, new information indicates that home oral irrigation can be considered an effective *alternative* to daily flossing.
    1. The addition of a water flosser once daily with plain water to either a manual or power brushing routine was an effective alternative to dental floss for the reduction of bleeding, gingivitis, and biofilm (7,19).
    2. The water flosser and a manual toothbrush were 29% more effective at plaque removal than a manual toothbrush and floss (15).

  C. **Individuals with Special Needs.** Home irrigation has been shown to be safe and effective for patients with special needs.
    1. Dental Implants. For improving the health of peri-implant tissues, daily irrigation using a tip with three soft filaments and water at medium pressure was significantly more effective at reducing bleeding than manual brushing and flossing (16).
    2. Individuals with Diabetes. For individuals living with diabetes, twice-daily water irrigation using the soft rubber tip provided a 44% better reduction in bleeding over routine oral hygiene (6).
    3. Individuals with Orthodontic Appliances. For those with orthodontic appliances, the dental water jet with the orthodontic tip provided 3.76 times better biofilm removal and 26% better bleeding reduction than flossing using a floss threader (20,25).
    4. Prosthetic Bridgework and Crowns. For individuals with bridgework and/or crowns, daily irrigation produced significant reductions in inflammation (26).

4. Patient Instruction
   A. Considerations for Irrigator Use: Product Safety
      1. Water flossers have been extensively studied on thousands of people with more than 60 studies since the 1960s. Examination with a scanning electron microscope of chronic periodontal pockets immediately following irrigation found no evidence of trauma or injury to the tissue (3).
      2. The incidence of bacteremia from a dental water jet is similar to other healthcare devices (27).
         a. The American College of Cardiology/American Heart Association 2008 Guideline Update on Valvular Heart Disease: Focused Update on Infective Endocarditis states "Maintenance of optimal oral health and hygiene may reduce the incidence of bacteremia from daily activities and is more important than prophylactic antibiotics for a dental procedure to reduce the risk of infective endocarditis" (28).
         b. Before recommending a water flosser or any device to a patient who is at high risk for infective endocarditis, it is imperative that dental healthcare providers consider both the patient's overall medical and oral health status. Consultation with a physician is advisable in order to assess the patient's overall risk for infective endocarditis.
   B. Irrigant Solutions. Most solutions can be used in a water flosser. The most effective agent is one that is acceptable to the patient.
      1. Water
         a. Simple tap water has been demonstrated as highly effective in numerous clinical trials (3,6,7,10,12,14–16,19,20). Therefore, the addition of any antimicrobial agent for home oral irrigation should be considered carefully.
         b. Water has several advantages; it is readily available, cost-effective, and has no side effects.
      2. Antimicrobial Solutions
         a. Chlorhexidine (CHX)
            1. For home irrigation, chlorhexidine can be diluted with water. Use of diluted solutions of chlorhexidine has been studied in concentrations from 0.02% to 0.06% (8,13,18,21).
            2. Because of better interproximal and subgingival penetration with irrigation compared to rinsing, a diluted solution of chlorhexidine is acceptable for daily irrigation. In some cases, dilution can minimize staining.
            3. CHX is available by prescription only. In the United States, the maximum strength is 0.12%. In Europe, it is available at 0.2%.
         b. Essential Oils
            1. For home irrigation, the effectiveness of an essential oil mouth rinse has been demonstrated only when used at full strength (9).
            2. Essential oil mouthrinses are available over the counter in both brand name and generic forms.
   C. Criteria for Equipment Selection. Selection of an irrigation device may be confusing because there are many types on the market. The commercial and scientific claims of some devices have yet to be evaluated. Only pulsating water flossers have clinical research supporting safety and efficacy. As each device operates differently in respect to pressure and pulsation, outcomes from studies on one brand of product cannot be transferred to another product brand. Therefore, before recommending any device, it is important to evaluate the research unique to that brand of product.

5. **Technique for Use of Irrigation Tips**
   A. **General Instructions**
      1. It is important for both dental healthcare providers and patients to read all instructions thoroughly before using a water flosser.
      2. The fluid reservoir can be filled with water, a solution of water and mouthwash, or a solution of an antimicrobial and water. The irrigating solution should be at warm temperature for maximum patient comfort.
      3. The unit should be flushed after using any solution other than water. After using a diluted solution, such as diluted chlorhexidine, the unit is cleaned by filling the reservoir with warm water and running the unit while holding the handle in the sink until the reservoir is empty.
      4. Most patients seem to comply with recommendations to use a water flosser and find a standard irrigation tip easy to use for supragingival irrigation (12). For subgingival irrigation, it is important to provide patients with clear instructions on its use including the specific areas where the tip should be used.
   B. **Irrigation Tips.** Irrigation is accomplished using a standard irrigation tip, a subgingival soft rubber tip, a soft-tapered brush orthodontic tip, or a tip with three fine filaments.

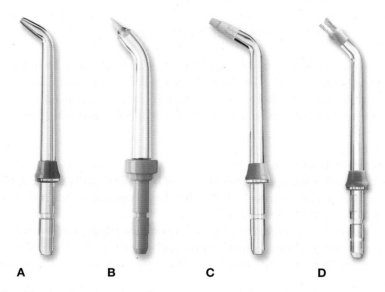

Figure 24-3. Irrigation Tips. Four examples of irrigation tip designs. **A:** Standard irrigation tip. **B:** Subgingival tip. **C:** Orthodontic tip. **D:** Filament-type tip.

   1. **Standard irrigation tips** are usually made of a plastic material (Fig. 24-3A).
      a. This type of tip is recommended for generalized, full-mouth irrigation.
      b. Water flosser devices with standard irrigation tips may deliver solution that penetrates a depth of 50% or more of the pocket (5).
   2. **Subgingival irrigation tips** usually have a soft rubber-tipped end (Fig. 24-3B).
      a. Subgingival irrigation tips are recommended for use in areas such as deep pockets, furcation areas, dental implants, or areas that are difficult to access with a standard tip.
      b. Subgingival placement of the tip allows the water or antimicrobial agent to penetrate deeper into a pocket.
         1. In periodontal pockets 6 mm or less in depth, the subgingival tip may deliver water that penetrates up to 90% of the pocket depth (4).

2. In deeper pockets—7 mm or more—depth of penetration is somewhat less at 64% of the depth of the pocket (4).

3. **Orthodontic irrigation tips** have a soft-tapered brush end that enhances biofilm removal and provides for simultaneous irrigation (Fig. 24-3C).
   a. Orthodontic tips can be used for full-mouth irrigation and are recommended for people with orthodontic appliances, implants, or who need additional help with biofilm removal.
   b. The bristles should come in light contact with the tooth or orthodontic appliances to facilitate biofilm removal.
      1. The orthodontic tip when used in conjunction with toothbrushing was 3.76 times as effective as dental floss at removing plaque.
      2. When compared to toothbrushing only, the toothbrushing and orthodontic tip combination was 5.83 times as effective (20).

4. **Filament-type irrigation tips** have three soft filaments surrounding a standard jet tip. This can enhance plaque removal and is safe for use around dental implants (Fig. 24-3D).
   a. The filament-type tip has also been shown to remove plaque biofilm (14).
   b. The filament-type tip used around an implant was 145% better at reducing bleeding than manual brushing and flossing (16).

C. **Procedure for Use of a Standard Tip**
   1. Initially the pressure setting should be adjusted to its lowest setting. Over time as the condition of the gingival tissue improves, pressure should be increased to at least the medium setting as this setting is where clinical efficacy has been demonstrated (1,2).
   2. The water spray is used to "trace" along the gingival margin with the tip positioned at a 90-degree angle almost touching the gingiva (Fig. 24-4). The tip should be held briefly at each interproximal area.

D. **Procedure for Use of a Subgingival Irrigation Tip**
   1. The dental hygienist should instruct the patient on the areas of his or her mouth where use of a subgingival irrigation tip would be beneficial, such as pockets, dental implants, or furcation areas. The patient should be instructed on use of the tip in each area or these areas.
   2. The pressure setting is adjusted to its lowest setting. *The subgingival tip is designed for use only at the lowest pressure setting.*
   3. The tip should be placed at the site before starting the irrigation unit. The subgingival tip is directed at a 45-degree angle and placed at the gingival margin or slightly beneath the gingival margin as recommended by the manufacturer (Fig. 24-5).
   4. Once the tip is in place, the irrigation unit is turned on and the fluid is allowed to flow briefly in the area.
   5. After a site has been irrigated, the unit is paused and the subgingival tip is repositioned in the next area of the mouth.

E. **Procedure for the Use of Orthodontic and Filament Tips**
   1. Initially, the pressure setting should be adjusted to its lowest setting. Over time as the condition of the gingival tissue improves, pressure should be increased to at least the medium setting as this setting is where clinical efficacy has been demonstrated (1,2).
   2. The water spray is used to "trace" along the gingival margin with the tip positioned at a 90-degree angle touching the gingiva (Figs. 24-6 and 24-7). The tip should be held briefly in each interproximal area.
   3. This tip can also be placed around orthodontic brackets or wires, or implants to enhance cleaning.

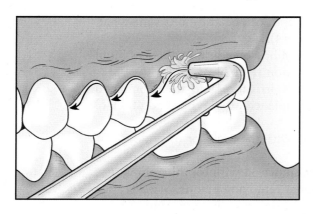

Figure 24-4. Placement of the Standard Irrigation Tip. The water spray is used to "trace" along the gingival margin with the tip positioned at a 90-degree angle almost touching the gingiva.

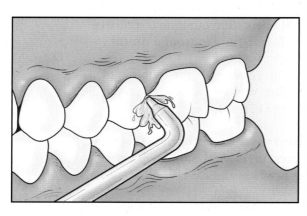

Figure 24-5. Placement of the Subgingival Irrigation Tip. The tip should be placed at the site before starting the irrigation unit. The subgingival tip is directed at a 45-degree angle and placed at the gingival margin or slightly beneath the gingival margin as recommended by the manufacturer.

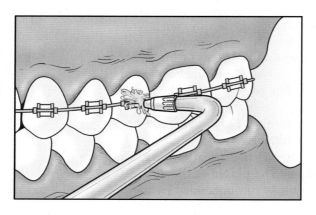

Figure 24-6. Placement of the Orthodontic Tip. The special orthodontic tip is used with the tip positioned at a 90-degree angle.

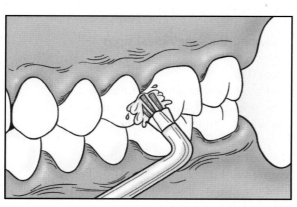

Figure 24-7. Placement of the Filament-Type Tip. The filament-type tip is used with the tip positioned at a 90-degree angle.

Section 2
Professional Subgingival Irrigation

1. **Introduction to Professional Irrigation**
   A. **Description of Subgingival Irrigation.** Professional subgingival irrigation is the in-office flushing of pockets performed by the dental hygienist or dentist using one of three systems:
      1. A blunt-tipped irrigating cannula that is attached to a handheld syringe (Fig. 24-8)
      2. Ultrasonic unit equipped with a reservoir (Fig. 24-9)
      3. A specialized air-driven handpiece that connects to the dental unit airline
   B. **Goal of Subgingival Irrigation.** The purpose of supragingival irrigation is the disruption and dilution of bacteria and their products from within periodontal pockets.

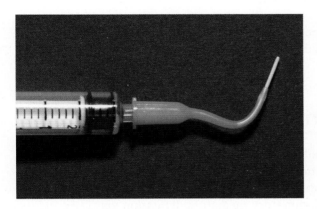

Figure 24-8. Handheld Syringe. Close-up view of the tip of a handheld syringe used for subgingival irrigation. The tip is positioned subgingivally for delivery of an antimicrobial solution.

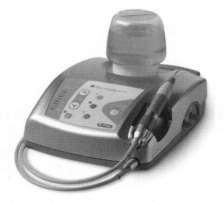

Figure 24-9. Reservoir for Ultrasonic Unit. This ultrasonic device has an optional reservoir system for dispensing irrigant solutions—such as chlorhexidine gluconate—to an ultrasonic tip. (Courtesy of Hu-Friedy, Mfg.)

   C. **Irrigant Solutions.** Solutions used for subgingival irrigation include chlorhexidine gluconate, povidone-iodine and water, stannous fluoride oral rinse, tetracycline dilutions, or Listerine.
2. **Effectiveness of Professional Subgingival Irrigation**
   A. **Single Professional Application**
      1. The status of professional subgingival irrigation in the treatment of periodontitis remains controversial (29,30).
      2. In-office subgingival irrigation with an antimicrobial agent has been shown to have only limited or no beneficial effects over nonsurgical periodontal instrumentation alone.
         a. Several research studies indicate that irrigation did not enhance the therapeutic effect over that attained by nonsurgical periodontal instrumentation alone (31–36).
         b. Other studies found a minimal improvement. However, after 6 months, there was no significant difference between irrigation and nonsurgical periodontal instrumentation regarding probing depths or inflammatory status (37–41).

3. There is no long-lasting substantivity of the antimicrobial agent in the periodontal pocket due to the continuous flow of gingival crevicular fluid from the pocket, and the presence of serum and proteins in the pocket. A substantive antimicrobial agent, such as chlorhexidine gluconate, would have to be retained in the pocket and be released slowly over a period of time to interfere with the repopulation of bacteria within the pocket.

B. **Conclusions Regarding Professional Irrigation.** A position paper (42) on the role of supra- and subgingival irrigation in the treatment of periodontal diseases concludes:

1. "... there currently is insufficient evidence to indicate that subgingival irrigation routinely should be used as a supplemental in-office procedure."

2. "However, preliminary data using high concentrations (37,40) and prolonged or multiple applications (31,34,35,40,43,44) of antimicrobials have shown some promise in improving periodontal status. Consequently, additional studies are needed to ascertain the full potential of subgingival irrigation as an adjunct to periodontal therapy" (42).

3. Subgingival irrigation performed before periodontal instrumentation may reduce the incidence of bacteremia and reduce the number of microorganisms in aerosols.

Chapter Summary Statement

When used daily for at home self-care, supragingival and subgingival irrigation via a water flosser can be beneficial for periodontal patients. A well-established body of evidence indicates that pulsating devices have the ability to remove biofilm and reduce bleeding, gingivitis, periodontal pathogens, and inflammatory mediators. Irrigation via a water flosser also benefits patients with special oral health needs and considerations including those in periodontal maintenance or with implants, crowns, bridges, orthodontic appliances, and diabetes.

The status of professional subgingival irrigation in the treatment of periodontitis remains controversial. In-office subgingival irrigation with an antimicrobial agent has been shown to have only limited or no beneficial effects over nonsurgical periodontal instrumentation alone.

Section 3
Focus on Patients

Clinical Patient Care

> **C A S E   1**
>
> You have just recommended a water flosser to your patient, and he has accepted, but he has no idea how to use the product. The patient is in periodontal maintenance, has two 5-mm pockets (#3M and #18D), one 6-mm pocket (#14M), and a furcation area on #30. He also has an implant replacing #19. What type of instructions would you provide for the patient?

Evidence in Action

> A new patient comes to your practice from another state. She has had periodontal therapy in the past. The patient uses a power toothbrush and flosses irregularly. Supragingival plaque control looks good, but several areas of the mouth bleed upon probing. The medical history indicates that the patient has had type 2 diabetes for 7 years. How would you make a recommendation for the water flosser to this patient?

Ethical Dilemma

> Your next patient is Darren, a 26-year-old male, who just recently returned from a 3-year stint in the Peace Corps. Prior to his Peace Corps experience, Darren had received routine and regular dental care but has not been to a dentist in the last 3 years. As you review his medical history, he states that he thinks that he may have suffered from a bout of "infective endocarditis" while away, but as he was working in an underdeveloped third world country, his definitive diagnosis was unclear.
>
> You start your periodontal assessment, and discover that his periodontal probe readings have significantly increased from 1 to 3 mm at his last appointment, to generalized 4- to 5-mm probe readings. His tissues appear moderately inflamed, as he presents with substantial supragingival biofilm and subgingival calculus. However, his radiographs show no signs of bone loss.
>
> You recently attended a continuing education course on the use of "water flossers," and feel that this will be an ideal adjunctive periodontal aid for Darren, based on your clinical findings. You start explaining the device and demonstrating its use to Darren, who becomes quite agitated and says that he absolutely refuses to use it. While working in the Peace Corps, clean water was extremely scarce and considered a luxury. There is no way, he states, that he will "waste water" in this fashion. You are not sure how to proceed.
>
> 1. What ethical principles are in conflict in this dilemma?
> 2. What is the best way for you to handle this ethical dilemma?
> 3. Do you have an ethical obligation to treat this patient?

References

1. Bhaskar SN, Cutright DE, Gross A, et al. Water jet devices in dental practice. *J Periodontol.* 1971;42(10):658–664.
2. Selting WJ, Bhaskar SN, Mueller RP. Water jet direction and periodontal pocket debridement. *J Periodontol.* 1972;43(9):569–572.
3. Cobb CM, Rodgers RL, Killoy WJ. Ultrastructural examination of human periodontal pockets following the use of an oral irrigation device in vivo. *J Periodontol.* 1988;59(3):155–163.
4. Braun RE, Ciancio SG. Subgingival delivery by an oral irrigation device. *J Periodontol.* 1992;63(5):469–472.
5. Eakle WS, Ford C, Boyd RL. Depth of penetration in periodontal pockets with oral irrigation. *J Clin Periodontol.* 1986;13(1):39–44.
6. Al-Mubarak S, Ciancio S, Aljada A, et al. Comparative evaluation of adjunctive oral irrigation in diabetics. *J Clin Periodontol.* 2002;29(4):295–300.
7. Barnes CM, Russell CM, Reinhardt RA, et al. Comparison of irrigation to floss as an adjunct to tooth brushing: effect on bleeding, gingivitis, and supragingival plaque. *J Clin Dent.* 2005;16(3):71–77.
8. Chaves ES, Kornman KS, Manwell MA, et al. Mechanism of irrigation effects on gingivitis. *J Periodontol.* 1994;65(11):1016–1021.
9. Ciancio SG, Mather ML, Zambon JJ, et al. Effect of a chemotherapeutic agent delivered by an oral irrigation device on plaque, gingivitis, and subgingival microflora. *J Periodontol.* 1989;60(6):310–315.
10. Cutler CW, Stanford TW, Abraham C, et al. Clinical benefits of oral irrigation for periodontitis are related to reduction of pro-inflammatory cytokine levels and plaque. *J Clin Periodontol.* 2000;27(2):134–143.
11. Drisko CL, White CL, Killoy WJ, et al. Comparison of dark-field microscopy and a flagella stain for monitoring the effect of a Water Pik on bacterial motility. *J Periodontol.* 1987;58(6):381–386.
12. Flemmig TF, Epp B, Funkenhauser Z, et al. Adjunctive supragingival irrigation with acetylsalicylic acid in periodontal supportive therapy. *J Clin Periodontol.* 1995;22(6):427–433.
13. Flemmig TF, Newman MG, Doherty FM, et al. Supragingival irrigation with 0.06% chlorhexidine in naturally occurring gingivitis. I. 6 month clinical observations. *J Periodontol.* 1990;61(2):112–117.
14. Gorur A, Lyle DM, Schaudinn C, et al. Biofilm removal with a dental water jet. *Compend Contin Educ Dent.* 2009;30 Spec No 1:1–6.
15. Goyal CR, Lyle DM, Qaqish JG, et al. Evaluation of the plaque removal efficacy of a water flosser compared to string floss in adults after a single use. *J Clin Dent.* 2013;24(2):37–42.
16. Magnuson B, Harsono M, Stark PC, et al. Comparison of the effect of two interdental cleaning devices around implants on the reduction of bleeding: a 30-day randomized clinical trial. *Compend Contin Educ Dent.* 2013;34 Spec No 8:2–7.
17. Newman MG, Cattabriga M, Etienne D, et al. Effectiveness of adjunctive irrigation in early periodontitis: multi-center evaluation. *J Periodontol.* 1994;65(3):224–229.
18. Newman MG, Flemmig TF, Nachnani S, et al. Irrigation with 0.06% chlorhexidine in naturally occurring gingivitis. II. 6 months microbiological observations. *J Periodontol.* 1990;61(7):427–433.
19. Rosema NA, Hennequin-Hoenderdos NL, Berchier CE, et al. The effect of different interdental cleaning devices on gingival bleeding. *J Int Acad Periodontol.* 2011;13(1):2–10.
20. Sharma NC, Lyle DM, Qaqish JG, et al. Effect of a dental water jet with orthodontic tip on plaque and bleeding in adolescent patients with fixed orthodontic appliances. *Am J Orthod Dentofacial Orthop.* 2008;133(4):565–571; quiz 628 e1–e2.
21. Walsh TF, Glenwright HD, Hull PS. Clinical effects of pulsed oral irrigation with 0.2% chlorhexidine digluconate in patients with adult periodontitis. *J Clin Periodontol.* 1992;19(4):245–248.
22. Felo A, Shibly O, Ciancio SG, et al. Effects of subgingival chlorhexidine irrigation on peri-implant maintenance. *Am J Dent.* 1997;10(2):107–110.
23. Lainson PA, Bergquist JJ, Fraleigh CM. A longitudinal study of pulsating water pressure cleansing devices. *J Periodontol.* 1972;43(7):444–446.
24. Offenbacher S, Heasman PA, Collins JG. Modulation of host PGE2 secretion as a determinant of periodontal disease expression. *J Periodontol.* 1993;64(5 suppl):432–444.
25. Tsai CC, Ho YP, Chen CC. Levels of interleukin-1 beta and interleukin-8 in gingival crevicular fluids in adult periodontitis. *J Periodontol.* 1995;66(10):852–859.
26. Krajewski J, Giblin J, Gargiulo AW. Evaluation of a water pressure cleaning device as an adjunct to periodontal treatment. *J Amer Soc Periodont.* 1964;2:76–78.
27. Wilson W, Taubert KA, Gewitz M, et al. Prevention of infective endocarditis: guidelines from the American Heart Association: a guideline from the American Heart Association Rheumatic Fever, Endocarditis, and Kawasaki Disease Committee, Council on Cardiovascular Disease in the Young, and the Council on Clinical Cardiology, Council on Cardiovascular Surgery and Anesthesia, and the Quality of Care and Outcomes Research Interdisciplinary Working Group. *Circulation.* 2007;116(15):1736–1754.
28. Nishimura RA, Carabello BA, Faxon DP, et al. ACC/AHA 2008 guideline update on valvular heart disease: focused update on infective endocarditis: a report of the American College of Cardiology/American Heart Association Task Force on Practice Guidelines: endorsed by the Society of Cardiovascular Anesthesiologists, Society for Cardiovascular Angiography and Interventions, and Society of Thoracic Surgeons. *Circulation.* 2008;118(8):887–896.
29. Hallmon WW, Rees TD. Local anti-infective therapy: mechanical and physical approaches. A systematic review. *Ann Periodontol.* 2003;8(1):99–114.
30. Shiloah J, Hovious LA. The role of subgingival irrigations in the treatment of periodontitis. *J Periodontol.* 1993;64(9):835–843.
31. Braatz L, Garrett S, Claffey N, et al. Antimicrobial irrigation of deep pockets to supplement non-surgical periodontal therapy. II. Daily irrigation. *J Clin Periodontol.* 1985;12(8):630–638.
32. Herzog A, Hodges KO. Subgingival irrigation with Chloramine-T. *J Dent Hyg.* 1988;62(10):515–521.
33. Krust KS, Drisko CL, Gross K, et al. The effects of subgingival irrigation with chlorhexidine and stannous fluoride. A preliminary investigation. *J Dent Hyg.* 1991;65(6):289–295.
34. Listgarten MA, Grossberg D, Schwimer C, et al. Effect of subgingival irrigation with tetrapotassium peroxydiphosphate on scaled and untreated periodontal pockets. *J Periodontol.* 1989;60(1):4–11.

35. MacAlpine R, Magnusson I, Kiger R, et al. Antimicrobial irrigation of deep pockets to supplement oral hygiene instruction and root debridement. I. Bi-weekly irrigation. *J Clin Periodontol.* 1985;12(7):568–577.

36. Shiloah J, Patters MR. DNA probe analyses of the survival of selected periodontal pathogens following scaling, root planing, and intra-pocket irrigation. *J Periodontol.* 1994;65(6):568–575.

37. Christersson LA, Norderyd OM, Puchalsky CS. Topical application of tetracycline-HCl in human periodontitis. *J Clin Periodontol.* 1993;20(2):88–95.

38. Khoo JG, Newman HN. Subgingival plaque control by a simplified oral hygiene regime plus local chlorhexidine or metronidazole. *J Periodontal Res.* 1983;18(6):607–619.

39. Rosling BG, Slots J, Webber RL, et al. Microbiological and clinical effects of topical subgingival antimicrobial treatment on human periodontal disease. *J Clin Periodontol.* 1983;10(5):487–514.

40. Southard SR, Drisko CL, Killoy WJ, et al. The effect of 2% chlorhexidine digluconate irrigation on clinical parameters and the level of Bacteroides gingivalis in periodontal pockets. *J Periodontol.* 1989;60(6):302–309.

41. Wolff LF, Bakdash MB, Pilhlstrom BL, et al. The effect of professional and home subgingival irrigation with antimicrobial agents on gingivitis and early periodontitis. *J Dent Hyg.* 1989;63(5):222–225, 241.

42. Greenstein G. Position paper: the role of supra- and subgingival irrigation in the treatment of periodontal diseases. *J Periodontol.* 2005;76(11):2015–2027.

43. Macaulay WJ, Newman HN. The effect on the composition of subgingival plaque of a simplified oral hygiene system including pulsating jet subgingival irrigation. *J Periodontal Res.* 1986;21(4):375–385.

44. Wennstrom JL, Dahlen G, Grondahl K, et al. Periodic subgingival antimicrobial irrigation of periodontal pockets. II. Microbiological and radiographical observations. *J Clin Periodontol.* 1987;14(10):573–580.

 STUDENT ANCILLARY RESOURCES

A wide variety of resources to enhance your learning and understanding of this chapter are available on thePoint®.

- Visit thePoint to access:
  - Audio Glossary
  - Animations
  - Suggested Readings
  - Answers to Review Questions
  - Case Studies

CHAPTER

25

Chemical Agents in Periodontal Care

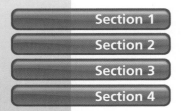
Clinical Application. As discussed in other chapters of this textbook, it is clear that periodontal diseases are caused by bacterial infections and that bacteria found in dental plaque biofilm are the primary causative agents in these diseases. Many bacterial infections that have affected mankind have been brought under control using various chemical agents to attack bacteria that cause those diseases. It is quite natural for researchers and clinicians alike to search for chemical agents or medications to help in the difficult task of controlling periodontal diseases. This chapter discusses some of the more important chemical agents that can be used in biofilm control.

Learning Objectives

• Describe the difference between systemic delivery and topical delivery of chemical agents.

• Explain the term systemic antibiotic.

• Explain why systemic antibiotics are not used routinely in the treatment of patients with plaque-associated gingivitis and patients with chronic periodontitis.

• Describe three examples of mouthrinse ingredients that can help reduce the severity of gingivitis.

• List three antimicrobial agents that can be delivered with controlled-release delivery devices.

• Explain why toothpastes are nearly ideal delivery mechanisms for chemical agents.

• List two toothpaste ingredients that can reduce the severity of gingivitis.

Key Terms

Systemic delivery
Topical delivery
Microbial reservoir
Systemic antibiotics
Antibiotic resistance

Conventional mechanical
   periodontal therapy
Controlled-release delivery
   device
Therapeutic mouth rinses
Efficacy

Stability
Substantivity
Safety
Active ingredient
Inactive ingredient
Essential oils

Section 1
Introduction to Chemical Agents in Biofilm Control

As discussed in other chapters of this textbook, it is clear that periodontal diseases are caused by bacterial infections, and that bacteria found in dental plaque biofilm are the primary causative agents in these diseases. Research indicates 1,000 species of bacteria have been found in dental plaque biofilm. Many bacterial infections that have affected mankind have been brought under control using various chemical agents to attack bacteria that cause those diseases.

1. **Delivery of Chemical Agents in Periodontal Patients.** Chemical agents useful in biofilm control can be delivered by using either systemic delivery or topical delivery.
   A. **Systemic Delivery**
      1. In dentistry, **systemic delivery** usually refers to administering chemical agents in the form of a tablet or capsule. When a tablet is taken by the patient, the chemical agent contained is released as the tablet dissolves, and the agent subsequently enters the blood stream—thus the chemical agent is circulated "systemically" throughout the body.
      2. As the chemical agent circulates throughout the body, it is also incorporated into the tissues of the periodontium including the gingival crevicular fluids where it can come into contact with bacteria causing periodontal diseases.
      3. An example of systemic delivery of a chemical agent would be for a patient to take a tablet or capsule of the antibiotic penicillin. The penicillin passes through the wall of the gastrointestinal tract and enters body tissues. In medical care, systemic delivery of chemical agents can also be administered by injection into a muscle or blood vessel, although this mode of systemic delivery has little to do with the control of dental biofilm.
   B. **Topical Delivery**
      1. In dentistry, **topical delivery** usually refers to intraoral placement of a chemical agent or local delivery using controlled-release devices into a periodontal pocket where the chemical agent then comes into contact with biofilm forming either on the teeth or in the periodontal pocket.
      2. Examples of topical delivery in dentistry would be using a mouth rinse or toothpaste that contains a chemical agent that can kill bacteria growing in dental biofilm. In this instance the chemical agent would come into contact with the teeth, oral mucous membranes, and the surface of dental biofilm.
      3. It should be noted that when chemical agents come into contact with oral mucous membranes, some of the agents enter the bloodstream by passing through the mucous membranes, but the bulk of the agent contacts the bacteria topically. See Table 25-1 for an overview of topical and systemic delivery mechanisms for chemical agents used in dental biofilm control.
2. **Considerations for Use of Chemical Agents in Periodontal Patients**
   A. **Resistance of the Biofilm to the Delivery of Chemical Agents**
      1. Research shows that the surface of dental plaque biofilm is covered by a slime layer that can act as a barrier preventing some chemical agents from actually contacting bacteria that are a part of the plaque biofilm.

TABLE 25-1. DELIVERY MECHANISMS FOR CHEMICAL AGENTS

Delivery Type	Specific Mechanisms	Possible Patient Benefits
Topical	Therapeutic mouth rinses	Reduce the severity of gingival inflammation
Topical	Therapeutic dentifrices	Reduction in dentinal hypersensitivity Reduction in gingival inflammation Reduction of supragingival calculus Reduction in surface stains
Topical	Subgingival irrigation	Disruption and dilution of bacteria within the dental biofilm
Topical	Controlled-release delivery devices	Subject subgingival bacteria to therapeutic levels of a drug for a period of a week or longer
Systemic	Tablets, capsules	Help control aggressive periodontitis Fight acute oral infections

Box 25-1. Microbial Reservoirs for Periodontal Pathogens

- Bacterial plaque biofilm in protected sites such as furcation areas
- Bacteria in residual calculus deposits that are not removed during nonsurgical therapy
- Bacteria living within the connective tissue adjacent to a periodontal pocket
- Bacteria that have penetrated dentinal tubules
- Bacteria protected by irregularities in tooth surfaces after mechanical treatment
- Bacteria protected by poorly defined restoration margins

2. Because of the protective nature of the surface slime layer, mechanical biofilm control—to disrupt the structure of the biofilm—is still important to allow the chemical agents to reach the bacteria themselves.

B. **Microbial Reservoirs for Periodontal Pathogens.** In the oral cavity, there are a variety of microbial reservoirs that can lead to rapid repopulation of bacterial pathogens in a treated periodontal patient.

   1. A **microbial reservoir** is a niche or secure place in the oral cavity that can allow periodontal pathogens to live undisturbed during routine therapy and subsequently repopulate periodontal pockets quickly.
   2. An example of a microbial reservoir would be a residual calculus deposit following periodontal instrumentation. Living bacteria found within the calculus deposit can reproduce in periodontal pockets and continue to promote disease even after what appears to be thorough nonsurgical therapy.
   3. Box 25-1 provides an overview of some of the many microbial reservoirs for periodontal pathogens in the oral cavity.

3. **Criteria for Effective Chemical Agents.** For chemotherapy to be effective, it must meet three requirements: (1) reach the site of disease activity, namely the base of the pocket, (2) be delivered at a bacteriostatic or bactericidal concentration, and (3) remain in place long enough to be effective (1). See Table 25-2 for a comparison of the effectiveness of common drug delivery systems for management of periodontitis.

4. **Chemical Agents Effective Against Periodontitis.** Periodontal instrumentation is an effective mechanical therapy for periodontitis (2,3). In deep or tortuous pockets or sites that do not respond to nonsurgical periodontal therapy, however, it may be beneficial to use adjunctive chemical agents (4,5). At this point, there is no biofilm control chemical agent that can halt periodontitis, but there are a number of different chemical agents that can be used as part of comprehensive treatment for patients with periodontal diseases. An overview of some of the types of chemical agents that have been suggested for use in biofilm control in periodontal patients is presented in Table 25-3.

TABLE 25-2. COMPARISON OF DRUG DELIVERY SYSTEMS FOR MANAGEMENT OF PERIODONTITIS

	Adequate Drug Concentration	Reaches Site of Disease Activity	Adequate Time in Place to be Effective
Mouth rinsing	Good	Poor	Poor
Subgingival irrigation	Good	Good	Poor
Systemic delivery	Fair	Good	Fair
Controlled-release delivery	Good	Good	Good

TABLE 25-3. OVERVIEW OF SOME OF THE CHEMICAL AGENTS USED IN BIOFILM CONTROL

Type of Agent	Example of Agent	Means of Administration
Antibiotics	Tetracyclines	Tablet/capsule Local delivery mechanism
Bisbiguanide antiseptics	Chlorhexidine	Mouth rinse Local delivery mechanism
Fluorides	Stannous fluoride	Mouth rinse Toothpaste
Metal salts	Tin/zinc	Mouth rinse Toothpaste
Oxygenating agents	Hydrogen peroxide	Mouth rinse
Phenolic compounds	Essential oils	Mouth rinse
Quaternary ammonium	Cetylpyridinium chloride	Mouth rinse
Tertiary amine surfactant	Delmopinol	Mouth rinse

Section 2
Use of Systemic Antibiotics to Control Biofilm

1. Overview of Systemic Antibiotics
   A. Definitions
      1. Antibiotics are medications used to help fight infections either because they kill bacteria or because they can inhibit the growth of bacteria.
      2. Systemic antibiotics refer to those antibiotics that can be taken orally or that can be injected and are in widespread use in fighting bacterial infections throughout the world. In North America, healthcare providers such as physicians and dentists have access to a broad range of antibiotic drugs for use in patients with infections. These drugs have been used for many years to help the body fight certain bacterial infections and have undoubtedly been responsible for saving countless lives.
   B. Systemic Antibiotics Studied for Use in Periodontal Diseases. Systemic antibiotics have also been studied for their use in controlling periodontal diseases. Box 25-2 lists some examples of systemic antibiotics that have been studied by researchers for use in periodontal patients.
   C. Plaque-Induced Gingivitis and Chronic Periodontitis
      1. For most patients with the more common forms of periodontal diseases (i.e., either plaque-induced gingivitis or chronic periodontitis), current recommendations are for clinicians to avoid the routine use of systemic antibiotic drugs to control these diseases. There are two major reasons for recommendations to avoid their routine use in these patients.
         a. One reason dentists do not use systemic antibiotics routinely to control the more common forms of periodontal diseases is antibiotic resistance (6–8). Antibiotic resistance refers to the ability of a bacterium to withstand the effects of an antibiotic by developing mechanisms to protect the bacterium from the killing or inhibiting effects of the antibiotic. Most species of subgingival bacteria are considerably more resistant in biofilms than in planktonic cultures. Resistance appeared to be age related because biofilms demonstrated progressive antibiotic resistance as they matured with maximum resistance coinciding with the steady-state phase of biofilm growth (9).
            1. According to the National Science Foundation and the Centers for Disease Control, antibiotic resistance is a serious public health problem throughout the world, and the problem is increasing in scope. When antibiotic resistant strains of bacteria develop, they are generally not affected by the antibiotic, survive, and continue to cause more damage.
            2. An example of how antibiotic resistance can be a public health problem is the high incidence of penicillin-resistant microorganisms that have already limited the usefulness of this important drug. As more and more bacteria develop resistance to the antibiotic penicillin, the usefulness of this antibiotic as a lifesaving drug will continue to decrease.

Box 25-2. Examples of Systemic Antibiotics Studied for Use in Periodontal Care

- Penicillin and amoxicillin
- Tetracyclines
- Erythromycin
- Metronidazole
- Clindamycin

   b. Another reason dentists do not use systemic antibiotics routinely to control periodontal diseases is that studies indicate that in most patients these diseases respond to conventional mechanical periodontal therapy just as well as they respond to the systemic administration of antibiotics. **Conventional mechanical periodontal therapy** is a term that refers to self-care, periodontal instrumentation (scaling and root planing), and control of local contributing factors.

2. When antibiotics are being considered for use in periodontal patients, careful patient selection is necessary.
   a. When tempted to use systemic antibiotics to control either plaque-induced gingivitis or chronic periodontitis, dental healthcare providers must weigh potential benefits and disadvantages. At this point, most clinicians have decided that the potential harm outweighs the benefits.
   b. In patients with chronic periodontitis the efficacy of using antibiotic therapy is not completely clear, and antibiotic therapy in these patients should usually be limited to those patients who have continued periodontal breakdown after thorough conventional mechanical periodontal therapy.
   c. It should be noted that even though systemic antibiotics are rarely indicated for routine treatment of patients with plaque-induced gingivitis or chronic periodontitis, they are frequently indicated in the treatment of patients with rarer forms of periodontitis, such as aggressive periodontitis.

3. Patient education. Even though systemic antibiotic drugs are not normally used for patients with plaque-induced gingivitis or chronic periodontitis, systemic antibiotics are discussed here because periodontal patients can ask why antibiotics are not being recommended for them.
   a. This question may arise when the patient learns that periodontitis is a bacterial infection. This is a natural question for a patient to ask given the widespread use of antibiotics in fighting infections of all sorts.
   b. When confronted with a question from a patient about why antibiotics are not being recommended, the dental hygienist can explain the following facts:
      1. Most cases of gingivitis and periodontitis can be readily controlled with treatments that do not require the use of systemic antibiotics.
      2. Overuse of systemic antibiotics often results in the development of antibiotic-resistant strains of bacteria, simply compounding a complex dental problem. This is a major public health concern, since many antibiotics can be rendered useless for lifesaving measures through the development of antibiotic resistance.

D. Aggressive Periodontitis
   1. The use of antibiotics in conjunction with mechanical therapy is usually indicated in patients with aggressive forms of periodontitis (10–13).
   2. When antibiotics are being considered for use, microbiologic analysis is a wise clinical step. Microbiologic analysis involves sampling the bacteria associated with the disease process and testing cultures of the bacteria for specific antibiotic susceptibility. Utilizing microbiologic analysis can avoid prescribing inappropriate antibiotics that can lead to a poor clinical response. Figure 25-1 illustrates the relationship between periodontal diagnoses and the use of systemic antibiotics.

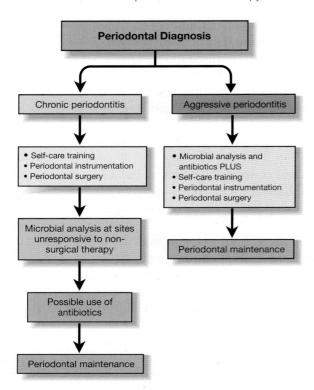

Figure 25-1. The Relationship Between Periodontal Diagnosis and the Use of Systemic Antibiotics.

2. **Use of Tetracyclines in Periodontal Patients.** One of the antibiotic groups, the group of drugs called tetracyclines, has received special attention by researchers because it has some specific properties that make it attractive to consider for use in selected periodontal patients.

   A. **Tetracyclines Tend to be Concentrated in the Gingival Crevicular Fluids.** When tetracycline drugs are administered orally, the drugs permeate body tissues and reach a certain concentration in the blood serum. The level of tetracycline drugs, however, is more concentrated within the gingival crevicular fluids flowing into periodontal pockets than the level found in the blood serum. This results in a higher concentration of the drug in exactly the site it might be needed in a periodontal patient.

   B. **The Tetracyclines are Effective Against Most Strains of *Aggregatibacter Actinomycetemcomitans*.** *Aggregatibacter actinomycetemcomitans* is one of the periodontal pathogens thought to be a primary player in many patients with periodontitis.

   C. **The Tetracyclines Have Other Effects in Addition to Their Antimicrobial Properties**
      1. Tetracyclines inhibit the action of collagenase—one of the enzymes responsible in part for breakdown of the periodontium in periodontitis patients.
      2. Any drug that can inhibit the action of collagenase can be expected to slow the progress of breakdown of the periodontium that is seen in periodontitis.

   D. **Certain Tetracyclines are Effective in Subantimicrobial Doses**
      1. A subantimicrobial dose (SDD) of the doxycycline (20 mg twice a day) significantly improved clinical parameters associated with periodontal health in patients with periodontitis when used as an adjunct to a maintenance schedule of periodontal instrumentation (10,11,13).
      2. Several studies accessed whether long-term SDD of doxycycline produces doxycycline-resistant oral microflora in adults with periodontitis. These studies found no evidence of antibiotic resistance in the SDD doxycycline treatment groups (11,13).

Section 3
Use of Topically Delivered Chemical Agents

1. Controlled Release of Antimicrobial Chemicals
   A. Overview of Controlled-Release Mechanisms
      1. A **controlled-release delivery device** usually consists of an antibacterial chemical that is imbedded in a carrier material. It is designed to be placed directly into the periodontal pocket where the carrier material attaches to the tooth surface and dissolves slowly, producing a steady release of the antimicrobial agent over a period of several days within the periodontal pocket (14).
      2. The earliest version of these products involved coating carrier fibers with chemical agents that would be released following placement of the fibers within periodontal pockets. Use of this early example of these products involved a return patient office visit for removal of the fibers.
      3. The latest versions of these products involve imbedding antimicrobial agents into carrier materials, which dissolve slowly over approximately 1 week. The carrier material can be placed into a periodontal pocket, and as it dissolves it slowly releases the antimicrobial agent.
      4. Antimicrobial agents currently used in controlled-release delivery devices include chlorhexidine and some of the antibiotic drugs such as the tetracyclines. In the future, other drugs may be used for this purpose.
   B. **Rationale for Use.** The goal of the use of these controlled-release delivery devices is to subject subgingival bacteria to therapeutic levels of an antibacterial drug for a sustained period. Most of these controlled-release devices continue to deliver chemicals into the pockets for approximately 1 week.
   C. Benefits of Controlled-Release Delivery Devices
      1. Use of controlled-release delivery devices has been shown to result in a small increase in attachment level in a periodontal pocket (about a 2-mm reduction found in probing depths).
      2. Controlled studies are available to guide dental healthcare providers in the appropriate use of these new devices.
         a. Controlled-release devices may be indicated for use in localized periodontal pockets that are nonresponsive after thorough nonsurgical and surgical periodontal therapy.
         b. When these products were used along with periodontal instrumentation, they can result in both an improvement in probing depth reduction and a clinical attachment gain. The clinical significance of the small amount of improvement is unclear at this point. Routine use of controlled-release delivery devices as an adjunct to periodontal instrumentation and periodontal maintenance may show improved results in future phase III designed clinical studies.
         c. Current guidelines support the use of controlled-release devices in combination with periodontal instrumentation (3–5,15–18).
   D. **Controlled-Release Mechanisms.** Several controlled-release delivery products have been introduced in the United States over the last few years, and it is likely that more will be available within the next few years. The chemical agents that have been incorporated into these devices and marketed over the past few years are outlined next.

1. Tetracycline Hydrochloride–Containing Fibers
   a. One of the first of these products released for use involved tetracycline hydrochloride–containing fibers that were to be inserted into the periodontal pocket to deliver a high concentration of tetracycline to the site for several days.
      1. Marketed under the brand name Actisite, *this product is no longer available in the United States.*
      2. *This mechanism represents the first successful product of this type, and is discussed here for historical purposes.*
   b. Technique for Fiber Placement and Stabilization
      1. A gingival retraction cord-packing instrument was used to insert the tetracycline-containing fibers into a pocket, but the insertion was time-consuming.
      2. The fiber was placed under the gingival margin around an entire tooth, and the pocket was filled by layering the fiber back and forth upon itself (Fig. 25-2).
      3. Finally, adhesive was applied along the gingival margin to keep the fiber in the pocket.
      4. A return patient visit to the dental office was needed for fiber removal.
   c. Adverse reactions that were reported for this product included discomfort on fiber placement, oral candidiasis, allergic response, gingival inflammation, and pain.
2. Minocycline Hydrochloride Microspheres
   a. Marketed under the brand name Arestin.
   b. Another example of a controlled-release mechanism delivers the antibiotic minocycline hydrochloride in a powdered microsphere form. Minocycline hydrochloride is a broad-spectrum, semisynthetic tetracycline derivative that is bacteriostatic.
   c. Application
      1. A cannula tip is used to expel the microspheres into the pocket (Fig. 25-3) where it binds to the tooth surface because of the sticky nature of the carrier material.
      2. Over 5 to 7 days, the powdered microspheres dissolve releasing the imbedded minocycline, so there is nothing to remove from the pocket.
   d. Studies demonstrate that repeated subgingival administration of minocycline microspheres in the treatment of adult periodontitis is safe and is more effective than periodontal instrumentation alone in reducing probing depths in periodontitis patients (19,20).
   e. Adverse reactions. Possible adverse reactions include oral candidiasis or an allergic response. In addition, the use of antibiotic preparations may result in the development of resistant bacteria.
   f. Contraindications for use. This product is a tetracycline derivative, and should not be used in patients who are hypersensitive to any tetracycline or in women who are pregnant or nursing.
3. Doxycycline hyclate gel
   a. Marketed under the brand name Atridox.
   b. This product is a gel system that delivers the antibiotic doxycycline (also a tetracycline derivative) to the periodontal pocket.

  c. Application of doxycycline hyclate gel

   1. The gel is expressed into the pocket with a cannula (Fig. 25-3), and after placement the gel solidifies into a wax-like substance.

   2. The cannula tip is placed near the pocket base and gel is expressed using a steady pressure until the gel reaches the top of the gingival margin.

   3. A limitation to this delivery system is that the gel tends to cling to the cannula when withdrawn from the pocket, which can be reduced by using a moistened dental hand instrument to hold the gel in place while slowly withdrawing the cannula tip from the pocket.

   4. The gel is biodegradable (it dissolves), so there is nothing to remove from the pocket.

  d. In a 6-month multicenter trial, results indicate that periodontal instrumentation combined with local application of doxycycline in deep periodontal sites can be considered as a justified approach for nonsurgical treatment of chronic periodontitis (21).

  e. Adverse reactions

   1. Possible adverse reactions include oral candidiasis or an allergic response.

   2. The use of antibiotic preparations may result in the development of resistant bacteria.

  f. Contraindications for use. This product is a tetracycline derivative, and should not be used in patients who are hypersensitive to any tetracycline or in women who are pregnant or nursing.

4. Chlorhexidine gluconate chip

  a. Marketed under the brand name PerioChip.

  b. Another example of a controlled-release device is a tiny gelatin chip containing the antiseptic chlorhexidine that is inserted into a periodontal pocket that is 5 mm or greater in depth (Fig. 25-4).

  c. Investigations indicate that the chlorhexidine gluconate chip, when used as an adjunct to periodontal instrumentation, significantly reduces loss of alveolar bone (22).

  d. Application

   1. The gelatin chip is inserted into the periodontal pocket.

   2. The gelatin chip can be difficult to insert into some pockets due to the size and shape of the chip.

   3. The gelatin chip is bioabsorbed, so there is no need to have it removed after placement.

  e. Since chlorhexidine is not an antibiotic, there is no risk of antibiotic resistance with the use of the chlorhexidine gluconate gelatin chip.

  f. A 1-year clinical trial by Henke et al. (23) suggest that a chlorhexidine chip may reduce periodontal surgical needs at little additional cost.

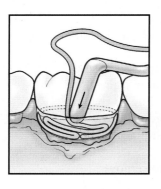

Figure 25-2. Fibers Inserted into the Pocket. One of the first local delivery mechanisms used involved a tetracycline-containing fiber. The tetracycline-containing fiber was inserted into the periodontal pocket, and the entire pocket was filled by layering the fiber back and forth upon itself. The fiber released the tetracycline slowly over several days, and required removal after 5 to 7 days. **This product is no longer available in the United States**.

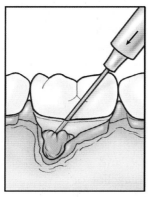

Figure 25-3. Products Expelled into the Pocket. Some local delivery mechanisms involve placing the carrier material into a periodontal pocket with a cannula tip. Minocycline hydrochloride–containing microspheres and doxycycline gel are examples of such products. These carrier materials adhere to the tooth surfaces and dissolve slowly—releasing the antimicrobial agents trapped in the carrier material.

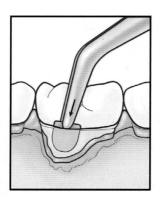

Figure 25-4. Gelatin Chip Inserted into Pocket. The gelatin chip is inserted into periodontal pockets 5 mm or greater in depth. The gelatin chip adheres to the tooth surface and dissolves slowly—releasing the chlorhexidine antimicrobial agent trapped in the gelatin.

2. Mouth Rinses as Aids in Biofilm Control

A. Introduction to Mouth Rinses

1. Many mouth rinses available today are therapeutic mouth rinses. **Therapeutic mouth rinses** are mouth rinses that have some actual benefit (provide some therapeutic action) to the patient in addition to the simple goal of breath freshening and halitosis reduction.

   a. In the context of this chapter therapeutic mouth rinses would be rinses that decrease dental biofilm enough to also decrease the severity of gingivitis. Figure 25-5 pictures two examples of therapeutic mouth rinses.

   b. Clinical studies support the effectiveness of therapeutic mouth rinses used in addition to proper home care for the reduction of dental biofilm and the control of gingivitis. Insufficient evidence is available to support the claim that therapeutic mouth rinses can reduce the risk of developing periodontitis or the rate of progression of periodontitis (24,25). Over the last few decades, researchers are still searching for chemicals that can be added to mouth rinses that might actually reduce or halt periodontitis.

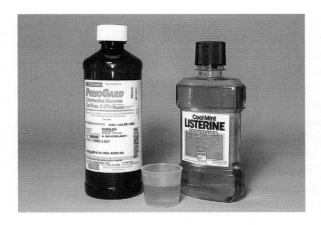

Figure 25-5. Therapeutic Mouth Rinses. Two examples of therapeutic mouth rinses used to aid in dental biofilm control. The mouth rinse pictured on the left contain chlorhexidine gluconate as its active ingredient. The mouth rinse pictured on the right contains essential oils as the active ingredient and is available over the counter.

2. It should be noted that in addition to therapeutic mouth rinses that can aid in the control of biofilm and gingivitis, there are other therapeutic mouth rinses available that can benefit the patient in a variety of ways such as decreasing the risk of developing dental caries and treatment of dentinal hypersensitivity.

B. **Characteristics That an Ideal Mouth Rinse Should Possess.** Investigations into chemical biofilm control have not yet produced a biofilm control mouth rinse that can be used as a total substitute for mechanical biofilm control. However, these investigations have indeed produced mouth rinses that can be useful components of a comprehensive program of patient self-care. An ideal mouth rinse would possess four characteristics that are described below.

1. **Efficacy.** The active ingredient in the rinse should be effective in inhibiting (bacteriostatic) or killing periodontal pathogens (bactericidal).

2. **Stability.** The ingredients in the mouth rinse should be stable at room temperature and have a reasonable shelf life.

3. **Substantivity** (sub-stan-tiv-ity). The active ingredient in the rinse should display the property of substantivity. This means that the active ingredient would be retained in the oral cavity for a while following rinsing and would be released slowly over time (usually several hours), resulting in a continuing antimicrobial effect against periodontal pathogens.

   a. Substantivity is an important characteristic, since dental biofilm grows and matures continuously.

   b. An active ingredient that displays the property of substantivity would continue to kill periodontal pathogens over an extended number of hours following rinsing.

4. **Safety.** The ingredients in the mouth rinse should not produce any harmful effects to the tissues in the oral cavity or systemically to the patient.

C. **Ingredients of Mouth Rinses**

1. Products such as mouth rinses contain both active ingredients and inactive ingredients.

   a. An **active ingredient** is a component that produces some benefit for the patient (such as a reduction in the severity of gingival inflammation associated with gingivitis).

   b. All mouth rinses also contain **inactive ingredients**.

      1. Inactive ingredients are included in mouth rinse formulations simply to add other properties such as color enhancement, taste improvements, increase in shelf life, or to keep components in a liquid state.

2. Though these ingredients are called "inactive," there can be associated side effects with some of these ingredients in certain patients. It is important that clinicians maintain familiarity with the inactive ingredients of rinses as well as the active ingredients.

2. Many chemicals that might be placed in mouth rinses have been investigated for their effect against both biofilm and gingivitis.

   a. Chemicals that reduce biofilm formation to only a minor degree usually have little or no clinically significant effect against gingivitis, and therefore may not be very useful in controlling a disease such as gingivitis. Many mouth rinses marketed today fall into this category.

   b. Among the many ingredients tested for efficacy against gingivitis, four mouthrinse ingredients that have some effect against gingivitis have been studied extensively. These ingredients are listed below.

      1. Chlorhexidine gluconate
      2. Essential oils
      3. Cetylpyridinium chloride
      4. Delmopinol

D. Mouth Rinses Containing Chlorhexidine Gluconate

1. One group of mouth rinses currently available contains chlorhexidine gluconate as the active ingredient. These rinses are only available through prescriptions in the United States, but they can be purchased over the counter in some other countries.

   a. Mouth rinses containing chlorhexidine gluconate as the active ingredient have been demonstrated to reduce the severity of gingivitis in numerous clinical studies.

   b. In the United States the concentration of chlorhexidine gluconate used in prescription mouth rinses is 0.12%, but it should be noted that a higher concentration is used in mouth rinses in some other countries.

2. At this point, chlorhexidine is the most effective antimicrobial agent for long-term reduction of biofilm and gingivitis. For this reason, it is often regarded as the standard against which all other topical chemical biofilm control agents are judged (26,27).

   a. The effectiveness of chlorhexidine gluconate mouth rinses is due to the following characteristics.

      1. Chlorhexidine is bactericidal agent that is effective against both gram-positive and gram-negative bacteria.
      2. Chlorhexidine binds with oral tissues in the mouth and is slowly released over time (several hours) in a concentration that will continue killing bacteria. Thus, these rinses display the property of substantivity (27).
      3. Chlorhexidine has a very low level of toxicity and shows no permanent retention in the body.

3. The primary mechanism of action for chlorhexidine gluconate is disruption of the integrity of the cell walls of bacteria.

4. Chlorhexidine-containing mouth rinses are useful adjuncts to biofilm control in many patients. Current recommendations for use of this mouth rinse (0.12% chlorhexidine gluconate) are to rinse with one-half ounce for 30 seconds twice daily, 30 minutes after toothbrushing.

5. There are several groups of patients that should be considered for use of chlorhexidine gluconate mouth rinse. Some of these are outlined below:

   a. Special needs patients. The use of a chlorhexidine mouth rinse is suggested for specific groups of patients who have special needs. Two examples of such patients are those with immunodeficiencies that might be more susceptible to infections in general and patients who are unable to perform biofilm control because of some impairment.

   b. Postsurgical care patients. Following periodontal surgery, it is frequently difficult for patients to perform adequate mechanical biofilm control during the healing period without damaging the surgical site. In these patients, chlorhexidine mouth rinses can be used for postsurgical rinsing as a temporary adjunct to mechanical biofilm control. Use of a chlorhexidine mouth rinse following periodontal surgery for 4 to 6 weeks can be effective in many patients to promote healing.

   c. Patients with Candida infections. It should be noted that a variety of medications are used to control Candida infections, but chlorhexidine mouth rinses can be used as a disinfectant for dental appliances such as complete dentures or partial dentures in patients with these infections.

   d. Patients with high caries risk. Chlorhexidine is also effective against the bacteria responsible for dental caries. Rinsing with chlorhexidine mouth rinses has been used to reduce the counts of caries causing bacteria in certain patients.

   e. Patients with oral piercings or dental implants. Chlorhexidine mouth rinses have also been recommended for use by patients for aftercare of oral piercings and dental implants.

   f. Patients who are immunocompromised. Chlorhexidine rinsing is recommended for patients being treated with radiation therapy or immunosuppressive drugs.

6. Chlorhexidine mouth rinses do have their limitations (27–29).

   a. Chlorhexidine is an antiplaque agent that can prevent plaque formation, but its mode of action does not allow it to remove plaque already present on tooth surfaces efficiently. In a randomized split-mouth study, Zanatta found that a 0.12% chlorhexidine gluconate mouth rinse had little antiplaque and antigingivitis effect on previously plaque-covered surfaces. These results confirm the diminished effect of chlorhexidine on structured biofilm and reinforce the necessity of mechanical biofilm disruption before the initiation of chlorhexidine mouth rinse (29).

   b. Also, the chlorhexidine molecule reacts with anionic surfactants (sodium lauryl sulfate) present in certain toothpaste formulations, thus reducing the effectiveness of the chlorhexidine (26).

7. Chlorhexidine mouth rinses have been evaluated related to their effectiveness as a preprocedural rinse for dental office procedures producing aerosols. Studies suggest that a preprocedural chlorhexidine rinse eliminates the majority of bacterial aerosols generated by the use of an ultrasonic unit (30,31).

E. **Mouth Rinses Containing Essential Oils**

1. Chemicals referred to as essential oils have been used as active ingredients in some mouth rinses for many years. Chemical agents included in the group of chemicals called essential oils include thymol, menthol, eucalyptol, and methyl salicylate.

2. Mouth rinses containing essential oils are available over the counter (i.e., available without a prescription). Listerine mouth rinse is one example of a rinse containing essential oils, but there are other products on the market with similar ingredients.

3. There are numerous investigations related to the efficacy of essential oils in controlling gingivitis published in the literature.

   a. This group of chemicals can indeed help control biofilm, and they have received the Seal of Acceptance from the American Dental Association for their effect against *gingivitis*.

   b. A 6-month controlled clinical study demonstrated that the essential oil mouth rinse and the chlorhexidine mouth rinse had comparable antiplaque and antigingivitis activity (32).

   c. Several investigations found no significant difference with respect to reduction of gingival inflammation between an essential oil mouth rinse and a chlorhexidine mouth rinse. In long-term use, the essential oil mouth rinse appears to be a reliable alternative to chlorhexidine mouthwash with respect to parameters of gingival inflammation (33,34).

   d. The mechanism of action of essential oils appears to be disruption of the integrity of the cell wall and inhibition of certain bacterial enzymes.

   e. Essential oil mouth rinses are much less expensive than chlorhexidine mouth rinses and can be purchased without a prescription. Insofar as the side effects associated with chlorhexidine mouth rinses—staining, taste alteration—may limit patient compliance, essential oil mouth rinses can have a distinct role in the management of patients with periodontal diseases.

F. **Mouth Rinses Containing Quaternary Ammonium Compounds**

   1. Some mouth rinses currently marketed contain the quaternary ammonium compound cetylpyridinium chloride as the active ingredient.

   2. This surface active agent also kills bacteria by disrupting bacterial cell walls.

   3. This chemical agent binds to oral tissues but is released so rapidly that it has very limited substantivity, limiting its effectiveness in controlling dental biofilm.

   4. Investigations have shown that cetylpyridinium chloride can reduce the severity of gingivitis and supragingival biofilm, but the level of reduction is less than either chlorhexidine gluconate or essential oils (35,36).

G. **Mouth Rinses Containing Delmopinol**

   1. Some mouth rinses currently marketed contain delmopinol as the active ingredient, which is a third-generation morpholinoethanol derivative and tertiary amine surfactant.

   2. This chemical agent forms a barrier preventing biofilm from adhering to the tooth surface and gingiva. Delmopinol interferes with the enzymes responsible for the formation of biofilm and inhibits biofilm.

   3. Tooth- and tongue-staining side effects have been reported with delmopinol but were not found to be comparable with the staining associated with chlorhexidine gluconate.

   4. Investigations have shown that delmopinol effectively reduces the severity of gingivitis and biofilm when used adjunctively with mechanical biofilm removal and is a good alternative to chlorhexidine gluconate for some patients who cannot tolerate the associated side effects and allergies (37,38).

H. Problems With Mouthrinse Ingredients
   1. No chemicals are completely safe for all patients, and most mouth rinses have produced unwanted side effects in some patients. Reported side effects for some of the active ingredients discussed above are outlined in Table 25-4.
   2. As already discussed, in addition to the active ingredients mouth rinses contain inactive ingredients such as flavoring agents and preservatives that can create problems for some patients. Two of these ingredients are listed below.
      a. Alcohol. Some mouth rinses have rather high levels of alcohol content, and these should be avoided in patients addicted to alcohol.
      b. Salt. Some mouth rinses have rather high levels of sodium, making them questionable for use in certain patients with hypertension (high blood pressure).

TABLE 25-4. POSSIBLE SIDE EFFECTS OF MOUTH RINSES

Essential Oils Rinses	Chlorhexidine Gluconate Rinses
• Burning sensation in the mouth • Bitter taste • Drying out of mucous membranes	• Allergic reaction • Extrinsic staining of teeth • Discoloration of tongue • Alterations of taste • Increase in calculus formation • Transient anesthesia

3. **Toothpastes as Delivery Mechanisms for Biofilm Control Agents.** Dentifrices such as toothpastes and gels would appear to be nearly ideal delivery mechanisms for chemical agents that might benefit patients, since most patients use these products daily. Originally dentifrices were simply aids to brushing, but today there are a variety of chemical agents that can be added to toothpastes that may actually benefit some patients in other ways.
   A. **Categories of Toothpastes.** The American Dental Association loosely classifies toothpastes as falling into one of the following categories:
      1. Antitartar activity
      2. Caries prevention
      3. Cosmetic effects
      4. Gingivitis reduction
      5. Biofilm formation reduction
      6. Reduction of tooth sensitivity
   B. **Active Chemical Ingredients.** This American Dental Association classification of toothpastes underscores the broad range of benefits that can be derived from active ingredient chemical agents added to some toothpastes.
      1. Some of these chemical agents are added to impart special benefits to periodontal patients. See Table 25-5 for some examples of the chemical agents that can be used as active ingredients in toothpastes for their periodontal benefits.
      2. Stannous fluoride has been used successfully as an anticaries agent for many years. Studies indicate that stannous fluoride also affects dental biofilm and can also reduce the severity of gingivitis when used as an active ingredient in toothpastes.

3. Triclosan is a topical antimicrobial agent used in many products and is now available as the active ingredient in toothpaste.
   a. Triclosan can be combined with copolymers to enhance its substantivity (binding and subsequent slow release), which has been found to be retained in the oral cavity for 12 hours.
   b. Studies indicate that when combined with copolymers, triclosan (when delivered in toothpaste form) can decrease the severity of gingivitis more than dentifrice with stannous fluoride (39,40).
   c. Triclosan can also be combined with zinc citrate to reduce dental calculus formation.
C. **The Future.** Toothpastes appear to be ideal delivery mechanisms for chemical agents that might be expected to control certain periodontal conditions, such as gingival inflammation. It is reasonable to expect that additional research in this area will result in additional toothpaste formulations that target periodontal conditions such as gingivitis.

TABLE 25-5. EXAMPLES OF TOOTH ACTIVE INGREDIENTS USED FOR PERIODONTAL BENEFITS

Ingredients	Actions
Pyrophosphates	Reduces *supra*gingival calculus
Stannous fluoride	Reduces *supra*gingival biofilm Reduces gingival inflammation
Triclosan	Reduces *supra*gingival calculus Reduces gingival inflammation
Zinc citrate	Reduces *supra*gingival calculus

Chapter Summary Statement

Chemical agents that can be used to control dental biofilm can be delivered both systemically and topically. Since dental biofilm is covered by a protective slime layer, chemical agents will not necessarily contact all of the targeted bacteria, and their use must be accompanied by mechanical biofilm control that can disrupt the structure of the biofilm.

Systemic antibiotics are not normally used to control dental biofilm in patients with the most common periodontal conditions (plaque-associated gingivitis and chronic periodontitis) because of the high risk of developing antibiotic-resistant strains. Mouth rinses can be useful adjuncts in the treatment of patients with periodontal diseases. Thus, far the most effective ingredients to control biofilm that can be incorporated into mouth rinses include chlorhexidine and the essential oils. Controlled-release delivery devices are also available to help control bacterial biofilm in periodontal patients. Toothpastes are widely used by patients and appear to be an ideal mechanism for delivery of chemical agents to aid in biofilm control.

In selecting the appropriate delivery system, the clinician has to weigh the efficacy of the products, ease of use, availability, and cost. Although local delivery systems do not replace existing periodontal therapies, they do have a place in the treatment of periodontitis and offer the dental team additional methods to aid in the control of periodontal diseases.

Section 4
Focus on Patients

Clinical Patient Care

CASE 1

A patient shows you a bottle of mouth rinse and asks you if it would be all right to use this mouth rinse instead of brushing and flossing so frequently. You study the label on the bottle of mouth rinse and find that the active ingredients are the essential oils. How should you respond to this patient about substituting this rinse for other self-care efforts such as brushing and flossing?

CASE 2

A patient being treated by the members of your dental team has generalized chronic periodontitis. Following your thorough explanation of the nature of chronic periodontitis and your emphasis that this disease is indeed a bacterial infection, the patient asks this question, "If periodontitis is an infection, can you ask the dentist to give me a prescription for an antibiotic?" How should you respond to this patient's question?

CASE 3

A new patient being seen by your dental team has recently moved into your city. She has previously been treated for chronic periodontitis and has been on periodontal maintenance for several years. She is now having trouble with mechanical biofilm control because of increasing dexterity problems. What chemical agents can you recommend that might help reduce the patient's gingival inflammation?

Ethical Dilemma

Your patient, Sandy L, is a 24-year-old woman who has come to your office for a second opinion. Her chief complaint is that she feels that her periodontal health is not improving, and if anything, getting worse.

You review her health history, and she states that she has been under the care of her uncle, who is a 70-year-old periodontist. She has been taking tetracycline for the last 5 years, and is concerned with her periodontal and overall health. She did not bring any radiographs, as she doesn't want her uncle to know about this appointment.

Your examination reveals that Sandy has relatively good oral hygiene, with slight supragingival visible calculus between her mandibular anterior teeth. However, she presents with generalized severe gingival recession, and her attachment level readings range from 3 to 6 mm, with localized 7-mm readings on her posterior teeth.

continued on next page

It is hard to get a full picture due to the lack of radiographs. Sandy's periodontal status is troubling and you are not sure if the antibiotics that she is taking are actually helping her. You ask if she ever had a microbiologic analysis, to sample her oral bacteria susceptibility. She is not sure of any procedures, as she "just left all of that stuff to her uncle, the periodontal expert."

1. What do you think have may caused the patient's generalized recession?
2. What factors may have contributed to the patient's disease progression?
3. What ethical principles are in conflict in this dilemma?

References

1. Finkelman RD, Polson AM. Evidence-based considerations for the clinical use of locally delivered, controlled-release antimicrobials in periodontal therapy. *J Dent Hyg.* 2013;87(5):249–264.
2. Cobb CM. Clinical significance of non-surgical periodontal therapy: an evidence-based perspective of scaling and root planing. *J Clin Periodontol.* 2002;29 (suppl 2):6–16.
3. Drisko CL, Cochran DL, Blieden T, et al. Position paper: sonic and ultrasonic scalers in periodontics. Research, Science and Therapy Committee of the American Academy of Periodontology. *J Periodontol.* 2000;71(11):1792–1801.
4. Hanes PJ, Purvis JP. Local anti-infective therapy: pharmacological agents. A systematic review. *Ann Periodontol.* 2003;8(1):79–98.
5. Greenstein G. The role of local drug delivery in the treatment of chronic periodontitis. Things you should know. *Dent Today.* 2004;23(3):110–115.
6. Mah TF, O'Toole GA. Mechanisms of biofilm resistance to antimicrobial agents. *Trends Microbiol.* 2001;9(1):34–39.
7. Rams TE, Degener JE, van Winkelhoff AJ. Antibiotic resistance in human chronic periodontitis microbiota. *J Periodontol.* 2014;85(1):160–169.
8. Walker CB. The acquisition of antibiotic resistance in the periodontal microflora. *Periodontol 2000.* 1996;10:79–88.
9. Sedlacek MJ, Walker C. Antibiotic resistance in an in vitro subgingival biofilm model. *Oral Microbiol Immunol.* 2007;22(5):333–339.
10. Caton JG, Ciancio SG, Blieden TM, et al. Treatment with subantimicrobial dose doxycycline improves the efficacy of scaling and root planing in patients with adult periodontitis. *J Periodontol.* 2000;71(4):521–532.
11. Ciancio S, Ashley R. Safety and efficacy of sub-antimicrobial-dose doxycycline therapy in patients with adult periodontitis. *Adv Dent Res.* 1998;12(2):27–31.
12. Slots J; Research, Science and Therapy Committee. Systemic antibiotics in periodontics. *J Periodontol.* 2004;75(11):1553–1565.
13. Thomas J, Walker C, Bradshaw M. Long-term use of subantimicrobial dose doxycycline does not lead to changes in antimicrobial susceptibility. *J Periodontol.* 2000;71(9):1472–1483.
14. Ciancio SG. Site specific delivery of antimicrobial agents for periodontal disease. *Gen Dent.* 1999;47(2):172–178.
15. Finkelman RD. Re: role of controlled drug delivery for periodontitis (position paper). The American Academy of Periodontology (2000;71:12–40). *J Periodontol.* 2000;71(12):1929–1933.
16. Greenstein G. Local drug delivery in the treatment of periodontal diseases: assessing the clinical significance of the results. *J Periodontol.* 2006;77(4):565–578.
17. Greenstein G, Tonetti M. The role of controlled drug delivery for periodontitis. The Research, Science and Therapy Committee of the American Academy of Periodontology. *J Periodontol.* 2000;71(1):125–140.
18. Killoy WJ. The clinical significance of local chemotherapies. *J Clin Periodontol.* 2002;29 Suppl 2:22–29.
19. van Steenberghe D, Rosling B, Soder PO, et al. A 15-month evaluation of the effects of repeated subgingival minocycline in chronic adult periodontitis. *J Periodontol.* 1999;70(6):657–667.
20. Williams RC, Paquette DW, Offenbacher S, et al. Treatment of periodontitis by local administration of minocycline microspheres: a controlled trial. *J Periodontol.* 2001;72(11):1535–1544.
21. Wennstrom JL, Newman HN, MacNeill SR, et al. Utilisation of locally delivered doxycycline in non-surgical treatment of chronic periodontitis. A comparative multi-centre trial of 2 treatment approaches. *J Clin Periodontol.* 2001;28(8):753–761.
22. Jeffcoat MK, Palcanis KG, Weatherford TW, et al. Use of a biodegradable chlorhexidine chip in the treatment of adult periodontitis: clinical and radiographic findings. *J Periodontol.* 2000;71(2):256–262.
23. Henke CJ, Villa KF, Aichelmann-Reidy ME, et al. An economic evaluation of a chlorhexidine chip for treating chronic periodontitis: the CHIP (chlorhexidine in periodontitis) study. *J Am Dent Assoc.* 2001;132(11):1557–1569.
24. Barnett ML. The role of therapeutic antimicrobial mouthrinses in clinical practice: control of supragingival plaque and gingivitis. *J Am Dent Assoc.* 2003;134(6):699–704.
25. Osso D, Kanani N. Antiseptic mouth rinses: an update on comparative effectiveness, risks and recommendations. *J Dent Hyg.* 2013;87(1):10–18.
26. Jones CG. Chlorhexidine: is it still the gold standard? *Periodontol 2000.* 1997;15:55–62.
27. Mathur S, Mathur T, Shrivastava R, et al. Chlorhexidine: the gold standard in chemical plaque control. *Natl J Physiol Pharm Pharmacol.* 2011;1(2):45–50.
28. Li W, Wang RE, Finger M, et al. Evaluation of the antigingivitis effect of a chlorhexidine mouthwash with or without an antidiscoloration system compared to placebo during experimental gingivitis. *J Investig Clin Dent.* 2014;5(1):15–22.

29. Zanatta FB, Antoniazzi RP, Rosing CK. The effect of 0.12% chlorhexidine gluconate rinsing on previously plaque-free and plaque-covered surfaces: a randomized, controlled clinical trial. *J Periodontol.* 2007;78(11):2127–2134.

30. Gupta G, Mitra D, Ashok KP, et al. Efficacy of preprocedural mouth rinsing in reducing aerosol contamination produced by ultrasonic scaler: a pilot study. *J Periodontol.* 2014;85(4):562–568.

31. Klyn SL, Cummings DE, Richardson BW, et al. Reduction of bacteria-containing spray produced during ultrasonic scaling. *Gen Dent.* 2001;49(6):648–652.

32. Charles CH, Mostler KM, Bartels LL, et al. Comparative antiplaque and antigingivitis effectiveness of a chlorhexidine and an essential oil mouthrinse: 6-month clinical trial. *J Clin Periodontol.* 2004;31(10):878–884.

33. Stoeken JE, Paraskevas S, van der Weijden GA. The long-term effect of a mouthrinse containing essential oils on dental plaque and gingivitis: a systematic review. *J Periodontol.* 2007;78(7):1218–1228.

34. Van Leeuwen MP, Slot DE, Van der Weijden GA. Essential oils compared to chlorhexidine with respect to plaque and parameters of gingival inflammation: a systematic review. *J Periodontol.* 2011;82(2):174–194.

35. Haps S, Slot DE, Berchier CE, et al. The effect of cetylpyridinium chloride-containing mouth rinses as adjuncts to toothbrushing on plaque and parameters of gingival inflammation: a systematic review. *Int J Dent Hyg.* 2008;6(4):290–303.

36. Versteeg PA, Rosema NA, Hoenderdos NL, et al. The plaque inhibitory effect of a CPC mouthrinse in a 3-day plaque accumulation model - a cross-over study. *Int J Dent Hyg.* 2010;8(4):269–275.

37. Addy M, Moran J, Newcombe RG. Meta-analyses of studies of 0.2% delmopinol mouth rinse as an adjunct to gingival health and plaque control measures. *J Clin Periodontol.* 2007;34(1):58–65.

38. Moran J, Addy M, Wade WG, et al. A comparison of delmopinol and chlorhexidine on plaque regrowth over a 4-day period and salivary bacterial counts. *J Clin Periodontol.* 1992;19(10):749–753.

39. Ciancio S, Panagakos FS. Superior management of plaque and gingivitis through the use of a triclosan/copolymer dentifrice. *J Clin Dent.* 2010;21(4):93–95.

40. Haraszthy VI, Zambon JJ, Sreenivasan PK. Evaluation of the antimicrobial activity of dentifrices on human oral bacteria. *J Clin Dent.* 2010;21(4):96–100.

 STUDENT ANCILLARY RESOURCES

A wide variety of resources to enhance your learning and understanding of this chapter are available on thePoint®.

- Visit thePoint to access:
  - Audio Glossary
  - Animations
  - Suggested Readings
  - Answers to Review Questions
  - Case Studies

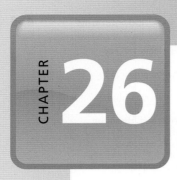

Host Modulation Therapy

Clinical Application. Host modulation therapy is currently one of the most exciting areas of research related to periodontal diseases. Though recommended clinical applications of this topic are limited, everyone who is involved in the care of patients with periodontal disease will read more and more publications devoted to this topic. To interpret these publications correctly, dental hygienists will need to understand what host modulation therapy can include and will need to be prepared to accept this modality as a valid part of patient care. This chapter provides an outline of the topic of host modulation therapy.

Learning Objectives

- Explain the term host modulation therapy.
- Explain the potential importance of host modulation therapy.
- Name some anti-inflammatory mediators.
- Name some proinflammatory mediators.
- List three types of drugs that have been studied for use as possible host modulating agents.
- Explain why low-dose doxycyclines are useful as host modulating agents.
- Explain the term subantibacterial dose.
- Make a list of treatment strategies for a periodontitis patient that includes host modulation.

Key Terms

Host modulation therapy
Osteoporosis
Biochemical mediators
Anti-inflammatory mediators

Proinflammatory
  mediators
Doxycycline
Subantibacterial doses

Nonsteroidal
  Anti-inflammatory Drugs
  (NSAIDs)
Bisphosphonates

Section 1
Introduction to the Host Modulation Therapy

For several decades the focus of therapy for patients with inflammatory periodontal diseases has been directed toward controlling the microbial etiology of these diseases; minimizing the bacterial challenge to the periodontium has been a successful strategy for the treatment of many patients with both gingivitis and periodontitis. Beyond any doubt, plaque biofilm control strategies will continue to play a major role in the therapy for patients with periodontal disease.

Based upon current knowledge of the underlying pathology involved in periodontal diseases, additional strategies for therapy are emerging that may also be employed for patients with inflammatory periodontal diseases. One of these additional strategies relates to the concept of host modulation therapy (1–4).

1. **Host Modulation Therapy Defined.** **Host modulation therapy** can be defined as altering a patient's (i.e., the host's) defense responses to help the body defenses limit damage caused by a disease. In dentistry the concept of host modulation therapy focuses on how the body responds to the bacterial challenge rather than simply reducing that bacterial challenge posed by plaque biofilm.

2. **Examples of Host Modulation Therapy in Medicine**
   A. Host modulation therapy is *not* a new concept in medicine, and it has been a part of the medical care for patients with a variety of systemic diseases for many years. One example of a common systemic disease for which physicians frequently use host modulation is osteoporosis.
   B. **Osteoporosis** is a progressive bone disease that is characterized by a decrease in both bone mass and bone density that can lead to an increased risk of bone fractures. Osteoporosis affects millions of patients in the United States.
   C. Treatments for osteoporosis can be broadly divided into two categories based upon how the treatment medications affect the bone. One group of medications *reduces bone resorption* while the second group of medications *stimulates bone formation*.
      1. Antiresorptive agents, which include medications such as estrogen, selective estrogen receptor modulators, and bisphosphonates, reduce bone resorption and help to preserve bone mineral density.
      2. Bone-forming agents stimulate bone formation, thereby increasing overall bone mineral density.
   D. Patients who receive the types of medications discussed above are said to be receiving host modulation therapy, that is, the host response to the disease (loss of bone mass and density) is modulated to minimize the effects of the disease to prevent bone fractures.

3. **Importance of Host Modulation Therapy in Dentistry.** The potential importance of host modulation as one strategy in managing periodontitis patients is huge.
   A. As already discussed in other chapters, many adults show signs of periodontal or gingival disease with severe periodontitis affecting approximately 15% of the adult population in the United States. Because so many patients have inflammatory periodontal diseases, there is a continuing need for cost-effective strategies for managing periodontitis patients.
   B. As the population in the United States ages, it is reasonable to expect the prevalence of periodontitis to increase, making the need for the most cost-effective therapy even greater.

C. In addition, there is mounting evidence that periodontal health and several systemic conditions (such as diabetes and cardiovascular disease) are linked, again making it likely that the demand for periodontal therapy will increase over the upcoming decades.

4. **Review of Host Responses That Can Be Modulated**

   A. The fundamental pathologic processes for periodontitis have been outlined in other chapters of this book; in those chapters the following issues have been discussed.

      1. Bacteria (and bacterial products) that are a part of the plaque biofilm initiate an inflammatory response in the periodontium. The bacteria stimulate the immune cells to produce **biochemical mediators** (i.e., biologically active compounds) that activate this inflammatory response.

      2. The inflammatory response functions as a protective response that keeps the bacterial infection from doing serious harm to the periodontium in many patients partly through the production of chemicals called anti-inflammatory mediators.

         Anti-inflammatory mediators are biochemical mediators that are protective and help keep the bacterial infection from doing serious harm to the periodontium. These anti-inflammatory mediators include the cytokines IL-4 (interleukin-4) and IL-10 (interleukin-10).

      3. Box 26-1 shows an overview of some of the anti-inflammatory biochemical mediators that have been discussed in other chapters.

      4. If the bacterial challenge is great enough, however, the nature of the protective responses changes, resulting in the production of additional biochemical mediators that can lead to actual damage within the periodontium.

         a. Some biochemical mediators (referred to as **proinflammatory mediators**) can damage the periodontium. These proinflammatory biochemical mediators include chemicals such as matrix metalloproteinases (MMPs), certain cytokines, prostanoids, and other less well-understood mediators (5–9).

         b. Specific examples of these proinflammatory mediators include prostaglandin E_2 IL-1α (interleukin-1 alpha), IL-1β (interleukin-1 beta), IL-6 (interleukin-6), and tumor necrosis factor alpha.

         c. For example, one of the MMPs is an enzyme called collagenase that can actually break down collagen. Collagen is one of the major building blocks in the periodontium, and its breakdown is part of the fundamental pathology in periodontitis.

         d. Box 26-2 shows some of the proinflammatory biochemical mediators.

      5. In the periodontium these altered host defense responses can result in both breakdown of connective tissue fibers and resorption of alveolar bone (the precise type of tissue destruction seen in periodontitis).

      6. Much of the destruction of the periodontium that accompanies periodontitis is thought to be a result of these altered processes that occur as part of the host defenses (the host inflammatory and immune responses).

   B. Fundamentally, the concept of host modulation therapy as a strategy in treating periodontitis patients is to limit the damaging effect of the altered host responses by modifying (or modulating) the effect of these destructive biochemical mediators. Modulation of host defenses is currently an important focus for periodontal research, and host modulation therapy will undoubtedly play a far larger part in periodontal therapy in the future.

Box 26-1. Examples of Anti-Inflammatory Biochemical Mediators

These biochemical mediators help the body fight off the effects of the bacterial challenge:
- IL-4 (interleukin-4)
- IL-10 (interleukin-10)
- IL-1ra (receptor antagonist)
- TIMPs (tissue inhibitors of matrix metalloproteinases)

Box 26-2. Examples of Proinflammatory Biochemical Mediators

These biochemical mediators can lead to destruction of the tissues of the periodontium:
- IL-1 (interleukin-1)
- IL-6 (interleukin-6)
- PGE_2 (prostaglandin E_2)
- $TNF\alpha$ (tumor necrosis factor alpha)
- MMPs (matrix metalloproteinases)

Section 2
Potential Host Modulating Therapies in Periodontal Patients

1. Use of Tetracycline Medications
   A. Doxycycline
      1. **Doxycycline** is a tetracycline antibiotic drug that has been used to treat a variety of infections.
         a. As with other antibiotic medications, doxycycline must be given in doses high enough to affect the targeted bacteria to help the body fight an infection.
         b. Antibiotic doses high enough to inhibit or kill bacteria are sometimes called antibacterial doses. A typical antibacterial dose for doxycycline would be 50 to 100 mg every 12 hours.
      2. Doxycycline has other effects besides its antibiotic effect that is seen with the higher doses described above.
         a. If this medication is given even at low doses (*below that needed for any antibacterial effect*), it decreases the effects of the enzyme collagenase (one of the matrix metalloproteinases or MMPs).
         b. As already discussed, MMPs (such as collagenase) can be released in inflamed periodontal tissues and can cause breakdown of the connective tissue. Prevention of the action of collagenase can inhibit the progress of periodontitis.
         c. Doses of an antibiotic that are below the normal bacterial killing or inhibiting doses are referred to as **subantibacterial doses**.
         d. Since doxycycline at low doses (or subantibacterial doses) alters the body defenses by inhibiting part of the destruction that can occur in periodontitis, it is considered one example of a host modulating agent (10–22).

e. The FDA (U. S. Food and Drug Administration) has approved subantibacterial doses of doxycycline (20-mg tablets) for use in treating patients with periodontitis.
1. Low doses of doxycycline must be taken twice daily in tablet form to be effective in periodontitis patients.
2. No antibacterial effects on the oral bacteria or bacteria in other parts of the body have been found with the use of low-dose doxycycline.
3. Studies of this drug have also shown a clinical benefit when used as an adjunct to periodontal instrumentation.
4. Though tetracyclines used at antibacterial doses can have side effects (including nausea, vomiting, photosensitivity, and hypersensitivity reactions), doxycycline at low doses appears to be accompanied by a very low incidence of adverse effects.
3. Studies have shown reductions in probing depths and gains in clinical attachment levels as well as the prevention of periodontal disease progression with the use of subantibacterial doses of doxycycline in periodontitis patients.
B. Use of Chemically Modified Tetracyclines
1. Chemically modified tetracyclines are derivatives of tetracycline group of drugs that lack antimicrobial action but have potent host modulating effects.
2. Though these drugs lack antimicrobial action, they can inhibit elevated matrix metalloproteinases, proinflammatory cytokines, and other destructive mediators (23).
3. Bone resorption can also be suppressed by these drugs.
4. Development of resistant bacteria and gastrointestinal toxicity seen with antibacterial doses of the tetracyclines is *not* produced by chemically modified tetracyclines (23).
5. Chemically modified tetracyclines are currently being investigated as potential host modulation therapeutic agents in the management of chronic diseases like periodontitis, but only further research may demonstrate their efficacy and safety in periodontal patients.
2. Use of Nonsteroidal Anti-inflammatory Drugs
A. Nonsteroidal anti-inflammatory drugs (NSAIDs) have been used for many years in medical care to treat pain, acute inflammation, and chronic inflammatory conditions.
1. Box 26-3 shows examples of drugs included in the group called NSAIDS.
2. NSAIDs can reduce tissue inflammation by inhibiting the action of prostaglandins including PGE_2.
B. In periodontal studies systemically administered NSAIDs have been evaluated for their effect on periodontitis (a disease intimately associated with inflammation).
1. In the periodontium NSAIDs can both reduce inflammation and inhibit osteoclast activity.
2. Some NSAIDs, when administered daily over 3 years, have been shown to slow the rate of alveolar bone loss associated with periodontitis.
3. More research is needed in this area to clarify the efficacy and safety of using NSAIDs as host modulating agents in periodontal patients.
C. Long-term use of NSAIDs in periodontitis patients is not recommended because of significant side effects that can develop with the use of these drugs.
1. Side effects from NSAIDs can include gastrointestinal problems, hemorrhage (bleeding), and kidney or liver impairment.
2. In addition, when a patient with periodontitis stops taking daily doses of NSAIDs, there can be an acceleration of bone loss seen before taking the drugs.
3. At present no NSAIDs are approved for the treatment of periodontal disease.

Box 26-3. Examples of NSAID Medications

- Salicylates (aspirin)
- Indomethacin
- Ibuprofen
- Flurbiprofen
- Naproxen

   D. Even though NSAIDs are not currently recommended for use in host modulation in periodontitis patients, they have been discussed here because of the extensive dental research that has involved these drugs.

   E. In addition to systemically administered NSAIDs, topically applied NSAIDs have been studied for their possible benefits to periodontitis patients.

      1. Topical NSAIDs have also been shown to reduce PGE_2 (prostaglandin E_2) in gingival crevicular fluid in periodontitis patients (24–27).

      2. Topically administered NSAIDs have not been approved for the management of periodontitis, but more study of the possible use of topical NSAIDs is warranted.

3. Use of Bisphosphonate Medications

   A. **Bisphosphonates** are drugs that can inhibit the resorption of bone by altering osteoclastic activity, though the mechanism of action for these drugs is not fully understood.

   B. Early research indicates there may be some benefit to periodontitis patients from the ability of bisphosphonates to alter osteoclastic activity (bone resorption activity) (25,28).

   C. Some of the bisphosphonates have side effects that may limit their use in periodontitis patients, but they are discussed in this section because of the interest that has been shown in these drugs over the last few years.

   D. One of the possible side effects of these drugs is osteonecrosis of the jaws following their extended use (29). Osteonecrosis is the destruction and death of bone tissue, in this case the bone tissue of the jaw. Studies are under way to clarify the precise risk and etiology of this serious side effect of bisphosphonates.

   E. *At present there are no bisphosphonate drugs that are approved for the treatment of periodontal disease.*

4. Use of Statin Medications

   A. Recently it has been suggested that statin drugs that are normally used to control elevated cholesterol levels may have an effect upon periodontitis.

   B. There are quite a few statin medications available, but only a few such as simvastatin and atorvastin have been suggested as possible host modulation agents in periodontal patients.

   C. Statin medications have several effects including offering some protection against systemic inflammation (30).

   D. At this point the efficacy of these drugs in periodontal patients needs to be clarified with additional research studies.

5. Dietary Supplementation

   A. Dietary supplementation is another avenue that may hold promise for developing strategies to modify the host response to chronic periodontitis, especially if it is possible to enhance the resolution of inflammation through dietary supplements.

    B. The possibility of supplementing the diet with specific biomolecules, such as essential fatty acids, is currently being investigated for its effect upon periodontitis (31–33).

    C. Using supplements of omega-3 fatty acids to modify the host response to chronic periodontitis and reduce the severity of periodontal disease would certainly be a straightforward strategy for host modulation therapy if studies demonstrate the efficacy of such supplements.

6. **Use of Other Types of "Host Modulation Agents"**

    A. Several potential agents have been investigated for use as adjuncts to periodontal surgical procedures.

    B. These drugs do not produce the same types of effects discussed for the other potential host modulating agents, but they are mentioned here because some authors have referred to them as "host modulating agents."

    C. These agents are generally applied topically during periodontal surgical procedures and have been suggested for use for possible enhancement of wound healing or possible enhancement of regeneration of periodontal tissues following the surgery.

    D. Some agents of this type that have been investigated are enamel matrix proteins, bone morphogenetic proteins (BMP-2, BMP-7), and certain growth factors.

    E. Currently the only local host modulation agent approved for adjunctive use during periodontal surgery is an enamel matrix protein called Emdogain, and this agent is under continuing study.

    F. Members of the dental team should expect additional host modulation products to be investigated and to appear on the market; careful evaluation of each of the products will be needed (2).

Section 3
Host Modulation Therapy as a Part of Comprehensive Periodontal Patient Management

1. Periodontal therapy based upon minimizing the bacterial challenge has been a primary therapeutic modality for many years, and this therapy has proved to be successful in many patients.
   A. Studies indicate, however, that markers of periodontal disease in patients with periodontitis undergo little change following conventional mechanical periodontal therapy, in spite of its successful outcomes.
   B. It appears that even though conventional periodontal therapy based upon minimizing the bacterial challenge is usually successful, the underlying disease processes may indeed be diminished in severity, but they may remain fundamentally unchanged.
   C. These observations should not distract from a clinician's enthusiasm for recommending conventional periodontal therapy, but they should make clinicians eager for more therapies to be developed and to be added to those currently available.
2. Employing host modulation therapy in the comprehensive management of some periodontal patients seems to be a promising strategy to employ in the future.
   A. It should be reemphasized that at present the only host modulation therapy agent currently being recommended is the low-dose tetracyclines, but as discussed, investigations have indicated that at least theoretically other possible host modulation therapies may one day be employed in periodontal patients.
   B. It must also be noted that when used in periodontitis patients, sound clinical practice dictates that the use of low-dose doxycycline therapy be accompanied by all of the usual treatment strategies such as risk factor reduction (i.e., smoking cessation counseling) and bacterial challenge reduction (i.e., self-care training and periodontal instrumentation).
3. Box 26-4 lists the array of therapeutic strategies that can be employed when managing a patient with periodontitis to illustrate that host modulation therapy may be viewed as another therapy among the long list of options available for a patient with periodontal disease.
4. Figure 26-1 shows some theoretical possibilities for host modulation as a part of overall management of periodontitis patients.

Box 26-4. Therapeutic Options for a Periodontitis Patient

1. Patient education and training in self-care.
2. Employment of motivational strategies for patient self-care.
3. Reduction of the bacterial challenge by periodontal instrumentation.
4. Use of local delivery systems for antimicrobial agents.
5. Elimination of local contributing factors.
6. Systemic risk factor reduction.
7. Host modulation therapy.
8. Periodontal surgery.
9. Periodontal maintenance.

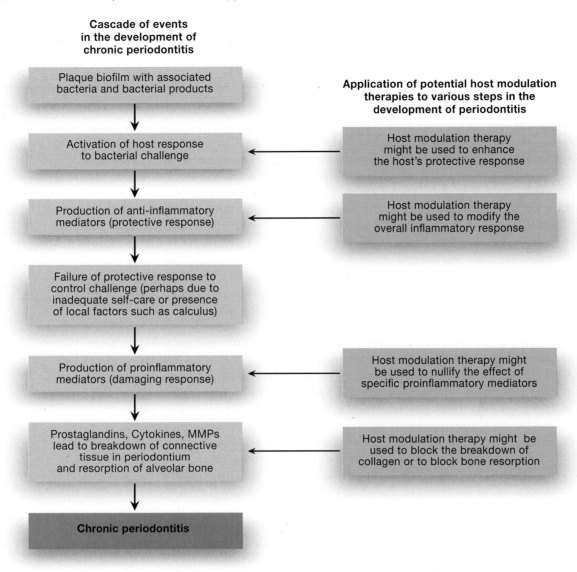

**Cascade of events
in the development of
chronic periodontitis**

Plaque biofilm with associated
bacteria and bacterial products

**Application of potential host modulation
therapies to various steps in the
development of periodontitis**

Activation of host response
to bacterial challenge

Host modulation therapy
might be used to enhance
the host's protective response

Production of anti-inflammatory
mediators (protective response)

Host modulation therapy
might be used to modify the
overall inflammatory response

Failure of protective response to
control challenge (perhaps due to
inadequate self-care or presence
of local factors such as calculus)

Production of proinflammatory
mediators (damaging response)

Host modulation therapy might
be used to nullify the effect of
specific proinflammatory mediators

Prostaglandins, Cytokines, MMPs
lead to breakdown of connective
tissue in periodontium
and resorption of alveolar bone

Host modulation therapy might be
used to block the breakdown of
collagen or to block bone resorption

Chronic periodontitis

Figure 26-1. Application of Potential Host Modulation Therapies. Potential host modulation therapies can be applied to a cascade of events starting with plaque biofilm and ending with chronic periodontitis. This figure shows the wide range of potential applications that research may make possible in the future.

Chapter Summary Statement

Host modulation therapy in periodontal patients (i.e., altering the body's defense mechanisms to limit damage from the oral bacterial challenge) is an interesting and ongoing line of investigation. Host modulation therapy has been suggested as an additional therapeutic strategy in periodontitis patients. At this point, low-dose doxycycline has been approved for use as a host modulating agent in humans with periodontitis. When used in subantimicrobial doses, this drug can help inhibit the progress of periodontitis. Members of the dental team will undoubtedly encounter much research activity related to additional host modulating therapies over the next several decades.

Section 4
Focus on Patients

Evidence in Action

CASE 1

A new patient in your dental team's office has a periodontal diagnosis of generalized severe chronic periodontitis. Explain how host modulation therapy might be included among other treatment strategies used to help control the damage to the periodontium that normally accompanies periodontitis.

Ethical Dilemma

Tammy is a 60-year-old artist, who you see every 3 months for periodontal maintenance, as she suffers from generalized chronic periodontitis. As you review her health history today, she states that she is now taking Fosamax, which was prescribed by her primary care physician, Dr. James. She states that she has been diagnosed with osteoporosis and has been taking Fosamax for the last 2 months. Dr. James also told Tammy that the medication would be helpful in stabilizing her periodontal disease, which was a side benefit. He assured her that there was no down side in taking the medication.

Tammy has done some research on line and has found some disturbing evidence of the possible side effects of Fosamax. She asks for your thoughts and opinion.

1. Are bisphosphonate drugs approved for the treatment of periodontal disease?
2. What would you tell Tammy about the possible side effects of the use of bisphosphonate drugs?
3. Are there ethical principles in conflict with this dilemma?

References

1. Bhatavadekar NB, Williams RC. New directions in host modulation for the management of periodontal disease. *J Clin Periodontol*. 2009;36(2):124–126.
2. Gokhale SR, Padhye AM. Future prospects of systemic host modulatory agents in periodontal therapy. *Br Dent J*. 2013;214(9):467–471.
3. Salvi GE, Lang NP. Host response modulation in the management of periodontal diseases. *J Clin Periodontol*. 2005;32 Suppl 6:108–129.
4. Tonetti MS, Chapple IL; Working Group 3 of Seventh European Workshop on Periodontology. Biological approaches to the development of novel periodontal therapies–consensus of the Seventh European Workshop on Periodontology. *J Clin Periodontol*. 2011;38 Suppl 11:114–118.
5. Birkedal-Hansen H. Role of matrix metalloproteinases in human periodontal diseases. *J Periodontol*. 1993;64(5 Suppl):474–484.
6. Deo V, Bhongade ML. Pathogenesis of periodontitis: role of cytokines in host response. *Dent Today*. 2010;29(9):60–62, 64–66; quiz 68–69.
7. Golub LM, Lee HM, Greenwald RA, et al. A matrix metalloproteinase inhibitor reduces bone-type collagen degradation fragments and specific collagenases in gingival crevicular fluid during adult periodontitis. *Inflamm Res*. 1997;46(8):310–319.
8. Kornman KS. Host modulation as a therapeutic strategy in the treatment of periodontal disease. *Clin Infect Dis*. 1999;28(3):520–526.
9. Offenbacher S, Heasman PA, Collins JG. Modulation of host PGE2 secretion as a determinant of periodontal disease expression. *J Periodontol*. 1993;64(5 suppl):432–444.

10. Caton J, Ryan ME. Clinical studies on the management of periodontal diseases utilizing subantimicrobial dose doxycycline (SDD). *Pharmacol Res.* 2011;63(2):114–120.

11. Choi DH, Moon IS, Choi BK, et al. Effects of sub-antimicrobial dose doxycycline therapy on crevicular fluid MMP-8, and gingival tissue MMP-9, TIMP-1 and IL-6 levels in chronic periodontitis. *J Periodontal Res.* 2004;39(1):20–26.

12. Emingil G, Atilla G, Sorsa T, et al. The effect of adjunctive low-dose doxycycline therapy on clinical parameters and gingival crevicular fluid matrix metalloproteinase-8 levels in chronic periodontitis. *J Periodontol.* 2004;75(1):106–115.

13. Golub LM, McNamara TF, Ryan ME, et al. Adjunctive treatment with subantimicrobial doses of doxycycline: effects on gingival fluid collagenase activity and attachment loss in adult periodontitis. *J Clin Periodontol.* 2001;28(2):146–156.

14. Golub LM, Suomalainen K, Sorsa T. Host modulation with tetracyclines and their chemically modified analogues. *Curr Opin Dent.* 1992;2:80–90.

15. Gu Y, Walker C, Ryan ME, et al. Non-antibacterial tetracycline formulations: clinical applications in dentistry and medicine. *J Oral Microbiol.* 2012;4.

16. Novak MJ, Dawson DR 3rd, Magnusson I, et al. Combining host modulation and topical antimicrobial therapy in the management of moderate to severe periodontitis: a randomized multicenter trial. *J Periodontol.* 2008;79(1):33–41.

17. Novak MJ, Johns LP, Miller RC, et al. Adjunctive benefits of subantimicrobial dose doxycycline in the management of severe, generalized, chronic periodontitis. *J Periodontol.* 2002;73(7):762–769.

18. Preshaw PM, Hefti AF, Bradshaw MH. Adjunctive subantimicrobial dose doxycycline in smokers and non-smokers with chronic periodontitis. *J Clin Periodontol.* 2005;32(6):610–616.

19. Preshaw PM, Hefti AF, Jepsen S, et al. Subantimicrobial dose doxycycline as adjunctive treatment for periodontitis. A review. *J Clin Periodontol.* 2004;31(9):697–707.

20. Subramanian S, Emami H, Vucic E, et al. High-dose atorvastatin reduces periodontal inflammation: a novel pleiotropic effect of statins. *J Am Coll Cardiol.* 2013;62(25):2382–2391.

21. Thomas JG, Metheny RJ, Karakiozis JM, et al. Long-term sub-antimicrobial doxycycline (Periostat) as adjunctive management in adult periodontitis: effects on subgingival bacterial population dynamics. *Adv Dent Res.* 1998;12(2):32–39.

22. Walker C, Preshaw PM, Novak J, et al. Long-term treatment with sub-antimicrobial dose doxycycline has no antibacterial effect on intestinal flora. *J Clin Periodontol.* 2005;32(11):1163–1169.

23. Agnihotri R, Gaur S. Chemically modified tetracyclines: novel therapeutic agents in the management of chronic periodontitis. *Ind J Pharmacol.* 2012;44(2):161–167.

24. Howell TH, Williams RC. Nonsteroidal antiinflammatory drugs as inhibitors of periodontal disease progression. *Crit Rev Oral Biol Med.* 1993;4(2):177–196.

25. Reddy MS, Geurs NC, Gunsolley JC. Periodontal host modulation with antiproteinase, anti-inflammatory, and bone-sparing agents. A systematic review. *Ann Periodontol.* 2003;8(1):12–37.

26. Salvi GE, Lang NP. The effects of non-steroidal anti-inflammatory drugs (selective and non-selective) on the treatment of periodontal diseases. *Curr Pharm Des.* 2005;11(14):1757–1769.

27. Williams RC, Jeffcoat MK, Howell TH, et al. Altering the progression of human alveolar bone loss with the non-steroidal anti-inflammatory drug flurbiprofen. *J Periodontol.* 1989;60(9):485–490.

28. Weinreb M, Quartuccio H, Seedor JG, et al. Histomorphometrical analysis of the effects of the bisphosphonate alendronate on bone loss caused by experimental periodontitis in monkeys. *J Periodontal Res.* 1994;29(1):35–40.

29. Thumbigere-Math V, Michalowicz BS, Hodges JS, et al. Periodontal disease as a risk factor for bisphosphonate-related osteonecrosis of the jaw. *J Periodontol.* 2014;85(2):226–233.

30. Price U, Le HO, Powell SE, et al. Effects of local simvastatin-alendronate conjugate in preventing periodontitis bone loss. *J Periodontal Res.* 2013;48(5):541–548.

31. Dawson DR 3rd, Branch-Mays G, Gonzalez OA, et al. Dietary modulation of the inflammatory cascade. *Periodontol 2000.* 2014;64(1):161–197.

32. Elkhouli AM. The efficacy of host response modulation therapy (omega-3 plus low-dose aspirin) as an adjunctive treatment of chronic periodontitis (clinical and biochemical study). *J Periodontal Res.* 2011;46(2):261–268.

33. Sculley DV. Periodontal disease: modulation of the inflammatory cascade by dietary n-3 polyunsaturated fatty acids. *J Periodontal Res.* 2014;49(3):277–281.

 ## STUDENT ANCILLARY RESOURCES

A wide variety of resources to enhance your learning and understanding of this chapter are available on thePoint®.

- Visit thePoint to access:
  - Audio Glossary
  - Animations
  - Suggested Readings
  - Answers to Review Questions
  - Case Studies

Periodontal Surgical Concepts for the Dental Hygienist

Clinical Application. As members of dental teams, dental hygienists must understand the fundamental concepts related to periodontal surgery so that they can discuss this important topic with both patients and other healthcare providers. In addition, hygienists often play a primary role in the management of patients following periodontal surgery. A basic understanding of periodontal surgical procedures can provide the framework for improved patient care during critical stages of healing of periodontal surgical wounds. This chapter provides foundation information about basic concepts associated with periodontal surgery.

Learning Objectives

- List the objectives for periodontal surgery.
- Explain the term relative contraindications for periodontal surgery.
- Define the terms repair, reattachment, new attachment, and regeneration.
- Explain the difference between healing by primary intention and secondary intention.
- Explain the term elevation of a flap.
- Explain two methods for classification of periodontal flaps.
- Describe two types of incisions used during periodontal flaps.
- Describe healing following flap for access and open flap debridement.

- Describe the typical outcomes for apically positioned flap with osseous surgery.
- Define the terms ostectomy and osteoplasty.
- Define the terms osteoinductive and osteoconductive.
- Explain the terms autograft, allograft, xenograft, and alloplast.
- Name two types of materials available for bone replacement grafts.
- Explain why a barrier material is used during guided tissue regeneration.
- Explain the term periodontal plastic surgery.
- List two types of crown lengthening surgery.
- List some disadvantages of gingivectomy.
- Describe the technique for a gingival curettage.
- Explain what is meant by biological enhancement of periodontal surgical outcomes.
- Name two broad categories of materials used for suturing periodontal wounds.
- Explain the term interrupted interdental suture.
- List general guidelines for suture removal.
- Describe the technique for periodontal dressing placement.
- List general guidelines for periodontal dressing management.
- Explain the important topics that should be covered in postsurgical instructions.
- List steps in a typical postsurgical visit.

Key Terms

Resective
Osseous defect
Relative contraindications
Repair
Reattachment
New attachment
Regeneration
Primary intention
Secondary intention
Tertiary intention
Periodontal flap
Elevation
Full-thickness flap
Blunt dissection
Partial-thickness flap
Sharp dissection
Nondisplaced flap
Displaced flap
Horizontal incision

Crevicular incision
Internal bevel incision
Vertical incision
Flap for access
Open flap debridement
Osseous resective surgery
Ostectomy
Osteoplasty
Apically positioned flap with
    osseous resective surgery
Bone replacement graft
Osteogenesis
Osteoconductive
Osteoinductive
Autograft
Allograft
Xenograft
Alloplast
Guided tissue regeneration

Periodontal plastic surgery
Mucogingival surgery
Free gingival graft
Subepithelial connective
    tissue graft
Laterally positioned flap
Coronally positioned flap
Semilunar flap
Frenectomy
Crown lengthening surgery
Functional crown lengthening
Esthetic crown lengthening
Gingivectomy
Gingivoplasty
Gingival curettage
Periodontal microsurgery
Nonabsorbable suture
Absorbable suture
Periodontal dressing

Section 1
Introduction to Periodontal Surgery

All busy general dental practices encounter many patients who can benefit from periodontal surgery. One fundamental overreaching goal for most periodontal surgical procedures is to provide an environment in the periodontium that can be maintained in health and comfort throughout the life of the patient. In most instances as the severity of periodontitis increases, controlling periodontal disease with nonsurgical therapy alone becomes more and more difficult, and the need for periodontal surgery as part of comprehensive patient care becomes increasingly likely.

EVOLUTION OF CONCEPTS RELATED TO PERIODONTAL SURGERY

1. **Historical Perspective for Periodontal Surgery.** Various types of periodontal surgery have been recommended for dental patients with periodontitis and other periodontal conditions for many years.
   A. Historically, periodontal surgery was recommended mainly to remove what was thought to be dead or infected tissue in the periodontium; these early periodontal surgical procedures were mainly **resective** procedures. The term resective surgery refers to those procedures that simply cut away and remove some of the periodontal tissues. This concept of resecting or cutting away tissues lead to a variety of surgical techniques that have little in common with most modern periodontal surgery.
   B. There are a few of the resective periodontal surgical procedures that still have a limited use in modern periodontal care (i.e., the gingivectomy as discussed in subsequent chapter sections), but most modern periodontal surgical procedures have moved away from this early concept of simply resecting tissues.
2. **Move Toward Modern Periodontal Surgical Techniques**
   A. During the past few decades, as more research data has become available, an evolution of both the objectives and techniques for periodontal surgery has taken place.
   B. The emphasis in periodontal surgery has shifted from the resective types of periodontal surgery to periodontal surgical procedures that rebuild or regenerate periodontal tissues damaged or lost because of disease.

INDICATIONS AND CONTRAINDICATIONS FOR PERIODONTAL SURGERY

1. **Indications for Periodontal Surgery.** Periodontal surgeons can employ an array of surgical techniques that are directed toward different outcomes. The most common indications for periodontal surgery are outlined below and in Box 27-1.
   A. **To Provide Access for Improved Periodontal Instrumentation of Root Surfaces**
      1. Periodontal surgery can provide access for more thorough periodontal instrumentation. Since instrumentation of root surfaces in the presence of deep periodontal pockets is so very difficult, the improved access that can be provided by periodontal surgery can be a huge advantage for clinicians.
      2. Even though clinicians can select from a wide array of hand and ultrasonic instruments, as probing depths in the dentition increase, it becomes more and more difficult to reach root surfaces for thorough periodontal instrumentation.
      3. Periodontal surgery involving carefully planned incisions through the gingiva can allow for temporary lifting of the soft tissue off the tooth surface. More

details about this type of surgery are presented under *flap for access* in the following descriptions of periodontal surgery.

Box 27-1. Indications for Periodontal Surgery

- To provide access for improved periodontal instrumentation of root surfaces
- To reduce pocket depths
- To provide access to periodontal osseous defects
- To resect or remove tissue
- To regenerate the periodontium lost due to disease
- To graft bone or bone-stimulating materials into osseous defects
- To improve the appearance of the periodontium
- To enhance prosthetic dental care
- To allow for the placement of a dental implant

B. **To Reduce Pocket Depths**
1. As pocket depth increases, it can become increasingly difficult for patients to perform effective self-care techniques, and plaque biofilms that thrive in the protected environment of the deep pocket can make it impossible to stop the progress of periodontitis.
2. Periodontal surgical procedures can reduce the pocket depths, so that a combination of daily self-care and periodic professional periodontal maintenance increases the chance of maintaining the periodontium in health throughout the life of the patient.

C. **To Provide Access to Periodontal Osseous Defects**
1. An **osseous defect** is a deformity in the tooth-supporting alveolar bone usually resulting from periodontitis. Figure 27-1 shows an example of an osseous defect as viewed during a periodontal surgical procedure.
    a. As periodontitis advances, alveolar bone loss results in changes in the normal contour and structure of the supporting alveolar bone.
    b. The pattern of bone loss can vary from one tooth to the next and even on different aspects of the same tooth, creating an array of defects in alveolar bone contours referred to as osseous defects.

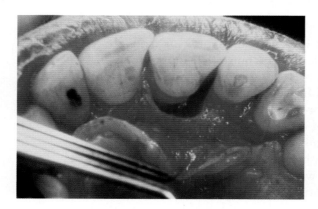

Figure 27-1. Periodontal Osseous Defect Exposed During Surgery. The soft tissues have been incised and temporarily moved away from the teeth to reveal the bone contour. Note the extensive alveolar bone loss around one of the central incisor teeth creating a moat-like defect around this tooth. This type of bone defect would be an ideal site for bone replacement graft discussed later in the chapter.

   2. Periodontal surgery to modify the alveolar bone level or contour is called periodontal osseous surgery.
      a. Bone defects can be managed surgically through a variety of techniques discussed later in this chapter.
      b. Information about how osseous defects can be managed using periodontal surgery is presented under the topics *osseous resective surgery, apically positioned flap with osseous surgery, bone replacement graft,* and *guided tissue regeneration* in other sections of this chapter.

D. **To Resect or Remove Tissue**
   1. Enlarged gingival tissues can be unsightly and can also interfere with proper self-care; in some patients, enlarged gingiva can even interfere with comfortable mastication.
   2. Even though the focus of most modern periodontal surgery is *not* resection of tissues, this surgical approach can still be indicated in some instances.
   3. Periodontal surgery can be used to remove and reshape enlarged gingiva; additional information on this type of periodontal surgery is found in the chapter section that discusses the *gingivectomy.*

E. **To Regenerate the Periodontium Lost Due to Disease**
   1. One of the long-range goals in periodontics is to be able to regenerate the periodontium predictably; the term regenerate implies growing back of lost cementum, lost periodontal ligament, and lost alveolar bone to reconstruct the periodontium damaged by periodontitis.
   2. Periodontal regenerative procedures can reconstruct some of the damage by periodontitis through regenerating lost bone and other tissues.
   3. Although it is not possible to regenerate the periodontium in all instances, it is possible to achieve this regeneration in many sites using some sophisticated periodontal surgical techniques; information on periodontal surgery that can be expected to regenerate the periodontium is presented under *guided tissue regeneration* in another section of this chapter.

F. **To Graft Bone or Bone-Stimulating Materials into Osseous Defects**
   1. Some periodontal osseous defects offer the opportunity for the periodontal surgeon to graft either bone or bone-stimulating materials into the defects.
   2. Although this surgery may seem quite similar to periodontal regeneration surgery, grafting bone does not necessarily imply regeneration of other parts of the periodontium such as cementum and periodontal ligament. More information on this interesting topic is located under *bone replacement graft* in another section of this chapter.

G. **To Improve the Appearance of the Periodontium**
   1. Some patients have gingival levels or gingival contours that result in an unattractive smile; periodontal surgery also includes a variety of techniques for improving the appearance of the gingiva and improving the quality of a patient's smile.
   2. There are, of course, many restorative techniques for improving the appearance of the teeth themselves, but in many patients, alteration of the appearance of the gingiva must be coordinated with restorative dentistry and orthodontics to achieve a truly pleasing appearance. More information on this topic is found in the other sections of this chapter under *periodontal plastic surgery* and *crown lengthening surgery.*

H. **To Enhance Prosthetic Dental Care**
   1. Modern prosthetic dental care has created the need for a variety of periodontal surgical procedures such as altering alveolar ridge contours, lengthening tooth

crowns, augmenting the amount of gingiva, or augmenting the bone in an edentulous site prior to implant placement.

2. Modern periodontal surgery includes many procedures directed toward enhancing some aspect of restorative dentistry and enhancing prosthetic dental care. These surgical procedures may involve combinations of all types of periodontal surgery.

I. **To Allow for the Placement of a Dental Implant**
  1. Replacement of missing teeth with a dental implant is an option that must be considered when natural teeth are lost. The topic of dental implants is discussed in Chapter 31 but is listed here as one of the indications for periodontal surgery for completeness.
  2. Periodontal surgery can also be used to prepare sites for dental implants.
     a. One of the basic tenets of dental implant placement is that the implant must be surrounded by sound alveolar bone.
     b. It is not at all unusual for edentulous sites—where implants are to be placed—to be deficient in the amount of alveolar bone needed to surround the implant. Such sites can require some type of bone grafting procedure prior to implant placement.

2. **Contraindications for Periodontal Surgery**
  A. **The Concept of Relative Contraindications.** Most contraindications for periodontal surgery are relative contraindications rather than absolute contraindications.
     1. **Relative contraindications** are conditions that may make periodontal surgery inadvisable for some patients when the conditions or situations are severe or extreme, but at the same time, these conditions may not be contraindications when the conditions are mild.
     2. An example of this concept of relative contraindications for periodontal surgery might be patients with hypertension (high blood pressure).
        a. A patient with uncontrolled severe hypertension would not be a candidate for periodontal surgery as long as the blood pressure remains *severely* elevated.
        b. At the same time, a patient with only mildly elevated blood pressure may be a suitable candidate for periodontal surgery.
  B. **Common Relative Contraindications for Periodontal Surgery.** Box 27-2 outlines a list of the more common *relative contraindications* for periodontal surgery; each of these relative contraindications is discussed briefly below.
     1. **Patients Who Have Certain Systemic Diseases or Conditions**
        a. Systemic diseases or conditions that can be relative contraindications for periodontal surgery include conditions such as the following:
           1. Uncontrolled hypertension
           2. Recent history of myocardial infarction (heart attack)
           3. Uncontrolled diabetes
           4. Certain bleeding disorders
           5. Kidney dialysis
           6. History of radiation to the jaws
           7. HIV infection
        b. It should be noted that consultation with a patient's physician is always indicated if there is any doubt about the patient's health status or if there is any doubt about how that status might affect planned periodontal surgical intervention.

Box 27-2. Common Relative Contraindications for Periodontal Surgery

- Patients who have certain systemic diseases or conditions
- Patients who are totally noncompliant with self-care
- Patients who have a high risk for dental caries
- Patients who have totally unrealistic expectations for surgical outcomes

2. Patients Who Are Totally Noncompliant with Self-Care
   a. The outcomes of many types of periodontal surgery are at least in part dependent upon the level of plaque biofilm control maintained by the patient's daily efforts at self-care following the surgical procedure.
   b. Lack of compliance with self-care instructions can be a relative contraindication for some types of periodontal surgery if that lack of compliance is so poor that it precludes the possibility of achieving acceptable periodontal surgical outcomes.
3. Patients Who Have a High Risk for Dental Caries
   a. Some types of periodontal surgery result in exposure of portions of tooth roots. In a patient with uncontrolled dental caries where the risk for dental caries will remain quite high, it may not be wise to perform the types of periodontal surgery that increase root exposure due to the potentially devastating effect of root caries.
   b. Most often, a high risk for dental caries can be altered, but when bringing the caries risk to an acceptable level is impossible, this risk can be a relative contraindication for some types of periodontal surgery.
4. Patients Who Have Totally Unrealistic Expectations for Surgical Outcomes
   a. Periodontitis damages the tissues that support the teeth, and surgical correction of that damage does not always result in a perfectly restored periodontium even when performed by the most skilled periodontal surgeon.
   b. If a patient cannot understand the nature of periodontal surgery and cannot develop realistic expectations for the outcomes of any planned periodontal surgery, it would not be wise to proceed with a plan for periodontal surgery. Thus, patient expectations can also be a relative contraindication for periodontal surgery.

POSSIBLE OUTCOMES FOR PERIODONTAL SURGERY

Table 27-1 illustrates possible outcomes that may result from successful periodontal surgery: (1) formation of a long junctional epithelium (as can be seen in response to nonsurgical therapy), (2) resolution of inflammation and the associated periodontal pocket (as can be seen in response to nonsurgical therapy), and (3) regeneration (which is an expectation for some types of periodontal surgery but not expected as a result of nonsurgical therapy alone).

TABLE 27-1. POSSIBLE OUTCOMES FROM SUCCESSFUL PERIODONTAL SURGERY

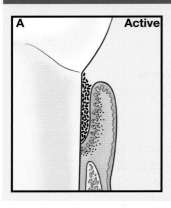

A: Periodontal Pocket Prior to Therapy. The periodontal pocket with bacterial plaque and inflammation within the tissues prior to therapy.

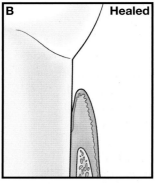

B: Healing by Long Junctional Epithelium. Healing in the area of the former pocket at the site by formation of a long junctional epithelium.

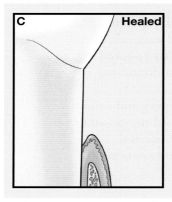

C: Healing with Tissue Shrinkage. Healing at the site by resolution of the inflammation in the tissues and shrinkage of the tissues.

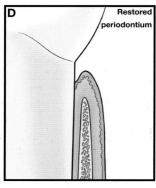

D: Healing by Regeneration. Healing at the site by regeneration of the periodontal tissues.

TERMINOLOGY USED TO DESCRIBE HEALING AFTER PERIODONTAL SURGERY

Terminology used to describe healing following periodontal surgery can be quite confusing. Two sets of terminology are frequently used to describe healing of periodontal surgical wounds. One set of terms attempts to describe the various types of wound healing that can result from the surgery, and the second set of terms describes the degree of wound closure achieved at the time of surgery. The dental hygienist needs to have an accurate understanding of both sets of terms, since all members of the dental team are likely to encounter some of these terms frequently.

1. **Terminology Describing Types of Wound Healing.** All periodontics textbooks present four terms that are used in describing the types of healing of the periodontium following periodontal surgery: *repair, reattachment, new attachment,* and *regeneration.* These terms are used to convey very specific concepts when describing the results of periodontal surgery.
   A. Healing by *REPAIR*
      1. Repair *is healing of a wound by formation of tissues that do not precisely restore the original architecture or original function of the body part.*
         a. An example of healing by repair would be the formation of a scar during the healing of an accidental cut involving a finger.
         b. Certainly the healing of the finger wound is complete following formation of the scar, but the scar tissue is not precisely the same type of tissue in appearance or function that existed on that part of the finger before the cut.
      2. Repair is a perfectly natural type of healing for many types of wounds, including some wounds created during periodontal surgery.
         a. An example of repair in the periodontium is the healing that occurs following periodontal instrumentation (scaling and root planing).
            1. The usual healing of the wound created by periodontal instrumentation results is a close readaptation of epithelium to the tooth root.
            2. This readaptation of epithelium has been referred to as formation of a long junctional epithelium and has been discussed and illustrated in Chapter 22.
         b. A long junctional epithelium is a perfectly legitimate type of healing, but it does not duplicate the precise periodontal tissues that were originally anatomically close to the tooth root. *With the formation of a long junctional epithelium, there is no formation of new bone, new cementum, or new periodontal ligament during the healing process.*
   B. Healing by *REATTACHMENT*
      1. Reattachment *is healing of a periodontal wound by the reunion of the connective tissue and roots where these two tissues have been separated by incision or injury but not by disease* (1).
      2. Frequently it is necessary to move *healthy tissue* away from the tooth root or bone temporarily during some types of periodontal surgery. For example, moving the tissue may be necessary to allow access to damaged parts of the periodontium on adjacent teeth. The expected healing for this type of incision is healing by reattachment.
   C. Healing by *NEW ATTACHMENT*
      1. New attachment *is a term used to describe the union of a pathologically exposed root with connective tissue or epithelium.*
      2. Healing by new attachment occurs when the epithelium and connective tissues are newly attached to a tooth root *where periodontitis had previously destroyed this attachment* (i.e., where attachment loss has occurred) (2,3).

3. New attachment differs from reattachment because new attachment only occurs in an area formerly damaged by disease, whereas reattachment occurs when tissues are separated in the absence of disease (frequently as a result of the surgical procedure).

4. Figure 27-2 illustrates the specific area on a tooth that must have newly attached epithelium and connective tissue for the healing to be called new attachment.

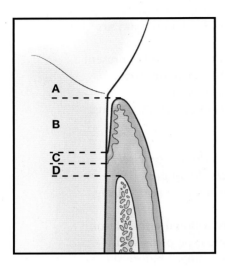

Figure 27-2. **Area of the Tooth Root Involved in New Attachment.** This drawing shows a site on a tooth where attachment loss has occurred. **A:** Enamel surface. **B:** Area of attachment loss. **C:** Junctional epithelium. **D:** Connective tissue attachment. To be qualified as new attachment the tissues must be attached to the tooth surface in the area labeled B in this drawing.

D. Healing by *REGENERATION*

1. **Regeneration** is the biologic process by which the architecture and function of lost tissue is *completely* restored.

2. Healing by regeneration results in the regrowth of the precise tissues that were present before the disease or damage occurred.

3. For healing of the periodontium to be described as regeneration, the healing would have to result in the reformation of lost cementum, lost periodontal ligament, and lost alveolar bone.

4. Regeneration of the periodontium is indeed possible with modern periodontal surgical procedures, but unfortunately the periodontium *cannot be regenerated predictably* in all sites with current periodontal surgical techniques.

2. **Terminology Describing the Degree of Wound Closure.** A second set of terms has also been used to describe events following periodontal surgery. These terms describe the degree of wound closure (i.e., how the margins or edges of the surgical wound relate to each other following the surgery but before healing). These terms include healing by primary intention, secondary intention, and tertiary intention.

A. **Healing by Primary Intention**

1. Healing by **primary intention** occurs when the wound margins or edges are closely adapted to each other.

2. An example of primary intention healing would be seen in a small wound in a finger that required stitches. To adapt the margins of the wound closely, a physician places stitches.

3. Healing by primary intention is usually faster than the other types of healing, but it is not always possible to create wounds where the wound margins are closely adapted when performing periodontal surgery.

4. It should be noted that healing by primary intention in the periodontium may pose challenges for the healing that differ from healing by primary intention in other sites in the body—such as, healing of a cut finger.

      a. One edge of a surgical wound in the periodontium may be a tooth root that is, of course, avascular and cannot contribute any living cells to the wound healing process.

      b. This would differ from healing by primary intention for a wound such as a cut finger, because both edges of the wound in finger would be able to contribute living cells to the healing process.

B. Healing by Secondary Intention

    1. Healing by **secondary intention** takes place when the margins or edges of the wound are not closely adapted (i.e., the two wound edges are not in close contact with each other).

    2. When healing by secondary intention takes place, granulation tissue must form to close the space between the wound margins prior to growth of epithelial cells over the surface of the wound.

    3. Healing by secondary intention is generally slower than healing by primary intention, since more vascular and cellular events are required in this type of healing.

    4. Ideally, all wounds created during periodontal surgery would be wounds that would be expected to heal by primary intention, but in reality, many of the wounds created during this type of surgery involve some wound healing by secondary intention.

C. Healing by Tertiary Intention

    1. An example of healing by **tertiary intention** would be healing of a wound that is temporarily left open with the specific intent of surgically closing that wound at a later date.

    2. Healing by tertiary intention is not normally a type of healing that applies to healing of periodontal surgical procedures and is mentioned here only for completeness.

Section 2
Understanding the Periodontal Flap

Many modern periodontal surgical techniques begin by performing a periodontal flap, and the periodontal flap is an important step in most periodontal surgical procedures. As periodontitis progresses, it damages the attachment of the connective tissue to tooth roots and it destroys supporting alveolar bone. Treating patients with periodontitis and repairing damage done to the underlying periodontium requires gaining access to both tooth roots and alveolar bone. As attachment loss associated with periodontitis progresses, access to tooth roots with conventional nonsurgical periodontal therapy becomes difficult if not impossible. Elevating a periodontal flap is the mechanism for gaining access to the underlying periodontal structures and to the tooth roots affected by the disease; any overview of periodontal surgery requires some understanding of the principles involved in performing a periodontal flap. This chapter section discusses the techniques and the associated terminology related to performing some of the many variations of a periodontal flap.

1. Introduction to Periodontal Flaps

  A. Description of Procedure

    1. A **periodontal flap** is a surgical procedure in which incisions are made in the gingiva or mucosa to allow for separation of the surface tissues (epithelium and connective tissue) from the underlying tooth roots and underlying alveolar bone.

    2. Separating the surface tissues from the underlying tooth root and alveolar bone is commonly referred to as **elevation** or raising of the flap; the term elevation is used to convey the concept of lifting the surface tissues away from the tooth roots and the alveolar bone.

3. Once the surface gingiva or mucosa is elevated off the underlying roots and bone, it can be replaced at its original position or it can be displaced to different locations that will be discussed in upcoming sections under some of the specific types of surgery.

4. Table 27-2 shows a series of drawings that illustrate a typical periodontal flap surgical procedure used to gain access to the underlying tooth roots and alveolar bone.

TABLE 27-2. TYPICAL PERIODONTAL FLAP SURGICAL PROCEDURE USED TO GAIN ACCESS TO UNDERLYING TOOTH ROOTS AND ALVEOLAR BONE

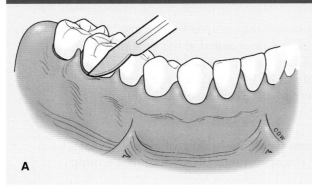

A: Making an incision to allow for separation of the soft tissue from the roots and alveolar bone.

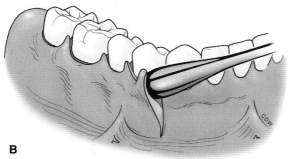

B: Elevating (or raising) the soft tissue flap from the roots of the teeth and alveolar bone.

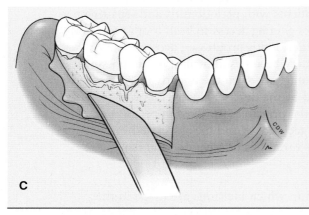

C: Improved visualization of both the tooth roots and alveolar bone contours with the flap elevated.

B. **Indications for a Periodontal Flap**
1. Most modern periodontal surgical procedures require performing periodontal flaps as a part of the procedure.
2. Basically, the flap elevation is done to provide access for some treatment either to tooth roots or the alveolar bone, or to both of these structures.
   a. Periodontal flaps can be elevated simply to provide access to tooth root surfaces for completion of meticulous periodontal instrumentation (scaling and root planing) that was begun as a part of nonsurgical periodontal therapy. Use of a periodontal flap for improved access to tooth roots is discussed in more detail later in this chapter under the heading *flap for access*.
   b. Periodontal flaps may also be used to provide access to reshape or treat alveolar bone defects resulting from periodontitis. In the following sections of this chapter, the topic of *apically positioned flaps with osseous resective surgery* provides an example of this type of procedure.
2. **Classification of Periodontal Flaps.** There are several classification schemes used to describe periodontal flaps. Two of the most common include (1) the degree of bone exposure provided by the flap and (2) the location of the margin (or edge) of the flap when it is sutured back into place.
   A. **Degree of Bone Exposure.** One method of classification of periodontal flaps is to describe the flap based upon the degree of exposure of alveolar bone following flap elevation. Using this method of classification, flaps would be described as being either full thickness or partial thickness.
   1. A **full-thickness flap**, or mucoperiosteal flap as it is also called, includes elevation of entire thickness of the soft tissue (including epithelium, connective tissue, and periosteum). The periosteum is a dense membrane composed of fibrous connective tissue that closely wraps the outer surface of the alveolar bone.
      a. The full-thickness flap provides the complete access to underlying bone that might be needed when bone replacement grafting or periodontal regeneration procedures are anticipated.
      b. The full-thickness flap is elevated with what is generally referred to as a **blunt dissection.**
         1. Blunt dissection means that the tools used to elevate (or raise) the flap are not sharpened on the edge (i.e., blunted or slightly rounded on the edge); blunt dissection minimizes the chance of accidental damage to the flap.
         2. In this type of flap elevation, the flap is lifted or pried up using surgical tools called periosteal elevators, and it is elevated in a manner quite similar to lifting the peeling off of an orange. Figure 27-3 illustrates a full-thickness flap (or mucoperiosteal flap) elevated during a periodontal surgical procedure.

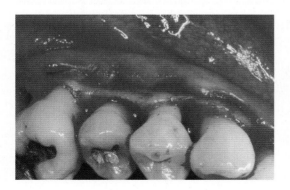

Figure 27-3. Full-Thickness or Mucoperiosteal Flap. This photograph taken during a typical periodontal flap surgery shows a full-thickness or mucoperiosteal flap (i.e., a flap of soft tissue that includes epithelium, underlying connective tissue, and the periosteum elevated off the teeth and alveolar bone). Note the exposure of the underlying alveolar bone margin and osseous defects associated with that bone interdentally.

2. A **partial-thickness flap**, or split-thickness flap as it is also called, includes elevation of only the epithelium and a thin layer of the underlying connective tissue rather than the entire thickness of the underlying soft tissues.

   a. The partial-thickness flap is elevated with **sharp dissection**; sharp dissection requires incising the underlying connective tissue in such a manner as to separate the epithelial surface plus a small portion of the connective tissue from the periosteum. *Use of this technique would leave the periosteal tissues covering the bone.*

   b. To perform the sharp dissection needed in a partial-thickness flap, a surgeon must limit this approach to areas of gingiva that are relatively thick; careful inspection of gingiva will reveal that gingiva is quite thin in some patients but somewhat thicker in others.

   c. Research data indicates that when alveolar bone is exposed during a flap procedure, there is a potential loss of a very small surface layer of the bone following the procedure. Whereas this change in the surface of the alveolar bone does not affect final healing, this fact can make use of a full-thickness flap inadvisable in certain instances.

B. **Location of the Soft Tissue Margin.** Another method of classifying periodontal flaps is to describe flaps based upon the location of the margin of the soft tissue when it is sutured back in place. Using this method of classification, flaps would be described as being either nondisplaced or displaced.

   1. A **nondisplaced flap** is a flap that is sutured with the margin of the flap at its original position in relationship to the CEJ on the tooth.

   2. A **displaced flap** is a flap that is sutured with the margin of the flap placed at a position other than its original position in relationship to the CEJ of the tooth. Note that a displaced flap can be positioned either apically, coronally, or laterally in relationship to its original position.

     a. For a displaced flap to be moved to a new position (such as coronally or laterally), the surgeon must perform the flap elevation in such a manner that the base of the flap extends into the movable mucosal tissues.

     b. Displaced flaps are generally not possible to perform on the palatal surface of the teeth because of the absence of movable mucosa in this anatomical location.

C. **Common Terminology.** Box 27-3 provides an overview of common terminology used to classify periodontal flaps.

Box 27-3. Common Terminology Used to Classify Periodontal Flaps

1. Terminology Based Upon Bone Exposure
   - Full-thickness flap
   - Partial-thickness flap
2. Terminology Based on Location of Flap Margin
   - Nondisplaced flap
   - Displaced flap

Box 27-4. Types of Incisions Utilized During Periodontal Flaps

1. Horizontal Incisions
   - Crevicular incisions
   - Internal bevel incisions
2. Vertical Incisions
   - Vertical releasing incision

3. **Types of Incisions Used During Periodontal Flap Surgeries.** Most of the incisions made prior to elevation of a periodontal flap are made with surgical scalpel blades, but there are a variety of special periodontal knives that can be used to perform some of these incisions. Several basic types of incisions are utilized during periodontal flap surgery. Some familiarization with terminology related to flap incisions could be useful to the dental hygienist in understanding specific types of periodontal surgery. These incisions can be broadly classified as either horizontal or vertical incisions. Box 27-4 provides an overview of the types of incisions utilized during periodontal flaps.

   A. **Horizontal Incisions.** Horizontal incisions run parallel to the gingival margins in a mesiodistal direction.

      1. One type of horizontal incision commonly employed during flap surgery is the crevicular incision (or sulcular incision as it is sometimes called).

      2. In the crevicular incision the surgical scalpel is carefully placed into the gingival crevice or sulcus and the tissues are incised apically to bone.

      3. A second type of horizontal incision is the internal bevel incision.

      4. In an internal bevel incision the surgical scalpel enters the marginal gingiva but is not placed directly into the crevice or sulcus; the scalpel blade enters the gingival margin approximately 0.5 to 1.0 mm away from the margin and follows the general contour of the scalloped marginal gingiva.

      5. Using an internal bevel incision results in leaving a small collar of soft tissue around the tooth root (including the lining of the pre-existing periodontal pocket); this collar of tissue is removed during most periodontal flap procedures.

      6. Terminology related to these incisions can be quite confusing.

         a. The internal bevel incision has also been referred to as a "reverse bevel incision" or the "initial incision," since it is usually made as a first step during a routine periodontal flap procedure.

         b. The sulcular incision has also been referred to as the "second incision," since it is usually made as the second step during a routine flap procedure.

   B. **Vertical Incisions.** Vertical incisions run perpendicular to the gingival margin in an apicoocclusal direction.

      1. Vertical incisions are primarily used to allow elevation of the flap during the surgical procedure without stretching or damaging the soft tissues during flap elevation.

      2. The primary type of vertical incisions have also been referred to as vertical releasing incisions, since once this type of incision passes the mucogingival junction, the flap is "released" or has possibilities for movement in relationship to the underlying bone and adjacent soft tissues.

Section 3
Descriptions of Common Types of Periodontal Surgery

1. **Flap for Access**
   A. **Procedure Description**
      1. **Flap for access** (or modified Widman flap surgery) is used to provide access to the tooth roots for improved root preparation (1,4–6). In this surgical procedure the gingival tissue is incised and temporarily elevated (lifted away) from the tooth roots. Figure 27-4 shows a flap for access with the flap elevated and partial removal of collar of tissue.
      2. There are two main advantages of flap for access.
         a. Flap for access surgery provides excellent access to the tooth roots for thorough instrumentation in sites where deep pocket depths may have hindered periodontal instrumentation during nonsurgical therapy.
         b. Flap for access surgery also provides an intimate adaptation of healthy connective tissues to the debrided tooth roots following suturing of the wound to allow for healing by primary intention.
      3. The tissues are elevated only enough to allow good access for periodontal instrumentation of the tooth roots. Following root treatment, the gingival tissue is replaced at its original position (i.e., a nondisplaced flap) and stabilized with sutures.
   B. **Steps in a Typical Flap for Access.** The usual steps followed during flap for access surgery are outlined below.
      1. An internal bevel incision is begun through the surface of the gingiva surrounding the teeth; the incision is made approximately 0.5 to 1 mm away from the gingival margin and follows the scallop of the marginal gingiva.
      2. The internal bevel incision that was begun as the first incision through the surface gingiva is retraced and extended apically all the way to the alveolar bone.
      3. The flap is elevated far enough to provide good access to the tooth roots.
      4. A crevicular or sulcular incision is then made from the base of the pocket to the bone to facilitate removal of the small collar of tissue remaining around the necks of the teeth.
      5. If needed, an incision may be made at the base of remaining tissue collar to completely free this tissue, and the tissue collar is removed.
      6. With the flap elevated tooth roots are instrumented to remove remaining plaque, calculus deposits, root contaminants, and root irregularities. While

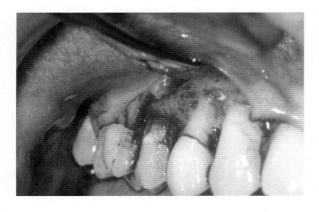

Figure 27-4. Flap for Access in Progress. This photograph was taken during a flap for access. In the photograph, the flap has been incised and elevated. Partial removal of the collar of tissue has been performed.

performing the debridement, residual periodontal ligament fibers adhering to the tooth root near the base of the pocket are left undisturbed.

7. The flaps may be thinned if needed to allow for intimate adaptation of the gingiva to the necks of the teeth; alveolar bone contour is not altered unless minor recontouring is needed to allow for proper adaptation of the flap.

8. The flap is repositioned and sutured at its original position (nondisplaced); special effort is made to insure that the tips of the facial and lingual papillae are in actual contact to promote healing by primary intention at this critical interdental site.

C. Healing After Flap for Access

1. The type of healing expected from flap for access surgery is *healing by repair* and usually involves formation of a *long junctional epithelium.*

2. Research shows that flap for access surgery can result in a stable dentogingival unit that can be maintained in health with periodic periodontal maintenance by the dental team and proper self-care by the patient.

D. Special Considerations for the Dental Hygienist

1. During routine nonsurgical periodontal instrumentation, it may not be possible to perform thorough calculus removal if the pocket depths are deeper than 6 mm. Flap for access surgery provides greatly improved access to root surfaces in areas of deeper pockets where the results of conventional nonsurgical periodontal instrumentation alone would be limited.

2. Even in patients where flap for access surgery is part of the treatment plan, every effort should be made to minimize the inflammation associated with chronic periodontitis by performing complete nonsurgical therapy prior to the surgical intervention.

   a. The dental hygienist plays a critical role in promoting patient understanding of how nonsurgical and surgical treatment are related—first, nonsurgical therapy followed by surgical therapy if needed.

   b. Thorough and meticulous nonsurgical therapy even in areas of deep pockets can reduce the extent of any planned periodontal surgical treatment and is always an important part of patient care.

2. Open Flap Debridement

A. Procedure Description

1. Open flap debridement is a term that describes a periodontal surgical procedure quite similar in concept and execution to flap for access surgery. In the periodontal literature another term that has been used interchangeably with open flap debridement is flap curettage.

2. Historically, the term open flap debridement was used to describe some of the original flap procedures that were first developed by periodontal surgeons many years ago.

3. Today open flap debridement (or flap curettage) is usually performed with steps quite similar to flap for access with the following exceptions:

   a. Exception #1. Open flap debridement usually includes more extensive flap elevation than flap for access—providing access not only to the tooth roots but also to all of the alveolar bone defects. Remember that during flap for access surgery the flap is elevated only far enough to provide good access to the tooth roots.

   b. Exception #2. Whereas flap for access includes a nondisplaced flap, open flap debridement may include displacing the flap margin to a new location (i.e., during an open flap debridement the flap margin may be sutured in a position more apical to its original position).

B. Steps in Typical Open Flap Debridement
 1. The procedure begins with horizontal incisions that can be either crevicular or internal bevel incisions; vertical releasing incisions can be included as needed to allow for atraumatic flap elevation.
 2. Full-thickness (mucoperiosteal) flaps are elevated to provide access to both tooth roots and the underlying alveolar bone defects.
 3. Granulation tissue is removed from existing osseous defects and interdental areas.
 4. Tooth roots are instrumented to remove remaining plaque, calculus deposits, root contaminants, and root irregularities.
 5. Osteoplasty, which is not normally included in open flap debridement, is performed only if it is needed to allow for readaptation of the tissues to the tooth roots.
 6. Flaps are sutured either at their original level (nondisplaced) or at a level more apical to their original position (displaced).
 7. Figure 27-5 illustrates critical steps in a typical open flap debridement.

C. Healing Expected After Open Flap Debridement
 1. Healing from open flap debridement is typically resolution of much of the existing inflammation within the periodontal tissues.
 2. The formation of a long junctional epithelium can occur along with slight remodeling of some of the osseous bone defects caused by periodontitis.
 3. Typically little if any bone regrowth occurs following open flap debridement.
 4. It is common for residual periodontal pockets to remain in some sites following this procedure—thus, complicating both patient self-care and professional periodontal maintenance.

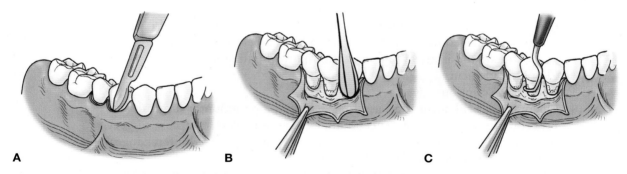

A   B   C

Figure 27-5. Critical Steps During a Typical Open Flap Debridement. A: Incisions being made to bone from within the crevice or pocket base. **B:** Flap elevation to expose tooth roots and alveolar bone. **C:** Periodontal instrumentation of the roots of the teeth.

3. Osseous Resective Surgery. The word "osseous" is defined as 'having to do with bone." Thus, periodontal osseous surgery is surgery involving the alveolar bone.
 A. Description of Procedure
  1. Periodontal osseous resective surgery (or periodontal osseous surgery) is a term used to describe periodontal surgery employed to correct many of the strange deformities of the alveolar bone that often result from advancing periodontitis (7,8).

2. The fundamental goal for this type of periodontal surgery is to eliminate periodontal pockets, and this goal can be achieved when osseous surgery is combined with an apically displaced flap as discussed in the next section.

B. Rationale for Periodontal Osseous Surgery

1. Gingiva has a tendency to follow its natural architecture with or without the support of underlying alveolar bone; the natural architecture of gingiva includes a scalloped contour where the gingiva over the facial and lingual surfaces of teeth is apical to the level of the interdental papillae.

2. As periodontitis progresses, the contours of alveolar bone are altered by the formation of osseous defects referred to with names such as osseous craters, one-walled, two-walled, and three-walled osseous defects, which have been discussed in other chapters of this textbook. In areas where these osseous defects form, attachment loss accompanies the alveolar bone contour changes and periodontal pockets form.

3. Osseous surgery attempts to reestablish alveolar bone contours that mimic the predictable eventual contours of the gingiva following healing from periodontal surgery. Thus, periodontal osseous surgery can be used to minimize the discrepancy between the bone contour and the gingival contour to eliminate periodontal pockets following complete healing.

4. Periodontal osseous resective surgery is commonly performed in patients with moderate periodontitis where the bone defects created by the periodontitis are primarily osseous craters; as discussed in other chapters of this book, osseous craters are the most common type of periodontal osseous defect in periodontitis patients.

C. Special Terminology Associated with Osseous Surgery—Ostectomy and Osteoplasty
Osseous surgery is frequently employed in the treatment of patients with moderate periodontitis, and this topic is discussed in detail in all periodontal textbooks. Two terms frequently arise during discussions of osseous surgery (ostectomy and osteoplasty), and these terms can be a bit confusing.

1. One of these terms is ostectomy. **Ostectomy** or osteoectomy refers to the removal of alveolar bone that is actually attached to the tooth (i.e., that is still providing some support for the tooth).

   a. Ostectomy results in the immediate loss of a small amount of attachment at certain sites, and for that reason ostectomy must be used with appropriate caution by the surgeon.

   b. In spite of the slight attachment loss that occurs during ostectomy, this is an excellent method of eliminating periodontal pockets associated with certain commonly occurring osseous defects such as osseous craters. The removal of small amounts of supporting bone is justified by the attainment of alveolar bone contours that are compatible with the natural contours of the gingiva.

   c. Figure 27-6 illustrates technique for ostectomy that might be performed during periodontal osseous resective surgery.

2. The second of these terms is osteoplasty. **Osteoplasty** refers to reshaping the surface of alveolar bone without actually removing any of the supporting bone.

3. In reality, most periodontal osseous resective surgery involves both ostectomy and osteoplasty, and when performed with precision, these procedures can result in alveolar bone contours that mimic the contours of the gingiva following complete healing.

4. Box 27-5 outlines the special terminology associated with periodontal osseous surgery.

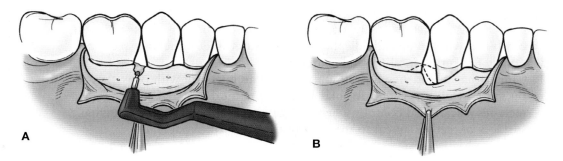

A   **B**

Figure 27-6. Ostectomy Technique. A: Following exposure of the interdental osseous crater, one of the crater walls (facial wall in this illustration) is being removed with a special surgical bur. **B:** Based upon the newly established bone level at the site, the surrounding bone is contoured in an attempt to reestablish a more natural bone contour.

Box 27-5. Special Terminology Associated with Periodontal Osseous Surgery

- Ostectomy—removal of some tooth-supporting bone
- Osteoplasty—reshaping of the surface bone contours

    D. **Steps in Periodontal Osseous Resective Surgery**
       1. Incisions are made and flaps are elevated to provide access to the osseous defects and the surrounding alveolar bone; these incisions typically are done on both the facial and lingual surfaces of the teeth and typically include both horizontal and vertical releasing incisions.
       2. Granulation tissue associated with the osseous defects is thoroughly debrided to allow full visualization to the extent and shape of the osseous defects.
       3. All remaining soft tissue tags in the surgical site are identified and removed usually using a combination of hand and ultrasonic instrumentation.
       4. Tooth root surfaces are debrided to remove all plaque, calculus, root contaminants, and root irregularities.
       5. Osteoplasty is performed to remove thick bone ledges where they exist on the facial and lingual surfaces of the alveolar bone.
       6. Ostectomy is performed to eliminate interproximal osseous defects.
       7. Bone contours are refined with hand instruments and surgical burs.
       8. The gingiva is sutured into place (usually at a more apical position than the original level as discussed in the next section).
    E. **Healing After Periodontal Osseous Resective Surgery**
       1. When periodontal osseous resective surgery is performed in areas of the dentition where osseous craters exist, it is normally possible for the surgeon to recreate a natural contour to the alveolar bone.
       2. When this osseous resective surgery is combined with the apically positioned flap as discussed in the next section of this chapter, it is frequently possible to reestablish a normal crevice or sulcus depth without the presence of residual periodontal pockets following the surgery.
       3. For most patients with moderate periodontitis, once periodontal pockets are eliminated using this type of surgery, with reasonable self-care by the patient and periodontal maintenance by the dental team, it is possible to maintain the dentition in health.

4. **Apically Positioned Flap with Osseous Resective Surgery**
   A. **Procedure Description**
      1. An **apically positioned flap with osseous resective surgery** is a periodontal surgical procedure involving a combination of a displaced flap (displaced in an apical direction) plus resective osseous surgery.
         a. As already discussed, correction of altered alveolar bone contours to mimic the contours of healthy alveolar bone is usually referred to as periodontal osseous resective surgery.
         b. Following contouring of the alveolar bone, the flap in this procedure is sutured at a position that is more apical to its original position in relationship to the tooth CEJs (apically positioned or apically displaced flap).
      2. This periodontal surgical procedure is ideal for minimizing periodontal pocket depths in patients with osseous craters caused by moderate periodontitis.
         a. An apically displaced flap can result in a gingival margin that is apical to the CEJ of the tooth. This new position of the gingival margin means that more of the root of the tooth is visible in the mouth.
         b. The reduced pocket depth can facilitate both self-care by the patient and periodontal maintenance by the dental team.
   B. **Steps in an Apically Positioned Flap with Osseous Resective Surgery**
      1. This procedure normally begins with an internal bevel incision. The internal bevel incision can preserve the width of keratinized tissue that is important to the overall procedure, because this width of keratinized tissue will be displaced apically as a final step.
      2. The internal bevel incision is followed by flap elevation and crevicular incision prior to removal of the collar of tissues around the necks of the teeth.
      3. Vertical releasing incisions are made as needed to avoid damage to the flap.
      4. Granulation tissues are debrided, and osseous defects are exposed as discussed in the previous section.
      5. Periodontal osseous resective surgery is performed to mimic the contours of healthy alveolar bone; this osseous surgery normally includes both ostectomy and osteoplasty.
      6. The flap is sutured at a position apical to its original position (usually near the tooth–bone junction).
      7. The surgical site is covered with periodontal dressing to stabilize the flap at its apical location.
      8. Table 27-3 illustrates the critical steps in an apically positioned flap with osseous resective surgery.

TABLE 27-3. CRITICAL STEPS IN AN APICALLY POSITIONED FLAP WITH OSSEOUS RESECTIVE SURGERY

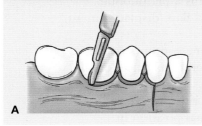

A: Internal bevel incision and vertical releasing incision being made around the teeth.

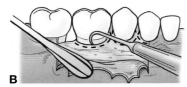

B: Removal of the collar of soft tissue following flap elevation.

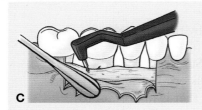

C: Ostectomy being performed after identification of osseous defects.

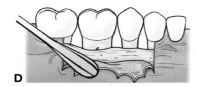

D: Inspection of the final bone contours after ostectomy and osteoplasty.

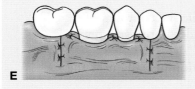

E: Suturing of both the flap margins and the vertical releasing incisions. Note that the level of the flap margin is displaced in an apical position compared to its original position.

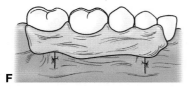

F: Placement of periodontal dressing to stabilize the flap at its new position during the early phase of healing.

C. Healing of an Apically Positioned Flap with Osseous Resective Surgery
1. Final healing of this type of surgery results in a normal attachment (both junctional epithelium and connective tissue attachment) at a position more apical on the tooth root.
2. It should be emphasized that apically positioned flap with osseous resection cannot eliminate all periodontal osseous defects, especially where the defects are quite severe.
3. Research has shown that an apically positioned flap combined with periodontal osseous surgery can result in a stable dentogingival junction

that can be maintained in health with reasonable self-care by the patient and periodic periodontal maintenance by the dental team.

    4. Figure 27-7 illustrates the results of a healed apically positioned flap used to treat a furcation involvement on a molar tooth.

D. Special Considerations for the Dental Hygienist

    1. During surgery to minimize periodontal pockets, it is common for the gingival margin to be positioned at a more apical level to the CEJ than it originally occupied.

        a. This apical positioning results in exposure of a portion of the root to the oral cavity.

        b. Visibility of a portion of the root may be an esthetic concern for the patient.

        c. In patients with a high caries risk, exposure of root surface in the oral cavity can lead to root caries. Therefore, this type of surgery may be contraindicated in patients with a high risk for dental caries.

    2. Temporary dentinal hypersensitivity is a frequent patient postsurgical complaint following this type of surgery. As discussed in other chapters, dentinal hypersensitivity usually diminishes over time if the patient maintains good plaque control.

    3. Before surgery, the members of the dental team should inform the patient about anticipated changes in appearance and about the potential for dentinal hypersensitivity. The dental hygienist should also assure the patient that if sensitivity does occur, measures could be taken to minimize the sensitivity.

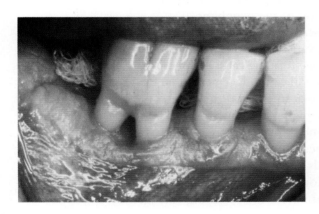

Figure 27-7. Results of an Apically Positioned Flap. This apically positioned flap was performed to treat a large furcation involvement on the molar tooth. Note that in this case the healed gingival margin leaves the tooth CEJ coronal to the gingival margin.

5. Bone Replacement Grafts
   A. Procedure Description
      1. **Bone replacement graft** is a surgical procedure used to encourage the body to rebuild alveolar bone that has been lost usually as a result of periodontal disease.
      2. Bone grafting has been commonplace in medicine for many years, but grafting bone replacement materials into the periodontium offers some unique challenges different from bone grafting in medicine.
         a. Bone grafts placed into periodontal defects are subject to constant contamination from bacteria and saliva traveling along the existing tooth roots adjacent to the graft site; this constant potential for contamination from bacteria would not be the case in many bone grafts in medicine (such as a bone graft done during a hip replacement).
         b. In addition, the healing of bone grafts in periodontal defects can be disrupted by the growth of epithelium into the wound that can lead to graft failure; this potential disruption by the growth of epithelium would also not be the case in most medical bone grafts.
   B. Terminology Associated with Bone Replacement Grafts
      1. **Osteogenesis** is the term that is used to describe the potential for new bone cells and new bone to form following bone grafting (9). Bone replacement graft materials frequently are referred to based on their osteogenic potential.
         a. Some grafting materials have been described as **osteoconductive**. Osteoconductive grafting materials are grafts where the grafting materials form a framework for bone cells existing outside the graft to use to penetrate the graft during the formation of the new bone.
         b. Other grafting materials have been described as **osteoinductive**. Osteoinductive grafting materials are grafts where the actual cells within the grafting material are converted into bone-forming cells, and these cells then form the new bone (i.e., when the material can induce new bone formation).
      2. Using this terminology, the ideal bone replacement graft material would be one that is osteoinductive and one that has a high osteogenic potential.
   C. **Broad Categories of Materials Used for Bone Replacement Grafting.** Many potential grafting materials have been studied in relationship to their osteogenic potential. In general, these grafting materials can be described as falling into one of the four broad categories: autografts, allografts, xenografts, and alloplasts. These four categories of bone graft material have widely varying osteogenic potentials.
      1. **Autografts** are bone replacement materials taken from the patient who is receiving the graft. Periodontal autografts can be taken from sites in the patient's own jaws or occasionally from other areas of the patient's body.
      2. **Allografts** are bone replacement grafts taken from individuals who are genetically dissimilar to the donor (i.e., another human). Of course when allografts are used, these grafting materials must be modified to eliminate the potential for rejection.
      3. **Xenografts** are bone replacement grafts taken from another species, such as bovine bone replacement graft material, which can be placed in a human. Again, these materials must be modified to eliminate the potential for rejection.
      4. **Alloplasts** are bone replacement grafts that are synthetic materials or inert foreign materials.
      5. Autografts have the highest osteogenic potential, and alloplasts have the least osteogenic potential with osteogenic potential for allografts and xenografts between those two extremes.

6. Though autografts have the most osteogenic potential, it is not always possible to obtain enough autogenous bone from a patient to fill all of the osseous defects that need grafting. This creates the need during many periodontal surgical procedures for a bone graft material from a source other than the patient being treated.

7. In some instances these grafting materials can be used in combinations such as mixing autogenous bone with an allograft material to obtain the needed volume of grafting material for a particular grafting site.

8. Box 27-6 provides an overview of materials used for bone replacement grafts.

Box 27-6 Materials Used for Bone Replacement Grafts

- Autograft—bone taken from patient's own body
- Allograft—bone taken from another human
- Xenograft—bone taken from another species
- Alloplast—synthetic bone-like material

D. **Examples of Specific Materials Used for Bone Replacement Grafting.** Numerous materials have been studied for possible use of bone replacement grafting over the past several decades. None of the materials is ideal, but many of them have been shown to have some osteogenic potential. The discussion below describes some examples of the types of bone replacement graft materials that have been studied.

1. Autogenous bone grafts from intraoral sites
   a. As already discussed, autografts are graft materials taken from the patient's own body.
   b. Autografts from intraoral sites have been used in periodontics for many years, and currently these autogenous grafts are considered the gold standard when comparing other grafting materials for their osteogenic potential.
   c. It should not be surprising that autogenous bone is the most effective grafting material, since it already contains living bone cells and viable bone growth factors from the patient—in contrast to some of the other grafting materials such as alloplasts, which are usually manufactured materials.
   d. Intraoral sources for the autograft material can be from sites such as bone removed during ostectomy or osteoplasty, exostoses removed during surgery, bone removed from edentulous ridges, bone taken from healing extraction sites, bone taken from the chin, and bone harvested from the jaws distal to the teeth in a dental arch.
   e. A variety of techniques for harvesting the graft material and insuring its osteogenic potential have been advocated. These techniques usually include exposing the alveolar bone by elevating a periodontal flap, removing granulation tissue associated with an osseous defect, treating the tooth root adjacent to the defect, placing the graft material into the defect, and closing the flap by suturing it at its original level on the teeth.
   f. In addition to harvesting particles or larger pieces of bone, autogenous bone grafts include the use of materials such as osseous coagulum. Osseous coagulum is a mixture of bone dust and blood taken from the patient made by removing small particles of cortical bone and mixing it with blood from the surgical site.

g. One technique for collecting autogenous graft material from a patient during a periodontal surgical procedure involves the bone blend technique. This technique involves collecting bone in a plastic capsule and pestle and triturating the material into a workable mass of bone blend that can be grafted into osseous defects.

h. Though small particles or pieces of cortical bone are usually selected as autogenous grafting material, cancellous bone marrow may also be used. One common intraoral site to harvest bone marrow is from a maxillary tuberosity.

i. One *disadvantage* to using autogenous bone grafts is that when they are used, they frequently require a second surgical site for harvesting the graft material, increasing the potential for postsurgical problems.

2. Autogenous bone from extraoral sites

a. Iliac (or hip) cancellous marrow has been studied as an autogenous bone replacement graft material.

b. When used in periodontal defects this material does result in bone formation in osseous defects. Today marrow from the hip is rarely used for autogenous grafting into periodontal defects, however, because of the potential for root resorption adjacent to the grafting site, the potential for postoperative problems associated with the donor site, and the difficulty in obtaining this type of donor material.

3. Freeze-dried bone allografts. Bone allografts (taken from another human and processed) are attractive surgical options as bone replacement graft materials. There has been a lot of interest in periodontics in identifying an ideal bone allograft. If the ideal bone allograft could be identified for use in periodontal patients, there would be no need for a second surgical site to obtain an autogenous graft. In addition, if the ideal bone allograft could be identified, there would be no worry about limitation of the availability of the amount of graft material needed.

a. As already discussed, allografts are graft materials taken from another individual of the same species (i.e., another human who is recently deceased).

b. Freeze-dried bone allografts (both calcified and decalcified) have been used successfully as bone replacement allografts, and bone allograft products have been available commercially for some time (10–16).

1. Bone allograft materials are obtained from the cortical bone of a donor within a few hours of death, defatted, washed in alcohol, and frozen.

2. The graft material is then demineralized, ground into particles, and stored in sterile vials until used in a clinical setting.

c. Since allografts are materials that are foreign to the body of the patient receiving the graft and since potential deceased donors may have diseases that could be transmitted to the patient being treated, steps must be taken to maximize the safety of this type of grafting material. These steps usually include the following:

1. Excluding potential donors that are members of disease high-risk groups,

2. Testing of cadaver tissues to exclude donors with infection or malignant disease, and

3. Treating the allograft with chemical agents or with other techniques to inactivate viruses.

d. Whereas the risk of disease transmission using allograft materials is not zero, the risk of viral transmission by the use of allograft bone replacement material has been described as highly remote.

  e. Allograft products for use in periodontal defects are available in two types based on how they are processed: freeze-dried bone allografts and decalcified freeze-dried bone allografts.

   1. Freeze-dried bone allograft (FDBA)

    a. Freeze-dried bone allograft or FDBA is an osteoconductive allograft graft material that has been reported to result in some bone fill.

    b. Bone fill from FDBA can be improved if the material is mixed with some autogenous bone at the time of placement.

   2. Decalcified freeze-dried bone allograft (DFDBA)

    a. Decalcified freeze-dried bone allograft or DFDBA is an osteoinductive graft material that has a higher osteogenic potential than FDBA, and DFDBA is preferred by many clinicians.

    b. The osteogenic potential for DFDBA has been shown to vary depending upon several factors such as the extent of demineralization as well as other factors.

4. Bovine-derived bone

 a. Bovine-derived bone is an example of a xenograft material; xenografts are materials taken from another species.

 b. Xenografts such as bovine-derived bone have also been used as bone replacement grafts in periodontal defects (17).

 c. An anorganic bovine bone has been tested and marketed, and studies have shown successful regrowth of some bone with this material.

  1. Anorganic bovine bone is bovine bone that has been treated to remove all of its organic components to eliminate the risk of rejection.

  2. Removing the organic components from bovine bone leaves a porous structure, similar in structure to human bone.

  3. It has been suggested that the porous structure of anorganic bovine bone can act as scaffolding for new bone and that it can act through this mechanism as an osteoinductive material.

5. Plaster of Paris

 a. Plaster of Paris has been used as an alloplastic bone replacement grafting material (18).

 b. Plaster of Paris is actually calcium sulfate, which is porous and biocompatible when placed in periodontal wounds; when calcium sulfate is placed in a periodontal wound, it resorbs within a few weeks.

 c. Though this material has been studied and used in humans as a bone replacement graft material, its efficacy related to osteogenic potential has not been proven.

6. Bioactive glass

 a. Bioactive glass ceramics have been studied and used as alloplastic bone replacement grafting materials (19–21).

 b. This ceramic material consists of calcium salts, phosphates, and silicone dioxide; when used as an alloplastic bone replacement graft, bioactive glass is used in particulate form.

 c. When bioactive glass comes in contact with periodontal tissues, the particulate surfaces can incorporate proteins and can attract osteoblasts that can subsequently form bone.

7. Calcium phosphate
   a. Calcium phosphate biomaterials have been used as alloplastic grafting materials for several decades. Calcium phosphate is osteoconductive and is well tolerated by body tissues.
   b. Two types of calcium phosphate materials have been used: hydroxyapatite and tricalcium phosphate.
   c. Though these materials can result in some clinical repair of periodontal defects, they are either poorly resorbable (tricalcium phosphate) or not resorbable at all (hydroxyapatite) and can remain encapsulated by collagen within the periodontal tissues.

E. Healing After Bone Replacement Grafting
   1. Final healing expected from bone replacement grafting usually includes a partial rebuilding of alveolar bone lost because of periodontitis.
      a. It is not known, however, if successful bone grafting always results in the reformation of cementum and periodontal ligament in addition to the alveolar bone.
      b. In spite of what appears to be good radiographic and clinical healing, the reformed bone in some cases may not actually be attached to the cementum by periodontal ligament fibers.
   2. Research has shown that a successful bone graft combined with reasonable self-care by the patient and periodic periodontal maintenance by the dental team can result in retaining a severely compromised tooth over time.

F. Special Considerations for the Dental Hygienist
   1. The site of a bone replacement graft should be left undisturbed for many months and should not be probed until an appropriate interval has elapsed. The dental hygienist should consult with the dentist to determine when a grafted site may be probed safely.
   2. Meticulous plaque control in any grafted site is critical. In the early stages of the healing, the dental team maintains some of the responsibility for plaque control at the site, because the patient may temporarily be unable to perform adequate self-care.

6. Guided Tissue Regeneration
   A. Procedure Description
      1. Guided tissue regeneration (GTR) is a periodontal surgical procedure employed to encourage regeneration of lost periodontal structures (i.e., to regrow lost cementum, lost periodontal ligament, and lost alveolar bone).
         a. When a periodontal surgical wound is created such as the elevation of a flap, the healing of the wound may involve cells from several different sources surrounding the wound.
         b. Figure 27-8 illustrates the potential sources of cells that could contribute to healing tissues within a periodontal surgical wound.
         c. Guided tissue regeneration techniques involve the use of a barrier membrane to delay the normally rapid ingrowth of epithelium into a healing periodontal wound; the rapid growth of epithelium into the wound can interfere with the slower growth of other cells critical to the healing process (22–35).
         d. Figure 27-9 illustrates how a barrier membrane might be placed under a periodontal flap at the time of surgery to delay the ingrowth of unwanted types of cells into the healing of the wound.
         e. Delay of the ingrowth of epithelium into a healing periodontal wound can allow for undifferentiated cells from the periodontal ligament to populate the root area and differentiate into the tissues that normally comprise the periodontium (i.e., cementum, PDL, and alveolar bone).

f. The barrier membranes used during a GTR procedure can also be used in conjunction with bone graft materials in some instances.

g. As the name implies, guided tissue regeneration can result in a true regeneration of the periodontium.

2. Goal of guided tissue regeneration

a. When the entire array of types of periodontal surgery is viewed, periodontal regeneration is the ultimate goal, and there is much ongoing research related to GTR.

b. Although regeneration of the cementum, periodontal ligament, and alveolar bone is the ultimate goal of periodontal therapy, regeneration of the periodontium is not completely predictable with techniques in use today.

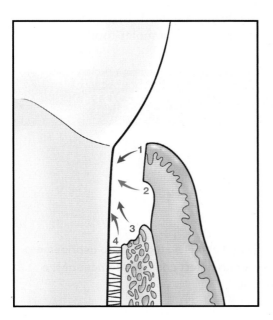

Figure 27-8. Potential Sources of Cells in a Healing Periodontal Surgical Wound. There are four potential sources of cells that can contribute to the healing of a periodontal surgical wound such as a flap:

1. Gingival epithelial cells,
2. Gingival connective tissue cells,
3. Bone cells, and
4. Periodontal ligament cells.

Of these four types of cells the most rapidly growing of them are the gingival epithelial cells.

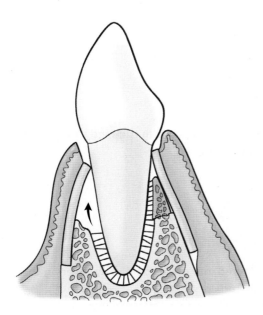

Figure 27-9. Use of Barrier Material to Inhibit the Rapid Growth of the Gingival Epithelial Cells. Note that the barrier has been placed to interfere with the growth of the epithelial cells from the flap margin along the tooth root to give the undifferentiated cells a chance to populate the wound and contribute to the healing.

B. Steps in a Typical Guided Tissue Regeneration Procedure

1. The first step in guided tissue regeneration is to make appropriate incisions and elevate a flap. In this procedure, the flap usually is elevated one to two teeth beyond the site of the osseous defects.
2. The osseous defects are thoroughly debrided and the roots in the site are planed.
3. The selected membrane is trimmed to the size needed for the site; during this membrane trimming, the membrane is allowed to extend several millimeters beyond the defect in all directions.
4. The membrane is sutured into place with a sling suture placed around the tooth.
5. The flap is sutured into place (frequently slightly coronally), so that the flap covers the membrane completely.
6. Table 27-4 illustrates the use of a barrier membrane during a guided tissue regeneration procedure used to treat a furcation involvement in a molar tooth.

TABLE 27-4. USE OF BARRIER MATERIAL DURING GUIDED TISSUE REGENERATION IN THE TREATMENT OF A MOLAR TOOTH WITH DEEP FURCATION INVOLVEMENT

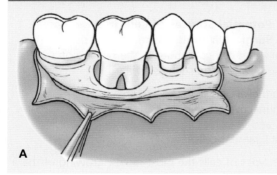

A: Flap is incised and elevated prior to debridement of the osseous defect and debridement of the tooth root.

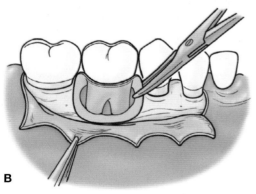

B: A barrier is selected, custom trimmed to size, and sutured into place.

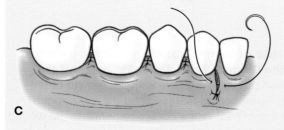

C: Flap is sutured into place completely covering the barrier material.

C. Barrier Materials Used During Guided Tissue Regeneration
   1. Some of the barrier materials in current use require removal following healing of the wound, so their use necessitates a second surgical procedure to remove the barrier material.
      a. Expanded polytetrafluoroethylene (ePTFE) is the most commonly used nonresorbable membrane material.
      b. These nonresorbable membranes are also available commercially with embedded titanium strips to prevent collapse of the membrane into larger osseous defects.
   2. Other barrier materials in current use are resorbable and thus do not require removal at some later date; bioresorbable membranes are preferred by many clinicians for most surgical applications.
      a. There are several types of bioresorbable membranes; these types include polyglycoside synthetic polymers, bovine and porcine collagen, and calcium sulfate.
      b. One disadvantage of bioresorbable membranes are that they lack rigidity that can be provided by titanium reinforcements available in some nonresorbable membranes.
D. Use of Guided Tissue Regeneration with Bone Replacement Grafts
   1. The simultaneous use of barrier membranes to promote regeneration along with bone replacement grafts is one clinical option.
   2. At this point, most of the studies have been directed toward the use of barrier materials combined either with decalcified freeze-dried bone allograft (DFDBA) or calcium sulfate.
   3. Available studies suggest that regeneration efforts can be improved by the combined use of both barrier materials and bone replacement grafting.
E. Healing Following Guided Tissue Regeneration
   1. The healing expected from guided tissue regeneration is *regeneration* of part or all of the periodontium that was destroyed by periodontitis.
   2. As already mentioned, guided tissue regeneration requires the use of a barrier material.
      a. During surgery, a barrier material is placed under the flap to stop the rapidly growing epithelium from migrating along the root surface and interfering with the connective tissue regrowth on the root. (It is the connective tissue components from the periodontal ligament space that actually provide the cells needed to regrow cementum, periodontal ligament, and alveolar bone.)
      b. *It is important to remember that if a barrier material were not used, the epithelial tissue would regrow very rapidly, covering the tooth root and blocking access to the root by the slower growing connective tissue and undifferentiated cells. The epithelial growth covering the root blocks the connective tissue cells of the periodontal ligament from making contact with the root surface.*
F. Special Considerations for the Dental Hygienist
   1. During the GTR surgical procedure, every effort is made to close the wound to cover the barrier material completely.
      a. If exposure of part of the barrier material is noted at any of the postsurgical visits, measures should be instituted to minimize bacterial contamination of the barrier material.
      b. For example, a patient with exposed barrier materials may need special self-care instructions for the topical application of antimicrobial agents to the surgical site.

2. Sites treated by guided tissue regeneration should not be probed for several months following the procedures. The dental hygienist should consult with the dentist to determine when each individual site can be probed safely.

7. Periodontal Plastic Surgery
   A. Description
      1. **Periodontal plastic surgery** is the term most commonly used in modern dentistry to describe periodontal surgery that is directed toward correcting problems with attached gingiva, aberrant frenum, or vestibular depth.
      2. The term periodontal plastic surgery includes an array of periodontal surgical procedures that can be used to improve esthetics of the dentition and to enhance prosthetic dentistry as well as to deal with damage resulting from periodontitis.
      3. Some of these procedures include techniques that have been used in medical plastic surgery for many years. Periodontal plastic surgery can be used to alter the tissues surrounding both natural teeth and dental implants (36–41).
   B. Terminology Relating to Periodontal Plastic Surgery
      1. Readers of periodontal literature can sometimes be confused by the terminology associated with periodontal plastic surgery, since some other terms have also been used to describe procedures currently included under this term.
      2. The term **mucogingival surgery** has been used in the past to describe periodontal surgical procedures that alter the relationship between gingiva and mucosa. Some of the periodontal plastic surgical procedures utilized in modern dentistry were previously described as mucogingival surgical procedures, and this older terminology can still be encountered.
      3. Another term that has been used to describe some of these types of procedures is reconstructive surgery; the term reconstructive surgery underscores that the goal of some of these procedures is to reconstruct (or rebuild) periodontal tissues such as gingiva.
   C. Goals of Periodontal Plastic Surgery
      1. Many periodontal plastic surgical procedures are designed to alter components of the attached gingiva, and that type of procedure can dramatically alter the appearance of the tissues. Most patients want a pleasing smile, and because the gingiva is readily visible in many patients, patients frequently seek improvements in the appearance of the gingiva.
      2. In addition to altering the appearance of the tissues, some periodontal plastic surgical procedures improve function. Function can be compromised when lack of attached gingiva on a tooth limits the options for restoration of a tooth by contraindicating the intracrevicular placement of restoration margins.
      3. This chapter part includes an overview of some of the more common types of procedures included under the heading periodontal plastic surgery. Box 27-7 provides an overview of the types of procedures commonly included in periodontal plastic surgery.

Box 27-7. Overview of Procedures Commonly Included in Periodontal Plastic Surgery

- Free gingival graft
- Subepithelial connective tissue graft
- Laterally positioned flap
- Coronally positioned flap
- Semilunar flap
- Frenectomy
- Crown lengthening surgery

8. **Free Gingival Graft**
   A. **Description of a Free Gingival Graft**
      1. A **free gingival graft** is a type of periodontal plastic surgery that was one of the first procedures used to augment the width of attached gingiva.
      2. The free gingival graft requires harvesting a donor section of tissue, usually from the palate, so there are two intraoral wounds that are created during this surgery: the donor site and the recipient site.
         a. The donor tissue for a free gingival graft includes both the *surface epithelium and some of the underlying connective tissue.*
         b. Taking the tissue for a free gingival graft from a donor site leaves a wound that is an open connective tissue surface that must be allowed to heal by secondary intention, and healing of this donor wound can be troublesome for the patient.
      3. Figure 27-10 shows a free gingival graft sutured in place on the facial surface of a mandibular incisor tooth root.
      4. The free gingival graft has been used to provide root coverage in areas of gingival recession but augmentation of the width of attached gingiva can also be performed without the need for obtaining any root coverage.
      5. The free gingival graft is an example of an autograft, since the donor tissue is taken from the same individual that is to receive that donor tissue.
      6. One complicating factor for the free gingival graft that is used for root coverage is that the graft is completely severed from its blood supply and at least a portion of the graft is then placed over an avascular root surface; special care is required to encourage diffusion of nutrients to the graft to maintain its viability during the early stages of healing.

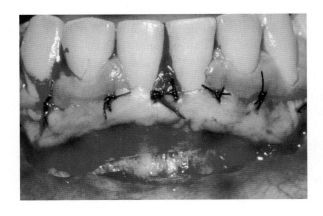

Figure 27-10. Free Gingival Graft Placed on Facial Surface of Tooth Root. The graft is placed over an area of root previously exposed by advanced gingival recession. Note the sutures that have been placed to immobilize the graft during healing.

   B. **Steps in a Typical Free Gingival Graft**
      1. The root surfaces in the area of gingival recession are planed to remove plaque, calculus, root contaminants, and root irregularities.
      2. Horizontal and vertical incisions are made at the recipient site after planning the precise location of the needed graft; surface epithelium is removed to prepare a firm connective tissue bed to receive the graft material.
      3. A template (frequently made from foil) is prepared to provide a pattern for the exact size and shape of the donor graft that will be needed.
      4. Using the template as a guide for the size and shape, the graft is obtained from the donor site (usually the palate) by incising through the epithelium and through a thin layer of connective tissue beneath the epithelium; the graft is removed from the site using sharp dissection.

5. The graft is sutured at the recipient site; during suturing, care is taken to prevent a blood clot from forming between the graft and the recipient vascular bed.

6. Both the donor site and recipient site are protected with periodontal dressing; in some instances the donor site on the palate is covered with a previously prepared acrylic retainer to hold the dressing over the donor site.

C. Healing Expected with a Typical Free Gingival Graft

1. Successful healing of a free gingival graft depends upon survival of the connective tissue part of the graft. In most instances, the epithelium sloughs off during the healing period, later to be replaced by new epithelium.

2. Survival of the tissues depends initially upon diffusion of nutrient-containing fluid from the vascular recipient tissues followed by growth of new blood vessels into the grafted material. Immobilization of the graft during the healing phase is a critical element in allowing the diffusion of nutrients, reconnection of existing blood vessels, and formation of new blood vessels.

3. Successful augmentation of gingiva as well as successful root coverage has been reported following the use of the free gingival graft.

4. Unfortunately, following complete healing of the free gingival graft, there is normally a less than ideal color match between the healed graft and the adjacent gingiva.

9. Subepithelial Connective Tissue Graft

A. Description of Subepithelial connective tissue graft

1. The subepithelial connective tissue graft is a periodontal plastic surgical procedure that can also be used to augment the width of attached gingiva and to cover areas of gingival recession.

2. In addition to gingival augmentation, the subepithelial connective tissue graft is used to alter the contour of alveolar ridges to improve the esthetics of some types of dental prostheses.

3. This procedure uses an autograft of connective tissue (without epithelium) that can be harvested from a variety of intraoral sites, but that is usually taken from the patient's **palate**.

B. Typical steps in a Subepithelial Connective Tissue Graft

1. A partial-thickness flap is elevated at the recipient site using sharp dissection; the flap normally extends one-half to one tooth to the mesial and distal of the site of recession to be covered.

2. The exposed tooth root is thoroughly planed to remove plaque, calculus, root contaminants, and root irregularities.

3. The connective tissue graft is obtained by incising through the epithelium of the palate and lifting a segment of connective tissue from beneath the epithelium using sharp dissection. The surface tissues at the donor site can then be sutured to allow for healing by primary intention.

4. The graft tissue is placed over the denuded tooth root and under the partial-thickness flap at the recipient site.

5. The outer portion of the partial-thickness flap is placed over the graft and sutured into place, making sure that at least half of the graft is covered by the outer portion of the flap.

6. Periodontal dressing is placed to protect the grafted site; since the donor site will heal by primary intention, normally no dressing is needed at the donor site.

C. Healing Expected After a Subepithelial Connective Tissue Graft

1. When root coverage is attempted with the subepithelial connective tissue graft, it is reasonable to expect coverage, though not all sites result in complete root coverage.

2. The subepithelial connective tissue graft results in excellent esthetics, since the color of the healed tissues often mimics the natural pre-existing tissue color precisely.

D. Acellular Dermal Matrix Allograft

1. As a substitute for autogenous connective tissue, an acellular dermal matrix allograft material is now available.

2. Following harvesting, the allograft is treated to remove cellular components, but it retains blood vessel channels, collagen, elastin, and proteoglycans.

3. This dermal matrix allograft material can be used in some periodontal surgical procedures in place of autogenous connective tissue, but when used it must be completely covered by a partial-thickness flap.

10. Laterally Positioned Flap

A. Description of a Laterally Positioned Flap

1. The laterally positioned flap is a periodontal plastic surgery technique that can be used to cover root surfaces with gingiva in isolated sites of gingival recession.

2. The laterally positioned flap involves a displaced flap (displaced laterally in this case).

3. Use of this technique requires an adequate donor tissue (gingiva) on a tooth root adjacent to the site of recession.

4. Since the gingiva to be displaced laterally will be taken from an adjacent tooth, the site of the donor tissue must have thick, healthy covering of gingiva to allow the donor tissue to be taken without resulting in harm to the donor site.

B. Steps in a Typical Laterally Positioned Flap

1. The recipient site is prepared by thoroughly planing the exposed tooth root and by removing epithelium from the surface of the gingiva surrounding the area of recession, thus exposing some connective tissue to serve as a vascular recipient bed for the displaced flap.

2. A partial-thickness flap is elevated from the donor site using a series of carefully planned vertical incisions to provide mobility in the flap after elevation.

3. The elevated flap is rotated laterally so as to cover the recipient site including both the prepared bed of connective tissue and the prepared tooth root.

4. The flap is stabilized at its new location using a combination of interrupted sutures and sling sutures.

5. The surgical site is covered with aluminum foil and periodontal dressing to protect the healing wound.

C. Healing Expected After a Laterally Positioned Flap

1. With careful selection of donor sites and skillful manipulation of the tissues, little recession will occur on the donor site.

2. The laterally positioned flap can result in excellent root coverage in many instances, since the flap maintains part of its own blood supply (unlike the free gingival graft, which is completely severed from its blood supply).

11. Coronally Positioned Flap

A. Description of a Coronally Positioned Flap

1. The coronally positioned flap is a periodontal plastic surgical procedure that can be used to repair gingival recession if the recession is not advanced.

2. As the name implies the coronally positioned flap is a displaced flap (displaced in a coronal direction in this case).

3. One advantage to this procedure compared to a free gingival graft or a subepithelial connective tissue graft is that it does not require a second surgical site to provide the donor tissue.

4. One disadvantage to this procedure is that it can be difficult to stabilize the flap with sutures at a more coronal position.

5. In some instances the coronally positioned flap requires a two-stage procedure.

   a. If the thickness of the gingiva at the proposed donor site is inadequate, gingiva must be augmented at the donor site with a surgical procedure prior to advancement of the coronally positioned flap.

   b. When indicated, this gingival augmentation may be accomplished with a free gingival graft prior to the coronal positioning.

B. **Steps in a Typical Coronally Positioned Flap**

   1. Exposed tooth roots are planed to remove plaque, calculus, root contaminants, and root irregularities.

   2. Internal bevel and vertical releasing incisions are made at the site to be coronally positioned; the vertical releasing incisions extend into the alveolar mucosa to allow for mobility of the flap margin in a coronal direction.

   3. Surface epithelium is removed from the site to create a vascular recipient bed.

   4. The flap is elevated; the elevation can be full thickness or split thickness or a combination of the two depending upon the overall thickness of the tissues being elevated.

   5. The flap is advanced in a coronal direction and sutured using a combination of interrupted and sling sutures.

   6. Periodontal dressing is placed to prevent movement of the flap during healing.

C. **Healing Expected with a Typical Coronally Positioned Flap.** The coronally positioned flap can be used successfully to cover areas of gingival recession when the gingival recession is not advanced.

12. **Semilunar Flap**

A. **Description of a Semilunar Flap.** The semilunar flap is a periodontal plastic surgical procedure that can be used to cover gingival recession where the recession is not far advanced and where the keratinized tissues have an adequate thickness. The semilunar flap is a variation of a coronally positioned flap.

B. **Steps in a Typical Semilunar Flap**

   1. The level of the alveolar bone is sounded (located) to insure that coronal positioning of the semilunar flap does not inadvertently expose alveolar bone at the base of the flap.

   2. A semilunar, curved incision is made from one interdental area to the adjacent interdental area over the tooth root.

   a. The interdental sites for the incisions are selected to be slightly coronal to the position anticipated for the flap advancement.

   b. This incision begins in the gingiva and arcs into the mucosa and then back into the gingiva.

   3. A split-thickness flap is performed using sharp dissection to free the surface of the flap from the underlying connective tissue.

   4. The semilunar flap is displaced coronally and stabilized with gentle pressure for several minutes; if needed, the flap can be stabilized with interrupted sutures, but sometimes suturing is not required.

13. Frenectomy
    A. Description of a Frenectomy
       1. Frenectomy is a periodontal plastic surgical procedure that results in removal of a frenum, including removal of the attachment of the frenum to bone.
          a. Some authors use the term frenotomy to indicate a variation of the frenectomy.
          b. The frenotomy includes only incision of the frenum but does not remove the attachment of the frenum from the bone surface.
       2. If a frenum is attached too close to the gingival margin, it can result in repeated pulling of the gingival margin away from the tooth surface and can contribute to persistent inflammation in the tissues; in addition, a frenum too close to the gingival margin can interfere with daily self-care.
          a. An aberrant frenum position that requires a frenectomy occurs most often in the frenum between the maxillary central incisors and mandibular central incisors.
          b. An aberrant frenum position can also occur in other locations such as on the facial surface of premolar and canine teeth and on the lingual surface of the mandibular central incisors.
    B. Steps in a Typical Frenectomy
       1. The frenum is grasped with a hemostat placed to the depth of the vestibule.
       2. Incisions are made through the tissues on both the under surface and the upper surface of the beaks of the hemostat.
       3. The triangular piece of tissue held by the hemostat is removed exposing connective tissue over the surface of the bone.
       4. The connective tissue covering the bone is incised and dissected.
       5. Periodontal dressing is applied to the wound.
    C. Alternative Techniques for the Frenectomy
       1. Frequently the frenectomy is performed in conjunction with other types of periodontal surgery, and a variety of techniques have been described.
       2. Other techniques for performing a frenectomy include removing the tissue of the frenum with electrosurgery or with a laser.
    D. Healing Following a Frenectomy. Expected healing following a frenectomy is elimination of the gingival margin movement caused by the frenum.
14. Crown Lengthening Surgery
    A. Description of Procedure. Crown lengthening surgery refers to periodontal plastic surgery designed to create a longer clinical crown for a tooth by removing some of the gingiva and usually by removing some alveolar bone from the necks of the teeth (42).
    B. Terminology. Two terms frequently used when describing crown lengthening surgery are functional crown lengthening and esthetic crown lengthening
       1. Functional crown lengthening refers to crown lengthening performed on a tooth where the remaining tooth structure is inadequate to support a needed restoration.
          a. Functional crown lengthening surgery can be used to make a restorative dental procedure (such as a crown) possible when the only sensible alternative might be to remove the tooth.
          b. Crown lengthening surgery may be necessary when a tooth is decayed or broken below the gingival margin.
             1. When a badly damaged tooth is to be restored, the dentist will evaluate the tooth and surrounding tissues to determine if the final restoration of the tooth will damage the soft tissue attachment (i.e., encroach upon the biologic width).
             2. If such damage can be expected, crown lengthening surgery is usually indicated prior to the placement of the final restoration.

2. **Esthetic crown lengthening** refers to crown lengthening performed on teeth to improve the appearance of the teeth where there is excessive gingiva or a "gummy smile" as it is sometimes called.
   a. Crown lengthening surgery can be used to improve the esthetics of the gingiva, especially on anterior teeth with short clinical crowns.
      1. An individual's smile may be unattractive because of the height or lack of symmetry of the gingiva surrounding the teeth.
      2. In some cases tooth crowns are actually the correct length, but they appear too short in the mouth because there is an excess of gingival tissue covering the teeth.
   b. During esthetic crown lengthening, the gingival tissues are incised and reshaped to expose more of the natural crown of the tooth; frequently some of the alveolar bone must also be removed to insure healing of the tissues at a more apical position.
C. **Surgical Procedure.** The actual surgical procedure followed during crown lengthening surgery usually involves an apically positioned flap (displaced flap) with osseous resective surgery much like that already discussed.
   1. Unlike the typical apically positioned flap with osseous surgery, crown lengthening surgery may be indicated in the presence of a perfectly healthy periodontium simply to allow for improved esthetics or to allow for exposure of more tooth structure prior to restoration.
   2. Also, unlike the typical apically positioned flap with osseous surgery, esthetic crown lengthening frequently requires the use of a template prepared to guide the surgeon in positioning the tissues during the surgery.
   3. Occasionally, esthetic crown lengthening may require only a gingivectomy type procedure to be discussed later in this chapter, but most often, esthetic crown lengthening requires some alveolar bone removal, so an apically positioned flap with osseous surgery is most often indicated instead of a gingivectomy.
D. **Healing After Crown Lengthening Surgery**
   1. Healing of crown lengthening surgery is similar to that described for the apically positioned flap with osseous surgery.
   2. Final healing of crown lengthening surgery results in a normal attachment (both junctional epithelium and connective tissue attachment) at a position more apical on the tooth root.
E. **Special Considerations for the Dental Hygienist**
   1. Since crown lengthening surgery usually involves exposure of additional tooth surface to the oral environment, temporary dentinal hypersensitivity is also a common result of this type of periodontal surgery; it is imperative for the dental team to warn patients in advance that they may experience temporary dentinal hypersensitivity following crown lengthening surgery.
   2. As already discussed, when dentinal hypersensitivity results, the dental hygienist may need to institute measures to help the patient deal with the sensitivity.
   3. Control of dentinal hypersensitivity requires meticulous plaque control during the healing phase, and this can be a problem, since mechanical plaque control must be restricted following most surgical procedures.
   4. It is the responsibility of the members of the dental team to aid the patient in plaque control until healing allows the patient to resume routine self-care.

15. Gingivectomy
    A. Description of a Gingivectomy
        1. The **gingivectomy** is a surgical procedure designed to excise and remove some of the gingival tissue. Historically, the gingivectomy was used for many years in periodontics as a primary treatment modality, but it plays a greatly reduced role in modern dentistry.
        2. When a gingivectomy is performed, the tissues are excised (cut away), removing some of the gingiva that would normally be attached to the tooth surface, thus the gingivectomy is a resective procedure.
        3. The gingivectomy results in a more apical position of the marginal gingiva in relationship to the CEJ of the tooth.
        4. Terminology related to gingivectomy can be confusing because of the overlapping use of two terms: gingivectomy and gingivoplasty.
            a. In contrast to the gingivectomy described above, **gingivoplasty** is a term used to describe a surgical procedure that simply reshapes the surface of the gingiva to create a natural form and contour to the gingiva.
            b. Unlike the gingivectomy, gingivoplasty implies reshaping the surface of the gingiva without removing any of the gingiva actually attached to the tooth surface.
            c. In reality, during almost all gingivectomy type procedures, a certain amount of gingivoplasty is also performed, so the precise distinction between these two companion terms can be a bit cloudy.
        5. There is still a limited place in modern dentistry for the gingivectomy procedure.
            a. Periodontal diseases can produce deformities of the gingiva including conditions such as gingival enlargements, gingival craters, and gingival clefts.
            b. Occasionally, even in the absence of periodontal pockets, these deformities occur and need to be altered to allow for improved esthetics, improved mastication, or enhanced ease of patient self-care.
        6. Figure 27-11 illustrates the types of incisions involved when performing a gingivectomy.

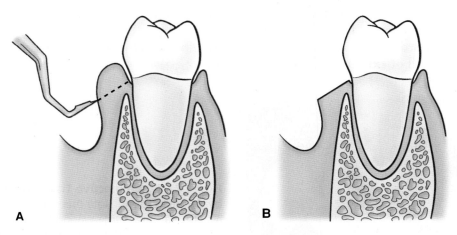

A   B

Figure 27-11. Gingivectomy Incisions. **A:** The placement of a special gingivectomy knife to incise the excess gingival tissue. Note that the direction of the tissue bevel being created is approximately 45 degrees to the tooth surface. **B:** The excess tissue has been excised and removed creating a more natural level and contour of the gingiva on the tooth surface.

B. **Disadvantages of Gingivectomy**
1. In modern periodontal therapy, the gingivectomy is usually limited to removing enlarged gingiva to improve esthetics or to allow for better access for self-care in isolated sites.
2. Though gingivectomy can be used to reshape more extensive areas of enlarged gingiva as might be seen in gingival overgrowth in response to certain medication use, periodontal surgeons have other more effective surgical options today.
3. As a surgical technique, gingivectomy has several *disadvantages*:
   a. One disadvantage to gingivectomy is that it leaves a large open connective tissue wound that results in a somewhat slower surface healing than most other periodontal surgical procedures; this generally results in the expectation of more discomfort for the patient during the healing phase.
   b. Figure 27-12 illustrates the type of connective tissue wound that occurs following a gingivectomy.
   c. Another disadvantage of gingivectomy is that following healing it invariably results in a longer appearing tooth because of the excision of some of the gingiva.
   d. A third disadvantage to the gingivectomy is that it does not provide access to the underlying alveolar bone, so when access to the alveolar bone is needed, the surgeon must select another type of surgical approach.
   e. A fourth disadvantage to the gingivectomy is that it does not conserve keratinized tissue (gingiva); in many surgical sites it is unwise to remove keratinized tissue, since it may already be minimal in width.
   f. In spite of these disadvantages, the gingivectomy can be a useful surgical procedure in selected sites.

C. **Steps in Performing a Typical Gingivectomy**
1. Existing periodontal pockets are explored and the levels of the bases of the pockets are marked on the surface of the gingiva by punching a hole through the surface of the gingiva.
2. Using special gingivectomy knives (both broad bladed and narrow bladed), gingiva is excised at the levels of the bases of the pockets.
3. As the incision is made, care is taken to produce a 45-degree bevel of the gingiva against the tooth to mimic the natural contour of the surface of the gingiva in relationship to the tooth.
4. The excised portion of the gingiva is removed (which also removes the soft tissue wall of existing periodontal pockets).

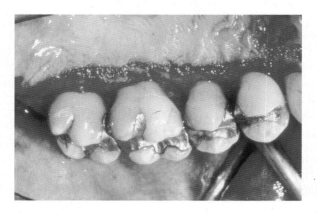

Figure 27-12. Connective Tissue Wound Created by Gingivectomy. Note that the gingivectomy results in a rather large wound that exposes connective tissue. This large wound usually results in protracted healing, since the healing requires that the epithelium grows across the wound created by the gingivectomy.

5. The wound surface is inspected, remaining tissue tags are removed and gingival contours are refined as needed.

6. The tooth surfaces are inspected and debrided to remove plaque, calculus, root contaminants, and root irregularities.

7. The surgical wound is covered with periodontal dressing.

D. Healing Expected After a Gingivectomy

1. Healing of the gingivectomy requires healing by secondary intention, since the gingivectomy incisions invariably leave an exposed connective tissue surface.

2. The approximate rate that gingiva grows across a connective tissue wound in the oral cavity is 0.5 mm each day; since the gingivectomy normally leaves many millimeters of connective tissue exposed, the healing time can be protracted.

3. The final healing of the wound created by a gingivectomy is a normal attachment of the epithelium and connective tissues to the tooth root at a level that is more apical in position than the original gingival level.

4. Following a gingivectomy, the teeth in the surgical area will appear to be longer since more of the root is exposed where the tissue was excised.

   a. Of course, if more tooth exposure is the desired result of the procedure, this procedure can result in an acceptable outcome.

   b. However, if the exposure of more root structure is not esthetically desirable in a particular site in the oral cavity, another surgical approach would be selected by the surgeon.

E. Special Considerations for the Dental Hygienist

1. As already mentioned, the gingivectomy wound leaves a broad connective tissue surface exposed that can be very uncomfortable for the patient during the healing phase.

2. Postsurgical discomfort can be managed by placing a periodontal dressing over the wound to provide protection and by prescribing analgesics (pain medications) for use following surgery.

3. At the time of the dressing removal at the first postsurgical visit following a gingivectomy, the dental hygienist will frequently need to replace the periodontal dressing to enhance wound comfort until total epithelialization of the wound has occurred.

4. Healing of the wound created by a gingivectomy procedure progresses in a predictable manner.

   a. As already discussed, research studies have shown that oral epithelium grows across the exposed connective tissue at an approximate rate of 0.5 mm per day.

   b. Thus, it is possible for the clinical team to predict approximate healing times by estimating the wound size; this of course is useful when counseling patients about what to expect during the postsurgical phase.

16. Gingival Curettage

A. Procedure Description

1. **Gingival curettage** is an older type of periodontal surgical procedure that involves an attempt to scrape away the lining of the periodontal pocket usually using a periodontal curet, often a Gracey curet.

   a. During periodontal instrumentation, some unintentional curettage of the gingiva always occurs, but the term gingival curettage refers to a separate surgical procedure performed after routine periodontal instrumentation has removed most of the plaque, calculus, and root contaminants.

    b. Research has demonstrated that normally the same benefits from gingival curettage can be derived from thorough periodontal instrumentation by the clinician plus meticulous self-care by the patient. Thus, curettage is rarely needed as a separate periodontal surgical procedure in modern dentistry.

  2. Variations of the gingival curettage. Although the gingival curettage is no longer routinely recommended as a separate periodontal surgical procedure, some clinicians have advocated variations on this technique.

    a. One variation is performing gingival curettage with caustic chemicals.

      1. Examples of some chemicals that have been used for a chemical curettage include sodium hypochlorite and phenol.

      2. The extent of tissue destruction that follows the use of caustic chemicals cannot be controlled, and studies have failed to show any efficacy for this type of curettage.

    b. Another variation is performing gingival curettage with ultrasonic devices.

      1. In this technique, ultrasound is used to debride the epithelial lining of periodontal pockets.

      2. Some authors have found the use of ultrasound as effective as manual curets in removing the pocket linings, but since the fundamental premise for gingival curettage is not sound, this technique is not advocated today either.

    c. A third variation of the gingival curettage is the excisional new attachment procedure (known as ENAP).

      1. The excisional new attachment procedure was developed as a definitive curettage performed with a surgical scalpel.

      2. During an ENAP, a surgical scalpel is used to incise away the lining of a periodontal pocket, including the linings of interproximal pockets.

      3. Sutures are placed only if the tissues do not rest against the necks of the teeth passively.

B. Indications for Gingival Curettage in Modern Dentistry

  1. Studies have shown that healing of soft tissues following periodontal instrumentation is not normally improved by subsequent gingival curettage, so the indications for this procedure today are quite limited.

  2. Though gingival curettage is not normally recommended as part of modern periodontal therapy, a few indications for this procedure still exist; these indications include the following:

    a. Gingival curettage can be performed in lieu of more definitive types of surgery when the more definitive procedures are contraindicated because of health concerns in the patient.

    b. Gingival curettage can be performed during periodontal maintenance in sites of persistent inflammation where definitive periodontal surgery has already been performed.

C. Steps in a Typical Gingival Curettage

  1. Curets are used to scrape away the lining of the soft tissue wall of the periodontal pockets.

  2. Care is taken to place the cutting edge of the curet in direct contact with the soft tissue rather than away from the soft tissue as might be done during routine periodontal instrumentation.

3. A horizontal stroke with the curet is used to engage the lining of the pocket.
4. Light finger pressure can be used against the surface of the gingiva to stabilize the tissue during the scraping motion.

D. Healing Following Gingival Curettage

1. Healing expected following gingival curettage would be healing by repair and the formation of a long junctional epithelium.
2. This is the same type of healing you would expect following thorough periodontal instrumentation.
3. Figure 27-13 illustrates the type of healing that would be expected following a gingival curettage.

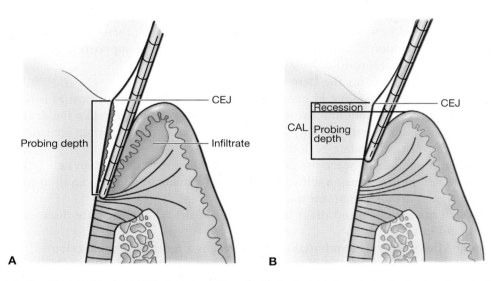

Figure 27-13. Healing Following Gingival Curettage. A: Periodontal pocket prior to treatment showing inflammation and calculus on the roots. **B:** Healing following gingival curettage and root instrumentation. Healing includes resolution of inflammation and readaptation of some junctional epithelium.

17. **Dental Implant Placement.** Dental implants are discussed in Chapter 31, but they are briefly mentioned in this section to underscore that the placement of dental implants can utilize many periodontal surgical techniques. The planning and surgical placement of dental implants is quite complex and the interested reader is directed toward the many excellent textbooks devoted to that topic. In addition to the surgery involved in placing dental implants, periodontal surgical procedures can help prepare sites for the placement of dental implants.

A. Description of Dental Implant Placement

1. As discussed in Chapter 31, a dental implant is an artificial tooth root that is placed into the alveolar bone to hold a replacement crown or prosthesis (denture or bridge).
2. Most dental implants in current use are endosseous implants that are placed in alveolar bone and protrude through the mucoperiosteum.
   a. Dental implant placement usually requires exposure of alveolar bone using the principles of periodontal flap surgery, drilling a precise hole in the alveolar bone, insertion of a metallic implant into the site, and suturing of the wound created.
   b. There are a variety of dental implants in current use including various lengths, diameters, and designs; most types of dental implants have threads much like a screw has threads.

3. Some dental implants are designed to be covered with gingiva during healing, and others are designed to leave a portion of the implant exposed in the oral cavity during healing. Those that are covered require a second surgical procedure following healing to expose the top of the implant.

4. When preparing a site to receive a dental implant and during dental implant placement any of the periodontal surgical procedures already discussed may be employed.

B. **Healing Expected Following Dental Implant Placement**

1. Healing following placement of a dental implant results in bone growth in such close proximity to the implant surface that the implant is stable enough to support a tooth-shaped restoration or a dental prosthetic appliance.

2. It should be noted that though dental implants are not surrounded by cementum and periodontal ligament (as are natural teeth), these implants are subject to periodontal disease that can result in the loss of supporting bone just like the natural tooth.

C. **Special Considerations for the Dental Hygienist**

1. Patient self-care following placement of a dental implant is as critical as it is following every periodontal surgical procedure, and the members of the dental team must assume responsibility for helping the patient with plaque control during the critical healing period.

2. Once an implant site heals, the gingiva surrounding the implant can be maintained in health using self-care techniques similar to what is required to keep tissues around a natural tooth healthy.

3. Implant maintenance and the role played by the dental hygienist are discussed in detail in Chapter 31.

18. **Periodontal Microsurgery. Periodontal microsurgery** is a term used to describe periodontal surgery performed with the aid of a surgical microscope. Principles of microsurgery have had a good deal of influence in medicine and will continue to influence the performance of certain periodontal surgical procedures, especially periodontal plastic surgery. Periodontal surgery performed using microsurgery techniques can result in procedures performed with increased precision on the part of the surgeon.

19. **Laser Therapy.** The use of lasers (light amplification by stimulated emission of radiation) to focus a beam of light of a single wavelength at periodontal site has become an important topic in dentistry and periodontics.

A. There is much debate related to some aspects of this topic among clinicians and scientists (43–50). Lasers can cut or coagulate soft tissues with efficiency, and this fact makes the use of lasers during some surgical procedures such as gingivectomy, gingivoplasty, biopsy of soft tissues, ablation of lesions, vestibuloplasty, and frenectomies useful adjuncts.

B. However, in periodontal patients lasers have also been used to remove pocket epithelium and decontaminate periodontal pockets in an effort to attain improved attachment levels, but the precise efficacy of these types of therapies in periodontitis patients is not clear at this point.

C. Current statements by the American Academy of Periodontology and the American Dental Association caution that there is insufficient evidence to support the use of lasers as a single form of treatment in periodontitis patients at this time (51,52). Studies that may clarify the efficacy of this type of treatment will continue to be published.

Section 4
Biological Enhancement of Surgical Outcomes

Many attempts have been made to enhance the outcomes of periodontal surgery by using chemical or biologic mediators to influence the healing following periodontal surgical procedures. This chapter section provides a brief overview of some of the biologic mediators that have been studied. There is much ongoing research into this topic, and it is reasonable to expect that this ongoing research will reveal fundamental mechanisms for enhancing periodontal surgical outcomes that will prove useful in a clinical setting.

1. Root Surface Modification
   A. Mechanical Root Preparation
      1. Many years of observation of the healing of periodontal surgical wounds demonstrate that gingival tissues adjacent to tooth roots—that have previously been exposed because of attachment loss—heal better when the roots are free of plaque, calculus, and root contaminants.
      2. These observations have lead to the incorporation of mechanical root preparation as a routine part of most periodontal surgical procedures. Hand and ultrasonic instruments have been used extensively for this purpose.
   B. Chemical and Biologic Mediators. Chemical and biologic mediators also have been used in attempts to enhance the healing of the gingiva adjacent to the tooth roots beyond what can be achieved by periodontal instrumentation alone. Several chemical mediators have been studied for possible benefits to the gingival healing process (53,54).
      1. EDTA (ethylenediamine tetraacetic acid) has been used to decalcify the surface of the root following mechanical root preparation.
         a. Possible benefits of using EDTA on roots include removal of the dentin smear layer, exposure of ends of embedded collagen fibers in remaining cemental surface, and removal of endotoxin buried deeper below the root surface.
         b. Though some clinicians have used this chemical to enhance root preparation, most of the evidence indicates that there is very little positive effect on the outcomes of any surgery by the use of this chemical to prepare tooth roots.
      2. A second chemical agent that has been referred to as a biologic mediator, again to enhance the outcomes of periodontal root preparation, is tetracycline.
         a. Tetracyclines are a family of antibiotics with varied properties in addition to their antibiotic effects. It has been suggested that tetracyclines applied to roots during surgery may enhance the migration of fibroblasts to the root surfaces during healing in addition to slightly decalcifying the surfaces of the roots.
         b. Most studies indicate that using this biologic mediator on root surfaces during surgery has little effect on the outcomes of the surgical procedures.
2. Growth Factors. Growth factors are naturally occurring proteins that regulate both cell growth and development. Several growth factors are being studied for their effect in enhancing the predictability of periodontal regeneration and studies of these potential biologic mediators are continuing (27,55). These growth factors include PDGF (platelet-derived growth factor) and IGF (insulin-derived growth factor). It is reasonable to expect that continued research into the use of growth factors to improve periodontal surgical outcomes might lead to clinical application of some of these factors in the future.

3. **Enamel Matrix Derivative (EMD)**
   A. **Periodontal Regeneration Factors**
      1. It is clear that periodontal regeneration depends upon the type of cells that first populate the periodontal surgical wound.
      2. As already discussed, using barrier materials to insure that the correct cells enter the healing surgical wound without the early interference of epithelium can result in more predictable periodontal regeneration. The use of barriers to insure periodontal regeneration, however, has not been very successful in all sites of more advanced osseous defects.
   B. **Protein Preparations.** Research into using protein preparations and growth factors to enhance periodontal regeneration by mimicking natural healing processes has shown some promising results.
      1. Enamel matrix derivative (EMD) has been used to enhance periodontal regeneration.
      2. Enamel matrix derivative (EMD) is a preparation of proteins extracted from porcine tooth buds; EMD is the tooth bud extract mixed with a propylene glycol alginate carrier (56–60).
      3. The major constituents of this extract appear to be proteins called amelogenins and enamelin.
      4. At this point it appears that EMD may indeed enhance periodontal regeneration and that the safety of this material is quite high when used in conjunction with periodontal surgery.
      5. EMD is currently being used by clinicians in an attempt to improve outcomes of some types of periodontal surgery.
      6. Studies into the precise constituents in this protein extract that can enhance healing are continuing.

4. **Platelet-Rich Plasma (PRP).** Another example of a biologic mediator is platelet-rich plasma (PRP). Using platelet-rich plasma requires obtaining a sample of the patient's blood and separating the blood sample into three separate fractions: platelet-rich plasma (PRP), red blood cells, and platelet poor plasma. The PRP fraction of blood contains high numbers of platelets plus PDGF (platelet-derived growth factor), TGF-β (transforming growth factor-beta), and fibrinogen. Clinically both calcium and thrombin are added to the PRP to activate the production of fibrin before the preparation is applied in the surgical site. Though some studies indicate some enhancement of the healing process following the use of this preparation, it is not clear that the growth factors are present in high enough concentrations to have much effect on the actual surgical outcomes, and additional studies of this material are underway (61,62).

5. **Bone Morphogenetic Proteins (BMP).** Bone morphogenetic proteins (BMPs) are a group of regulatory glycoproteins that have been studied for possible use in the field of periodontal regeneration because of their known osteoinductive effects. Both purified and recombinant BMPs are currently being studied, and early results indicate possible enhancement of regeneration in some treated sites. Unfortunately using BMP to enhance surgical outcomes has resulted in tooth ankylosis and much further study of this material is indicated. Investigations into the use of bone morphogenetic proteins to enhance periodontal regeneration are continuing.

Section 5
Patient Management Following Periodontal Surgery

The dental hygienist plays a major role in supporting the management of patients following periodontal surgery. This chapter section discusses components of postsurgical management including use of sutures, use of periodontal dressings, delivery of postsurgical instructions, and organizing postsurgical visits. It is important to realize that the management of the patient during the healing phase following periodontal surgery can be as important to the surgical outcomes as the skill of the surgeon performing the surgery.

USE OF SUTURES IN PERIODONTAL SURGICAL WOUNDS

1. Overview of the Use of Sutures in Periodontal Wounds. Many periodontal surgical procedures such as periodontal flaps require the placement of sutures to stabilize the position of the soft tissues during the early phases of healing; a suture, or stitch as it is sometimes called, is a device placed by a surgeon to hold tissues together during healing.
   A. Characteristics of Suture Material
      1. To be useful in periodontal wounds suture materials need to be nontoxic, flexible, and strong.
      2. Some suture materials have been reported to have a "wicking" effect (i.e., they can allow bacteria to travel down the suture and contaminate the surgical wound); this wicking effect is believed to have a negative effect on the surgical outcomes.
      3. When placing sutures, periodontal surgeons take great care not to put tension on a flap with sutures (i.e., to insure that the flap lies passively at the intended position before suturing); sutures are used to stabilize the flap in its passive position.
      4. If a suture places tension on a flap, the suture material will pull out of the tissues during healing and will fail to serve the purpose of stabilizing the tissues.
   B. Types of Suture Material. In general two types of suture material are used: nonabsorbable and absorbable. Box 27-8 provides an overview of some of the suture materials available for use in periodontal wounds.
      1. Nonabsorbable suture is a suture made from a material that does not dissolve in body fluids. A clinician must remove the nonabsorbable sutures after some healing of the wound has occurred.
      2. Absorbable suture is a suture made from a material designed to dissolve harmlessly in body fluids over time; though absorbable sutures do not normally require removal by the dental team, some absorbable sutures do not dissolve particularly well in saliva.

Box 27-8. Examples of Suture Materials

Nonabsorbable:
- Braided silk
- Monofilament nylon
- Expanded polytetrafluoroethylene (ePTFE)
- Braided polyester

Absorbable:
- Plain and chromic gut
- Polyglactin 910
- Polyglecaprone 25

Box 27-9. Overview of General Indications for Common Suture Techniques

1. Interrupted suture: closure of vertical incisions, closure of nondisplaced flaps
2. Sling suture: closure of displaced flaps
3. Continuous sling suture: closure of displaced flaps, closure of nondisplaced flaps

2. **Suture Placement Techniques.** Familiarity with some general techniques for suturing can guide the hygienist assigned the task of suture removal at a postsurgical appointment. Box 27-9 provides an overview of general indications for some of the more common suturing techniques for periodontal surgical wounds. Three of the most common suture placement techniques are discussed and illustrated below.

A. **Interrupted Interdental Suture**
   1. During most periodontal flap surgery, flaps are elevated on both the facial and lingual (or palatal) surfaces of the teeth; an interrupted interdental suture usually involves suturing the facial and lingual papillae together, but this technique is also ideal for closing vertical incisions.
   2. When interrupted interdental sutures are placed to close a periodontal flap procedure, a separate suture is placed and tied in each of the interdental sites.
   3. An interrupted interdental suture that might be utilized during a periodontal flap for access procedure is illustrated in Figures 27-14 and 27-15.
   4. When removing interrupted interdental sutures, the clinician must cut each of the interdental sutures before pulling out the suture material.

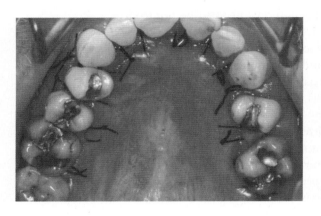

Figure 27-14. Interrupted Interdental Sutures. Interrupted interdental sutures have been placed in each interdental site on the maxillary arch. Note that there is a knot associated with each of these interrupted sutures that would need to be cut prior to removal. (Courtesy of Dr. John S. Dozier, Tallahassee, FL.)

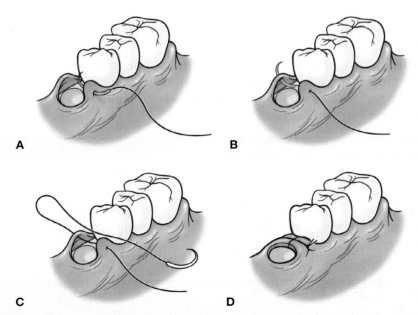

Figure 27-15. Interrupted Interdental Suture. In these drawings the most mesial tooth has been removed to allow for visualization of the path of the interrupted interdental suture. **A:** Suture placed through papilla on the facial. **B:** Suture placed through the papilla on the lingual. **C:** Suture returned to facial surface. **D:** Knot tied in suture on the facial.

B. **Continuous Loop Suture**
1. The continuous loop suture is preferred by many clinicians for suturing many types of periodontal flaps.
2. When continuous loop sutures are used, following placing the suture material through two interdental papillae, the end of the suture is looped around the teeth to reach the next interdental site rather than being tied at each interdental site; the suture is tied following placement of the loop around the terminal tooth.
3. A continuous loop suture that might be utilized during an apically positioned flap is illustrated in Figures 27-16 and 27-17.
4. Removal of a continuous loop suture can frequently be accomplished with a single cut through the suture near the knot before pulling out the suture material.

C. **Sling Suture**
1. Some periodontal surgical wounds require the placement of a sling suture; the sling suture is used to sling or suspend the tissues around the cervical area of a tooth rather than to tie soft tissue to other soft tissue.
2. The sling suture is frequently used when a flap is displaced in an apical direction. Figure 27-18 illustrates a sling suture.
3. It should be noted that when facial and lingual flaps are sutured using the sling suture technique, a separate sling suture must be placed on both the facial and lingual surfaces.
4. Removal of the sling suture only requires locating the individual knots, cutting the suture near the knot, and careful extraction of the suture.

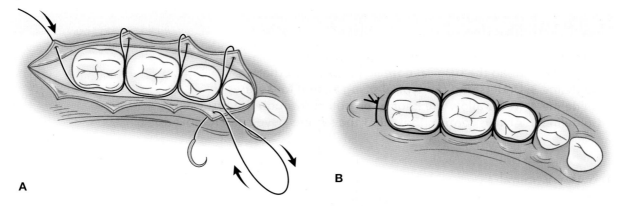

A   **B**

Figure 27-16. Continuous Loop Suture. Note that the suture is looped around each of the cervical areas of the teeth and passed through the tissues associated with each interdental area **(A)**, but that it is tied only at the end of the continuous loop **(B)**.

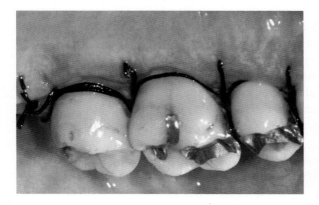

Figure 27-17. Continuous Loop Suture.
Continuous loop suture has been placed on the segment of teeth in maxillary arch. Note that the only knot visible is associated with the most distal tooth. (Courtesy of Dr. Don Rolfs, Periodontal Foundations, Wenatchee, WA.)

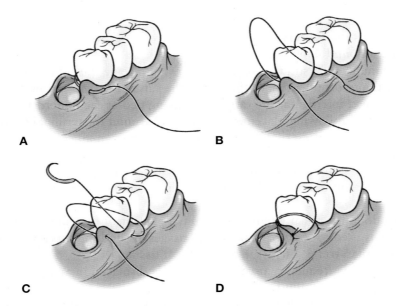

Figure 27-18. Sling Suture. In these drawings the most mesial tooth has been removed to allow for visualization of the path of the sling suture. **A:** Suture placed through the facial papilla. **B:** Suture looped around the lingual surface of the tooth without engaging the lingual soft tissues. **C:** Suture continues back to the facial surface under the contact and engages the facial papilla on the distal of the tooth. **D:** Suture continues back on same path and is tied on the surface where it first penetrated the facial papilla.

Box 27-10. General Guidelines for Suture Removal

Guideline 1: Remove sutures in a timely manner.
Guideline 2: Read the surgical note in the patient's chart.
Guideline 3: Understand the typical sizing system for sutures.
Guideline 4: Never allow the knot to be pulled through the tissues.
Guideline 5: Always confirm that all of the sutures have been removed.

---

3. Suture Removal
   A. Removal of Nonabsorbable Sutures
      1. Nonabsorbable sutures placed during surgical procedures are removed as part of routine postsurgical visits. Frequently remnants of absorbable sutures can also be removed at the routine postsurgical visits to avoid unnecessary tissue inflammation that can be caused by retained absorbable suture material that does not dissolve in a timely manner.
      2. Guidelines for timing of removal vary, but in general, sutures should be removed when wound healing has progressed to the point at which the sutures are no longer needed to stabilize the tissues. Many sutures are loose and no longer needed to stabilize the tissues at the time of the 1-week postsurgical visit.
      3. Most periodontal sutures should not be left in place longer than 2 weeks because they can act as irritants if the suture material remains in the tissues too long. It should be noted that sutures in some periodontal wounds are routinely left in place for much longer periods.
      4. Each periodontal surgical procedure is unique, and removal procedures can vary, but some general guidelines for suture removal are outlined below and in Box 27-10.

B. **General Guidelines for Suture Removal**
   1. Guideline 1: Remove sutures in a timely manner. Nonabsorbable sutures are generally removed after 1 week of healing; most absorbable sutures can be left in place 1 to 3 weeks.
   2. Guideline 2: Read the surgical note in the patient's chart prior to suture removal.
      a. The number and type of sutures placed should be a routine part of the chart entry recorded for each periodontal surgery.
      b. Knowing the number of sutures placed during the actual surgical procedure can help the dental hygienist confirm that all sutures have been located and removed during a postsurgical visit.
   3. Guideline 3: Understand the typical sizing system used for periodontal sutures.
      a. Though there are numerous sizes of sutures used in a medical setting, typical designations for suture sizes used in periodontal surgery are sizes 3-0, 4-0, and 5-0.
         1. In this sizing system, the 3-0 size is larger than the 4-0 size, and 4-0 is larger than 5-0.
         2. In the mouth, 5-0 can be more difficult to locate than a 4-0 size, especially in the posterior part of the mouth.
      b. The dental hygienist should learn the precise abbreviations used in the chart entries in the individual clinical setting. A typical example of an abbreviation would be "4-0 BSS." This would mean the size of the suture is 4-0, and BSS stands for black silk suture, a commonly used nonabsorbable suture material.
      c. Table 27-5 outlines designations for typical suture sizes used during periodontal surgery as they might appear in a patient's chart.
   4. Guideline 4: Never allow the knot to be pulled through the tissues.
      a. Sutures should be removed by cutting the suture material near the knot and grasping the knot with sterile cotton pliers.
      b. When the suture is gently pulled from the tissue, care should be taken not to force the knot itself through the tissue. This technique is illustrated in Figure 27-19.
      c. It should be noted that suture removal is rarely painful for the patient if care is taken not to create unnecessary tissue movement.
   5. Guideline 5: Always confirm that all of the sutures have been removed.
      a. Following suture removal, it is imperative to inspect the wound with care to insure that all of the sutures have indeed been located and removed.
      b. Remember that the patient chart entry made on the day of the surgery usually will contain information about how many sutures were actually placed.

TABLE 27-5. TYPICAL DESIGNATIONS FOR SUTURE SIZES USED IN PERIODONTAL SURGERY	
Suture Size	**Approximate Diameter of Suture**
3-0	0.20 mm
4-0	0.15 mm
5-0	0.10 mm

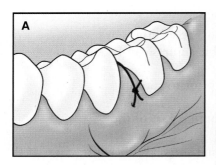 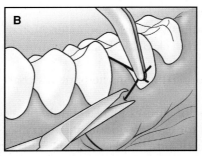 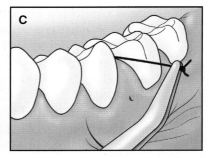

Figure 27-19. Suture Removal. A: Suture in place. **B:** Grasp the suture material and cut it near the knot. **C:** Gently pull the suture material from the tissue taking care not to pull the knot through the tissue.

USE OF PERIODONTAL DRESSING

1. **Purpose of Periodontal Dressing**
   A. **Periodontal dressing**, or periodontal pack as it sometimes called, is a protective material applied over a periodontal surgical wound. Periodontal dressings are used somewhat like using a bandage to cover a finger wound.
   B. Though the placement of periodontal dressings following periodontal surgery used to be routine, modern surgical techniques may or may not require placement of a periodontal dressing.
      1. The surgical wound created by the gingivectomy procedure leaves a raw connective tissue surface exposed that always requires a periodontal dressing.
      2. Periodontal flaps that are well adapted to the alveolar bone and tooth roots may not always require a periodontal dressing.
      3. Periodontal dressings can be placed to facilitate flap adaptation and are frequently indicated when the surgical procedures have created varying tissue levels or when displaced flaps are used.
      4. The periodontal surgeon will determine the need for dressing placement at the time of the surgical procedure.
2. **General Guidelines for Management of Periodontal Dressings**
   A. **Proper Placement**
      1. Remember that the periodontal dressing does not normally adhere to the teeth or gingiva and is retained primarily by pushing some of the material into the embrasure spaces to lock the dressing around the necks of the teeth mechanically.
      2. The use of less periodontal dressing is better than more dressing during placement; the proper amount of dressing is only enough to cover the wound.
      3. The dressing should be placed, so that there is no contact between the dressing and the teeth in the opposing arch when the patient bites down; occlusal contact with teeth in the opposing arch will quickly dislodge the dressing.
      4. Table 27-6 illustrates the proper placement of a periodontal dressing.
      5. It should be noted that suture material could accidentally become trapped within the periodontal dressing. When removing dressings, it may be necessary to loosen the dressing slightly and cut the suture before completely removing the dressing from the necks of the teeth.
      6. Periodontal dressings should be replaced every 5 to 7 days until the surgical wound is healed enough to be exposed.

TABLE 27-6. STEPS IN PERIODONTAL DRESSING PLACEMENT

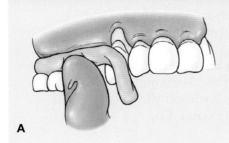

A

A: Dressing is pressed into the interdental spaces with gentle finger pressure on the facial.

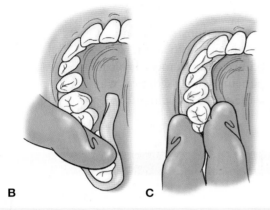

B   **C**

B: Dressing is looped around the most distal tooth and pressed into the interdental spaces on the palatal.

C: Gentle finger pressure is continued to join the dressing interdentally on the facial and palatal aspects.

D

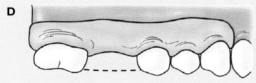

D: Dressing can be bridged across edentulous areas.

E

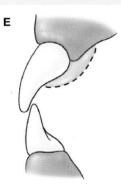

E: Dressing amount should be minimal to avoid contact of the dressing with the teeth in the opposite arch.

3. **Types of Periodontal Dressing.** There are two types of modern periodontal dressings commonly available for use today. Both types of periodontal dressing are held in place primarily by mechanical retention around the necks of the teeth.

   A. **Chemical Cure Paste.** One type is a two-paste chemical cure material that requires the mixing of paste from two tubes to form a dressing with a putty-like consistency.

   1. This type usually contains zinc oxide, mineral oils, and rosin plus a bacteriostatic or fungicidal agent.

   2. Mixing of these two-paste dressings is either by hand or in an automix cartridge.

   3. Examples of two-paste dressings are Coe-Pak manufactured by GC America, Inc. and PerioCare manufactured by Pulpdent Corp.

B. **Light-Cured Paste.** A second type is a light-cured gel that contains polyether urethane dimethacrylate resin.
   1. The dental hygienist must study the manufacturer's instructions with care and must practice placement of the dressing on a typodont (model) before using it in a patient's mouth.
   2. This type of dressing is available as a clear, translucent material that is preferred for use by some clinicians in esthetic areas of the dentition.
   3. An example of a light-cured gel periodontal dressing is Barricaid VLC periodontal surgical dressing manufactured by Dentsply Caulk Co.

POSTSURGICAL INSTRUCTIONS AND FOLLOW-UP VISITS

A member of the dental team should provide postsurgical instructions to the patient following periodontal surgery. Usually the patient is provided with both written and verbal instructions to minimize confusion and to maximize compliance. Typical postsurgical instructions are outlined in Box 27-11. For patients where sedation was required, the companion who accompanied the patient to the office is included when postsurgical instructions are given.

Box 27-11. Typical Postsurgical Instructions

1. If you have questions or concerns, call the office or the office emergency number right away. Office: 555-1111; emergency 555-2222.
2. *Do* take medications as prescribed. Report any problems with the medications immediately.
3. *Do* take it easy for several days. Limit your activity to mild physical exertion.
4. *Expect* some bleeding following the procedure. If heavy bleeding persists, call the office emergency number.
5. *Expect* some swelling. Intermittent use of an ice pack on the face in the area of the surgery during the first 8 to 10 hours following surgery can minimize swelling.
6. Diet Recommendations:
   a. Soft food only on the day of the surgery
   b. No hot beverages on the day of surgery
   c. Avoid chewing on the surgical site
7. Oral Self-Care:
   a. Rinse with recommended mouth rinse starting the day after surgery
   b. If dressing was placed, it may also be brushed lightly

---

1. **Postsurgical Instructions to the Patient**
   A. **Restrictions on Self-Care.** Most periodontal surgical procedures require some restrictions on self-care during the early phase of healing.
      1. It is common practice to prescribe 0.12% chlorhexidine mouth rinse to be used twice daily to aid with self-care until the patient can safely resume mechanical plaque control.
      2. In most cases following routine flap surgery and gingivectomy, manual self-care can be resumed by the patient in 10 to 14 days.

   3. For selected surgical procedures (such as guided tissue regeneration or bone grafting procedures) the surgical sites should not be cleaned with routine mechanical plaque control for up to 4 to 6 weeks.
   4. Areas of the dentition not involved by the periodontal surgery may be cleaned with routine self-care techniques.
B. **Postsurgical Medications.** Patients should be encouraged to take medications as prescribed.
   1. If systemic antibiotics are prescribed, it is particularly important for the patient to understand that all of this prescribed antibiotic medication should be taken.
   2. Common postsurgical medications include either nonsteroidal or narcotic pain medications, but usually, these pain medications should only be taken as long as needed.
C. **Dietary Changes.** Chewing frequently must be limited to areas not involved by the surgery until healing has progressed to an acceptable level.
   1. Many of these periodontal procedures require that the surgical site be undisturbed for an extended period of time.
   2. Recommendations for a soft or liquid diet for 24 to 48 hours are routine following most periodontal surgical procedures.
   3. Chewing should be limited to the side of the mouth not involved by the surgery, especially during the early phases of healing.
2. **Postsurgical Complications**
A. Facial swelling: It is common for the patient to experience some facial swelling following most types of periodontal surgery.
   1. Swelling can arise from the tissue trauma incurred during the procedure and can even occur during the second and third day following the surgery.
   2. Although this swelling can be disconcerting to the patient, it is usually not a sign that healing is compromised.
   3. Swelling can be minimized by the intermittent use of ice packs for the first 8 to 10 hours following the surgery.
B. Postsurgical bleeding: Some bleeding following periodontal surgery is to be expected.
   1. Patients should be reassured that minor bleeding is not a cause for alarm.
   2. Postsurgical instructions should be clear, however, that if excessive bleeding occurs the emergency number should be contacted immediately.
C. Smoking: Surgical patients, who have elected to continue smoking, should be cautioned to refrain during the healing phase.
3. **Organizing Postsurgical Visits.** It is the dentist's responsibility to manage postsurgical problems, such as extreme pain or infection. The dental hygienist, however, can perform much of the routine postsurgical patient management. Following periodontal flap surgery, the patient is most often reappointed in 5 to 7 days for the first postsurgical visit. Postsurgical care for the various types of periodontal surgery varies; however, steps to be followed at a typical postsurgical visit are outlined below.
A. **Steps Involved in a Typical Postsurgical Visit**
   1. Step 1. Patient interview: An interview is conducted with the patient to determine what the patient experienced during the days following the surgery. The patient interview should be detailed enough to provide the dental hygienist with an overview of possible problems to investigate and solve at the postsurgical visit. The following are some of the items that would normally be included in this interview. It is imperative that the dental hygienist alerts the dentist if any unusual conditions are reported by the patient or are observed during the postsurgical visit.

a. Analgesics: Following periodontal surgery, analgesics (pain control medications) are used to control patient discomfort. The patient should be asked about the current level of discomfort and if another prescription is needed.

b. Antibiotics: If antibiotics were needed following a surgical procedure, remind the patient that all of the antibiotic tablets should be taken. It is also important to find out if the patient experienced any unusual reactions to the antibiotic.

c. Antimicrobial mouth rinse: An antimicrobial mouth rinse such as 0.12% chlorhexidine gluconate may have been prescribed for the patient to use during healing, since mechanical plaque control must be restricted at the surgical site following periodontal surgery. Ask about the amount of mouth rinse remaining. During the course of the visit, it may be necessary to provide the patient another prescription for this mouth rinse.

d. Swelling: Following periodontal surgery, it is common for the patient to experience some facial swelling. Remember that although this swelling can be disconcerting to the patient, it is common and usually not a sign that healing is compromised.

e. Postsurgical bleeding: Inquire about postsurgical bleeding. It is common for patients to experience a little bleeding following periodontal surgery, but heavy bleeding should not have occurred following the procedure. If abnormal bleeding is suspected, the dentist should be alerted before planning any additional periodontal surgical intervention.

f. Sensitivity to cold: Sensitivity to cold following root exposure during many types of periodontal surgery is quite common. Although this is an annoying postsurgical occurrence, the sensitivity normally disappears within the first few weeks following the surgery if excellent plaque control is maintained.

2. Step 2. Vital signs: The patient's vital signs including blood pressure, pulse, and temperature are assessed. An elevated temperature at the first postsurgical visit can indicate a developing infection.

3. Step 3. Periodontal dressing: Any periodontal dressing placed at the time of surgery is removed, so that the surgical site can be examined. The surgical site is rinsed with warm sterile saline and cotton-tipped applicators are used to remove any debris adherent to the teeth, soft tissues, or sutures. Suture material can become trapped within the periodontal dressing. When removing dressings, it might be necessary to loosen the dressing slightly and cut the suture before completely removing the dressing from the necks of the teeth. Figure 27-20 shows interrupted interdental sutures ready for removal at the 1-week postsurgical visit.

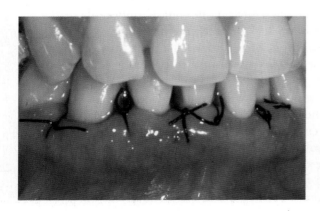

Figure 27-20. Interrupted Interdental Sutures Ready for Removal. At the 1-week postsurgical visit the periodontal dressing has been removed, the sutures have been cleaned with sterile saline, and the sutures are ready for removal.

4. Step 4. Examination of surgical site: Examine the surgical site with care. Tissue swelling or exudate such as pus can indicate a developing infection. Excessive granulation tissue that occasionally forms in the surgical site should be removed with a sharp curet.

5. Step 5. Suture removal: The sutures are cut and removed using sterile scissors and cotton pliers. Remember to pull the suture out of the tissue *without drawing the knot through the tissue.*

6. Step 6. Plaque removal: All plaque on the teeth in the area of the surgery is removed. It is usual that patients cannot perform perfect plaque control during the days following periodontal surgery, so plaque accumulation is likely. Part of the responsibility of the dental team is to help the patient with plaque control during the critical stages of healing.

7. Step 7. Replacement of periodontal dressing: If indicated, the periodontal dressing is replaced. For most surgical procedures, the periodontal dressing should be discontinued as soon as the patient can resume some mechanical plaque control. In a few instances the tissues will not be well adapted to the necks of the teeth, and replacement of the periodontal dressing should be considered to protect the continuing healing of the wound for at least another week.

8. Step 8. Self-care instructions: The patient is instructed in self-care. Mechanical plaque control should be resumed as soon as possible following periodontal surgery, but special instructions may be necessary during the first few weeks following the surgery.

   a. Special tools such as brushes with very flexible bristles may be required during early stages of healing.

   b. During postsurgical healing, it is frequently necessary to continue to modify the patient's plaque control techniques as the tissues heal and mature. Gingival margin contours usually are altered to some degree by the surgery, and this may necessitate the introduction of additional self-care aids that were not necessary prior to the surgery. Monitoring and modification of the patient's self-care efforts during the healing phase is one of the most important responsibilities of the dental team and can help assure success of the surgical procedure.

9. Step 9. Reappointment: The patient is reappointed for the second postsurgical visit. This second visit should occur 2 to 3 weeks following the surgery.

B. Follow-Up Visits

1. Following the initial postsurgical visit, additional postsurgical visits must be scheduled based upon the extent of healing of the surgical wound.

2. Professional tooth polishing should be performed every 2 weeks until the patient can safely resume routine self-care.

3. When healing is deemed complete by the dental team, the patient is always placed on a program of periodontal maintenance.

4. Attachment of the flap back to the alveolar bone is usually complete within 3 weeks following the surgery, and for many surgical procedures it is safe to proceed with restorative care in the surgical site after at least 6 weeks of healing. Note that some periodontal surgical procedures (such as bone replacement graft and periodontal regeneration) will require much longer periods of healing prior to restoration placement.

5. Remodeling of the soft tissue can continue, however, for up to 6 months, so the dentist may wait quite a while prior to final restoration placements in esthetic zones such as on anterior teeth.

Chapter Summary Statement

Periodontal surgery is a critical element in the care of most patients with moderate to severe periodontitis and a critical element in the care of many patients in need of restorative dental procedures. The periodontal flap is a fundamental part of most periodontal surgical procedures, and a basic understanding of the principles of periodontal flap surgery is important to the dental hygienist. The healing of periodontal surgical wounds is a complex process, and the terminology that has been used to describe the various types of healing that can occur in the periodontium can be confusing. A variety of specific types of periodontal surgery are being used; these techniques include procedures such as flap for access, osseous resective surgery, bone replacement grafting, periodontal regeneration, and periodontal plastic surgery among others; the dental hygienist should be familiar with the common types of periodontal surgery employed. Current research into enhancing the outcomes of periodontal surgery by using biologic mediators is ongoing. Postsurgical care following periodontal surgery is vital to successful surgical outcomes, and dental hygienists play a key role in the management of patients following periodontal surgery.

Section 6
Focus on Patients

CASE 1

You are assigned the task of providing nonsurgical therapy for a periodontitis patient. During routine nonsurgical periodontal therapy, you encounter multiple sites where the probing depths exceed 6 mm. During periodontal instrumentation, you are unable to instrument the root surfaces thoroughly in the areas of the deepest pockets. What should you tell the patient related to this clinical observation?

CASE 2

During nonsurgical periodontal therapy, a patient with chronic periodontitis informs you that the dentist had previously discussed the possibility of periodontal surgery. The patient expresses deep concern and fear over the thought of agreeing to any periodontal surgery. The patient tells you about an aunt who had periodontal surgery many years ago and had many problems following the surgery. How should you proceed?

CASE 3

At the time of the first week postsurgical visit, you note that a patient who had undergone flap for access surgery has a temperature of 101.5°F and a pulse rate of 70 beats/min. Clinical examination of the surgical site reveals that the sutures are in place, but there appears to be a good deal of swelling in one part of flap. How should you proceed?

CASE 4

You are assigned the task of managing the first week postsurgical visit for a patient who had an apically positioned flap with osseous resective surgery. Following removal of the periodontal dressing and removal of the sutures, you note that there are several areas where the healing is progressing by secondary intention because the flap could not be adapted to the teeth perfectly at the time of surgery. Though healing is progressing satisfactorily, it is apparent that not all of the connective tissue wound around the teeth is completely covered by epithelium yet. How should you proceed?

References

1. Caton, J. and S. Nyman, Histometric evaluation of periodontal surgery. I. The modified Widman flap procedure. *J Clin Periodontol,* 1980. 7(3): p. 212-23.
2. Nyman, S., et al., New attachment following surgical treatment of human periodontal disease. *J Clin Periodontol,* 1982. 9(4): p. 290-6.
3. Polson, A.M., S. Ladenheim, and P.J. Hanes, Cell and fiber attachment to demineralized dentin from periodontitis-affected root surfaces. *J Periodontol,* 1986. 57(4): p. 235-46.
4. Gantes, B.G. and S. Garrett, Coronally displaced flaps in reconstructive periodontal therapy. *Dent Clin North Am,* 1991. 35(3): p. 495-504.
5. Graziani, F., et al., Clinical performance of access flap surgery in the treatment of the intrabony defect. A systematic review and meta-analysis of randomized clinical trials. *J Clin Periodontol,* 2012. 39(2): p. 145-56.
6. Ramfjord, S.P. and R.R. Nissle, The modified widman flap. *J Periodontol,* 1974. 45(8): p. 601-7.
7. Caton, J. and S. Nyman, Histometric evaluation of periodontal surgery. III. The effect of bone resection on the connective tissue attachment level. *J Periodontol,* 1981. 52(8): p. 405-9.
8. Ochsenbein, C., A primer for osseous surgery. *Int J Periodontics Restorative Dent,* 1986. 6(1): p. 8-47.
9. Reynolds, M.A., et al., The efficacy of bone replacement grafts in the treatment of periodontal osseous defects. A systematic review. *Ann Periodontol,* 2003. 8(1): p. 227-65.
10. Bowen, J.A., et al., Comparison of decalcified freeze-dried bone allograft and porous particulate hydroxyapatite in human periodontal osseous defects. *J Periodontol,* 1989. 60(12): p. 647-54.
11. Guillemin, M.R., J.T. Mellonig, and M.A. Brunsvold, *Healing in periodontal defects treated by decalcified freeze-dried bone allografts in combination with ePTFE membranes (I). Clinical and scanning electron microscope analysis. J Clin Periodontol,* 1993. 20(7): p. 528-36.
12. Guillemin, M.R., et al., Healing in periodontal defects treated by decalcified freeze-dried bone allografts in combination with ePTFE membranes. Assessment by computerized densitometric analysis. *J Clin Periodontol,* 1993. 20(7): p. 520-7.
13. Mellonig, J.T., Freeze-dried bone allografts in periodontal reconstructive surgery. *Dent Clin North Am,* 1991. 35(3): p. 505-20.
14. Oreamuno, S., et al., Comparative clinical study of porous hydroxyapatite and decalcified freeze-dried bone in human periodontal defects. *J Periodontol,* 1990. 61(7): p. 399-404.
15. Rummelhart, J.M., et al., A comparison of freeze-dried bone allograft and demineralized freeze-dried bone allograft in human periodontal osseous defects. *J Periodontol,* 1989. 60(12): p. 655-63.
16. Sanders, J.J., et al., Clinical evaluation of freeze-dried bone allografts in periodontal osseous defects. Part III. Composite freeze-dried bone allografts with and without autogenous bone grafts. *J Periodontol,* 1983. 54(1): p. 1-8.
17. Mellonig, J.T., Human histologic evaluation of a bovine-derived bone xenograft in the treatment of periodontal osseous defects. *Int J Periodontics Restorative Dent,* 2000. 20(1): p. 19-29.
18. Bier, S.J. and M.C. Sinensky, The versatility of calcium sulfate: resolving periodontal challenges. *Compend Contin Educ Dent,* 1999. 20(7): p. 655-61; quiz 662.
19. Froum, S.J., M.A. Weinberg, and D. Tarnow, Comparison of bioactive glass synthetic bone graft particles and open debridement in the treatment of human periodontal defects. A clinical study. *J Periodontol,* 1998. 69(6): p. 698-709.
20. Lovelace, T.B., et al., Clinical evaluation of bioactive glass in the treatment of periodontal osseous defects in humans. *J Periodontol,* 1998. 69(9): p. 1027-35.
21. Low, S.B., C.J. King, and J. Krieger, An evaluation of bioactive ceramic in the treatment of periodontal osseous defects. *Int J Periodontics Restorative Dent,* 1997. 17(4): p. 358-67.
22. Caton, J., S. Nyman, and H. Zander, Histometric evaluation of periodontal surgery. II. Connective tissue attachment levels after four regenerative procedures. *J Clin Periodontol,* 1980. 7(3): p. 224-31.
23. Chambrone, L., et al., Root-coverage procedures for the treatment of localized recession-type defects: a Cochrane systematic review. *J Periodontol,* 2010. 81(4): p. 452-78.
24. Christgau, M., et al., Periodontal regeneration of intrabony defects with resorbable and non-resorbable membranes: 30-month results. *J Clin Periodontol,* 1997. 24(1): p. 17-27.
25. Cortellini, P., et al., Guided tissue regeneration with different materials. *Int J Periodontics Restorative Dent,* 1990. 10(2): p. 136-51.
26. Cortellini, P., G. Pini Prato, and M.S. Tonetti, Periodontal regeneration of human intrabony defects with titanium reinforced membranes. A controlled clinical trial. *J Periodontol,* 1995. 66(9): p. 797-803.
27. Darby, I.B. and K.H. Morris, A systematic review of the use of growth factors in human periodontal regeneration. *J Periodontol,* 2013. 84(4): p. 465-76.
28. Eickholz, P. and E. Hausmann, Evidence for healing of interproximal intrabony defects after conventional and regenerative therapy: digital radiography and clinical measurements. *J Periodontal Res,* 1998. 33(3): p. 156-65.
29. Garrett, S., Periodontal regeneration around natural teeth. *Ann Periodontol,* 1996. 1(1): p. 621-66.

30. Gottlow, J., Guided tissue regeneration using bioresorbable and non-resorbable devices: initial healing and long-term results. *J Periodontol*, 1993. 64(11 Suppl): p. 1157-65.

31. Khojasteh, A., et al., The effectiveness of barrier membranes on bone regeneration in localized bony defects: a systematic review. *Int J Oral Maxillofac Implants*, 2013. 28(4): p. 1076-89.

32. McClain, P.K. and R.G. Schallhorn, Long-term assessment of combined osseous composite grafting, root conditioning, and guided tissue regeneration. *Int J Periodontics Restorative Dent*, 1993. 13(1): p. 9-27.

33. Murphy, K.G. and J.C. Gunsolley, Guided tissue regeneration for the treatment of periodontal intrabony and furcation defects. A systematic review. *Ann Periodontol*, 2003. 8(1): p. 266-302.

34. Stoecklin-Wasmer, C., et al., Absorbable collagen membranes for periodontal regeneration: a systematic review. *J Dent Res*, 2013. 92(9): p. 773-81.

35. Tu, Y.K., et al., A Bayesian network meta-analysis on comparisons of enamel matrix derivatives, guided tissue regeneration and their combination therapies. *J Clin Periodontol*, 2012. 39(3): p. 303-14.

36. Consensus report. Mucogingival therapy. *Ann Periodontol*, 1996. 1(1): p. 702-6.

37. Cairo, F., M. Nieri, and U. Pagliaro, Efficacy of periodontal plastic surgery procedures in the treatment of localized facial gingival recessions. A systematic review. *J Clin Periodontol*, 2014. 41 Suppl 15: p. S44-62.

38. Camargo, P.M., P.R. Melnick, and E.B. Kenney, The use of free gingival grafts for aesthetic purposes. *Periodontol 2000*, 2001. 27: p. 72–96.

39. Harris, R.J., Root coverage with connective tissue grafts: an evaluation of short- and long-term results. *J Periodontol*, 2002. 73(9): p. 1054-9.

40. Langer, B. and L. Langer, Subepithelial connective tissue graft technique for root coverage. *J Periodontol*, 1985. 56(12): p. 715-20.

41. Miller, P.D., Jr. and E.P. Allen, The development of periodontal plastic surgery. *Periodontol 2000*, 1996. 11: p. 7–17.

42. Bragger, U., D. Lauchenauer, and N.P. Lang, Surgical lengthening of the clinical crown. *J Clin Periodontol*, 1992. 19(1): p. 58-63.

43. Aoki, A., et al., In vitro evaluation of Er:YAG laser scaling of subgingival calculus in comparison with ultrasonic scaling. *J Periodontal Res*, 2000. 35(5): p. 266-77.

44. Christensen, G.J., Soft-tissue cutting with laser versus electrosurgery. *J Am Dent Assoc*, 2008. 139(7): p. 981-4.

45. Frentzen, M., A. Braun, and D. Aniol, Er:YAG laser scaling of diseased root surfaces. *J Periodontol*, 2002. 73(5): p. 524-30.

46. Gold, S.I. and M.A. Vilardi, Pulsed laser beam effects on gingiva. *J Clin Periodontol*, 1994. 21(6): p. 391-6.

47. Israel, M. and J.A. Rossmann, An epithelial exclusion technique using the CO2 laser for the treatment of periodontal defects. *Compend Contin Educ Dent*, 1998. 19(1): p. 86-8, 90, 92-5.

48. Neill, M.E. and J.T. Mellonig, Clinical efficacy of the Nd:YAG laser for combination periodontitis therapy. *Pract Periodontics Aesthet Dent*, 1997. 9(6 Suppl): p. 1-5.

49. Sgolastra, F., et al., Efficacy of Er:YAG laser in the treatment of chronic periodontitis: systematic review and meta-analysis. *Lasers Med Sci*, 2012. 27(3): p. 661-73.

50. Yukna, R.A., R.L. Carr, and G.H. Evans, Histologic evaluation of an Nd:YAG laser-assisted new attachment procedure in humans. *Int J Periodontics Restorative Dent*, 2007. 27(6): p. 577-87.

51. American Academy of Periodontology statement on the efficacy of lasers in the non-surgical treatment of inflammatory periodontal disease. *J Periodontol*, 2011. 82(4): p. 513-4.

52. Affairs, C.o.S. Statement on lasers in dentistry.

53. Mariotti, A., Efficacy of chemical root surface modifiers in the treatment of periodontal disease. A systematic review. *Ann Periodontol*, 2003. 8(1): p. 205-26.

54. Oliveira, G.H. and E.A. Muncinelli, Efficacy of root surface biomodification in root coverage: a systematic review. *J Can Dent Assoc*, 2012. 78: p. c122.

55. Cochran, D.L. and J.M. Wozney, Biological mediators for periodontal regeneration. *Periodontol 2000*, 1999. 19: p. 40–58.

56. Esposito, M., et al., Enamel matrix derivative (Emdogain) for periodontal tissue regeneration in intrabony defects. A Cochrane systematic review. *Eur J Oral Implantol*, 2009. 2(4): p. 247-66.

57. Hammarstrom, L., Enamel matrix, cementum development and regeneration. *J Clin Periodontol*, 1997. 24(9 Pt 2): p. 658-68.

58. Heijl, L., et al., Enamel matrix derivative (EMDOGAIN) in the treatment of intrabony periodontal defects. *J Clin Periodontol*, 1997. 24(9 Pt 2): p. 705-14.

59. Koop, R., J. Merheb, and M. Quirynen, Periodontal regeneration with enamel matrix derivative in reconstructive periodontal therapy: a systematic review. *J Periodontol*, 2012. 83(6): p. 707-20.

60. Okuda, K., et al., Enamel matrix derivative in the treatment of human intrabony osseous defects. *J Periodontol*, 2000. 71(12): p. 1821-8.

61. Lynch, S.E., et al., A combination of platelet-derived and insulin-like growth factors enhances periodontal regeneration. *J Clin Periodontol*, 1989. 16(8): p. 545-8.

62. Marx, R.E., et al., Platelet-rich plasma: Growth factor enhancement for bone grafts. *Oral Surg Oral Med Oral Pathol Oral Radiol Endod*, 1998. 85(6): p. 638-46.

 ## STUDENT ANCILLARY RESOURCES

A wide variety of resources to enhance your learning and understanding of this chapter are available on the**Point®**.

- Visit thePoint to access:
  - Audio Glossary
  - Animations
  - Suggested Readings
  - Answers to Review Questions
  - Case Studies

Periodontal Emergencies

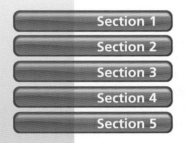
Clinical Application. There are several periodontal conditions that can bring a patient to a dental office on an emergency basis for relief of pain or discomfort. Occasionally in the early stages of some of these conditions, dental hygienists may encounter them during a routine patient appointment. Dental hygienists need to be familiar with these conditions, so that the patient's needs can be managed in a timely manner. This chapter outlines some of the more common periodontal emergency conditions and offer suggestions for management of the patients with these conditions.

Learning Objectives

- Name and describe the three types of abscesses of the periodontium.
- List the possible causes of abscesses of the periodontium.
- Compare and contrast the abscess of the periodontium and the pulpal abscess.
- Outline the typical treatment steps for a gingival abscess and a periodontal abscess.
- Describe the clinical situation that can result in a pericoronal abscess.
- Outline the typical treatment for a pericoronal abscess (pericoronitis).
- Describe the characteristics of necrotizing ulcerative gingivitis.
- Outline the typical treatment steps for necrotizing ulcerative gingivitis.
- Describe the symptoms of primary herpetic gingivostomatitis.

Key Terms

Acute periodontal
  conditions
Abscess of the
  periodontium
Pus
Suppuration
Circumscribed

Pulpal abscess
Gingival abscess
Periodontal abscess
Pericoronal abscess
Pericoronitis
Operculum
Trismus

Necrosis
Ulceration
Punched-out papillae
Pseudomembrane
Sequestrum
Primary herpetic
  gingivostomatitis

Section 1
Introduction to Acute Periodontal Conditions

1. Most periodontal diseases are chronic in nature and progress rather slowly; they can take years or decades to destroy the periodontium and lead to tooth loss. These diseases are rarely painful, especially in their earlier stages. There are a few periodontal diseases, such as aggressive periodontitis, that progress more rapidly. However, even aggressive periodontitis can take several years to lead to tooth loss, and it is not usually associated with pain in the early stages.
   A. There are several periodontal conditions that can bring patients to a dental office or hospital emergency room for relief of pain or other more dramatic symptoms (1).
   B. The emergency conditions described in this chapter are normally considered examples of acute periodontal conditions.
   C. The term "acute periodontal conditions" refers to conditions that are commonly characterized by having a sudden onset and a rapid course of progression. These acute conditions are frequently accompanied by pain and discomfort, and they may be unrelated to the presence of any pre-existing gingivitis or periodontitis (Box 28-1).
   D. It is imperative that all members of the dental team be alert for these conditions because their recognition and early intervention can limit subsequent permanent damage to the periodontium (2,3).
   E. Some of these acute conditions can be encountered in their earliest stages by the dental hygienist during routine treatment or recall appointments.
2. This chapter outlines some of the more common periodontal emergency conditions and briefly describes the treatment that may be recommended and performed by the dentist or the dental hygienist or by other healthcare providers.

Box 28-1. Characteristics of Acute Periodontal Conditions

- Sudden onset of the condition
- Rapid course of progression
- Accompanied by pain and discomfort
- May be unrelated to pre-existing gingivitis or periodontitis

---

Section 2
Abscesses of the Periodontium

1. Overview of Abscesses of the Periodontium
   A. Abscesses of the Periodontium Defined
      1. An abscess of the periodontium may be defined as an acute infection involving a circumscribed collection of pus in the periodontium.
      2. Abscesses of the periodontium are collections of pus within the periodontal tissues. Pus consists primarily of dead and dying neutrophils, bacteria, cellular debris, and fluid leaked from blood vessels; pus can result when body defense mechanisms are involved in attempting to control an infection. The process of forming pus is called suppuration.

3. In its earliest stages, the abscess of the periodontium can be discovered by the dental hygienist during an oral inspection at a routine treatment visit; but in more advanced stages, the abscess of the periodontium can bring the patient to the dental office for relief of pain.

4. Abscesses of the periodontium are usually described as being circumscribed. The term **circumscribed** means that the abscess is localized or confined to a specific site (i.e., the facial surface of a single tooth or perhaps the gingival margin on a specific tooth). Figure 28-1 illustrates a typical example of an abscess of the periodontium.

5. The precise bacterial etiology of the abscess of the periodontium is not clear, but it is known that most of these lesions contain microflora that are predominantly gram negative and anaerobic. Most studies indicate that the bacteria seen in these abscesses are similar to the bacteria seen in periodontitis patients with deeper pockets.

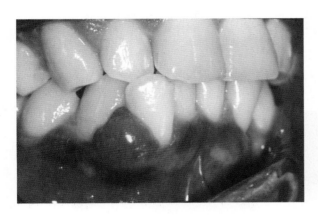

Figure 28-1. Abscess of the Periodontium. Note the localized swelling between the mandibular right canine and lateral incisor. Palpation of the swelling would reveal what feels like a fluid-filled sack. Pus can be found in this site.

Box 28-2. Characteristics of an Abscess of the Periodontium

- Pain that is constant and localized
- Circumscribed (localized) swelling in the periodontium
- Possible increase in tooth mobility
- Radiographic loss of alveolar bone not involving the tooth apex
- Tooth usually has a vital pulp

B. Characteristics of an Abscess of the Periodontium
1. Typical patient complaints related to an abscess of the periodontium include dental pain and swelling in the gingiva at a specific location (Box 28-2).
   a. Pain resulting from an abscess of the periodontium is usually described by the patient as a constant pain (as opposed to intermittent). Patients frequently report that the pain is easy for them to localize (i.e., the patient can point to the exact spot that hurts). Note that in some other conditions, a patient can report pain that is not at all localized to a specific location.
   b. In addition to pain and swelling, the patient may report difficulty in mastication and a bad taste in the mouth.

2. Oral examination will usually reveal the presence of a circumscribed swelling of the soft tissue. This swelling may involve the gingiva only, or it may involve both the gingiva and the mucosa.

3. Many teeth with an abscess of the periodontium can also exhibit a temporary increase in mobility.

4. Dental radiographs of a tooth with an abscess of the periodontium frequently reveal alveolar bone loss in the area of the abscess, but the bone loss does not usually involve the tooth apex. Figure 28-2 is a radiograph of a tooth with an abscess of the periodontium.

    a. Alveolar bone loss resulting from an abscess of the periodontium can occur extremely rapidly when compared with the rate of alveolar bone loss usually associated with all forms of either chronic or aggressive periodontitis.

    b. Although a dental radiograph of an abscess of the periodontium may reveal alveolar bone loss, in a periodontitis patient, it is not always possible to tell what part of the missing bone actually resulted from the acute infection and what part of the missing bone was caused by chronic periodontitis that was present before the abscess formed.

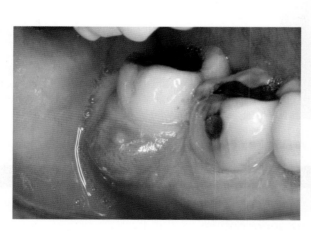
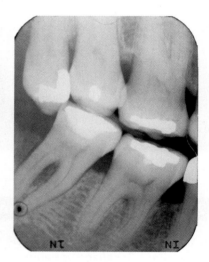

Figure 28-2. Abscess if the Periodontium Involving Mandibular Second Molar Tooth. The clinical photograph shows circumscribed swelling and inflammation of the gingival tissue on the facial surface of a mandibular second molar with an abscess of the periodontium. The radiograph of the site reveals loss of bone density between the roots of the molar tooth affected by the abscess. (Courtesy of Dr. Richard Foster, Guilford Technical Community College, Jamestown, NC.)

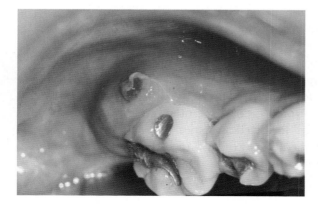

Figure 28-3. Path of Drainage. The abscess of the periodontium shown in this figure has broken through the surface tissues, establishing a path of drainage for the pus on its own.

5. Teeth affected by an abscess of the periodontium are usually vital (have healthy pulp tissue) and respond positively if pulp testing is performed.

6. Another clinical sign of an abscess of the periodontium can be an elevated body temperature; an elevated body temperature would not normally be present unless the abscess of the periodontium is spreading, so this would represent a serious sign if present. Since many abscesses of the periodontium are circumscribed (localized), they are not associated with an elevated body temperature.

7. When there is delay in treating an abscess of the periodontium, there can be additional oral changes (4). The collection of pus can break through the surface tissues, thus establishing a path of drainage for the pus on its own. Figure 28-3 illustrates an abscess of the periodontium that has drained spontaneously by breaking through the surface tissues.

C. **Causes of Abscesses of the Periodontium.** Several causes of abscesses of the periodontium have been reported (5,6). Theories about the origin of the abscess of the periodontium vary, but most investigators attribute formation of this type of abscess to one of the following scenarios.

1. **Blockage of the Orifice of a Pocket.** Blockage of the orifice (or opening) of a pre-existing periodontal pocket has been suggested as a cause of some abscesses of the periodontium. Most periodontal pockets have readily accessible openings that give easy access to a periodontal probe. Some authors have theorized that in certain instances, the opening of a periodontal pocket can become restricted in size because of temporary improvement of the surface tissue tone. This improvement of tissue firmness could result in trapping bacteria and fluids in a pre-existing periodontal pocket, leading to an abscess that begins within this existing periodontal pocket.

2. **Accidentally Forcing a Foreign Object into the Tissues.** It has also been suggested that an abscess of periodontium can be caused by accidentally forcing a foreign object into the supporting tissues of a tooth.
   a. A variety of foreign objects have been implicated in the formation of some abscesses of the periodontium. For example, an abscess could result when a patient accidentally punctures the gingiva with a toothpick, forcing bacteria into the tissue.
   b. Another common event that can result in an abscess of the periodontium is accidentally forcing some food product like a husk from a kernel of popcorn or a peanut skin into the tissues associated with the tissue inflammation as part of a periodontal pocket.

3. **Incomplete Calculus Removal in a Periodontal Pocket.** Incomplete calculus removal in a periodontal pocket has also been suggested as one cause of an abscess of the periodontium.
   a. When this occurs, it is usually thought to be in a site with a very deep probing depth where the calculus deposits are removed only in the most coronal aspects of the pocket near the gingival margin, but the calculus deposits deeper in the pocket are not completely removed because of difficulty of access for instrumentation of the tooth surface.
   b. It is theorized that removal of the more coronal calculus deposits allows the gingival margin to heal somewhat and to tighten around the tooth, like a drawstring of a pouch, preventing drainage of bacterial toxins and other waste products from the pocket. Bacteria remaining in the deeper aspects of the periodontal pocket could result in the formation of an abscess of the periodontium.

2. **Comparison Between the Periodontal Abscesses and the Pulpal Abscesses.** The clinical recognition and diagnosis of a periodontal abscess can be complicated in some instances because of the possible overlap of signs of a periodontal abscess with the signs of a pulpal abscess.

A. Abscesses affecting the tissues around a tooth can result for two different sources: (1) the periodontium itself, which surrounds the tooth or (2) the pulpal tissues that are within the pulp chamber of the tooth (7).

1. It is helpful for the dental hygienist to be familiar with the characteristics of these two types of abscesses, since the periodontal abscess and the pulpal abscess sometime appear to have somewhat similar clinical characteristics.

2. The characteristics of each of these types of abscesses are outlined in Table 28-1.

B. As already discussed, a periodontal abscess is an abscess that results from an acute infection of the periodontium.

C. On the other hand, a **pulpal abscess** is an abscess that results from an infection of the tooth pulp that can sometimes extend into the periodontium.

1. A pulpal abscess can be caused by death of the tooth pulp from trauma to the tooth or from deep dental decay; a dead tooth pulp is frequently referred to as a nonvital pulp.

2. Management of a patient with a pulpal abscess usually requires root canal treatment and will not be discussed in this chapter.

TABLE 28-1. DIFFERENTIATION OF THE TYPES OF ABSCESS

Characteristic	Periodontal Abscess	Pulpal Abscess
Vitality test results	Usually vital pulp	Usually nonvital pulp
Radiographic appearance	Bone loss present (not at apex)	Bone loss at tooth root apex
Symptoms	Localized, constant pain	Difficult to localize, intermittent pain

3. **Types of Abscesses of the Periodontium.** Authors generally describe three types of periodontal abscesses: (1) the gingival abscess, (2) the periodontal abscess, and (3) the pericoronal abscess, but there is considerable overlap in this very loose classification system.

A. **Gingival Abscess.** The **gingival abscess** refers to an abscess of the periodontium that is primarily limited to the gingival margin or to the interdental papilla without involvement of the deeper structures of the periodontium.

1. The gingival abscess can occur in a previously periodontally healthy mouth when some foreign object is forced into a healthy gingival sulcus. An abscess of the periodontium that is limited to the gingival margin area can follow this traumatic event.

2. Figure 28-4 illustrates a typical gingival abscess where the swelling is limited to the marginal gingiva of a single tooth.

B. **Periodontal Abscess.** The true **periodontal abscess** refers to an abscess of the periodontium that affects the deeper structures of the periodontium as well as the gingival tissues.

1. The periodontal abscess usually occurs in a site with pre-existing periodontal disease including pre-existing periodontal pockets.
2. The periodontal abscess usually affects the deeper structures of the periodontium and is not limited to the gingiva only.

C. **Pericoronal Abscess.** The pericoronal abscess refers to an abscess of the periodontium that involves tissues around the crown of a partially erupted tooth. The pericoronal abscess is also referred to as **pericoronitis**.

1. This type of abscess is seen in teeth where some of the soft tissues surrounding the teeth actually cover part of the occlusal surface of the teeth. Figure 28-5 illustrates a patient with a pericoronal abscess under a soft tissue flap partially covering a third molar tooth.

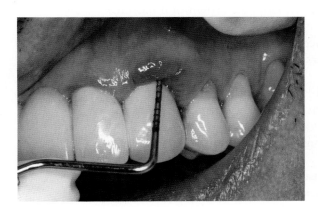

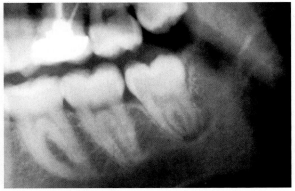

Figure 28-4. Gingival Abscess. Note that this abscess is limited to the gingival margin on the facial surface of this maxillary canine. (Courtesy of Dr. Richard Foster, Guilford Technical Community College, Jamestown, NC.)

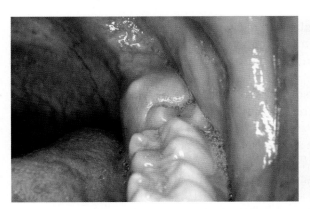

Figure 28-5. Pericoronal Abscess Involving a Mandibular Third Molar Tooth. The clinical photograph shows the typical clinical appearance of a mandibular third molar tooth with a pericoronal abscess. Note the swelling of the tissue that is partially covering the crown of the third molar. The radiograph of the site illustrated the position of the third molar in close relationship to the mandibular ramus. (Courtesy of Dr. Richard Foster, Guilford Technical Community College, Jamestown, NC.)

Box 28-3. Signs and Symptoms of a Pericoronal Abscess

- Pain at the site
- Swelling of operculum
- Possible trismus (limited mouth opening)
- Possible elevated body temperature
- Possible lymphadenopathy

---

2. The pericoronal abscess (or pericoronitis) is most frequently seen around mandibular third molar teeth. Since many third molar teeth do not have space to erupt fully, these teeth can have a flap of tissue covering part of the occlusal surface.

3. The flap of gingival tissue that covers a portion of the crown of a partially erupted tooth can become infected, and it is this type of infection under this flap of tissue that is referred to as a pericoronal abscess. The flap of soft tissue is called an **operculum**, and some authors also refer to the pericoronal abscess as an operculitis.

4. *Streptococci milleri* group bacteria, well-known for their ability to cause suppurative infections, are most likely involved in the pathogenesis of acute severe pericoronitis of the lower third molar (8).

5. The signs and symptoms of the pericoronal abscess are discussed below and outlined in Box 28-3.

6. Pain is common with the pericoronal abscess. The pain can arise from the tissue swelling itself, but pain can also arise when an opposing tooth occludes with the infected, swollen operculum.

7. Soft tissue swelling (edema) and redness (erythema) also usually accompany the pericoronal abscess.

8. As damage to tissue covering the partially erupted tooth progresses and the tissue swelling increases, the opposing tooth can frequently be seen to impinge (press) on the swollen tissue, creating additional tissue damage and additional patient discomfort.

9. Limited mouth opening is also seen in some cases of advanced pericoronal abscess; limited mouth opening is referred to as **trismus**.

10. Elevated body temperature (fever) and swollen lymph nodes (lymphadenopathy) also can be seen in advanced cases of pericoronitis.

4. Management of Patients with Abscesses of the Periodontium

   A. Treatment of a Gingival or Periodontal Abscess. The treatment of a patient with either a gingival or a periodontal abscess is similar.

      1. Fundamental treatment steps include (1) establishment of a path of drainage for the pus, (2) thorough periodontal debridement of the adjacent tooth surfaces in the area of the abscess, and (3) relief of pain.

      2. Steps commonly followed in treatment of patients with a gingival or a periodontal abscess are discussed below and are outlined in Box 28-4.

         a. It is normally necessary to anesthetize the site to be treated, since manipulation of the tissues involved by an abscess can be quite uncomfortable.

         b. Drainage of the pus from the abscess is critical. The abscess can be drained either through the pocket itself or by performing periodontal surgery (as discussed in Chapter 27). When drainage is established through the pocket, the toe of a *sterile* curet is used to puncture the soft tissue wall of the pocket to allow the drainage.

In some cases, drainage can be accomplished by incising through the surface tissues.

c. Thorough periodontal instrumentation of the tooth surfaces in the site of the abscess is important in bringing this type of abscess under control.

d. Some adjustment of the tooth occlusion is usually also indicated, since inflammation resulting from the abscess can force a tooth to extrude slightly from its socket, leading to trauma from occlusion and pain when masticating.

e. In more advanced cases of abscesses, antibiotics may also be needed, as with any other serious oral infection.

f. Some clinicians recommend using warm saline (salt water) rinses several times each day to help keep the abscess draining until it has healed completely.

g. A prescription for pain medication should always be considered, but over-the-counter pain medications can be adequate in many patients once the abscess has been drained.

h. Following emergency treatment of a patient with any abscess of the periodontium, the dental team should appoint the patient for a thorough periodontal assessment, since the abscess of the periodontium frequently occurs in a patient with existing untreated periodontal disease, and routine periodontal therapy may be needed.

B. **Treatment of a Pericoronal Abscess.** Treatment of patients with pericoronal abscess differs slightly from treatment of patients with other types of abscesses of the periodontium because of the difference in the anatomical location of these abscesses.

1. Fundamental treatment steps for a patient with pericoronitis include (1) establishment of a path of drainage for the pus, (2) irrigation of the undersurface of the operculum, (3) thorough periodontal debridement of the tooth surfaces in the area of the abscess, and (4) relief of pain (9).

2. Steps commonly followed in treatment of patients with a pericoronal abscess are discussed below and outlined in Box 28-5.

   a. It is normally necessary to anesthetize the site to be treated, since manipulation of the tissues involved by an abscess can be quite uncomfortable.

   b. Drainage of the pus from the abscess is critical. The abscess can be drained either through the pocket itself or by performing periodontal surgery (as discussed in Chapter 27). When drainage is established through the pocket, the toe of a *sterile* curet is used to puncture the soft tissue wall of the pocket to allow drainage. Abscesses around the crown of a partially erupted third molar tooth may be difficult to drain because of the anatomy of the region.

   c. Thorough periodontal instrumentation of the tooth surfaces in the site of the abscess is important in bringing this type of abscess under control.

   d. The area under the operculum that partially covers the tooth crown should be irrigated thoroughly. This irrigation can be done with sterile saline.

   e. In more advanced cases of abscesses antibiotics may be needed, as with any other serious oral infection.

   f. Some clinicians recommend using warm saline (salt water) rinses several times each day to help keep the abscess draining until it has healed completely.

   g. A prescription for pain medication should always be considered, but over-the-counter pain medications can be adequate in many patients once the abscess is drained.

h. Following emergency treatment of a patient with any abscess of the periodontium, the dental team should appoint the patient for a thorough periodontal assessment, since the abscess of the periodontium frequently occurs in a patient with existing untreated periodontal disease.

i. In some cases following resolution of the abscess, it is wise to excise the operculum that was involved in the pericoronal abscess. This removal can prevent recurrence of the abscess. In some cases following resolution of the abscess, the dentist may recommend extraction of malposed third molar teeth if there is inadequate jaw space for the third molar teeth to fully erupt.

Box 28-4. Steps in Treatment of a Gingival or Periodontal Abscess

- Administer local anesthesia
- Drain pus
- Thorough periodontal instrumentation
- Adjust occlusion if needed
- Prescribe antibiotics if needed
- Recommend warm saline rinses
- Prescribe pain medications if needed
- Follow up appointments

Box 28-5. Common Steps in Treatment of Patient with Pericoronal Abscess

- Administer local anesthesia
- Drain pus
- Thorough periodontal instrumentation
- Irrigate under operculum
- Prescribe antibiotics if needed
- Recommend warm saline rinses
- Prescribe pain medications if needed
- Evaluate the need for third molar extractions
- Establish follow-up appointments

Section 3
Necrotizing Periodontal Diseases

Necrotizing periodontal diseases include necrotizing ulcerative gingivitis (often referred to as NUG) and necrotizing ulcerative periodontitis (often referred to as NUP) (10). NUG and NUP also are discussed in Chapter 9. Both of these diseases are acute infections of the periodontium that can bring patients to the dental office for emergency treatment. NUG is an acute infection affecting the gingival tissues only. NUP is an acute infection that mimics NUG but can also affect the deeper structures of the periodontium such as the alveolar bone. Both conditions have been reported to occur in patients with compromised immune systems who therefore may have limited host defense mechanisms.

1. Necrotizing Ulcerative Gingivitis
   A. Overview of Necrotizing Ulcerative Gingivitis (NUG)
      1. Necrotizing ulcerative gingivitis or NUG is an acute infection of the periodontium that is limited to gingival tissues (11–13). Other names for this condition are Vincent infection, trench mouth, ulceromembranous gingivitis, and acute necrotizing ulcerative gingivitis (ANUG). As the name necrotizing ulcerative gingivitis implies, patients with NUG exhibit *necrosis* and *ulceration* of the gingiva.
         a. The term **necrosis** refers to cell death, in this instance referring to the death of the cells comprising the gingival epithelium.
         b. The term **ulceration** refers to the loss of the epithelium normally covering underlying connective tissue. In NUG, ulceration results from death of the epithelial cells and the subsequent loss of the epithelium that normally covers the underlying gingival connective tissue.
      2. An impaired host response appears to be associated with the development of NUG in many patients (14). This impaired response may be related to any of several factors such as poor nutrition, fatigue, psychosocial factors, systemic disease, alcohol abuse, or drug abuse. It should be noted that NUG also may be associated with the immunosuppression seen in HIV infection.
      3. It is not known if bacteria are the primary cause of NUG, but studies indicate that certain bacteria including spirochetal organisms and fusiform bacilli are always associated with the disease. Other organisms have also been reported to be present in NUG.
      4. NUG occurs in patients of all ages, but the highest incidence of NUG is seen in patients between 20 and 30 years of age (15). In the United States, NUG in children is not common, but it has been reported in children in underdeveloped countries.
      5. There are several clinical signs that distinguish NUG from other forms of gingivitis.
         a. One of those clinical signs is the presence of **punched-out papillae** (Fig. 28-6). In NUG, the necrosis associated with this condition can destroy the papillae between the teeth, resulting in the clinical appearance that the papillae are missing or "punched out." The term punched-out papillae is used to underscore the crater-like appearance left by the absence of the papillae.
         b. Another clinical sign is the formation of a **pseudomembrane**. The necrotic areas of gingiva are covered with a gray-white layer sometimes referred to as a pseudomembrane.
            1. This pseudomembrane actually consists of dead cells, bacteria, and oral debris; underlying this pseudomembrane is raw connective tissue.

2. Patients with NUG usually exhibit bleeding with the slightest manipulation of the gingival tissues. This bleeding results from breakage of some of the tiny blood vessels in the connective tissues exposed under the pseudomembrane.

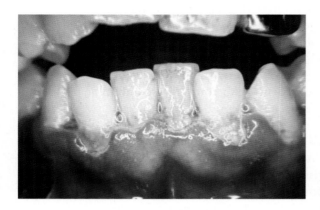

Figure 28-6. Necrotizing Ulcerative Gingivitis. Note that the necrotic areas have extended from the papillae onto the facial surfaces. The necrotic areas of the gingiva are covered with gray-white layer called the pseudomembrane. The necrosis has destroyed the papillae leading to what is called punched-out papillae that can be hidden by the pseudomembrane.

Box 28-6. Characteristics of NUG

- Oral pain
- Necrotic or punched-out gingival papillae
- Gingival bleeding with even slight manipulation of the gingival tissues
- Presence of pseudomembrane on affected sites
- Swollen lymph nodes (lymphadenopathy)
- Vague feeling of discomfort (malaise)
- Elevated body temperature
- Extreme halitosis (fetid breath)

B. **Characteristics of Necrotizing Ulcerative Gingivitis.** The characteristics of NUG are described below and outlined in Box 28-6.
1. Patients with NUG experience oral pain and frequently seek emergency care for that oral pain; the ulceration associated with the infection results in exposure of connective tissue, which can be quite uncomfortable for the patients. Because of the exposure of connective tissue, bleeding from the area can appear to be spontaneous.
2. The tissue necrosis can lead to destruction of the interdental papillae resulting in punched-out papillae; areas are normally covered with a collection of dead tissue cells and debris called a pseudomembrane.
3. Patients with NUG can display swollen lymph nodes (lymphadenopathy), a vague feeling of discomfort (malaise), and an elevated body temperature.
4. Because of the necrosis or death of cells involved with this disease, there is usually noticeable halitosis or bad breath in NUG patients. Some authors have described this halitosis as a fetid breath.
5. Certain associated behaviors or conditions are frequently present in patients who develop NUG; these include a history of smoking, a history of poor nutrition, and a history of severe stress.

6. It has also been reported that some patients who develop NUG have a human immunodeficiency virus (HIV)-positive status. NUG has also been reported to occur in some patients with HIV infection.

C. **Typical Treatment Steps for NUG.** The treatment of patients with NUG is summarized below and outlined in Box 28-7.

1. At the first appointment.
   a. The pseudomembrane should be removed carefully with irrigation and moist cotton.
   b. Supragingival periodontal instrumentation is performed. Instrumentation is limited because of the discomfort elicited by tissue manipulation.
   c. The patient is instructed regarding a gentle self-care regimen. Toothbrushing may need to be restricted to removal of debris with soft brushes.
   d. Patients may need to use standard regimens of twice daily rinses of chlorhexidine. Some authors have suggested using 3% hydrogen peroxide with equal parts of warm water every 2 to 3 hours.

2. At the first follow-up appointment 2 days after initial visit.
   a. Subgingival periodontal instrumentation usually can be begun at this appointment.
   b. Further instruction in self-care should be included at this visit.

3. At the second follow-up appointment approximately 5 days after initial visit, subgingival instrumentation usually can be completed.

4. In more advanced cases of NUG, antibiotics may be needed as in any other severe oral infection.

5. Following the resolution of the infection. The patient should be appointed for a comprehensive clinical assessment to identify any underlying chronic periodontal disease. Figure 28-7 illustrates before and after treatment photographs of a typical patient with early stages of NUG. Following complete resolution of the infection, some NUG patients require periodontal surgery to re-establish natural gingival contours.

Box 28-7. Typical Treatment Steps for a Patient with Necrotizing Ulcerative Gingivitis

1. At the first appointment.
   - The pseudomembrane should be removed carefully.
   - Supragingival periodontal instrumentation is performed. Instrumentation is limited because of the discomfort elicited by tissue manipulation.
   - The patient is instructed regarding a gentle self-care regimen.
2. At the first follow-up appointment 2 days after initial visit.
   - Subgingival periodontal instrumentation usually can be begun at this appointment.
   - Further instruction in self-care should be included at this visit.
3. At the second follow-up appointment approximately 5 days after initial visit.
   - Subgingival instrumentation usually can be completed.
4. Following the resolution of the infection, the patient should be appointed for a comprehensive clinical assessment to identify any underlying chronic periodontal disease or the possible need for surgical reshaping of the gingiva.

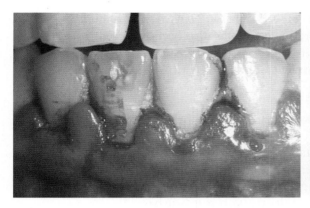 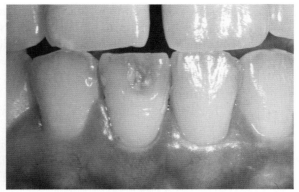

Figure 28-7. Necrotizing Ulcerative Gingivitis: Before and After Treatment. A: Necrotizing ulcerative gingivitis before treatment. **B:** The same patient after treatment. (Courtesy of Dr. Don Rolfs, Periodontal Foundations, Wenatchee, WA.)

2. Necrotizing Ulcerative Periodontitis
   A. Overview of Necrotizing Ulcerative Periodontitis (NUP)
      1. Symptoms of necrotizing ulcerative periodontitis or NUP can be similar to those of NUG but necrotizing ulcerative periodontitis also affects the deeper structures of the periodontium such as the alveolar bone (10,16,17). Necrotizing ulcerative periodontitis can occur in patients with NUG who go untreated.
      2. One unusual finding in NUP is that it can be accompanied by the formation of bone sequestra. A **sequestrum** is a fragment of necrotic (dead) bone. Sequestration is the process of forming a sequestrum.
      3. Figure 28-8 illustrates a patient with NUP.
   B. Typical Treatment of Necrotizing Ulcerative Periodontitis. Treatment of patients with NUP is complex and may require medical consultation, since the patients who develop this condition can have serious underlying medical compromising conditions that must be managed simultaneously with dental therapy (18–20). When patients with NUP are encountered in a general dental office, immediate referral to a periodontist is indicated.

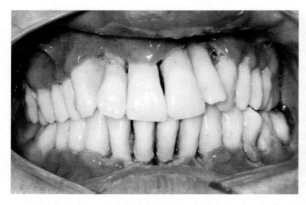 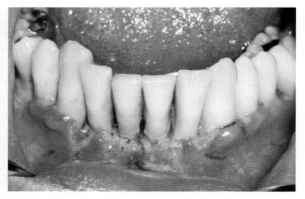

Figure 28-8. Necrotizing Ulcerative Periodontitis. A: A patient with NUP. **B:** Close-up of the mandibular arch showing bone sequestration. (Courtesy of Dr. Don Rolfs, Periodontal Foundations, Wenatchee, WA.)

Section 4
Primary Herpetic Gingivostomatitis

1. Overview of Primary Herpetic Gingivostomatitis.
   A. **Etiology of Primary Herpetic Gingivostomatitis.** Primary herpetic gingivostomatitis is actually a medical condition resulting from a viral infection. It is listed here as a periodontal emergency condition, since patients with this condition can first seek care in a dental office because of the nature of the oral symptoms that may develop in some cases.
   B. **Characteristics of Primary Herpetic Gingivostomatitis**
   1. Primary herpetic gingivostomatitis is a painful oral condition that can result from the initial infection with the herpes simplex virus (HSV) (21–23).
      a. There are two types of herpes simplex virus, oral herpes virus (HSVI) and genital herpes virus (HSVII) (24). Primary herpetic gingivostomatitis is usually caused by initial infection with HSVI but can also be caused by initial infection with HSVII.
      b. In the majority of patients, the initial infection with these viruses produces no noticeable clinical signs and can go undetected clinically. In other patients, however, the oral symptoms resulting from this initial infection can be quite severe, and it is these severe oral symptoms that are known as primary herpetic gingivostomatitis (Fig. 28-9).

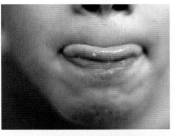

Figure 28-9. Primary Oral Infection with Herpes Simplex Virus. These three children demonstrate the spectrum of primary oral infection with the herpes simplex virus, which ranges from nearly asymptomatic to severe.

A: The first patient has a single vesicle on his tongue.

B: The second patient manifests widespread labial and gingival lesions. The parent's fingers are shown in the photograph; however, touching the infected area with bare fingers is *not* recommended. The dental hygienist should advise parents that contact with open sores or saliva can spread the virus.

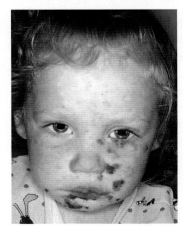

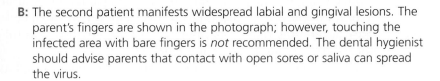

C: The third patient shows a severe infection with lesions on the face. (From Fleisher GR, Ludwig W, Baskin MN. *Atlas of Pediatric Emergency Medicine*. Philadelphia, PA: Lippincott Williams & Wilkins; 2004.)

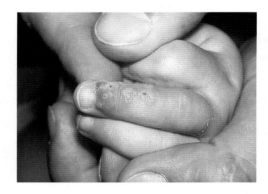

Figure 28-10. Primary Herpes Simplex Virus Infection in Infancy. Finger sucking likely caused the spread of the infection from the mouth to the hand of this infant. The parent's fingers are shown in the photograph; however, touching the infected area with bare fingers is not recommended. (From Goodheart HP. *Goodheart's Photoguide of Common Skin Disorders*. 2nd ed. Philadelphia, PA: Lippincott Williams & Wilkins; 2003.)

2. *Primary herpetic gingivostomatitis is contagious and requires careful attention to prevent its spread.*
   a. Infections caused by HSV are contagious during the vesicular stage when the virus is contained in the clear fluid in the vesicles.
   b. HSV1 is primarily spread by direct contact through kissing and contact with open sores or by contact with infected saliva.
   c. HSV1 can also spread from one part of the body to another, such as from saliva to the fingers, then to the eye. Touching the eye can result in a painful and dangerous herpetic infection of the cornea (herpes keratitis).
3. The initial infection with HSVI usually occurs in children or in young adults, but it can occur at any age (25).
4. Once a patient is infected with this virus, the infection can recur periodically throughout the life of the patient in the form of herpes labialis (fever blisters or cold sores).

2. **Clinical Signs and Treatment of Primary Herpetic Gingivostomatitis**
   A. **Clinical Signs.** As already mentioned, the clinical signs of primary herpetic gingivostomatitis can range from subclinical (no noticeable signs at all) to rather severe; the severe clinical signs are discussed below and outlined in Box 28-8.
      1. Severe oral pain can be associated with primary herpetic gingivostomatitis, and this discomfort results in difficulty in eating and drinking.
      2. The gingival tissues appear swollen (edematous), red (erythematous), and bleed quite easily when disturbed.
      3. Primary herpetic gingivostomatitis is accompanied by painful oral ulcers. Careful inspection of the gingival tissue can reveal small clusters of blisters (vesicles) on the tissues that burst, leaving numerous, painful oral ulcers. The ulcers are surrounded by a red halo.
         a. The ulcers can occur on lips, palate, and tongue as well as the gingival tissue.
         b. Pain caused by these ulcers can be such a major problem that eating and drinking can be impaired. Restricting fluids can even lead to dehydration, and dehydration in a child can be a serious medical emergency.
      4. In the more severe clinical manifestation, this infection is associated with signs and symptoms such as elevated body temperature, a vague feeling of discomfort (malaise), headache, and swollen lymph nodes (lymphadenopathy).
   B. **Treatment.** Treatment of patients with primary herpetic gingivostomatitis is primarily supportive (i.e., designed to keep the patient as comfortable as possible until the viral infection runs its course). Typical steps in the management of a patient with primary herpetic gingivostomatitis are discussed below and outlined in Box 28-9.

1. *The dental hygienist should keep in mind that primary herpetic gingivostomatitis is contagious,* and any plan for periodontal debridement of the teeth should be postponed until the initial infection regresses (26,27).

2. In young children, herpes simplex virus is transmitted primarily by contact with infected saliva. Precautions should be taken to protect others in the home, daycare center, or other environment in which the patient may encounter other children. Contact should be avoided with the child's mouth, as a painful cross-infection can occur on the fingers or nail cuticle if infected oral membranes are touched (Fig. 28-10). Dental assistants and hygienists must maintain universal precautions for infection control, and parents or guardians should be informed as well.

3. Primary herpetic gingivostomatitis usually regresses spontaneously (goes away without treatment) in approximately 2 weeks. Controlling discomfort and ensuring fluid intake are the main focus for supportive treatment.

4. Topical oral anesthetics can be used to control oral discomfort temporarily to allow the patient to eat or drink fluids. Examples of topical anesthetics that can be used are (1) 2% Lidocaine viscous and (2) Orabase with benzocaine (28,29).

5. In some patients, treatment will include antiviral medications (acyclovir), medications to reduce fever (antipyretics), and systemic medications to control pain (analgesics) (30,31).

6. In 2007, over 20,000 patients had hospital emergency department visits with a diagnosis of herpetic gingivostomatitis. Physicians should be trained to diagnose, manage, and refer patients. Improving access to dental care is crucial to managing this problem (32).

Box 28-8. Clinical Signs of Primary Herpetic Gingivostomatitis

- Oral pain with difficulty in eating and drinking
- Edematous gingival tissues (swollen gingival tissue)
- Bleeding from gingival tissue
- Vesicles (blisters) and ulceration of the gingival tissue and sometimes the lips, tongue, and palate; ulcerations surrounded by red halo
- Elevated body temperature
- Malaise (vague feeling of discomfort)
- Swollen lymph nodes

Box 28-9. Typical Steps in Management of Primary Herpetic Gingivostomatitis

1. Keep in mind that this disease is highly contagious.
2. Primary herpetic gingivostomatitis regresses spontaneously in about 2 weeks.
3. Control oral discomfort. Topical oral anesthetics can be used for temporary relief of oral discomfort, so that the patient can eat and drink fluids.
4. Recommend frequent fluid intake to avoid dehydration.
5. Refer the patient to a physician if systemic symptoms are severe or if the patient is unable to tolerate fluid intake.

Chapter Summary Statement

This chapter discussed some acute periodontal conditions that can bring patients to the office for an emergency visit. All members of the dental team should be on alert for these conditions. The dental hygienist may encounter some of these conditions in their earliest stages during routine treatment visits. Acute periodontal conditions include abscesses of the periodontium, necrotizing periodontal diseases, and primary herpetic gingivostomatitis.

Section 5
Focus on Patients

Clinical Patient Care

CASE 1

During a routine patient visit for periodontal maintenance, you note that there is swelling in the interdental papilla between a patient's two central incisors. The swelling is quite localized to the area between the incisors. As you manipulate the tissues, you note pus coming from the sulcus of one of the central incisors. You also note some mobility of one of the incisor teeth. When questioned, the patient informs you that she is aware that these tissues are swollen and that she has been flossing more in hope that the swelling would go down. In view of these clinical findings, how should you proceed at this maintenance visit?

CASE 2

A patient with necrotizing ulcerative gingivitis (NUG) is referred to you by the dentist for calculus removal. Your examination of the patient reveals ulceration of most interdental papillae with the typical punched-out papillae often seen with this disease. The necrotic tissue pseudomembrane is present covering the ulcerations, and heavy calculus deposits are evident. The patient is quite uncomfortable. How should you proceed with the calculus removal?

Evidence in Action

A concerned mother, who is one of your maintenance patients, brings her 3-year-old daughter to the office. An examination reveals that the child has primary herpetic gingivostomatitis.

Her mouth is very painful to the touch and she has an elevated temperature. What patient education would you provide to the child's mother? What treatment recommendations should the dental team make?

Ethical Dilemma

You are in your last semester of dental hygiene school, and the clinic has booked your morning appointment. Your patient is Josh K, a 21-year-old senior premed student who attends your university. As you review Josh's health history, he tells you that he is extremely stressed, as he has been studying for his MCATS, for entrance to medical school, as well as completing all of his papers and projects that are due before he graduates. He admits to eating poorly, due to his busy schedule, as well as feeling very fatigued. He is getting very little sleep, only about 3 hours per night, just trying to keep up and get everything done. He has scheduled his appointment today as his gums have become very sore and are bleeding. He tells you that he is just very uncomfortable.

Your clinical examination reveals that Josh's interdental papilla seem to have a "punched-out" appearance. There also appears to be a gray-white layer covering his gingival tissue. During your examination, even the slightest manipulation of his gingival tissues causes bleeding. Josh also presents with swollen lymph nodes, an elevated temperature, and extreme halitosis.

Although the clinical dentist is on vacation this week and did not examine Josh, you remember from your Periodontology class that these classic symptoms and appearance of his tissue appear to be consistent with a necrotizing periodontal disease. You excitedly tell Josh your diagnosis, and once you have finished his assessments, reappoint him for treatment next week.

You meet your roommate Maeve, who is also a dental hygiene student, for dinner in the cafeteria after clinic. You tell her all about Josh, and his classic textbook case of NUG. You decide to become "Poster Presentation" partners, and NUG will be your topic. You plan to take before and after photographs of Josh's gingiva for your poster.

1. How would you explain necrotizing periodontal disease to Josh?
2. What are the typical treatment steps for a patient with Necrotizing Ulcerative Gingivitis?
3. Are there ethical principles are in conflict in this dilemma?

References

1. Elangovan S, Nalliah R, Allareddy V, et al. Outcomes in patients visiting hospital emergency departments in the United States because of periodontal conditions. *J Periodontol.* 2011;82(6):809–819. doi:10.1902/jop.2010.100228.
2. Parameter on acute periodontal diseases. American Academy of Periodontology. *J Periodontol.* 2000;71(5 suppl):863–866. doi:10.1902/jop.2000.71.5-S.863.
3. Ahl DR, Hilgeman JL, Snyder JD. Periodontal emergencies. *Dent Clin North Am.* 1986;30(3):459–472.
4. Silva GL, Soares RV, Zenobio EG. Periodontal abscess during supportive periodontal therapy: a review of the literature. *J Contemp Dent Pract.* 2008;9(6):82–91.
5. Herrera D, Roldan S, Sanz M. The periodontal abscess: a review. *J Clin Periodontol.* 2000;27(6):377–386.
6. Valyi P, Gorzo I. [Periodontal abscess: etiology, diagnosis and treatment]. *Fogorv Sz.* 2004;97(4):151–155.
7. Antonelli JR. Acute dental pain, Part II: diagnosis and emergency treatment. *Compendium.* 1990;11(9):526, 528, 530–533.
8. Peltroche-Llacsahuanga H, Reichhart E, Schmitt W, et al. Investigation of infectious organisms causing pericoronitis of the mandibular third molar. *J Oral Maxillofac Surg.* 2000;58(6):611–616.
9. Blakey GH, White RP Jr, Offenbacher S, et al. Clinical/biological outcomes of treatment for pericoronitis. *J Oral Maxillofac Surg.* 1996;54(10):1150–1160.
10. Wade DN, Kerns DG. Acute necrotizing ulcerative gingivitis-periodontitis: a literature review. *Mil Med.* 1998;163(5):337–342.
11. Campbell CM, Stout BM, Deas DE. Necrotizing ulcerative gingivitis: a discussion of four dissimilar presentations. *Tex Dent J.* 2011;128(10):1041–1051.
12. Horning GM, Cohen ME. Necrotizing ulcerative gingivitis, periodontitis, and stomatitis: clinical staging and predisposing factors. *J Periodontol.* 1995;66(11):990–998.doi:10.1902/jop.1995.66.11.990.
13. Rowland RW. Necrotizing ulcerative gingivitis. *Ann Periodontol.* 1999;4(1):65–73; discussion 78. doi:10.1902/annals.1999.4.1.65.
14. Hooper PA, Seymour GJ. The histopathogenesis of acute ulcerative gingivitis. *J Periodontol.* 1979;50(8):419–423. doi:10.1902/jop.1979.50.8.419.

15. Kumar A, Masamatti SS, Virdi MS. Periodontal diseases in children and adolescents: a clinician's perspective part 2. *Dent Update.* 2012;39(9):639–642, 645–646, 49–52.

16. Berres F, Marinello CP. [Necrotizing ulcerative periodontitis. Diagnosis, treatment and follow-up–a case report]. *Schweiz Monatsschr Zahnmed.* 2004;114(5):479–495.

17. Novak MJ. Necrotizing ulcerative periodontitis. *Ann Periodontol.* 1999;4(1):74–78. doi:10.1902/annals.1999.4.1.74.

18. Barr CE, Robbins MR. Clinical and radiographic presentations of HIV-1 necrotizing ulcerative periodontitis. *Spec Care Dentist.* 1996;16(6):237–241.

19. Feller L, Lemmer J, Wood NH, et al. Necrotizing gingivitis of Kaposi sarcoma affected gingivae. *SADJ.* 2006;61(7):314–317.

20. Gowdey G, Alijanian A. Necrotizing ulcerative periodontitis in an HIV patient. *J Calif Dent Assoc.* 1995;23(1):57–59.

21. Kolokotronis A, Doumas S. Herpes simplex virus infection, with particular reference to the progression and complications of primary herpetic gingivostomatitis. *Clin Microbiol Infect.* 2006;12(3):202–211. doi:10.1111/j.1469–0691.2005.01336.x.

22. Mohan RP, Verma S, Singh U, et al. Acute primary herpetic gingivostomatitis. *BMJ Case Rep.* 2013;2013. doi:10.1136/bcr-2013-200074.

23. Tovaru S, Parlatescu I, Tovaru M, et al. Primary herpetic gingivostomatitis in children and adults. *Quintessence Int.* 2009;40(2):119–124.

24. Usatine RP, Tinitigan R. Nongenital herpes simplex virus. *Am Fam Physician.* 2010;82(9):1075–1082.

25. Chauvin PJ, Ajar AH. Acute herpetic gingivostomatitis in adults: a review of 13 cases, including diagnosis and management. *J Can Dent Assoc.* 2002;68(4):247–251.

26. Browning WD, McCarthy JP. A case series: herpes simplex virus as an occupational hazard. *J Esthet Restor Dent.* 2012;24(1):61–66. doi:10.1111/j.1708–8240.2011.00469.x.

27. Lewis MA. Herpes simplex virus: an occupational hazard in dentistry. *Int Dent J.* 2004;54(2):103–111.

28. Faden H. Management of primary herpetic gingivostomatitis in young children. *Pediatr Emerg Care.* 2006;22(4):268–269. doi:10.1097/01.pec.0000218982.46225.f5.

29. Stoopler ET, Balasubramaniam R. Topical and systemic therapies for oral and perioral herpes simplex virus infections. *J Calif Dent Assoc.* 2013;41(4):259–262.

30. Blevins JY. Primary herpetic gingivostomatitis in young children. *Pediatr Nurs.* 2003;29(3):199–202.

31. Nasser M, Fedorowicz Z, Khoshnevisan MH, Shahiri Tabarestani M. Acyclovir for treating primary herpetic gingivostomatitis. *Cochrane Database Syst Rev.* 2008;(4):CD006700. doi:10.1002/14651858.CD006700.pub2.

32. Elangovan S, Karimbux NY, Srinivasan S, et al. Hospital-based emergency department visits with herpetic gingivostomatitis in the United States. *Oral Surg Oral Med Oral Pathol Oral Radiol.* 2012;113(4):505–511. doi:10.1016/j.oooo.2011.09.014.

 ## STUDENT ANCILLARY RESOURCES

A wide variety of resources to enhance your learning and understanding of this chapter are available on thePoint®.

- Visit thePoint to access:
  - Audio Glossary
  - Animations
  - Suggested Readings
  - Answers to Review Questions
  - Case Studies

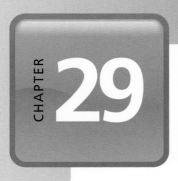

CHAPTER

29 Using Motivational Interviewing to Enhance Patient Behavior Change

Clinical Application. Behaviors such as effective plaque biofilm removal, adherence to regular professional periodontal maintenance visits, periodontal risk factor reduction, and healthy lifestyle habits are crucial issues for dental hygienists to address in their patient encounters. Effective management of the periodontal patient requires both knowledge of the disease process and understanding of human behavior and motivation to foster healthy oral self-care practices in patients. Motivational interviewing as discussed in this chapter can be a useful tool for hygienists to employ when attempting to enhance behavior change in patients.

Learning Objectives

- Recognize the role of ambivalence in patient behavior change and explain the goal of motivational interviewing with respect to ambivalence.
- Describe the primary difference between how hygienists often approach patient education and the motivational interviewing approach.
- Be able to identify the four key elements of the motivational interviewing philosophy, the five core skills and the four overlapping processes.
- Give examples of specific motivational interviewing methods and how they are used to enhance patient motivation for change.

Key Terms

Motivational interviewing
Patient-centered
Guiding style
Ambivalence
Partnership
Acceptance
Compassion

Evocation
Open-ended questions
Reflective listening
Affirm
Summarize
Elicit, Provide, Elicit
Engaging

Focusing
Evoking
Planning
Change talk
Sustain talk
Developing discrepancy

Section 1
Introduction to Human Behavior Change

Patients with periodontal disease often are advised to change certain behaviors—use tuft-end toothbrushes or stop smoking—in order to promote periodontal health. The dynamics of behavior change are among the most rewarding and most challenging encounters for dental hygienists. Chronic periodontitis is largely preventable, but prevention often requires that the patient becomes actively involved in making and maintaining changes in his or her lifestyle habits.

It is very common for the dental hygienist to encounter periodontal patients who do not use effective oral self-care measures or adhere to recommendations for professional periodontal maintenance. In order to persuade patients to improve, the dental hygienist often attempts to educate patients regarding the importance of these recommendations. Unfortunately the provision of education and expert advice alone are rarely sufficient to activate the patient and bring about the desired patient behavior change. All too often a dynamic develops in which the dental hygienist takes on the role of "the persuader" arguing for change while the patient takes on the role of "the resistor," shooting down all suggestions, and providing a long list of reasons why he or she can't follow the recommendations. Patients may also resist passively by not engaging and simply ignoring the attempt to persuade them. In the end, patients may become more resistant while dental hygienists may become frustrated and even convinced that addressing behavior change is futile (Fig. 29-1).

Although it is tempting to blame the patient for being resistant, a wealth of research suggests the explanation for why patients struggle with health behavior change is far more complex. Patients' motivation is a function of numerous factors ranging from past life experiences (e.g., attitudes, beliefs, and habits developed over time); to current situational constraints (e.g., lack of time, financial resources, health literacy and knowledge); to a lack of confidence and skills to make the necessary behavior change (1,2). Furthermore, the interpersonal communication style of a healthcare provider can play an important role in fostering or undermining patient motivation (3,4).

Dental hygienists typically approach patient education in a persuasive, directive manner offering facts about oral disease and unsolicited advice on prescriptive strategies to encourage oral health behavior change. The dental hygienist is the "expert" and the patient is the "recipient" of the expertise. When patients are not ready for behavior change, this directive, persuasive style can often induce feelings of embarrassment, guilt, or even shame, if they are not willing or able to make the change being recommended. Not surprisingly the patient response is often defensive (Fig. 29-2) and he/she may tune out the hygienist's recommendations, or delay return for professional therapy (5–8). Studies have shown that approximately 30% to 60% of health information provided in the clinician/patient encounter is forgotten within an hour and that patients and providers differ significantly in their recall about dental advice given and agreed upon actions for the future (9,10). Not surprisingly 50% of health recommendations provided by clinicians are not followed (10). For patients lacking in readiness or motivation, alternatives to the expert-oriented, directive, educational approach are needed. One empirically supported alternative is motivational interviewing (6).

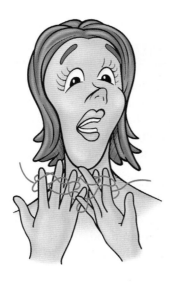

Figure 29-1. The Self-Care Struggle. Patients often struggle with professional recommendations for self-care—such as flossing—leading to frustration or even resistance to oral self-care routines.

Dental hygienists typically approach patient education in a persuasive, directive manner offering facts about oral disease and unsolicited advice on prescriptive strategies to encourage oral health behavior change. The dental hygienist is the "expert" and the patient is the "recipient" of the expertise. When patients are not ready for behavior change, this directive, persuasive style can often induce feelings of embarrassment, guilt, or even shame, if they are not willing or able to make the change being recommended. Not surprisingly the patient response is often defensive (Fig. 29-2) and he/she may tune out the hygienist's recommendations, or delay return for professional therapy (5–8). Studies have shown that approximately 30% to 60% of health information provided in the clinician/patient encounter is forgotten within an hour and that patients and providers differ significantly in their recall about dental advice given and agreed upon actions for the future (9,10). Not surprisingly 50% of health recommendations provided by clinicians are not followed (9). For patients lacking in readiness or motivation, alternatives to the expert-oriented, directive, educational approach are needed. One empirically supported alternative is motivational interviewing (5).

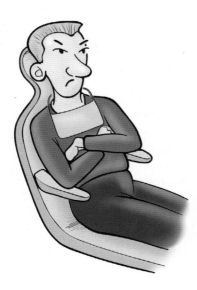

Figure 29-2. Defensive Patient Response. Health education advice alone usually creates defensiveness in the patient.

WHAT IS MOTIVATIONAL INTERVIEWING?

Motivational interviewing (MI) is defined as "a patient-centered counseling style for addressing the common problem of ambivalence about change" (6). At its core, the motivational interviewing (MI) approach to counseling is "patient-centered," which means that the consideration of behavior change is viewed from the patient's perspective rather than the clinician's perspective. For example, the clinician may wish that a patient did not smoke, as smoking is a major risk factor for periodontitis. The patient, on the other hand, might like to have healthier gums but enjoys smoking too much to quit. The clinician's reasons why the patient should make a change—though they may be excellent—are considered far less important than the reasons the patient sees for and against change.

The clinician's goal is to develop a clear understanding of the patient's perspective on the possibility of change. Although the approach is patient-centered, MI is not "nondirective" because the clinician DOES attempt to influence or encourage the patient toward healthy behavior change. One might think of this patient-centered approach as being somewhere along a continuum between "following," where the clinician mainly listens to the patient, and "directing," where the clinician tells or prescribes what the patient should do differently (11).

In MI, a guiding style is used to explore the ambivalence or pros and cons of change that the patient sees. Patients often feel ambivalent about behavior change—that is, they have mixed feelings and attitudes toward behavior change. Specific methods are used to foster the patient's intrinsic or "internal" motivation. Fostering the patient's internal motivation increases the likelihood that his or her ambivalence about changing will be resolved in the direction of change.

One of the underlying assumptions of MI is that ambivalence is typical in ANY change process (e.g., how do you feel about the need to eat at least five servings of fruit and vegetables every day, or exercise for 40 minutes 5 to 7 days a week?). It also assumes in MI that, when possible, patients tend to move naturally toward health. In other words the assumption is that most people WANT to be healthy, though they may not always feel motivated enough or capable enough of achieving it at any particular point in time. In MI the clinician attempts to tap into and enhance any natural internal desire for healthy change in patients.

EMPIRICAL SUPPORT FOR MOTIVATIONAL INTERVIEWING

Meta-analyses indicate that MI is effective for a range of behavioral outcomes including various health promoting behaviors, smoking cessation, and treatment engagement (12,13).

Recent studies have addressed MI related to oral care behavior change. One of the first studies published compared MI to traditional health education among mothers of young children at high risk for dental caries. This study found a significant reduction in early childhood caries among those receiving MI counseling at 1 year; however, at the 2-year evaluation, results were not significantly different despite a trend in caries rate difference of 35% for MI compared to 52% for traditional education (14,15).

Evidence for MI effectiveness with periodontal patients has been largely positive. Almomani et al. (16) examined the efficacy of MI for improving oral self-care in a sample of individuals with severe mental illness. Results revealed that at a single MI session prior to an oral health education session significantly enhanced motivation for regular brushing, increased oral health knowledge, and reduced plaque scores compared to oral health education alone. Similar effects were achieved in two studies of chronic periodontal patients. In a proof-of-concept, case study design over time, two patients, with bleeding on probing values of 68% and 83%, respectively, were provided with an MI intervention that included oral care practice in multiple sessions. Results showed statistically significant reductions in plaque and gingival index scores for both patients, with changes being maintained over a 24-month period (17). These authors used a similar MI intervention in an evaluator blind, randomized clinical trial with 113 subjects compared to usual care. Results at 1 year showed that gingival index and plaque index scores for the MI intervention group were significantly improved compared to a usual care control (18).

In contrast, two separate randomized clinical trials, both of which used a single MI session with periodontal patients, failed to show superiority of MI adjunctive to oral health education compared to oral health education, alone (19,20). In both of these studies, participants showed an improvement in periodontal measures, irrespective of group assignment. The reason hypothesized for the lack of superiority of MI adjunctive to health education was twofold. First the periodontal patients who were referred for specialty periodontal care and successfully followed up had already demonstrated motivation to improve their oral health; additionally, for some patients, multiple sessions may be needed to induce sustainable behavior change. A recent meta-analysis that examined the effect of MI across multiple health behaviors concluded that there does appear to be a dose–response effect to MI, with increased MI sessions or increased treatment time related to improved outcomes (13). Given that hygienists often see periodontal patients for multiple appointments during the active treatment phase, and then again at regular intervals for periodontal maintenance, implementing multiple sessions of MI may be ideally suited to periodontal care.

One concern of many health practitioners is whether MI can be effective in a healthcare setting where clinicians are not trained counselors and time is short. Teaching MI skills to dental hygiene students as an integral part of the curriculum is increasing in the United States and abroad. A recent report on the experience of implementing a new curriculum that teaches MI for behavior change showed that teaching MI skills is viewed as positive by faculty and students alike. More critically, standardized patient assessment of the students' ability to activate patients was significantly greater for students who received MI training compared to those that had traditional health education training (21). A meta-analysis also indicates that noncounselors can be effective when using MI with a significant effect in 80%of studies where MI was delivered by physicians (22). With respect to time, as little as 15 minutes has been shown to be effective in the majority of studies (12,22).

Section 2
Components of Motivational Interviewing

The philosophy or "spirit" of MI is captured in four key elements. The first element is **partnership** between the patient and clinician. In the MI approach, the clinician actively attempts to diminish his or her expert role. It is necessary to collaborate because the patient, not the clinician, is viewed as the expert on his or her life and the challenges of the behavior change in question. The second element is deep **acceptance** of the patient and their behavioral choices. Acceptance includes avoiding judgment, supporting the patient's autonomy, understanding the patient's perspective, and affirming their strengths and efforts. Third, MI is used only for the welfare of patients, which is referred to as **compassion**. The fourth element is **evocation**, in which the clinician encourages the patient to disclose their perspective and internal motivation rather than attempting to persuade or instill motivation "from the outside."

Although it is sometimes easy for a healthcare provider to feel responsible for a patient's decisions, it is ultimately not the clinician's choice or life. Patients are far more likely to choose and succeed with behavior change when they have voiced their own reasons for change and made their own decision to commit. In MI, the focus of the clinician is not on the desired healthcare outcome but on facilitating a meaningful conversation that provides the greatest opportunity for a patient to consider change. The final decision for change rests with the patient. The clinician may communicate respect for the patient's autonomy directly such as "*So how would you like to proceed?*" or indirectly such as at the beginning of the visit by asking permission to talk about oral self-care (Fig. 29-3).

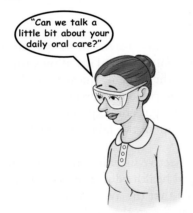

Figure 29-3. Asking Permission. Starting with asking the patient's permission can help foster a collaborative partnership.

CORE SKILLS OF MOTIVATIONAL INTERVIEWING

MI requires skill in a set of core communication skills that are used in strategic ways throughout the conversation.

Open-Ended Questions

Open-ended questions (questions that are framed to avoid a simple yes/no response) are preferred in MI. For example, "*How do you feel about using dental floss?*" "*How does brushing and flossing fit into your routine*" rather than "*Do you use dental floss?*" or "*Do you brush twice a day?*" The open-ended style of questioning encourages patients to elaborate and provides much more information to the clinician regarding the patient's perspective (Fig. 29-4).

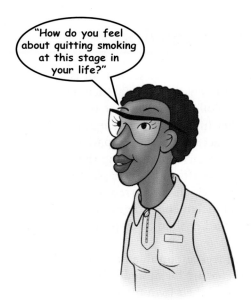

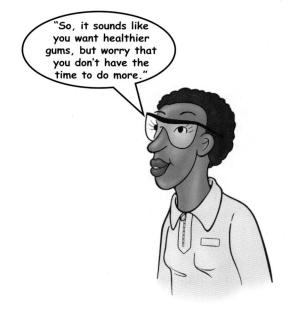

Figure 29-4. Use of Open-Ended Questions. Open-ended questions—that cannot be answered with a simple "yes" or "no" response—encourage the patient to provide additional information.

Figure 29-5. Reflecting Listening. By paraphrasing the patient's remarks, the clinician can double check if she understands the meaning of the patient's comments correctly.

Reflective Listening

Reflective listening is the process in which the healthcare provider listens to the patient's remarks and then paraphrases what the clinician heard the patient say. This allows the clinician to check with the patient that he or she is "getting the patient's message right," ensuring that the clinician is developing a good picture of the patient's perspective (Fig. 29-5). Reflective listening has the effect of validating the patient, expressing understanding (or empathy), and typically encourages the patient to elaborate, so that the clinician can learn more.

Through the process of open-ended questioning and reflective listening, the clinician can begin to shift from a clinician-centered approach to oral health education to a patient-centered view of oral health education. Research has shown that the average healthcare provider interrupts patient disclosures after 18 seconds (10). When this occurs, it sends a clear message that the patient's input is not respected nor seen as relevant. Affirming the patient's efforts and interest or willingness to seek care increases the patient's sense of trust. Once trust is established the patient can honestly express him/herself and begin to openly resolve ambivalence (mixed feelings) about change.

Affirm

In MI, the patient's strengths and efforts should be affirmed (acknowledged) to communicate support to the patient for discussing something difficult (i.e., a change about which they may feel embarrassment, guilt, and ambivalence). Expressing appreciation for the patient taking the time to be there, or being willing to discuss their smoking, or taking some small steps toward change can enhance the therapeutic relationship and encourage the patient to engage further in the counseling process.

Summarize

Brief **summaries** are used in MI to link and reinforce what has been discussed and provide an opportunity for the clinician to demonstrate empathy (e.g., *"So I think I now have a fairly good picture of how you view your smoking…."*). Summaries can be used to move the conversation in a new direction (e.g., the summary can lead to a statement like *"So given what we've talked about so far, what are your thoughts about the next step…?"* or tie different elements of the conversation together (e.g., after summarizing the patient's perspective on the difficulties of brushing regularly, the clinician might link to an earlier part of the conversation on the patient's dislike of the pain that he is experiencing: *"So it sounds like it's a real challenge to get a good brushing routine but at the same time you are really unhappy with the pain you are experiencing…."*).

Providing Information and Advice

Although the provision of information and advice should be done with caution—to avoid taking the expert role and to avoid the pitfall of pressing for change—there are nevertheless occasions when providing information is appropriate. For example, providing information may be necessary when the patient asks for information, or when motivation might be enhanced by new information that might help in overcoming obstacles to change. To avoid "taking on the expert role," the clinician can ask permission first: *"Would you be interested in hearing some more information about the benefits of quitting smoking for your oral health?"* (Fig. 29-6). The clinician avoids the "expert role" by referring to other sources for the information such as *"Many patients tell me…."* or *"Research seems to indicate…"* rather than saying *"I have found…"* or *"I would recommend…"*

A three-step process known as "**Elicit, Provide, Elicit**" is also a useful method for delivering information and advice in an MI consistent manner. The first step (Elicit) involves enquiring what the patient already knows. For example, *"What have you heard about the benefits of flossing on a daily basis?"* The second step (Provide) involves providing relevant information and advice: *"Yes you are right, those are some good reasons to floss daily. There are also some other reasons dental hygienists encourage flossing for cases like yours, such as…."* The final step (Elicit) involves checking back with the patient to see what they have taken from the information or advice provided. For example, *"So I'm wondering what you think about that research and how it applies to you?"*

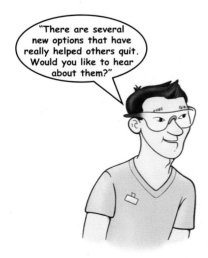

"There are several new options that have really helped others quit. Would you like to hear about them?"

Figure 29-6. Providing information or advice. In this example the clinician supports the patient's autonomy by asking permission before providing information.

FOUR PROCESSES OF MOTIVATIONAL INTERVIEWING

The method of MI involves four overlapping processes. The method begins with engaging in which a helpful rapport is established that serves as the foundation for everything that follows. Engaging leads to the process of focusing or establishing a direction or goal for behavior change. With the goal in mind the process of evoking is used to elicit the patient's motivation for change. When patients become sufficiently interested in making change the process of planning can begin involving the fostering of commitment and developing a specific plan of action for change. The processes are not a rigid sequential roadmap. Any of the processes can be engaged in throughout the conversation as needed.

Engaging

Patient engagement can be encouraged or discouraged depending on the clinician approach. For example, asking a series of specific questions that the patient is obliged to answer discourages their involvement in a collaborative dialog. In MI the clinician is encouraged to focus on eliciting and listening to the patient's perspective. An open-ended question can be used to initiate the discussion (e.g., *"What kinds of problems have you been having with your teeth lately?"*). Reflective listening can then be used to encourage the patient to elaborate while at the same time communicating empathy and acceptance (e.g., *"You've noticed that your gums are bleeding a lot."*). During the listening process the clinician pays attention to any opportunities to affirm the patient for any strengths or efforts (e.g., *"You've really been making an effort to try to brush more regularly."*). Summaries can be used to tie the conversation together highlighting the most relevant parts of the patient's story.

Focusing

To employ MI effectively, it is essential to have the behavior change goal or goals in mind. Focusing is the process of clarifying, in collaboration with the patient, what direction the conversation should take. A guiding style can be used to explore the patients' preferences, concerns, and priorities while considering the clinicians' concerns and priorities. For example, taking into account both patient and clinician perspectives the clinician may offer a range of alternative options for discussion (e.g., *"Based on what you have told me it sounds like we should decide what is most important to focus on today. We could talk about some of the challenges you're having with your brushing and flossing routine, we could discuss how to go about changing some of your eating habits to protect your teeth and gums, or we could talk about your smoking and how I could perhaps be of some help."*). During focusing it can also be necessary to provide information to the patient that can inform the direction that should be taken. The clinician can use the "elicit, provide, elicit" method to accomplish this in an MI consistent style.

Evoking

The assumption in MI is that most patients are ambivalent about change and the role of the clinician is to elicit or evoke their internal motivation as well as their confidence for making a change. Integral to this process is the encouragement or evoking of statements in the direction of change, referred to as change talk (e.g., *"I know smoking is bad for me; I would like to do a better job with taking care of my teeth."*). Research indicates that change talk is predictive of actual behavior change (6,23). As indicated above, the assumption is that most individuals have mixed feelings about change. Those patients having mixed feelings (pros and cons) about change implies that they do have some reasons or desire for change. The task of the clinician is to evoke, facilitate, and strengthen this desire for change. Change talk can be elicited with simple open-ended questions such as "*What advantages do you see of cutting back on sugary foods?*"

Another approach is to use the "motivation" or "importance ruler" in which the clinician asks "On a scale of 0 to 10 with 10 being most important, how important is to you to improve your oral self-care habits?" (Fig. 29-7).

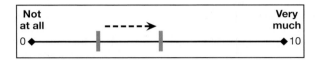

Figure 29-7. A Motivation Ruler. A motivation ruler is a method for facilitating change talk.

Once the patient identifies the self-rated importance of change, the clinician elicits change talk by asking, "*What made you pick three rather than zero?*" Rather than asking why the patient is NOT at 10, this open-ended question encourages the patient to express any importance that he or she DOES place on improving oral self-care behaviors. After eliciting and reflecting change talk, barriers to change can also be explored by asking, "*What would it take for you to increase the importance two or three additional levels?*" This approach can also be used to evoke confidence (or self-efficacy) in engaging in a new behavior, which is also often a key contributor to an individual's motivation to change.

In general, once the clinician has elicited change talk the goal is to encourage even more change talk. Reflective listening is very effective means of achieving this goal and the skilled MI clinician can encourage elaboration of a particular aspect of change talk by ending the reflective statement on that topic. For example, a reflection that ends with the change talk such as "*On the one hand you really love sugary foods, but on the other hand you really want to set a good example to your children.*" encourages elaboration by the patient of the desire to set a good example rather than the love of sugary foods because the change talk is reflected at the end of the reflective statement.

This example highlights another element of MI, which is how to respond to the opposite of change talk or "**sustain talk**" (e.g., "*I don't have enough time to floss every day.*"). These statements are often thought of as "resistance" but from an MI perspective they are merely an indication of the ambivalence that is assumed to be a normal part of behavior change. When the patient expresses reasons not to change, this is an ideal opportunity to listen well and explore the patient's perspective rather than attempting to persuade or provide counter arguments. This can be accomplished in various ways but most simply by using reflective listening (Fig. 29-8). Typically patients who have been validated after expressing their reasons for not changing are then much more ready to talk about reasons why they might want to change.

Evoking confidence is also essential for encouraging behavior change because individuals do not make efforts to change unless they believe they can succeed (2). Confidence can be evoked in various ways including brainstorming possible solutions, providing information and advice, or reviewing past successes.

Evoking may also involve "**developing discrepancy**" in which inconsistencies between a patient's values and goals and their current behavior is explored to enhance motivation for change. For example, most patients want to be healthy even though they may have chronic periodontitis and poor oral self-care. Similarly, they may want to avoid painful or unpleasant visits for dental care yet have poor oral self-care habits. The discrepancy between what would be ideal (e.g., be healthy or have no pain) and the status quo (poor self-care that results in periodontitis or pain and unpleasant visits for dental care) represents internal motivation for change that can be elicited or highlighted through open-ended questions and reflective listening (Fig. 29-9). For example, the hygienist might highlight the discrepancy with this reflection: "*It sounds like you find it hard to stick with the thorough brushing and flossing each day, but you would really like to have healthy gums.*"

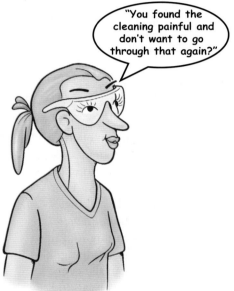

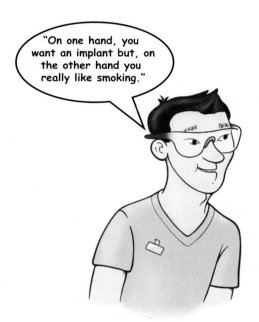

Figure 29-8. Reflecting Sustain Talk. When a patient expresses hesitation about change, the clinician should listen well and explore the patient's point of view rather than attempting to persuade the patient that change is needed.

Figure 29-9. Develop Discrepancy. Open-ended questions and reflective listening can highlight discrepancies between what would be ideal (e.g., improved periodontal health) and the status quo (continuing to smoke).

Planning

The process of planning for change can begin when there are signs of patient readiness such as increased change talk, less sustain talk, small steps taken toward change, and questions about change. With sensitivity to any renewed patient ambivalence that might call for a return to one of the earlier processes, the clinician guides the patient to consider whether they want to make a change and how that change will occur. Effective planning involves discussing with the patient the precise "how?" and "when?" of making the change. For example, rather than simply agreeing with the patient that they will "try to do a better job of brushing" the clinician might help the patient to work out a specific plan that will increase the likelihood of brushing (e.g., to brush right after eating dinner rather than waiting until just before going to bed when they feel too tired to do even one more thing). Once the plan is developed the clinician will attempt to strengthen commitment to the plan by evoking intention and commitment from the patient (e.g., "*What do you think of that strategy?* or *"Does it sound like something you want to try?"*).

Section 3
Implications for Dental Hygiene Practice

Moving from the clinician-centered perspective of oral health education to the patient-centered view of behavior change can enhance the patient's internal motivation for healthy behavior change. If the hygienist judges, lectures, and directs, the patient ceases to engage in dialog and be part of the solution. Ironically, this can result in yet more directive advice giving from the clinician. Using MI, the hygienist can engage in a more productive interaction in which he or she no longer feels responsible (and frustrated!) about the patient's decisions. Instead, the hygienist focuses on encouraging the patient to examine his or her attitudes about periodontal disease or the periodontal maintenance schedule.

MOTIVATIONAL INTERVIEWING: EXAMPLE 1

Mrs. J. is a 50-year-old attorney who has been referred to your periodontal dental office for evaluation and treatment. Mrs. J. has type 2 diabetes, a glycosylated hemoglobin value (HbA1c) of 8, and moderately severe chronic periodontitis. Mrs. J. has been sporadic in visiting her regular dentist and the letter from the referring dentist states that after a 1-year absence Mrs. J. presented recently with increased bleeding on probing and evidence of increasing attachment loss. The general dentist is concerned that without periodontal therapy, Mrs. J. will likely lose several teeth.

> **Hygienist:** I see that your general dentist has referred you here for periodontal treatment. Can you tell me a little about your past dental care and why you are here today?
>
> **Mrs. J.:** Yes, Dr. Smith thinks that if I don't get specialty treatment I'm going to lose some of my back teeth. I take care of my teeth and I think he's overreacting to my gums bleeding a bit more than usual.
>
> **Hygienist:** I am very happy you followed up with Dr. Smith and came in to see us (Affirmation). So if it's okay with you, I'd like to spend a little time talking about the health of your gums (Getting permission).
>
> **Mrs. J.:** That's fine with me.
>
> **Hygienist:** Good. So, if you would, can you tell me what is a typical day like for you and how taking care of your teeth fits into your normal day? (Open-ended question.)
>
> **Mrs. J.:** Sure. Most days I need to be at my office by 8:30, so I generally get up around 7, shower, have some coffee and toast, check emails, brush my teeth, and drive my 20-minute commute to the office. Once I'm at my office, my schedule is really full. I'm currently working on three really difficult cases that take up most of my time. I'm pretty stressed out! I don't eat a regular lunch but will usually snack on a granola bar to hold me over to dinner. I'm usually home around 6:30, have dinner, and then catch up on reading documents for the next day. Sometimes I brush my teeth before bed, but mostly I'm just too exhausted to care at night. I do try, but don't always succeed. The dental hygienist at Dr. Smith's is always on my case about not brushing enough, not flossing enough, and not coming in every 3 months.
>
> **Hygienist:** It sounds like you have a really busy schedule that makes it difficult for you to keep up with recommendations given by Dr. Smith's hygienist. If I

understand you, though, you do make a concerted effort to brush at least every morning (Reflective listening).

Mrs. J.: Yes, I am very good about brushing in the morning.

Hygienist: That's great. It's important to have a routine that works well for you (Affirmation). You mentioned that the hygienist at Dr. Smith's office is concerned about your not flossing enough or coming in every 3 months. Tell me about that (Open-ended questioning).

Mrs. J.: Shelley, that's her name, says that if I don't floss every day and come in to have my teeth scraped every 3 months that I'll end up losing my teeth. She lectures me every time I go in, and I really dread going to see her. I don't think she understands how busy my schedule is. The only reason I agreed to come here was that Dr. Smith thought you might be able to do something to get rid of my pockets.

Hygienist: So, it sounds like you are interested in improving your gum health but don't like being lectured when you go to the dentist (Reflective listening).

Mrs. J.: That's right. I also read in a magazine that diabetes might make my gum disease worse, so I figured it's worth finding out. Is that true? Can my diabetes make my gums worse? Can you get rid of my pockets, so this gum disease will stop?

Hygienist: There is quite a bit of new information about diabetes and periodontal disease, and there are some things that we can do at our office to reduce pockets. Research has shown that controlling gum disease, especially in diabetics, requires professional care but also requires patients to be actively involved in helping control the disease on a day-to-day basis. We have had many patients who have had very good success using this approach. Would you like to know more about it? (Providing information that was requested/Supporting autonomy.)

Mrs. J.: I would like to know more, but I'm skeptical that it's going to be more of the same that I hear from Shelley--"brush, floss, come to see me; brush, floss, come to see me."

Hygienist: Right... you want help but worry that it will still involve more effort on your part than you really have time for (Reflect).

Mrs. J.: Exactly!

Hygienist: Well, I want to emphasize that how we move forward is up to you. The time and effort you put in brushing and flossing is something you will need to determine based on what's most important to you (Support autonomy). If it's ok with you (Support autonomy/Ask permission), I'd like to try to go slowly, try to work with your busy schedule, and help you keep your teeth. After I conduct my exam, I'd also like to give you some information on diabetes and gum disease that you can read before your next visit and then we can talk more about how that might be contributing to your gum disease. Are you interested in that? (Support autonomy/Ask permission.)

Mrs. J.: That sounds good--the magazine article didn't give much detail, but it did say that diabetes can make gum disease worse. I'll make it a point of adding it to my evening reading tonight.

Hygienist: Excellent! I think you might find the information helpful as we work toward getting your gum disease under control.

MOTIVATIONAL INTERVIEWING: EXAMPLE 2

Mr. A. is a 58-year old banker who has come to the dental office wanting an implant for a first molar that was lost to periodontal disease last year. At the time, he was not interested in discussing a replacement but has made an appointment today, as he wants to get an implant for replacement. Although he contends that he brushes and flosses regularly, his oral self-care has only been fair for many years, he has a 30-year tobacco habit, and is currently smoking about 1½ pack of cigarettes a day.

> **Hygienist:** Good morning Mr. A. What brings you in today? (Open-ended questioning.)
>
> **Mr. A.:** Well, you know, I have this missing tooth here and when I chew it really bothers me. You know, food gets stuck up in there and on top of that it just doesn't look good when I smile. A buddy at work told me about implants and I'm seriously interested in getting one.
>
> **Hygienist:** So where that tooth is missing is causing you some problems and you aren't happy with the appearance of that gap (Reflective listening).
>
> **Mr. A.:** Yeah, every time I eat I get food caught. It doesn't hurt, but it's gotten really irritating. I know we talked about it when you took the tooth out, but I don't want a partial. I really want the implant. You mentioned then that my smoking might be a problem with getting an implant.
>
> **Hygienist:** Your friend told you about dental implants and you think it's the right choice for replacing that tooth (Reflective listening).
>
> **Mr. A.:** That's right. I know when I was here before you said that my smoking might be a problem with getting an implant.
>
> **Hygienist:** Yes, smoking is a major barrier for using implants because it makes it much harder for healing to occur and then maintain the health of tissues around the implant. But it sounds like you are really interested in getting an implant (Providing information in response to an implied question/Reflective listening).
>
> **Mr. A.:** I am!
>
> **Hygienist:** Well, can we spend a few minutes talking about your smoking, and what your thoughts and feelings about smoking are? (Asking permission.)
>
> **Mr. A.:** Sure, I'm a smoker and not ashamed of it.
>
> **Hygienist:** Okay, let me put it another way. On the one hand you want an implant but on the other hand you really like smoking? (Developing discrepancy.)
>
> **Mr. A.:** Well I've tried to quit before and it wasn't any fun. I'm not sure I could quit if I wanted to.
>
> **Hygienist:** Okay. You have tried to stop before without any luck, so you have the sense that even if you wanted to try to quit again, you don't think you could. It's something that is very hard for you (Reflective listening).
>
> **Mr. A.:** I went through that agony before and it didn't work. I don't want to put myself through that again.
>
> **Hygienist:** Trying to quit would be too painful and it's not important enough to you to stop right now (Rolling with resistance).
>
> **Mr. A.:** Yes, I enjoy it and haven't had any ill effects from smoking. I'm pretty happy to continue as I am.
>
> **Hygienist:** Well, other than the possible disadvantage that smoking has to getting this implant, are there any other disadvantages that you see to smoking? (Evoking change talk.)
>
> **Mr. A.:** Taxes keep going up, and it's an expensive habit, but I'm willing to pay the price. It's one of my luxuries in life.

Hygienist: Anything else? (Evoking change talk.)

Mr. A.: Only one thing--my kids really want me to quit. They are afraid I'm going to end up with something bad, but I haven't had any ill effects from smoking.

Hygienist: So, it sounds like the cost of smoking bothers you, but not too much, but you really haven't had any health problems. Your family worries though (Reflective listening to evoke more change talk).

Mr. A.: Yes, that's right.

Hygienist: I have the sense that you're not ready to quit right now, but I'd like to learn more regarding your thoughts about smoking if that's ok with you. Where would you put yourself on a scale of 0 to 10 where 0 is "no motivation at all to quit" and 10 is "very motivated"? I know you aren't a 10, but where would you be? (Evoking change talk using the motivation ruler.)

Mr. A.: Hmmmm. I'd probably put myself at a 2 or 3, somewhere in there.

Hygienist: So you have some small amount of motivation to quit--what gives you that level of motivation? (Evoking change talk using the motivation ruler.)

Mr. A.: Well I know that smoking isn't good for me, I'm not dumb. And like I said before, my family really wants me to quit. It would be a nice gesture to do that for my family. They really do have my best interests in mind.

Hygienist: You mentioned that you know smoking isn't good for you and your family worries about health effect. Can you tell me what ill health effects worry you? (Evoking change talk.)

Mr. A.: Sure--cancer and lung disease.

Hygienist: So, there are some disadvantages besides the implant that you've thought about, but you still aren't sufficiently motivated to quit. Earlier, though, you mentioned that you weren't sure that you would be able to quit even if you wanted to (Reflective listening to explore influence of confidence on motivation). How motivated would you be if you were more confident that you could quit?

Mr. A.: I guess if I knew I could succeed with quitting I'd be more motivated.

Hygienist: If we could help you with improving your confidence in quitting, would you find that helpful? (Evoking change talk/Assess interest before providing information or advice to support autonomy.)

Mr. A.: Yes, it might.

Hygienist: There are several options that we could work on to improve your confidence to quit smoking. We could focus on doing that while also discussing the feasibility of the implant. Do you think you might be interested in pursuing this? (Evoke commitment/change talk while supporting autonomy.)

Mr. A.: Sure. I guess I don't have anything to lose.

MOTIVATIONAL INTERVIEWING: EXAMPLE 3

Ms. S. is a 35-year-old administrative assistant at the local community college. She has come to the dental office as a new patient and desires tooth whitening for her "yellowed teeth." During the routine dental evaluation no caries are found; however, there is generalized moderate gingival inflammation with slight bone loss in the interproximal posterior regions. The patient reports that she had a partial "deep cleaning" 2 years ago at her previous dentist but had really sensitive teeth and didn't return for completing treatment.

Hygienist: Hello Ms. S. What brings you to our office? (Open-ended questioning)

Ms. S.: My friend recently came to see you to have his teeth whitened and they look terrific. I haven't been happy with the color of my teeth for a long time, so I thought you could make my smile whiter too.

Hygienist: Okay. Can we first spend a few minutes talking about your mouth and oral health? (Getting permission.)

Ms. S.: Sure, that's fine.

Hygienist: Good. Can you tell me a little about problems you have had and how taking care of your teeth fits into your regular day's events? (Open-ended questioning)

Ms. S.: I have really healthy teeth and have never had any cavities. I'm really not happy with the yellow color of my teeth and want to do something about that.

Hygienist: Anything else?

Ms. S.: Well, the last dentist I went to said I had some gum disease. My gums have always bled when I brush, but they made a big deal out of it. I had to see the hygienist for a deep cleaning, but my teeth got so sensitive afterward, I didn't go back.

Hygienist: Tell me a little more about your gum treatment (Open-ended questioning).

Ms. S.: The dentist and hygienist told me I had to have that deep cleaning or I could lose my teeth. Everyone in my family has gum disease and they still have most of their teeth. I must have inherited it. I'm really only interested in tooth whitening. I don't want any more deep cleanings.

Hygienist: It sounds like the deep cleaning you had was unpleasant and your gum disease is not very important to you (Reflective listening).

Ms. S.: I didn't say it wasn't important--I just want my teeth to look better. My teeth were so sensitive after having half of my mouth deep cleaned, I could barely drink anything with ice in it. If that is what it takes to have healthy gums, I'm happy just as I am.

Hygienist: The effects of the deep cleaning treatment were so bad that you don't want to go through it again even if it means not having healthy gums (Responding to sustain talk with reflective listening).

Ms. S.: It's not that it isn't important. I don't want to lose my teeth, but I also don't want all of that sensitivity. I was thinking that getting my teeth whitened will make me look better and wouldn't hurt as much.

Hygienist: Avoiding pain is really important to you (Responding to sustain talk with reflective listening).

Ms. S.: Yeah, I guess I sound pretty wimpy. My teeth are important but if I have to be in pain for a long time afterward it's not worth it to me.

Hygienist: You want healthy teeth and if you could get your teeth whitened and gum disease treated without a lot of pain afterward, it might be worth doing (Reflective listening).

Ms. S.: If I knew that I could get my gums healthy and not have to go through what I did before, I might be willing to discuss gum treatments. Is that possible?

Hygienist: There are several things that have worked for others to reduce the temperature sensitivity after deep cleaning. Are you interested in learning a little bit more? (Ask permission before providing information.)

Ms. S.: I might be.

Hygienist: All right, let me give you some information and we can talk about strategies for controlling the sensitivity after treatment. We can also talk about a plan for whitening your teeth once we get the gum disease under control. How would that meet your need for appearance and health? (Support autonomy.)

Chapter Summary Statement

A key challenge for dental hygiene practitioners is working with patients to foster behavior change to improve oral self-care. MI provides an empirically supported approach to the challenges of counseling patients for health behavior change. It rests on a foundation of partnership, acceptance, and compassion and uses specific methods such as open-ended questions and reflective listening to evoke patients' own reasons for change. Use of this patient-centered approach to behavior change can enhance the quality of encounters between hygienists and their patients by fostering greater patient motivation for change, and strengthening the patient–provider relationship.

Section 4
Focus on Patients

Clinical Patient Care

CASE 1

Refer to the case of Mrs. J. the 50-year-old attorney to answer the following questions:

1. Why does the hygienist begin with the question "Can you tell me a little about… why you are here today?"
2. Describe Mrs. J's ambivalence regarding behavior change (i.e., what cons AND pros for change does SHE see?).
3. What examples of "change talk" can you identify in the dialog?

CASE 2

Refer to the case of Mr. A. the 58-year-old banker to answer the following questions:

1. When the conversation first turns to smoking the hygienist asks Mr. A. *"Are you sufficiently motivated about the implant to consider stopping smoking?"* This is labeled as an example of "developing discrepancy." What discrepancy does this refer to and how is this meant to foster motivation for change?
2. What is Mr. A's ambivalence regarding behavior change (i.e., what cons AND pros for change does HE see?)
3. Mr. A. provided lots of change talk in the dialog but what turns out to be the key barrier for change that, if the hygienist can help address, will significantly increase his motivation?

CASE 3

Using the information in the case of Ms. S., the 35-year-old administrative assistant, try the following:

1. With a classmate take turns assuming the role of Ms. S. and the hygienist. Practice asking an open-ended question to begin the visit followed by a reflection of Ms. S's response.
2. Ms. S. could benefit from information on how to get her gums healthy while reducing sensitivity. With a classmate practice using the three step "Elicit, Provide, Elicit" process to give her some relevant information.

Ethical Dilemma

Dr. Jasper Greene hired Eden—a recent dental hygiene graduate—to work 4 days a week in his busy dental practice. Dr. Greene employs three other hygienists on a full-time basis, as well as three other dentists.

Dr. Greene was very pleased, as the patients really liked Eden, and he thought that she had excellent clinical skills, especially for a new graduate. Eden was quite happy too and enjoyed the office staff as well as the variety of patients she was treating. She was particularly excited to utilize the method of motivational interviewing, as a means to enhance patient behavior change, specifically as it related to patient self-care. While a student, Eden was praised by her clinical faculty for her exceptional mastery of this technique.

Approximately 3 months later, Dr. Greene had a cancellation and was walking by Eden's operatory while she was using motivational interviewing, and he stopped to listen to the conversation. Eden was working with a new patient, who was scheduled for periodontal instrumentation of deep periodontal pockets, but had a fear of needles, and refused anesthesia. She spent a significant amount of time counseling in a patient-centered manner. Dr. Greene was not familiar with this approach, and quite frankly, disagreed with the patient "calling the shots."

Later that day, Dr. Greene asked Eden to come to his office. He told her that she was to stop all this "mumbo jumbo," and tell each patient what was best for him/her, as she was the expert. He further told her that none of the other hygienists or dentists in the office utilizes this technique, and he requires continuity among his office staff.

Eden was very upset and did not know what to do. On the one hand she loved working for Dr. Greene, but on the other hand, she realized that she was not comfortable compromising her belief of patient-centered counseling and moving her patients naturally toward health.

1. Are there advantages to motivational interviewing?
2. Are there ethical principles in conflict in this dilemma?
3. What is the best way for Eden to handle this ethical dilemma?

References

1. Bandura A. *Self-Efficacy: the Exercise of Control*. New York: W.H. Freeman; 1997. ix: 604.
2. Fishbein M. Factors influencing behavior and behavior change. In: Baum A, Revenson T, Singer J, eds. *Handbook of Health Psychology*. Mahwah, NJ: Lawrence Erlbaum Associates; 2001: xx, 961.
3. Ryan RM, Deci EL. Self-determination theory and the facilitation of intrinsic motivation, social development, and well-being. *Am Psychol*. 2000;55(1):68–78.
4. Williams GC, McGregor HA, Zeldman A, et al. Testing a self-determination theory process model for promoting glycemic control through diabetes self-management. *Health Psychol*. 2004;23(1):58–66.
5. Freeman R. The psychology of dental patient care. 10. Strategies for motivating the non-compliant patient. *Br Dent J*. 1999;187(6):307–312.
6. Miller WR, Rollnick S; MyiLibrary. *Motivational Interviewing Helping People Change*. New York: Guilford Press; 2013. Available from: http://libproxy.temple.edu/login?url = http://lib.myilibrary.com/detail.asp?id = 394471 Connect to MyiLibrary resource.
7. Resnicow K, DiIorio C, Soet JE, et al. Motivational interviewing in health promotion: it sounds like something is changing. *Health Psychol*. 2002;21(5):444–451.
8. Shinitzky HE, Kub J. The art of motivating behavior change: the use of motivational interviewing to promote health. *Public Health Nurs*. 2001;18(3):178–185.
9. Misra S, Daly B, Dunne S, et al. Dentist-patient communication: what do patients and dentists remember following a consultation? Implications for patient compliance. *Patient Prefer Adherence*. 2013;7:543–549.
10. Prounis C. Doctor-patient communication. *Pharmaceutical Executive [Internet]*. 2005. Available from: http://www.pharmexec.com. Accessed April 3, 2015.
11. Rollnick S, Miller WR, Butler C. *Motivational Interviewing in Health Care: Helping Patients Change Behavior*. New York: Guilford Press; 2008: xiv, 210.
12. Lundahl B, Moleni T, Burke BL, et al. Motivational interviewing in medical care settings: a systematic review and meta-analysis of randomized controlled trials. *Patient Educ Couns*. 2013;93(2):157–168.
13. Lundahl W, Kunz C, Brownell C, et al. A meta-analysis of motivational interviewing: twenty-five years of empirical studies. *Res Social Work Prac*. 2010;20(2):137–160.
14. Weinstein P, Harrison R, Benton T. Motivating parents to prevent caries in their young children: one-year findings. *J Am Dent Assoc*. 2004;135(6):731–738.
15. Weinstein P, Harrison R, Benton T. Motivating mothers to prevent caries: confirming the beneficial effect of counseling. *J Am Dent Assoc*. 2006;137(6):789–793.
16. Almomani F, Williams K, Catley D, et al. Effects of an oral health promotion program in people with mental illness. *J Dent Res*. 2009;88(7):648–652.
17. Jonsson B, Ohrn K, Oscarson N, et al. An individually tailored treatment programme for improved oral hygiene: introduction of a new course of action in health education for patients with periodontitis. *Int J Dent Hyg*. 2009;7(3):166–175.
18. Jonsson B, Ohrn K, Oscarson N, et al. The effectiveness of an individually tailored oral health educational programme on oral hygiene behaviour in patients with periodontal disease: a blinded randomized-controlled clinical trial (one-year follow-up). *J Clin Periodontol*. 2009;36(12):1025–1034.
19. Brand VS, Bray KK, MacNeill S, et al. Impact of single-session motivational interviewing on clinical outcomes following periodontal maintenance therapy. *Int J Dent Hyg*. 2013;11(2):134–141.
20. Stenman J, Lundgren J, Wennstrom JL, et al. A single session of motivational interviewing as an additive means to improve adherence in periodontal infection control: a randomized controlled trial. *J Clin Periodontol*. 2012;39(10):947–954.
21. Bray KK, Catley D, Voelker MA, et al. Motivational interviewing in dental hygiene education: curriculum modification and evaluation. *J Dent Educ*. 2013;77(12):1662–1669.
22. Rubak S, Sandbaek A, Lauritzen T, et al. Motivational interviewing: a systematic review and meta-analysis. *Br J Gen Pract*. 2005;55(513):305–312.
23. Amrhein PC, Miller WR, Yahne CE, et al. Client commitment language during motivational interviewing predicts drug use outcomes. *J Consult Clin Psychol*. 2003;71(5):862–878.

 STUDENT ANCILLARY RESOURCES

A wide variety of resources to enhance your learning and understanding of this chapter are available on thePoint°.

- Visit thePoint to access:
  - Audio Glossary
  - Animations
  - Suggested Readings
  - Answers to Review Questions
  - Case Studies

Clinical Application. Periodontal maintenance is generally thought to be one of the most important phases of therapy that can be provided for patients with periodontal disease, yet patient cooperation with this aspect of periodontal therapy is not good. Since the dental hygienist often plays a major role in periodontal maintenance, this topic is of critical importance to the dental hygienist as well as other members of the dental team. This chapter outlines some of the fundamental aspects of periodontal maintenance for all members of the dental team to consider during patient care.

Learning Objectives

- Explain the term periodontal maintenance.
- List three objectives of periodontal maintenance.
- Describe how periodontal maintenance relates to other phases of periodontal treatment.
- List the usual procedures performed during an appointment for periodontal maintenance.
- Explain the term baseline data.
- Describe guidelines for determining whether the general practice office or the periodontal office should provide periodontal maintenance.
- Describe how to establish an appropriate interval between maintenance appointments.
- Define the term recurrence of periodontitis.
- List clinical signs of recurrence of periodontitis.
- List reasons for recurrence of periodontitis.
- Explain the term compliance.
- Define the terms compliant patient and noncompliant patient.
- List reasons for noncompliance with periodontal maintenance recommendations.

- Explain some strategies that can be used to improve patient compliance.
- Explain the term root caries.
- List recommendations for use of fluorides in the prevention of root caries.

Key Terms

Periodontal maintenance
Baseline data
Periodontal disease
  recurrence

Refractory periodontitis
Compliance
Compliant patient
Noncompliant patient

Root caries
Caries management
  by risk assessment
  (CAMBRA)

Section 1
Introduction to Periodontal Maintenance

1. **Description of Periodontal Maintenance.** Periodontal maintenance is a term that refers to the continuing patient care provided by members of the dental team to help a patient maintain periodontal health following the completion of nonsurgical or surgical periodontal therapy (1–5).
   - A. Periodontal therapy is performed at selected intervals to assist the patient in maintaining oral health; the precise intervals are selected to meet the needs of the individual patient.
   - B. Once begun, periodontal maintenance is normally continued for life of the natural dentition (or the life of the dental implants).
   - C. Periodontal maintenance can be discontinued temporarily if surgical or nonsurgical therapy must be reinstituted because of recurrent periodontal disease.
   - D. Periodontal maintenance is performed on both natural teeth and dental implants.
   - E. Though periodontal maintenance is the preferred term, other terms that have been used for periodontal maintenance are supportive periodontal therapy (SPT) and periodontal recall.
   - F. It is important to realize that periodontal maintenance is not synonymous with a dental prophylaxis.

2. **Importance of Periodontal Maintenance**
   - A. Periodontal maintenance is one of the most important phases of periodontal treatment.
     1. With good periodontal maintenance, most periodontitis patients can retain their teeth or implants in function and comfort throughout their lives (3,5).
     2. In the absence of periodontal maintenance, patients frequently exhibit a recurrence of periodontal disease (6–10).
     3. Periodontal maintenance can be successful regardless of the specific type of periodontal treatment (surgical or nonsurgical) needed by the patient.
     4. The success of periodontal maintenance in reducing tooth loss is well documented in the literature (9,11,12). Figure 30-1 illustrates some of the outcomes possible with periodontal maintenance.

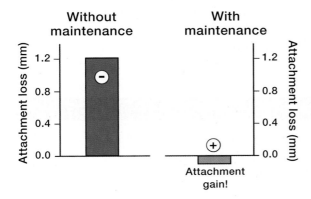

Figure 30-1. Attachment Loss With and Without Maintenance. A study by Axelsson and Lindhe assessed the efficacy of a periodontal maintenance care program to prevent the recurrence of disease in patients treated for advanced periodontitis. Patients who were not in a periodontal maintenance program had progressive attachment loss over a 6-year period. Similar patients in the study who were placed on maintenance care every 2 to 3 months over the 6-year period *exhibited some attachment gain.* (Data from Axelsson P, Lindhe J. The significance of maintenance care in the treatment of periodontal disease. *J Clin Periodontol.* 1981;8:281–294.)

3. **Goals of Periodontal Maintenance.** There are several overlapping goals of periodontal maintenance; these goals are discussed below and are summarized in Box 30-1.
   A. **To Minimize the Recurrence and Progression of Periodontal Disease.** There are several reasons that periodontal disease tends to recur.
      1. Of course, the primary risk factor for inflammatory periodontal disease is bacterial plaque biofilm.
         a. In spite of a patient's best self-care efforts, it is common for plaque biofilms to form at some sites and for some calculus to reform at some sites. Periodic professional biofilm and calculus removal is an important part of periodontal maintenance.
         b. It is common for a patient's self-care efforts to become less effective over time. Reinforcement or improvement of self-care techniques is also an important part of periodontal maintenance.
      2. Secondary risk factors for inflammatory periodontal diseases include plaque-retentive areas (such as restorations with overhangs), smoking, and certain systemic factors.
         a. Whereas these secondary risk factors should always be addressed as part of nonsurgical periodontal therapy, the condition of most patients changes over time. For example, restorative dental procedures can alter plaque-retentive sites or a patient's systemic condition can change.
         b. Continuing reassessment of the impact of secondary risk factors is also an important part of periodontal maintenance (11,13–15).
   B. **To Reduce the Incidence of Tooth Loss.** One of the primary overall goals of all phases of periodontal therapy (including periodontal maintenance) for most patients is to reduce the incidence of tooth loss (or reduce the incidence of implant loss).
      1. In a study by Wilson et al. (16), of tooth loss in maintenance patients in a private periodontal practice, tooth loss was shown to be inversely proportional to the frequency of periodontal maintenance.
      2. Other studies have also shown that patients who maintain regular periodontal maintenance lose fewer teeth than patients who receive less periodontal maintenance (11,17).
   C. **To Increase the Probability of Detecting and Treating Other Oral Conditions**
      1. As members of the healthcare community, members of the dental team need to be vigilant for the development of any oral condition that can affect patient welfare.
      2. Periodontal maintenance offers an ideal opportunity for ongoing monitoring of the overall oral health of a patient.

Box 30-1. Goals of Periodontal Maintenance

- Minimize the recurrence and progression of periodontal disease
- Reduce the incidence of tooth loss
- Increase the probability of detecting and treating other oral conditions

4. Patient/Clinician Roles in Periodontal Maintenance
   A. Periodontal maintenance is a team effort that requires commitment from everyone involved. The periodontal maintenance team includes the members of the dental team plus the patient and occasionally other healthcare providers such as the patient's physician.
   B. Periodontal maintenance requires considerable effort from the patient in sustaining meticulous self-care and cooperating with regular ongoing professional periodontal maintenance care. Patients must be made aware of the need for this ongoing effort even before receiving nonsurgical periodontal therapy.
   C. In addition, periodontal maintenance requires considerable effort on the part of the dental health team for professional care at regular intervals, renewal of patient motivation, instruction in self-care techniques, and elimination or reduction of primary and secondary risk factors.
5. **Relationship of Periodontal Maintenance to Other Phases of Therapy.** It is important for a clinician to understand how periodontal maintenance for a patient who has been treated for periodontal disease relates to other phases of comprehensive periodontal therapy; this relationship is summarized in Figure 30-2.

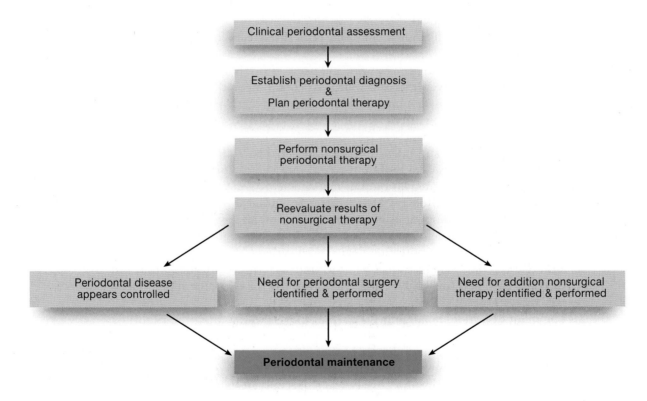

Figure 30-2. Phases of Periodontal Therapy. This flowchart illustrates how periodontal maintenance relates to other phases of periodontal therapy that are frequently provided for patients with periodontal disease.

Section 2
Planning Periodontal Maintenance

1. **When to Implement Periodontal Maintenance.** Following nonsurgical periodontal therapy, a reevaluation of the patient's periodontal status is performed with a particular emphasis on the results obtained from nonsurgical therapy.
   A. Based upon the findings of this reevaluation, additional therapy such as periodontal surgery might be recommended.
   B. At the reevaluation, the dental team must also decide what periodontal maintenance care will be needed.
   C. For most patients periodontal maintenance will begin following this reevaluation, since for many patients no further active therapy is needed at least in selected sites in the dentition.
   D. Even though periodontal surgery may be recommended in some sites, the maintenance phase begins following nonsurgical therapy at least for those sites where no further active periodontal therapy is indicated.
2. **Procedures for Professional Biofilm Removal**
   A. Traditionally, hand and/or ultrasonic instrumentation has been used for professional biofilm removal.
      1. In the hands of a well-trained clinician, both these techniques are effective in biofilm removal.
      2. The subgingival biofilm removal process using either hand and/or ultrasonic instrumentation, however, is a technically demanding and time-consuming procedure for the clinician and uncomfortable for many patients (18,19). Unpleasant feelings toward dental procedures may have a negative effect on patient compliance.
   B. Biofilm formation occurs rapidly in periodontal pockets following instrumentation. Professional biofilm removal must be performed frequently at regular intervals for subgingival biofilm management.
   C. **A Recent Innovation in Biofilm Management: Subgingival Air Polishing**
      1. **Air polishing technology** uses a combination of an abrasive powder with water and compressed air delivered to the tooth surface through an air polishing nozzle. Recently an air polishing device – Hu-Friedy Manufacturing's *Air-Flow Perio* – has been introduced in the United States and Canada that uses a specially designed subgingival nozzle and low-abrasive glycine-based powder to remove subgingival biofilms.
      2. The main objective of subgingival air polishing is to maintain the health of the periodontium by decreasing inflammation caused by the host response to plaque biofilms in the periodontal pocket.
      3. **The unique technology for subgingival air polishing**
         a. Subgingival air polishing devices use a specially designed disposable nozzle to deliver a low-abrasive powder to the subgingival environment.
            1. By using the newly designed nozzle, the jet spray has a lower flow and pressure than nozzles designed for supragingival polishing.
            2. The subgingival nozzle directs the powder and air mainly toward the root surface while the water exits at the tip of the nozzle.
         b. Subgingival air polishing uses a glycine-based powder that is biocompatible and gentle on the soft tissues of the oral cavity, subgingival epithelium, and cementum (20–22).
         c. *Before using this new technology, clinicians require special training in the proper use of the subgingival air polishing device.* Explaining the

techniques for use of subgingival glycine powder air polishing is beyond the scope of this chapter, but clinicians should be aware of this emerging technology and seek formal training in its use.

4. **Clinical evidence for subgingival air polishing with glycine-based powders**
   a. Subgingival air polishing for the removal of biofilm from root surfaces is a relatively new technology with clinical research supporting its safety and efficacy for use in nonsurgical periodontal therapy and treatment of peri-implant disease.
      1. Although subgingival air polishing is an emerging technology in the United States and Canada, this technology has been used and researched for several years in Europe.
      2. In June 2012, during the *EuroPerio 7 Conference in Vienna* (23), a consensus conference on mechanical biofilm management took place to review the current evidence from the literature on the clinical relevance of subgingival use of air polishing and to make practical recommendations for the clinician.
   b. Box 30-2 summarizes these recommendations, as well as, additional current evidence from the literature on subgingival biofilm management.

Box 30-2. Summary of Current Evidence on Subgingival Air Polishing

- Indications for the use of air polishing devices have been expanded from supragingival to subgingival air polishing in the past few years. In particular, the development of new low-abrasive glycine-based powders and devices with subgingival nozzles provides better access to subgingival and interdental areas (23).
- In periodontal pockets 5 mm or greater in depth, subgingivally applied low-abrasive powders—using a subgingival nozzle—remove subgingival biofilm significantly more efficaciously than curets (21,24).
- Clinical and microbiologic outcomes up to 2 months were not significantly different following subgingivally applied glycine powder air polishing, ultrasonic instrumentation, or instrumentation with curets (25,26).
- Full-mouth glycine powder air polishing results in a significantly decreased load of *Porphyromonas gingivalis* in the oral cavity (24).
- Using subgingivally applied glycine powder air polishing, subgingival biofilm removal can be achieved in a considerably shorter period of time compared to subgingival instrumentation using hand and/or ultrasonic instrumentation (25,26).
- ***Patients generally perceive glycine-based air polishing as more comfortable than hand and/or power-driven instrumentation*** (20,21,25–28).
- ***Air polishing does NOT remove calculus deposits***. For calculus removal, hand or ultrasonic instruments are still needed (27).
- Glycine-based powders result in noncritical loss of cemental substance (22,29).
- Glycine powder polishing causes less gingival erosion than hand instrumentation (20).
- Glycine powder polishing is safe and effective on titanium surfaces of dental implants (30,31).
- Glycine powder is safe on a variety of restorative materials and orthodontic brackets.
- Clinical, microbiologic, and histologic studies have confirmed subgingival glycine powder air polishing is safe, efficient, and comfortable when used as recommended by a trained professional (21,23–25,27,28,32).

> ## Box 30-3. Overview of Procedures Performed During a Periodontal Maintenance Appointment
>
> - Update medical status
> - Patient interview
> - Clinical assessment
> - Evaluation of effectiveness of patient self-care
> - Identification of treatment needs
> - Periodontal instrumentation
> - Patient counseling
> - Application of fluorides

3. **Procedures Performed During Periodontal Maintenance.** Successful periodontal maintenance requires the active participation of the patient as well as all members of the dental team. In most dental offices the dental hygienist plays a major role in procedures performed during periodontal maintenance. A typical patient office visit for periodontal maintenance includes procedures discussed below and outlined in Box 30-3 (33–35).

   A. **Update of Medical Status.** An update of a patient's medical status is always the first step in any clinical appointment.

   B. **Patient Interview**
      1. A patient interview is part of a periodontal maintenance appointment; during the interview, changes in the social or dental status of the patient should be explored and documented.
      2. Examples of social status issues that should be explored would be changes in lifestyle, bereavement, and work status.
      3. The patient interview should also include a review of dental care provided by other clinicians since the previous maintenance visit.
      4. In addition, the patient interview should clarify the patient's perception of his/her oral status including the patient's thoughts about problems encountered during self-care efforts.

   C. **Clinical Assessment**
      1. Following the patient interview, a thorough clinical assessment should be performed. Results of the clinical assessment should then be compared with previous baseline data. The term **baseline data** refers to clinical data gathered at the beginning of the periodontal treatment that is subsequently used for comparison.
      2. The actual clinical assessment usually includes steps such as those listed below.
         a. Extraoral and Intraoral Examination
         b. Dental Examination
         c. Radiographic Examination if indicated
         d. Periodontal Examination including the following features:
            1. Probing depths
               a. Probing depths should be recorded with the same attention to detail that was employed during the initial examination.
               b. Disease progression (continuing attachment loss) should be suspected when a 2-mm increase in probing depth is noted at a site.

2. **Bleeding on probing**
   a. When present, bleeding on probing is generally visible within a few seconds after gentle periodontal probing.
   b. Research suggests that after a few years of maintenance, a high frequency of bleeding on probing is a predictor of increased risk for progressive attachment loss (36).
   c. Bleeding sites should be charted because these sites may need more attention during periodontal instrumentation.
3. **Attachment level**
   a. Attachment levels should be recorded at critical sites in the dentition.
   b. The most reliable way to evaluate periodontal disease control is by sequential comparison of clinical attachment level measurements.
   c. Disease progression is thought to be indicated by a 2-mm increase in clinical attachment loss at a specific site *as measured with a manual periodontal probe.*
4. **Tooth mobility**
   a. In the assessment of tooth mobility, mobility can be stable or increasing. Increasing mobility over time is one of the important clinical features to note.
   b. The more severe the mobility measured in a tooth, the greater the risk of eventual tooth loss.
5. **Furcation involvement**
   a. Periodontal disease control is more difficult in areas of furcation involvement.
   b. The more advanced the furcation involvement, the greater the risk of tooth loss over time.
6. **Mucogingival involvement**
7. **Levels of plaque biofilm and calculus**

D. **Evaluation of Effectiveness of Self-Care**
   1. Patients often spend considerable time on self-care and justifiably expect to be informed about the effectiveness of their efforts.
      a. Plaque scores recorded after using a disclosing solution are good indications of the patient's level of self-care compliance, and disclosing solution can be used to allow patients to see biofilm accumulation.
      b. Plaque scores may reveal that the patient is in need of renewed instruction in self-care methods.
   2. Biofilm accumulation can be related to many factors; examples of these factors are listed below.
      a. Patients may lack the manual dexterity needed to carry out the self-care regimen that was recommended previously. When manual dexterity is a problem, alternative self-care techniques should be considered. Older patients can loose skills that they were perfectly capable of performing at a previous maintenance visit.
      b. Unfortunately it is common for patients to discontinue the use of one or more of the self-care methods recommended previously.
      c. Gingival recession or shrinkage may have occurred following periodontal surgery; introduction of new interdental aids may be indicated for plaque biofilm removal on proximal root surfaces.

E. Identification of Treatment Needs

1. It is a routine part of periodontal maintenance to perform thorough periodontal instrumentation to remove biofilm and calculus, but other treatment needs can also be identified.

2. Examples of other treatment needs can include local delivery of antimicrobials, restoration of dental caries, and reinstitution of active periodontal therapy.

3. Selective tooth polishing may be indicated for removal of tooth stains that are visible when the patient smiles.

F. Biofilm Removal

1. Biofilms are resistant to topical chemical control; therefore, frequent professional removal of plaque biofilm is an essential component of successful nonsurgical periodontal therapy.

2. Professional biofilm may be accomplished by hand and/or ultrasonic instrumentation or subgingival glycine powder air polishing.

G. Periodontal Instrumentation

1. The goal of periodontal instrumentation is to create an environment that is biologically acceptable to the tissues of the periodontium.

2. Thorough removal of all calculus deposits should be accomplished using hand/ and or ultrasonic instrumentation.

3. The main adverse effect of frequent mechanical instrumentation of the root surface is disturbance of the epithelial attachment and cumulative, irreversible root substance removal (37–42) and gingival recession (43,44).

   a. Hard tissue loss is one of the major causes of dentin sensitivity to hot and cold stimuli, as well as sensitivity to toothbrushing (45–48).

   b. Because periodontal instrumentation is a routine part of nonsurgical periodontal therapy, it is important that removal is accomplished in an efficient manner with minimal hard tissue damage (25).

      1. Following periodontal therapy, some patients will present for periodontal maintenance with little or no subgingival calculus deposits. In these patients, firm stroke pressure with the instrument against the tooth is not necessary and should be avoided.

      2. Ultrasonic instrumentation with a precision-thin tip has been shown to remove less root substance than hand instrumentation and offers the added benefit of the antimicrobial effect created by the vibrating ultrasonic tip (49–51).

      3. Plastic curets (such as those used to debride dental implants) can be effective for deplaquing root surfaces and minimize trauma to the root during maintenance care when no calculus is present or when implants are involved.

H. Patient Counseling

1. As already discussed, maintenance patients should always be counseled related to the effectiveness of self-care efforts since biofilm control by the patient is a critical element in preventing recurrence of periodontitis.

   a. Failure to provide this information may give a patient the impression that the dental team is not truly interested in the patient's dental health status.

   b. Most patients will need some reinforcement of motivation for biofilm control in addition to retraining in the complex skills involved.

2. It is also wise to include counseling that explains the need for compliance with the periodontal maintenance regimen, since compliance with the periodontal maintenance regimen will always remain a problem for some patients.

3. Other counseling may be indicated for specific patients. Examples of counseling that may be needed are caries prevention counseling, smoking cessation, or dietary changes.

I. Application of Fluorides

1. Professional application of fluoride treatments during periodontal maintenance care is normally indicated to promote remineralization of tooth surfaces, aid in the prevention of root caries, and aid in the control of dentinal hypersensitivity.

2. Research studies suggest that high concentrations of topical fluorides may also have some antimicrobial properties and may be of some benefit in decreasing plaque biofilm accumulation.

3. The use of fluorides is discussed in detail in Section 5 of this chapter.

4. Decisions Related to Periodontal Maintenance

A. Office Guidelines for Provision of Periodontal Maintenance. For patients treated in a periodontal office, the general dental team should discuss guidelines for how periodontal maintenance should be provided (i.e., either in the general dental practice office or in the periodontal practice). This decision is of course dependent in part on the experience and comfort levels of the members of the dental team, but some general guidelines are outlined below.

1. Patients who have been treated for mild chronic periodontitis can usually receive periodontal maintenance in a general dental practice.

2. Patients who have been treated for moderate chronic periodontitis can usually be managed by alternating periodontal maintenance visits between the general dental practice and the periodontal practice.

3. Patients with severe chronic periodontitis should receive periodontal maintenance in a periodontal practice. In addition, annual or semiannual visits should be scheduled with a general dentist who will provide restorative and other general dental care.

4. Patients who have been treated for aggressive periodontitis should receive all phases of periodontal therapy including periodontal maintenance in a periodontal practice. In addition, annual or semiannual visits should be scheduled with a general dentist who will provide restorative and other general dental care.

B. Establishing Appropriate Periodontal Maintenance Intervals

1. Establishing a periodontal maintenance interval that is appropriate for the patient can be challenging. The frequency of periodontal maintenance visits must be determined on an individual basis (52). Some factors to consider in determining the interval between maintenance visits include the following:

   a. Severity of periodontitis. In general the more severe the periodontitis, the shorter the intervals should be between periodontal maintenance visits.

   b. Adequacy of patient self-care. In general the more effective the patient's self-care, the less frequently the patient needs to be seen. For patients with less than optimal self-care the intervals between maintenance visits should be shorter.

   c. Host response. Systemic or genetic factors may negatively affect the host response. For example, a patient who continues to smoke or one with poorly controlled diabetes should be seen at shorter intervals (11,13).

2. An important guide for determining the frequency of maintenance care is based on the time interval for the repopulation of periodontal pathogens following thorough periodontal instrumentation.

   a. Studies indicate that following periodontal instrumentation the subgingival pathogens return to preinstrumentation levels in approximately 9 to 11 weeks in most patients, though times can vary (53).

b. Research evidence shows that periodontal maintenance should be performed at least every 3 months or less for the removal and disruption of subgingival periodontal pathogens. *This 3-month interval is the one most frequently recommended, though this interval may need to be adjusted based on clinical observation* (52).

c. Patients who receive frequent periodontal maintenance will experience less attachment loss and tooth loss than patients who have less frequent maintenance care.

Section 3
Periodontal Disease Recurrence

1. Understanding Periodontal Disease Recurrence
    A. Periodontal Disease Recurrence Defined
        1. The term periodontal disease recurrence refers to the return of the disease in *a patient who has been previously, successfully treated for periodontitis.*
        2. The term disease recurrence implies that the periodontitis was indeed brought under control during nonsurgical periodontal therapy (or nonsurgical periodontal therapy plus periodontal surgery), but that at some later time the periodontitis is once again resulting in progressive attachment loss.
        3. It should be noted that in spite of having received excellent treatment, patients who have been treated for periodontitis are at risk for recurrence of periodontitis for as long as teeth (or implants) are present.
        4. Recurrence of periodontitis can occur at specific sites only (not necessarily throughout the dentition). For example, it would be possible for a patient treated for periodontitis to experience disease recurrence on the mesial surface of a single premolar tooth and for all other teeth in the dentition to continue to show good disease control. It is also possible for disease recurrence to be noted throughout the dentition.
    B. Clinical Recognition of Recurrence of Periodontitis. At present the most effective way to identify sites of recurrence of periodontitis (i.e., sites of progressive attachment loss) is through thorough periodic clinical assessments. The usual clinical signs of recurrence of periodontitis are listed in Box 30-4.

Box 30-4. Clinical Signs of Recurrence

- Progressive clinical attachment loss
- Pockets that get deeper over time
- Pockets that bleed upon probing
- Pockets that exhibit exudate
- Radiographic evidence of progressing bone loss
- Increasing tooth mobility

C. Reasons for Disease Recurrence. Periodontitis recurs in patients for a variety of reasons, and the members of the dental team should be aware that it is not always possible to determine a specific reason for disease recurrence. However, the most common reasons for recurrence of periodontitis are the following:
    1. Inadequate self-care by the patient

2. Incomplete professional treatment
   a. Incomplete periodontal instrumentation
   b. Failure to control all local risk factors
3. Failure to control systemic factors
4. Inadequate control of occlusal contributing factors
5. Improper periodontal surgical technique
6. Attempting to treat teeth with a poor prognosis

D. **Refractory Disease Differentiated From Recurrent Disease.** Refractory periodontal disease should be differentiated from recurrent periodontal disease. Unfortunately periodontitis in certain patients is difficult or impossible to control even with all the modern therapies currently available and in spite of the efforts of the most skilled clinicians.

   1. As already discussed, the term recurrence of periodontal disease refers *to the return of the disease in a patient who has been previously, successfully treated for periodontitis.*
   2. The term **refractory periodontitis**, however, refers to periodontitis that is resistant to treatment from the outset of therapy even with what appears to be appropriate periodontal therapy.
   3. Referral to a periodontal practice is usually indicated when refractory periodontitis is suspected in a patient.

2. **Options for Management of Patients With Disease Recurrence.** The members of the dental team should be alert for the need for retreatment that may be identified at any time during periodontal maintenance. When periodontal disease recurrence is identified, planning of the needed retreatment can usually include several options:

   A. If inadequate patient self-care appears to be the fundamental cause of the disease recurrence, then nonsurgical therapy should be reinstituted followed by a reevaluation of the patient's periodontal status after an appropriate healing time.
   B. If failure to comply with the schedule of periodontal maintenance appears to be the fundamental cause of the disease recurrence, then nonsurgical therapy should be reinstituted along with further patient education about the need for maintenance followed by a reevaluation of the patient's periodontal status after an appropriate healing time.
   C. If there appears to be disease recurrence in limited individual sites in the presence of *adequate* patient self-care, treatment options can include localized periodontal instrumentation, local delivery of antimicrobial agents, or localized surgical therapy.
   D. If there appears to be disease recurrence in multiple sites in the presence of adequate patient self-care, periodontal surgical therapy is frequently indicated.
   E. If generalized attachment loss has recurred, the systemic condition of the patient should be reassessed with emphasis on the possible need for periodontal surgical intervention, for possible microbial analysis, or for possible local or systemic antimicrobial therapy. Patients of this type should be managed by a specialist in periodontics.

Section 4
Patient Compliance with Periodontal Maintenance

1. **Overview of Patient Compliance.** The term compliance is defined as the extent to which a person's behavior coincides with medical or health advice. Compliance has also called adherence or therapeutic alliance, but compliance is the most common term used in the literature.
   A. A patient is sometimes described as being a compliant patient if he/she follows recommendations for healthcare advice. Examples of compliant patients would be a patient who faithfully takes antihypertensive medications as prescribed by a physician or a patient who cooperates in meeting regularly scheduled periodontal maintenance appointments as recommended by the dental team.
   B. A patient is sometimes described as being a noncompliant patient if he/she does *not* follow recommendations for healthcare advice. Examples of noncompliant patients would be a patient who does not take prescribed medications daily to control diabetes or a patient who does not perform adequate daily self-care that has been recommended as part of a maintenance program.

2. **Patient Compliance During Periodontal Maintenance.** Patient compliance with a program of periodontal maintenance is not easy to achieve. It would require that a patient faithfully adhere to a strict program of recall appointments several times each year and follow very specific recommendations for meticulous daily self-care.
   A. Overall, patient compliance with most medical advice is poor, and it should not be surprising that patient compliance with periodontal maintenance is also poor.
   B. Studies of compliance exhibited by periodontal maintenance patients indicate that only 16% to 30% of the patients are fully compliant with periodontal maintenance (54–56).
   C. Reasons for noncompliance with periodontal maintenance are complex, and those reasons can be different for each patient and even for the same patient at different times (17,57–61).
   D. Examples of some reasons that have been suggested for noncompliance with recommended programs of periodontal maintenance include the following:
      1. Patient fear of receiving dental treatment
      2. The expense of the dental treatment involved
      3. The low priority for dental care for some patients in the face of competing demands for time
      4. Denial on the part of some patients related to the periodontal challenges they face
      5. Failure for some patients to understand the implications of noncompliance
      6. Perceived indifference on the part of the dental healthcare providers

3. **Strategies for Improving Compliance.** The thoughtful dental team will investigate and adopt strategies for improving patient compliance with periodontal maintenance (57). Some strategies for improving compliance are discussed below and outlined in Figure 30-3.
   A. Give a patient printed self-care instructions, and make sure to supply the instructions written in the patient's native language.
   B. Simplify self-care recommendations as much as possible for each patient.
      1. Patients often perceive self-care instructions as being difficult to follow and as too time-consuming in their busy lives.
      2. Self-care instructions should be as clear and as simple as possible while addressing the specific needs of the patient.

3. Caution should be exercised when recommending multiple types of self-care aids. Patients are less likely to comply with self-care when they are instructed to use multiple aids on a daily basis.

4. When possible, alternatives to traditional dental floss should be considered, since compliance with flossing is generally poor.

C. Vary the office approach to patient education and self-care instructions from appointment to appointment. Patients often complain about having to listen to the "same old lecture" from the dental hygienist at each periodontal maintenance appointment.

D. Seek out patient concerns and provide opportunities for communication by asking patients open-ended questions. Examples of open-ended questions appear below.

1. "What are your concerns about this suggestion or treatment?"

2. "How do you think you will fit this self-care recommendation into your daily schedule?"

3. "How would you compare using this powered flossing device to using traditional dental floss?"

E. Accommodate the individual patient's needs whenever possible. A satisfied patient is more likely to comply with self-care and maintenance appointments.

F. Keep patients fully informed about their periodontal condition.

1. At each visit counsel the patients about their periodontal health status.

2. Explain the benefits of having regularly scheduled periodontal maintenance visits and the risks of infrequent professional care.

G. Monitor compliance with the maintenance appointments and contact patients promptly when compliance seems to become a problem.

H. Provide positive feedback to patients as frequently as possible. Positive reinforcement can help improve compliance.

1. Areas of improvement should be pointed out to the patient (e.g., less biofilm accumulation, fewer bleeding sites, or less inflamed tissue).

2. Positive reinforcement should be used to convey a motivational message rather than criticism.

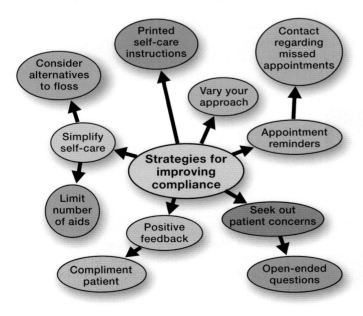

Figure 30-3. Suggestions for Improving Patient Compliance. An idea map of various strategies for improving patient compliance with recommendations for periodontal maintenance.

Section 5
Root Caries as a Complication During Maintenance

1. Introduction to Root Caries
    A. Occurrence of Root Caries in Patients With Periodontitis
        1. Whereas dental caries frequently occurs on enamel surfaces, the term root caries refers to tooth decay that occurs on the root surfaces of the teeth.
        2. According to the *1999–2004 National Health and Nutrition Examination Survey,*
            a. root caries is a significant problem for adults: 21.6% of adults aged 50 to 64 years and 31% of adults aged 65 to 74 years had unrestored or restored root caries.
            b. the percentage of adults with root caries increases to 42.3% at age 75 (62).
        3. The Northwest Practice-based Research Collaborative in Evidence-based Dentistry research network recently reported
            a. a total of 19.6% of adults had root caries.
            b. the factors associated with increased prevalence of root caries in middle-aged adults are being of the male sex, dry mouth, root surfaces exposed to the oral environment, and increased frequency of eating or drinking between meals (63).
        4. A 2004 systematic review on root caries incidence found that 23.7% of older adults *develop at least one new lesion annually* (64).
        5. Root caries occurs only if the root surface is exposed to the oral environment due to loss of attachment (65).
            a. In health, the root surface is protected by the periodontal attachment apparatus and is not exposed to the oral environment.
            b. The root may be exposed to the oral environment due to gingival recession or within a periodontal pocket.
    B. Clinical Appearance of Root Caries
        1. Active root caries lesions, usually, look yellowish to light brown and may be covered with biofilm. Inactive lesions appear dark brown or black (65,66). Figure 30-4 shows a typical clinical appearance of root caries.
        2. Root caries usually begins at or is slightly coronal to the free gingival margin. The carious lesions can spread laterally and can even extend circumferentially around the root surface (67).

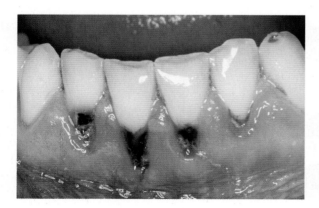

Figure 30-4. Root Caries. Root caries on the mandibular incisors of an individual with periodontitis. (Courtesy of Dr. Richard J. Foster, Guilford Technical Community College, Jamestown, NC.)

C. Etiology of Root Caries
   1. No specific microorganisms have been proven to cause root caries. Root caries is most likely the result of a mixed infection or a succession of bacterial populations, such as *Streptococcus mutans* and *Lactobacillus*. Recent studies, with few exceptions, fail to find association between *Actinomyces* and root caries (68).
   2. Like enamel caries, root caries requires a susceptible tooth surface, plaque biofilm, and time to initiate and progress. However, root caries differs from enamel caries in some aspects:
      a. Root surfaces are more vulnerable to demineralization than enamel surfaces. Root surfaces demineralize at a pH of 6.2 to 6.7 (69).
      b. Mineral loss for the root surface during the process of demineralization is up to 2.5 times greater than enamel (70).
   3. Risk factors for the development of root caries include attachment loss, inadequate patient self-care, a cariogenic diet, infrequent dental visits, past caries experience, inadequate salivary flow, lack of fluoride exposure, and removable partial dentures.
   4. In addition, individuals who have coronal caries are 2 to 3.5 times more likely to develop root caries (71).

2. **General Recommendations for the Prevention of Root Caries.** Root caries is a common problem in patients with periodontitis. Managing root caries from a restorative standpoint can be quite difficult, and the best strategy for managing root caries is to prevent the root caries from forming.

A. **Prevention of Periodontitis.** The prevention of periodontitis and its associated attachment loss is the most effective way to prevent root caries. In patients with existing periodontal disease, prevention of further attachment loss will reduce the surface area susceptible to decay.

B. **Fluoride for the Prevention of Root Caries**
   1. Root lesions can be arrested by remineralization. A 2007 systematic review of fluoride interventions for root caries concluded that fluoride appears to be a preventive and therapeutic treatment for root caries (72,73).
   2. A variety of fluoride products can be helpful in preventing root caries. Figure 30-5 depicts some of these products. A 2011 systematic review recommended 1.1% NaF pastes/gels and fluoride varnishes as the most effective modalities for root caries remineralization (74).
      a. **Fluoridated Drinking Water.** Several studies have demonstrated that the presence of fluoridated drinking water throughout the lifetime of an individual reduces the development of root surface caries (75).
      b. **Fluoride Toothpaste**
         1. The use of an 1,100 ppm sodium fluoride (NaF) dentifrice results in a significant decrease in root surface caries of 67% (76).
         2. A recent randomized clinical trial demonstrates that prescription strength fluoride toothpaste, containing 5,000 ppm NaF, is effective in reversing root caries (77).
         3. Patients using fluoride toothpastes should avoid rinsing with large volumes of water after the use of fluoride toothpaste (78).
      c. **Fluoride Mouthrinses.** Fluoride mouthrinses containing 0.05% NaF have been shown to significantly reduce root caries incidence (79).

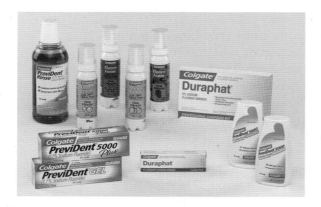

Figure 30-5. Fluoride Products. There are a variety of fluoride products for professional or home use that are helpful in the control of root caries. These include toothpastes, gels, foams, rinses, and varnishes. (Courtesy of Colgate-Palmolive company.)

    d. **Professional Application of Fluoride**
       1. A large long-term clinical study showed that semiannual applications of 1.23% APF gel significantly reduced the formation of new root caries. The number of remineralized lesions was significantly increased by daily rinsing with a 0.05% NaF rinse (80).
       2. Fluoride varnish applied every 3 months has been shown to reduce new root caries formation by over 50% (81).
    e. **New Fluoride Agents.** New fluoride agents, such as silver diamine fluoride are available in some countries and show promise as root caries preventive agents.

C. **Antimicrobial and Supplemental Remineralization Therapies**
    1. A recent systematic review found no benefit from the use of chlorhexidine varnish in reducing root caries (82). There is limited evidence of benefit from the use of a chlorhexidine mouthrinse (83). High and extreme caries risk adults should rinse with 10 mL of 0.12% chlorhexidine once daily for 1 wk/mo.
    2. Xylitol-containing gums and mints are recommended for high and extreme caries risk patients.
      a. The therapeutic dose of xylitol is 6 to 10 g spread throughout the day.
      b. A recent randomized clinical trial found 40% fewer root caries lesions in the xylitol group compared to placebo. The xylitol group received five lozenges containing 1 g of xylitol. The lozenges were consumed across the day (84).
    3. Casein phosphopeptide (CPP)-amorphous calcium phosphate (ACP) pastes are recommended for extreme caries risk patients.
      a. The paste can be applied with a fingertip on a daily basis.
      b. Most research on CPP-ACP is laboratory based rather than in vivo. However, CPP-ACP may promote remineralization in patients with low salivary flow.
      c. A 2008 systematic review concluded that there is insufficient evidence to make conclusions regarding the effectiveness of CPP-ACP in preventing caries (85).
    4. In a clinical practice guideline from the American Dental Association, application of a 1:1 mixture of chlorhexidine and thymol varnish (Cervitec Gel), every 3 months was recommended to reduce the incidence of root caries (86).

3. **Caries Management by Risk Assessment (CAMBRA)**
    A. **Caries Risk Assessment**
      1. Recent research clearly demonstrates that assigning caries risk assessment levels facilitates the effective management of patients for dental caries (87).

2. Subsequent to this research, protocols for clinical management of caries risk factor level were developed and employed at a number of dental schools (88). While complete consensus on these protocols continues to develop, there is strong agreement about treating patients for dental caries based on risk level (88).

3. These protocols for clinical management of caries risk are known as "Caries Management by Risk Assessment (CAMBRA)" (76,87).

4. The CAMBRA protocols seek to provide practical clinical guidelines for managing dental caries based upon risk group assessment. The protocols are based upon the best evidence at this time and can be used in planning effective caries management for any patient (87,89).

B. CAMBRA Treatment Recommendations

1. A caries risk assessment form
   a. In 2002, a group of experts from across the United States produced a caries risk assessment form (89).
   b. In 2006, outcomes research based upon the use of the form in a large cohort of patients was published, validating the form (90). The results from this study are the basis for the current version of the caries risk assessment form shown in Figure 30-6.

2. Caries risk determination. Assigning a "caries risk level" to a patient is the first step in managing the disease process. Table 30-1 presents the four risk levels groups (low, moderate, high, and extreme) and the recommendations for caries management procedures for each level.
   a. Low or moderate caries risk is assigned based on clinical judgment following an evaluation of the risk factors and protective factors of the patient.
   b. High caries risk is signified by the presence of any one of the following: visible cavities or radiographic penetration of the dentin, radiographic interproximal enamel lesions, white spots on smooth surfaces, or restorations in the last 3 years.
   c. Extreme caries risk is high caries risk and severe salivary gland hypofunction (salivary flow rate of less than 0.5 mL/min).

3. Evidence-based treatment plan. Following caries risk determination, the next step is to develop an evidence-based treatment plan based upon the patient's risk level.
   a. Low-risk patients should use fluoride toothpaste twice daily and professional topical fluoride applications are optional. Bacterial and salivary tests are not necessary. Most periodontal maintenance patients are not considered low risk because exposed roots are a primary risk factor for root caries.
   b. Moderate caries risk patients should use fluoride toothpaste twice daily, rinse with a 0.05% sodium fluoride mouthrinse, and receive fluoride varnish applications at maintenance appointments. Bacterial and salivary test are optional.
   c. High caries risk patients should use a prescription of 1.1% sodium fluoride toothpaste twice daily and receive one to three fluoride varnish applications during initial therapy. Fluoride varnish should be applied at 3-month intervals. Bacterial and salivary tests are recommended.
   d. Extreme caries risk patients receive the same CAMBRA therapies as high risk. In addition baking soda rinses, 0.5% sodium fluoride rinses and calcium/phosphate pastes may be recommended.

Caries Risk Assessment Form - Children Age 6 and Over/Adults

Patient Name: _____ Chart #: _____ Date: _____

Assessment Date: Is this (please circle) baseline   or   recall

Disease Indicators (Any one "YES" signifies likely "High Risk" and to do a bacteria test**)	YES = CIRCLE	YES = CIRCLE	YES = CIRCLE
Visible cavities or radiographic penetration of the dentin	YES		
Radiographic approximal enamel lesions (not in dentin)	YES		
White spots on smooth surfaces	YES		
Restorations last 3 years	YES		
Risk Factors (Biological or predisposing factors)			
MS and LB both medium or high (by culture**)		YES	
Visible heavy plaque on teeth		YES	
Frequent snack (>3x daily between meals)		YES	
Deep pits and fissures		YES	
Recreational drug use		YES	
Inadequate saliva flow by observation or measurement (***If measured, note the flow rate below)		YES	
Saliva reducing factors (medications/radiation/systemic)		YES	
Exposed roots		YES	
Orthodontic appliances		YES	
Protective Factors			
Lives/work/school flouridated community			YES
Fluoride toothpaste at least once daily			YES
Fluoride toothpaste at least 2x daily			YES
Fluoride mouthrinse (0.05% NaF) daily			YES
5,000 ppm F fluoride toothpaste daily			YES
Flouride varnish in last 6 months			YES
Office F topical in last 6 months			YES
Chlorhexidine prescribed/used one week each of last 6 months			YES
Xylitol gum/lozenges 4x daily last 6 months			YES
Calcium and phosphate paste during last 6 months			YES
Adequate saliva flow (>1 mL/min stimulated)			YES
Bacteria/Saliva Test Results: MS: LB: Flow Rate: mL/min. Date:			

VISUALIZE CARIES BALANCE
(Use circled indicators/factors above)
(EXTREME RISK = HIGH RISK + SEVERE SALIVARY GLAND HYPOFUNCTION)
CARIES RISK ASSESSMENT (CIRCLE): EXTREME   HIGH   MODERATE   LOW

Signature: _____ Date: _____

Figure 30-6. Caries Risk Assessment Form. (Used with permission from Featherstone JD, Domejean-Orliaguet S, Jenson L, et al. Caries risk assessment in practice for age 6 through adult. *J Calif Dent Assoc.* 2007;35(10):703–707, 710–713, Table 1.)

TABLE 30-1. CARIES MANAGEMENT BY RISK ASSESSMENT: CLINICAL GUIDELINES

Risk Level[a,b]	Frequency of Caries Radiographs	Frequency of Caries Recall	Saliva Test (Saliva Flow and Bacterial Culture)	Antibacterials Chlorhexidine Xylitol[c]	Fluoride	pH Control	Calcium Phosphate Topical Supplements
Low risk	Bitewing radiographs every 24–36 mo	Every 6–12 mo to reevaluate caries risk	May be done as a baseline reference for new patients	Per saliva test if done	OTC fluoride-containing toothpaste twice daily; Optional NaF varnish if excessive root exposure or sensitivity	Not required	Not required; Optional for excessive root exposure or sensitivity
Moderate risk	Bitewing radiographs every 18–24 mo	Every 4–6 mo to reevaluate caries risk	May be done as a baseline reference for new patients or if there is a suspicion of high bacterial challenge	Per saliva test if done; Xylitol (6–10 g/d) of gum or candies	OTC fluoride-containing toothpaste twice daily plus 0.05% NaF rinse daily. Initially 1–2 app of NaF varnish; 1 app at 4–6 mo recall	Not required	Not required; Optional for excessive root exposure or sensitivity
High risk[d]	Bitewing radiographs every 6–18 mo or until no cavitated lesions are evident	Every 3–4 mo to reevaluate caries risk and apply fluoride varnish	Saliva flow test and bacterial culture initially and at every caries recall app. to assess efficacy and patient cooperation	Chlorhexidine gluconate 0.12%; 10 mL rinse for 1 min daily for 1 wk each month. Xylitol (6–10 g/d)	1.1% NaF toothpaste twice daily instead of regular fluoride toothpaste; Optional 0.2% NaF rinse daily (1 bottle) then OTC 0.05% NaF rinse 2× daily. Initially 1–3 app of NaF varnish; 1 app at 3–4 mo recall	Not required	Optional; apply calcium/phosphate paste several times daily
Extreme risk[e] (High risk plus dry mouth or special needs)	Bitewing radiographs every 6 mo or until no cavitated lesions are evident	Every 3 mo to reevaluate caries risk and apply fluoride varnish	Saliva flow test and bacterial culture initially and at every caries recall app. to assess efficacy and patient cooperation	Chlorhexidine gluconate 0.12% (preferably CHX in water base rinse) 10 mL rinse for 1 min daily for 1 wk each month. Xylitol (6–10 g/d)	1.1% NaF toothpaste twice daily instead of regular fluoride toothpaste. OTC 0.05% NaF rinse when mouth feels dry, after snacking, breakfast, and lunch. Initially 1–3 app. NaF varnish; 1 app at 3-mo recall	Acid-neutralizing rinses as needed if mouth feels dry, after snacking, bedtime, and after breakfast. Baking soda gum as needed	Required. Apply calcium/phosphate paste twice daily

[a]For all risk levels: patients must maintain good self-care and a diet low in frequency of fermentable carbohydrates.
[b]All restorative work to be done with minimally invasive philosophy in mind.
[c]Xylitol is not good for pets (especially dogs). Used with permission from Featherstone JD, Domejean-Orliaguet S, Jenson L, et al. Caries risk assessment in practice for age 6 through adult. *J Calif Dent Assoc.* 2007;35(10):703–707, 710–713, Table 1.
[d]Patients with one (or more) cavitated lesion(s) are high-risk patients.
[e]Patients with one (or more) cavitated lesion(s) and severe hyposalivation are extreme-risk patients.

Chapter Summary Statement

Periodontal maintenance refers to continuing patient care provided by the dental team to help the periodontitis patient maintain periodontal health following complete nonsurgical or surgical periodontal therapy. In most dental offices the dental hygienist plays a major role in procedures performed during periodontal maintenance visits. Procedures in a typical office visit for periodontal maintenance include patient interview, clinical assessment, evaluation of effectiveness of self-care, identification of treatment needs, periodontal instrumentation, patient counseling, and application of fluorides. Currently the most frequently recommended interval for periodontal maintenance is every 3 months. Recurrence of periodontitis in treated patients with the need for additional active periodontal treatment is always a possibility. Patient compliance with periodontal maintenance recommendations is poor, but strategies can be employed to improve compliance. Root caries is a complication in many treated periodontitis patients.

Section 6
Focus on Patients

Clinical Patient Care

CASE 1

Your dental team has just completed a reevaluation of the results of nonsurgical therapy for a patient with generalized slight chronic periodontitis. The findings of the reevaluation reveal that the periodontitis appears to be under control and that periodontal maintenance is the next logical step. When should the first maintenance appointment be scheduled and what factors should be considered when assigning this maintenance interval?

CASE 2

One of your dental team's chronic periodontitis patients has recently undergone periodontal surgery and now has several sites of gingival recession exposing tooth roots. Unfortunately, this patient has had a high incidence of both coronal and root caries over the past few years. What measures might your team take to minimize the risk of further root caries in this patient?

CASE 3

A patient who has been treated for chronic periodontitis by your team has been followed for periodontal maintenance for more than 3 years. During each maintenance visit, there have been no indications of recurrence of the periodontitis. The patient calls you before her next maintenance visit to inform you that she has just been diagnosed with diabetes mellitus. She looked up diabetes on the Internet and now wants to know if this will affect her periodontal condition. How should your dental team respond to the patient's concern?

References

1. Allen E, Ziada H, Irwin C, et al. Periodontics: 10. Maintenance in periodontal therapy. *Dent Update.* 2008;35(3):150–152, 154–156.
2. Ramfjord SP. Maintenance care and supportive periodontal therapy. *Quintessence Int.* 1993;24(7):465–471.
3. Shumaker ND, Metcalf BT, Toscano NT, et al. Periodontal and periimplant maintenance: a critical factor in long-term treatment success. *Compend Contin Educ Dent.* 2009;30(7):388–390, 392, 394 passim; quiz 407, 418.
4. Tan AE. Periodontal maintenance. *Aust Dent J.* 2009;54(suppl 1):S110–S117.
5. Wilson TG Jr, Valderrama P, Rodrigues DB. The case for routine maintenance of dental implants. *J Periodontol.* 2014;85(5):657–660.
6. Bostanci HS, Arpak MN. Long-term evaluation of surgical periodontal treatment with and without maintenance care. *J Nihon Univ Sch Dent.* 1991;33(3):152–159.
7. Costa FO, Cota LO, Lages EJ, et al. Periodontal risk assessment model in a sample of regular and irregular compliers under maintenance therapy: a 3-year prospective study. *J Periodontol.* 2012;83(3):292–300.
8. Jansson L, Lagervall M. Periodontitis progression in patients subjected to supportive maintenance care. *Swed Dent J.* 2008;32(3):105–114.
9. Lorentz TC, Cota LO, Cortelli JR, et al. Tooth loss in individuals under periodontal maintenance therapy: prospective study. *Braz Oral Res.* 2010;24(2):231–237.
10. Soolari A. Compliance and its role in successful treatment of an advanced periodontal case: review of the literature and a case report. *Quintessence Int.* 2002;33(5):389–396.
11. Costa FO, Miranda Cota LO, Pereira Lages EJ, et al. Progression of periodontitis and tooth loss associated with glycemic control in individuals undergoing periodontal maintenance therapy: a 5-year follow-up study. *J Periodontol.* 2013;84(5):595–605.
12. Nibali L, Farias BC, Vajgel A, et al. Tooth loss in aggressive periodontitis: a systematic review. *J Dent Res.* 2013;92(10):868–875.
13. Chambrone L, Chambrone D, Lima LA, et al. Predictors of tooth loss during long-term periodontal maintenance: a systematic review of observational studies. *J Clin Periodontol.* 2010;37(7):675–684.
14. Costa FO, Lages EJ, Cota LO, et al. Tooth loss in individuals under periodontal maintenance therapy: 5-year prospective study. *J Periodontal Res.* 2014;49(1):121–128.
15. Ravald N, Johansson CS. Tooth loss in periodontally treated patients: a long-term study of periodontal disease and root caries. *J Clin Periodontol.* 2012;39(1):73–79.
16. Wilson TG Jr, Glover ME, Malik AK, et al. Tooth loss in maintenance patients in a private periodontal practice. *J Periodontol.* 1987;58(4):231–235.
17. Lorentz TC, Cota LO, Cortelli JR, et al. Prospective study of complier individuals under periodontal maintenance therapy: analysis of clinical periodontal parameters, risk predictors and the progression of periodontitis. *J Clin Periodontol.* 2009;36(1):58–67.
18. Axtelius B, Soderfeldt B, Edwardsson S, et al. Therapy-resistant periodontitis (II). Compliance and general and dental health experiences. *J Clin Periodontol.* 1997;24(9 Pt 1):646–653.
19. Croft LK, Nunn ME, Crawford LC, et al. Patient preference for ultrasonic or hand instruments in periodontal maintenance. *Int J Periodontics Restorative Dent.* 2003;23(6):567–573.
20. Petersilka G, Faggion CM Jr, Stratmann U, et al. Effect of glycine powder air-polishing on the gingiva. *J Clin Periodontol.* 2008;35(4):324–332.
21. Petersilka GJ, Tunkel J, Barakos K, et al. Subgingival plaque removal at interdental sites using a low-abrasive air polishing powder. *J Periodontol.* 2003;74(3):307–311.
22. Sahrmann P, Ronay V, Schmidlin PR, et al. Three-dimensional defect evaluation of air polishing on extracted human roots. *J Periodontol.* 2014;85(8):1107–1114.
23. Sculean A, Bastendorf KD, Becker C, et al. A paradigm shift in mechanical biofilm management? Subgingival air polishing: a new way to improve mechanical biofilm management in the dental practice. *Quintessence Int.* 2013;44(7):475–477.
24. Flemmig TF, Arushanov D, Daubert D, et al. Randomized controlled trial assessing efficacy and safety of glycine powder air polishing in moderate-to-deep periodontal pockets. *J Periodontol.* 2012;83(4):444–452.
25. Moene R, Decaillet F, Andersen E, et al. Subgingival plaque removal using a new air-polishing device. *J Periodontol.* 2010;81(1):79–88.
26. Wennstrom JL, Dahlen G, Ramberg P. Subgingival debridement of periodontal pockets by air polishing in comparison with ultrasonic instrumentation during maintenance therapy. *J Clin Periodontol.* 2011;38(9):820–827.
27. Petersilka GJ. Subgingival air-polishing in the treatment of periodontal biofilm infections. *Periodontol 2000.* 2011;55(1):124–142.
28. Petersilka GJ, Steinmann D, Haberlein I, et al. Subgingival plaque removal in buccal and lingual sites using a novel low abrasive air-polishing powder. *J Clin Periodontol.* 2003;30(4):328–333.
29. Petersilka GJ, Bell M, Haberlein I, et al. In vitro evaluation of novel low abrasive air polishing powders. *J Clin Periodontol.* 2003;30(1):9–13.
30. Sahrmann P, Ronay V, Sener B, et al. Cleaning potential of glycine air-flow application in an in vitro peri-implantitis model. *Clin Oral Implants Res.* 2013;24(6):666–670.
31. Schwarz F, Ferrari D, Popovski K, et al. Influence of different air-abrasive powders on cell viability at biologically contaminated titanium dental implants surfaces. *J Biomed Mater Res B Appl Biomater.* 2009;88(1):83–91.
32. Graumann SJ, Sensat ML, Stoltenberg JL. Air polishing: a review of current literature. *J Dent Hyg.* 2013;87(4):173–180.
33. Parameters of Care. American Academy of Periodontology. *J Periodontol.* 2000;71(5 suppl):i–ii, 847–883.
34. American Academy of Periodontology. Comprehensive periodontal therapy: a statement by the American Academy of Periodontology *. *J Periodontol.* 2011;82(7):943–949.
35. Cohen RE; Research, Science and Therapy Committee, American Academy of Periodontology. Position paper: periodontal maintenance. *J Periodontol.* 2003;74(9):1395–1401.
36. Lang NP, Joss A, Tonetti MS. Monitoring disease during supportive periodontal treatment by bleeding on probing. *Periodontol 2000.* 1996;12:44–48.

37. Flemmig TF, Petersilka GJ, Mehl A, et al. Working parameters of a magnetostrictive ultrasonic scaler influencing root substance removal in vitro. *J Periodontol*. 1998;69(5):547–553.

38. Flemmig TF, Petersilka GJ, Mehl A, et al. The effect of working parameters on root substance removal using a piezoelectric ultrasonic scaler in vitro. *J Clin Periodontol*. 1998;25(2):158–163.

39. Flemmig TF, Petersilka GJ, Mehl A, et al. Working parameters of a sonic scaler influencing root substance removal in vitro. *Clin Oral Investig*. 1997;1(2):55–60.

40. Kocher T, Fanghanel J, Sawaf H, et al. Substance loss caused by scaling with different sonic scaler inserts–an in vitro study. *J Clin Periodontol*. 2001;28(1):9–15.

41. Ritz L, Hefti AF, Rateitschak KH. An in vitro investigation on the loss of root substance in scaling with various instruments. *J Clin Periodontol*. 1991;18(9):643–647.

42. Schmidlin PR, Beuchat M, Busslinger A, et al. Tooth substance loss resulting from mechanical, sonic and ultrasonic root instrumentation assessed by liquid scintillation. *J Clin Periodontol*. 2001;28(11):1058–1066.

43. Badersten A, Nilveus R, Egelberg J. Effect of nonsurgical periodontal therapy. I. Moderately advanced periodontitis. *J Clin Periodontol*. 1981;8(1):57–72.

44. Badersten A, Nilveus R, Egelberg J. Effect of nonsurgical periodontal therapy. II. Severely advanced periodontitis. *J Clin Periodontol*. 1984;11(1):63–76.

45. Chabanski MB, Gillam DG. Aetiology, prevalence and clinical features of cervical dentine sensitivity. *J Oral Rehabil*. 1997;24(1):15–19.

46. Fischer C, Wennberg A, Fischer RG, et al. Clinical evaluation of pulp and dentine sensitivity after supragingival and subgingival scaling. *Endod Dent Traumatol*. 1991;7(6):259–265.

47. Tammaro S, Wennstrom JL, Bergenholtz G. Root-dentin sensitivity following non-surgical periodontal treatment. *J Clin Periodontol*. 2000;27(9):690–697.

48. von Troil B, Needleman I, Sanz M. A systematic review of the prevalence of root sensitivity following periodontal therapy. *J Clin Periodontol*. 2002;29 Suppl 3:173–177; discussion 195–196.

49. Dragoo MR. A clinical evaluation of hand and ultrasonic instruments on subgingival debridement. 1. With unmodified and modified ultrasonic inserts. *Int J Periodontics Restorative Dent*. 1992;12(4):310–323.

50. Jacobson L, Blomlof J, Lindskog S. Root surface texture after different scaling modalities. *Scand J Dent Res*. 1994;102(3):156–160.

51. Mishra MK, Prakash S. A comparative scanning electron microscopy study between hand instrument, ultrasonic scaling and erbium doped: Yttirum aluminum garnet laser on root surface: a morphological and thermal analysis. *Contemp Clin Dent*. 2013;4(2):198–205.

52. Darcey J, Ashley M. See you in three months! The rationale for the three monthly periodontal recall interval: a risk based approach. *Br Dent J*. 2011;211(8):379–385.

53. Shiloah J, Patters MR. Repopulation of periodontal pockets by microbial pathogens in the absence of supportive therapy. *J Periodontol*. 1996;67(2):130–139.

54. Famili P, Short E. Compliance with periodontal maintenance at the University of Pittsburgh: retrospective analysis of 315 cases. *Gen Dent*. 2010;58(1):e42–e47.

55. Ojima M, Hanioka T, Shizukuishi S. Survival analysis for degree of compliance with supportive periodontal therapy. *J Clin Periodontol*. 2001;28(12):1091–1095.

56. Wilson TG Jr. Compliance. A review of the literature with possible applications to periodontics. *J Periodontol*. 1987;58(10):706–714.

57. de Carvalho VF, Okuda OS, Bernardo CC, et al. Compliance improvement in periodontal maintenance. *J Appl Oral Sci*. 2010;18(3):215–219.

58. Mendoza AR, Newcomb GM, Nixon KC. Compliance with supportive periodontal therapy. *J Periodontol*. 1991;62(12):731–736.

59. Novaes AB Jr, Novaes AB. Compliance with supportive periodontal therapy. Part 1. Risk of non-compliance in the first 5-year period. *J Periodontol*. 1999;70(6):679–682.

60. Novaes AB Jr, Novaes AB. Compliance with supportive periodontal therapy. Part II: risk of non-compliance in a 10-year period. *Braz Dent J*. 2001;12(1):47–50.

61. Umaki TM, Umaki MR, Cobb CM. The psychology of patient compliance: a focused review of the literature. *J Periodontol*. 2012;83(4):395–400.

62. Dye BA, Tan S, Smith V, et al. Trends in oral health status: United States, 1988–1994 and 1999–2004. *Vital Health Stat*. 2007;(248):1–92.

63. Chi DL, Berg JH, Kim AS, et al., Northwest Practice-based RCiE-bD. Correlates of root caries experience in middle-aged and older adults in the Northwest Practice-based REsearch Collaborative in Evidence-based DENTistry research network. *J Am Dent Assoc*. 2013;144(5):507–516.

64. Griffin SO, Griffin PM, Swann JL, et al. Estimating rates of new root caries in older adults. *J Dent Res*. 2004;83(8):634–638.

65. Pitts NB, Ekstrand KR, ICDAS Foundation. International Caries Detection and Assessment System (ICDAS) and its International Caries Classification and Management System (ICCMS) - methods for staging of the caries process and enabling dentists to manage caries. *Community Dent Oral Epidemiol*. 2013;41(1):e41–e52.

66. Shivakumar K, Prasad S, Chandu G. International Caries Detection and Assessment System: a new paradigm in detection of dental caries. *J Conserv Dent*. 2009;12(1):10–16.

67. Berry TG, Summitt JB, Sift EJ Jr. Root caries. *Oper Dent*. 2004;29(6):601–607.

68. Zambon JJ, Kasprzak SA. The microbiology and histopathology of human root caries. *Am J Dent*. 1995;8(6):323–328.

69. Atkinson JC, Wu AJ. Salivary gland dysfunction: causes, symptoms, treatment. *J Am Dent Assoc*. 1994;125(4):409–416.

70. Ogaard B, Arends J, Rolla G. Action of fluoride on initiation of early root surface caries in vivo. *Caries Res*. 1990;24(2):142–144.

71. Papas A, Joshi A, Giunta J. Prevalence and intraoral distribution of coronal and root caries in middle-aged and older adults. *Caries Res*. 1992;26(6):459–465.

72. Griffin SO, Regnier E, Griffin PM, et al. Effectiveness of fluoride in preventing caries in adults. *J Dent Res*. 2007;86(5):410–415.

73. Heijnsbroek M, Paraskevas S, Van der Weijden GA. Fluoride interventions for root caries: a review. *Oral Health Prev Dent.* 2007;5(2):145–152.
74. Gibson G, Jurasic MM, Wehler CJ, et al. Supplemental fluoride use for moderate and high caries risk adults: a systematic review. *J Public Health Dent.* 2011;71(3):171–184.
75. Brustman BA. Impact of exposure to fluoride-adequate water on root surface caries in elderly. *Gerodontics.* 1986;2(6):203–207.
76. Jensen ME, Kohout F. The effect of a fluoridated dentifrice on root and coronal caries in an older adult population. *J Am Dent Assoc.* 1988;117(7):829–832.
77. Ekstrand KR, Poulsen JE, Hede B, et al. A randomized clinical trial of the anti-caries efficacy of 5,000 compared to 1,450 ppm fluoridated toothpaste on root caries lesions in elderly disabled nursing home residents. *Caries Res.* 2013;47(5):391–398.
78. Sjogren K, Birkhed D. Factors related to fluoride retention after toothbrushing and possible connection to caries activity. *Caries Res.* 1993;27(6):474–477.
79. Ripa LW, Leske GS, Forte F, et al. Effect of a 0.05% neutral NaF mouthrinse on coronal and root caries of adults. *Gerodontology.* 1987;6(4):131–136.
80. Wallace MC, Retief DH, Bradley EL. The 48-month increment of root caries in an urban population of older adults participating in a preventive dental program. *J Public Health Dent.* 1993;53(3):133–137.
81. Schaeken MJ, Keltjens HM, Van Der Hoeven JS. Effects of fluoride and chlorhexidine on the microflora of dental root surfaces and progression of root-surface caries. *J Dent Res.* 1991;70(2):150–153.
82. Slot DE, Vaandrager NC, Van Loveren C, et al. The effect of chlorhexidine varnish on root caries: a systematic review. *Caries Res.* 2011;45(2):162–173.
83. Featherstone JD, White JM, Hoover CI, et al. A randomized clinical trial of anticaries therapies targeted according to risk assessment (caries management by risk assessment). *Caries Res.* 2012;46(2):118–129.
84. Ritter AV, Bader JD, Leo MC, et al. Tooth-surface-specific effects of xylitol: randomized trial results. *J Dent Res.* 2013;92(6):512–517.
85. Azarpazhooh A, Limeback H. Clinical efficacy of casein derivatives: a systematic review of the literature. *J Am Dent Assoc.* 2008;139(7):915–924.
86. Rethman MP, Beltran-Aguilar ED, Billings RJ, et al. Nonfluoride caries-preventive agents: executive summary of evidence-based clinical recommendations. *J Am Dent Assoc.* 2011;142(9):1065–1071.
87. Featherstone JD, Domejean-Orliaguet S, Jenson L, et al. Caries risk assessment in practice for age 6 through adult. *J Calif Dent Assoc.* 2007;35(10):703–707, 710–713.
88. Young DA, Featherstone JD, Roth JR. Curing the silent epidemic: caries management in the 21st century and beyond. *J Calif Dent Assoc.* 2007;35(10):681–685.
89. Featherstone JD, Adair SM, Anderson MH, et al. Caries management by risk assessment: consensus statement, April 2002. *J Calif Dent Assoc.* 2003;31(3):257–269.
90. Domejean-Orliaguet S, Gansky SA, Featherstone JD. Caries risk assessment in an educational environment. *J Dent Educ.* 2006;70(12):1346–1354.

 STUDENT ANCILLARY RESOURCES

A wide variety of resources to enhance your learning and understanding of this chapter are available on thePoint®.

- Visit thePoint to access:
  - Audio Glossary
  - Animations
  - Suggested Readings
  - Answers to Review Questions
  - Case Studies

Periodontal Maintenance of Dental Implants

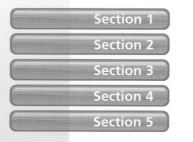

Clinical Application.
All dental healthcare providers will encounter patients with dental implants, and dental hygienists are at the forefront of providing maintenance care for patients with dental implants. This chapter provides an overview of dental implants and guidance for establishing appropriate maintenance to insure periodontal health of implants.

Learning Objectives

- Describe the components of a typical dental implant and restoration.
- Compare and contrast the periodontium of a natural tooth with the peri-implant tissues that surround a dental implant.
- Define the terms osseointegration and biomechanical forces as they apply to dental implants.
- Compare and contrast the terms peri-implant mucositis and peri-implantitis.
- Discuss the special considerations for periodontal instrumentation of a dental implant.
- Describe an appropriate maintenance interval for a patient with dental implants.
- In the clinical setting, select appropriate self-care aids for a patient with dental implants.

Key Terms

Dental implant
Implant body
Implant abutment
Biocompatible

Peri-implant tissues
Biological seal
Osseointegration
Peri-implant mucositis

Peri-implantitis
Biomechanical forces

Section 1
Anatomy of the Dental Implant

A **dental implant** is a nonbiologic (artificial) device surgically inserted into the jawbone to (1) replace a missing tooth or (2) provide support for a prosthetic denture. Over the past 30 years, research has validated the success of implant placement as a feasible option to replace missing teeth in partially or fully edentulous patients (1–7). The dental hygienist plays an important role in patient education and professional maintenance of the dental implant. Understanding the basic concepts of implantology and the anatomy of the peri-implant tissues is a prerequisite to understanding the maintenance of dental implants.

1. The Dental Implant System
    A. **Introduction to Dental Implant Systems.** Dental implant systems are used to replace individual teeth or support a fixed bridge or removable denture (Fig. 31-1). The components of a dental implant system are the (1) implant body, (2) the abutment, and (3) a prosthetic crown or prosthesis (Fig. 31-2).
    B. **The Implant Body**
        1. An **implant body** is the portion of the implant system that is surgically placed into the living alveolar bone (Fig. 31-3–31-5). This is sometimes referred to as the implant fixture or implant.
        2. The implant body acts as the "root" of the implant restoration. The implant body usually is threaded like a screw. These threads provide a greater surface area for contact with the alveolar bone.
            a. The metal used for dental implants is titanium or titanium alloy. Titanium is an ideal material for dental implants because it is a bone-friendly metal that is biocompatible and because it is a poor conductor of heat and electricity.
            b. The major disadvantage of titanium is that it is softer than other dental restorative metals and thus it scratches easily.
    C. **The Abutment**
        1. The **implant abutment** is a titanium post that attaches to the implant body and protrudes partially or completely through the gingival tissue into the mouth (Fig. 31-4).
        2. The abutment supports the restorative prosthesis (crown or denture).
        3. The titanium abutment is extremely **biocompatible** (not rejected by the body) and allows tissue healing around the abutment.

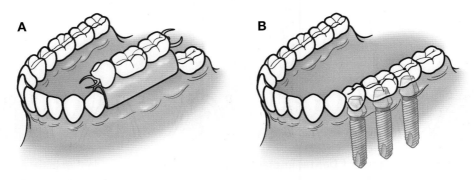

Figure 31-1. Replacement of Missing Teeth. A: Extracted teeth replaced by a traditional removable partial denture. **B:** Missing teeth replaced by three individual dental implants.

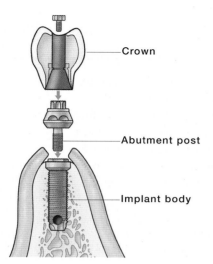

Figure 31-2. The Dental Implant System. The components of a dental implant system are the implant body and the abutment post. The implant body is placed into living alveolar bone. The abutment post extends into or through living gingival tissue into the mouth. A crown or other prosthesis is connected to the abutment either by a screw or by dental cement.

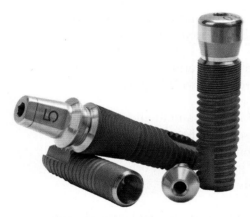

Figure 31-3. Implants and Components. Examples of screw-shaped titanium implant bodies and abutment posts.

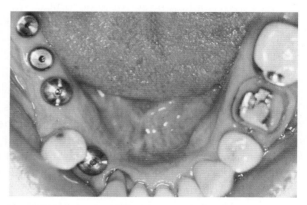

Figure 31-4. Abutments. This photograph shows the healing abutments for four implants.

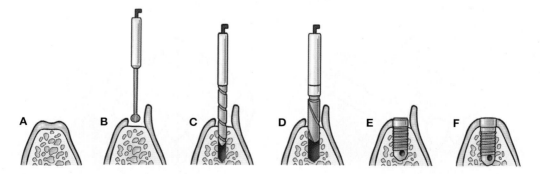

Figure 31-5. Surgical Placement of Dental Implants. A: Edentulous alveolar ridge. **B:** Initial osteotomy site established. **C, D:** Drills of increasing diameters used to prepare osteotomy to the size of the planned implant. **E:** Implant body seated in the osteotomy. The top of the implant body may be placed slightly above, level with, or slightly below the crest of the bone. **F:** Implant body seated in bone with cover screw attached. At the end of placement surgery, the implant can be covered with gingiva or left exposed to the oral cavity, as shown here. A healing time of several weeks to months is allowed, so that osseointegration can occur.

2. **The Peri-implant Tissues.** The peri-implant tissues are the tissues that surround the dental implant (Fig. 31-6). The peri-implant tissues are similar in many ways to the periodontium of a natural tooth, but there are some important differences (Table 31-1).
   A. Implant-to-Epithelial Tissue Interface
      1. The epithelium adapts to the titanium abutment post, or to the implant itself, creating a **biological seal**. The union of the epithelial cells to the abutment or implant surface is very similar to that of the epithelial cells to the natural tooth surface.
      2. The biological seal functions as a barrier between the implant and the oral cavity.
      3. As with a natural tooth, a sulcus lined by sulcular epithelium and junctional epithelium surrounds the abutment or in some cases, the top of the implant body.
   B. Implant-to-Connective Tissue Interface
      1. *The implant-to-connective tissue interface is significantly different from that of connective tissue of a natural tooth.*
      2. The implant surface lacks cementum, so the gingival fibers and the periodontal ligament cannot insert into the titanium surface as they do into the cementum of a natural tooth.
         a. On a natural tooth:
            1. The supragingival fibers brace the gingival margin against the tooth and strengthen the attachment of the junctional epithelium to the tooth. The supragingival fibers insert into the cementum.
            2. The periodontal ligament suspends and maintains the tooth in its socket.
            3. The periodontal ligament fibers also serve as a physical barrier to bacterial invasion.
         b. On an implant:
            1. The connective tissue fiber bundles support the healthy gingiva against the abutment. The connective tissue fiber bundles in the gingiva around an implant have been shown to be either (1) oriented parallel to the implant surface or (2) encircling the implant abutment (8). The fibers do not attach to the dental implant.
            2. There are no periodontal ligament fibers to provide protection for the dental implant. *Therefore, periodontal pathogens can create inflammation and destroy bone much more rapidly along a dental implant than along a natural tooth with its protective barrier of periodontal ligament fibers* (9–12).
            3. Since there are no gingival or periodontal ligament fibers inserting into the titanium surfaces, a periodontal probe will pass more easily through the tissues to the alveolar bone surrounding the implant.
      3. Keratinized gingival tissue may or may not be present around the dental implant.
   C. Implant-to-Bone Interface
      1. **Osseointegration** is the direct contact of the living bone with the surface of the implant body (with no intervening periodontal ligament). Osseointegration is the major requirement for implant success.
      2. Clinically, osseointegration is regarded as successful if there is
         a. an absence of clinical mobility of the implant
         b. no discomfort or pain when the implant is in function
         c. no increased bone loss or radiolucency surrounding the dental implant on a radiograph
         d. less than 0.2 mm of bone loss annually after the first year in function (13).

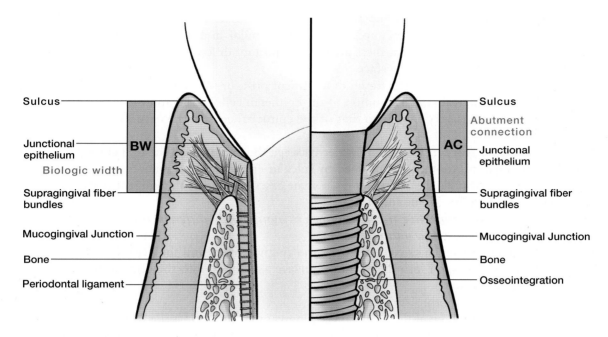

Figure 31-6. Comparison of Periodontium Interface with a Natural Tooth Versus a Dental Implant. The implant lacks the periodontal ligament connection to the alveolar bone and the gingival fibers do not insert into the titanium.

TABLE 31-1. TISSUES SURROUNDING A DENTAL IMPLANT	
Tissues	**Peri-implant Tissues**
Junctional epithelium	Attaches to the implant surface or abutment surface (biological seal)
Connective tissue fibers	Run parallel to or encircle the implant and abutment surface
Periodontal ligament	No periodontal ligament
Cementum	No cementum
Alveolar bone	In direct contact with the implant surface (osseointegration)

Section 2
Failing Implants: Peri-implant Disease

1. **Pathologic Changes in Implant Tissues**
   A. **Peri-implant Tissue Inflammation**
      1. Plaque biofilm can accumulate on the surfaces of teeth, restorations, oral appliances, and also on implants and abutments.
      2. The continuous presence of bacterial deposits can result in inflammation of the soft tissues around the implant.
      3. When the disease process progresses further, partial or total loss of osseointegration can occur.
   B. **Peri-implant Disease.** Pathologic changes of the peri-implant tissues can be referred to as peri-implant disease (Fig. 31-7). Peri-implant disease presents in two forms—peri-implant mucositis and peri-implantitis.
      1. **Peri-implant mucositis** (also called peri-implant gingivitis) is plaque-induced inflammation of the soft tissues—with no loss of supporting bone—that is localized in the mucosal tissues surrounding a dental implant.
         a. Peri-implant mucositis is reversible if the etiologic factors are removed (14). Peri-implant mucositis *may* progress to peri-implantitis.
         b. Peri-implant mucositis has been reported to occur in about 80% of subjects and 50% of implant sites, while peri-implantitis has been reported to occur in 28% to 56% of subjects and 12% to 43% of sites (15). However, the reported prevalence varies widely and change as implant designs evolve.
      2. **Peri-implantitis** is essentially chronic periodontitis affecting the soft and hard tissues surrounding a functioning osseointegrated dental implant, resulting in loss of supporting alveolar bone (8).
         a. Peri-implantitis begins at the coronal portion of the implant while the apical portion continues to be osseointegrated.
         b. An advanced peri-implantitis lesion can be diagnosed by the detection of radiographic bone loss around the implant (Fig. 31-8).
            1. The implant does not become mobile until the final stages of peri-implantitis.
            2. Implants that show mobility and signs of loss of osseointegration should be removed (16,17).
         c. Differences in the prevalence of peri-implantitis have been reported by a number of research studies. The prevalence reported in these studies ranges from 6.61% to 47% (18–21).

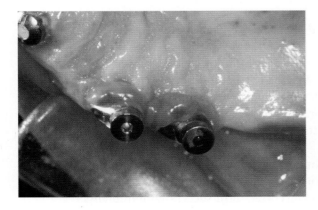

Figure 31-7. Peri-implant Disease. Inflammatory enlargement of peri-implant tissue resulting from poor daily self-care of the abutments and implant supported removable denture.

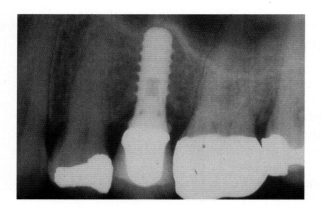

Figure 31-8. Peri-implantitis. This radiograph shows a titanium implant supporting a single crown. Note the residual cement near the crown margin. This has become a contributing factor for peri-implantitis since bone loss is evident on the radiograph.

2. **Etiology of Peri-implant Disease.** The major etiological factors associated with peri-implant disease are bacterial infection and biomechanical factors. Smoking is an additional factor that has been implicated in implant failure.
   A. **Bacterial Infection**
      1. Peri-implantitis—like periodontitis—occurs primarily as a result of an overwhelming bacterial infection and the subsequent host immune response (22).
      2. It appears that periodontal disease in both the peri-implant tissues and periodontium in natural teeth progresses in a similar fashion. *The rate of tissue destruction, however, tends to be more rapid in peri-implant tissues than in periodontal tissues.*
      3. Human cross-sectional studies found that peri-implantitis is associated with similar bacterial species to those associated with periodontitis (23–28).
         a. It is theorized that the natural teeth in a partially edentulous mouth act as a reservoir of periodontal pathogens that colonize the implants.
         b. This finding makes meticulous self-care of dental implants even more critical for the partially edentulous patient than for the fully edentulous patient.
   B. **Risk Factors.** The risk factors identified for each patient are essential in the estimation of the prognosis for the implants and these factors should be included in the determination of the appropriate maintenance interval. As in the treatment of periodontal disease, each patient must be assessed for the presence of risk factors that may help lead to peri-implant disease or its progression. Risk factors that should be considered include previous history of periodontal disease, ineffective self-care, residual cement, smoking, and biomechanical overload (22).
      1. **History of Previous Periodontal Disease.** Several systematic reviews indicated that peri-implantitis is a more frequent finding in patients with a history of periodontitis (29–32).
      2. **Poor Plaque Biofilm Control** (22)
      3. **Smoking.** Four systematic reviews concluded that there is an increased risk for peri-implantitis in smokers (30,33–35).
      4. **Residual Cement.** Implant-supported crowns are commonly held in place with cement. Residual cement (Fig. 31-9) may be left behind because of implant positioning that may hamper access to the subgingival space (36). Residual cement may induce inflammation due to its rough surface topography providing an environment for bacterial attachment (37).
      5. **Biomechanical Overload**
         a. Collectively, the forces placed on an implant have been called "biomechanical forces" to underscore the importance of both "biological" and "mechanical" aspects of controlling those forces to achieve long-term success with implants.

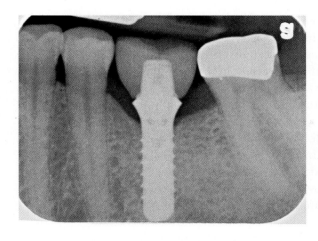

Figure 31-9. Residual Cement. The gap between the implant body and the crown exposes cement. Cement deposits typically are located subgingivally and are challenging to detect, especially if the cement is not visible radiographically. (Courtesy of Natalie A. Frost, DDS, MS, Omaha, NE.)

   b. Biomechanical forces on implants are influenced by a variety of factors that must be assessed by the clinician. Factors that influence the biomechanical forces include how much the occlusion is placed on the implant(s), the position of the implant, the number of implants supporting a prosthesis, and the distribution of the occlusal forces among the implants and remaining teeth.

   c. Since dental implants do not have a periodontal ligament, forces placed on an implant are transmitted directly to the alveolar bone (38,39). It is critical to minimize forces placed on an implant to avoid damage to the surrounding alveolar bone.

      1. Around a natural tooth the periodontal ligament helps absorb some of the forces placed on the tooth. These forces placed on natural teeth can arise from chewing food, supporting a dental appliance, or perhaps from habits such as bruxing.

      2. Dental implants lack the protective structure of the periodontal ligament that is found on natural teeth. If osseointegrated, the dental implant is in direct contact with the alveolar bone that completely supports it.

   d. Both bacterial plaque-related causes and excess biomechanical forces can contribute to the development of peri-implant disease. Both should be assessed and managed during implant maintenance appointments.

3. Detection of a Failing Implant

  A. Clinical Signs of a Failing Implant

    1. Soft Tissue Indictors. Clinical signs of a failing implant include the presence of a peri-implant pocket, bleeding after gentle probing, and/or suppuration from the pocket. The surrounding gingival tissue may or may not be swollen. Pain is usually not present.

    2. Implant Mobility. Absence of mobility is a very important clinical criterion for dental implants. ***The presence of mobility presently is the best indicator for diagnosis of implant failure*** (12).

      a. Implants should not move if osseointegrated and healthy (40,41).

        1. Implant mobility may indicate a lack of osseointegration.

        2. In some instances, mobility of an implant restoration may indicate the presence of a loose abutment or the rupture of the cement seal on cemented restorations. Mobility also can result from a loosening of the internal screw that attaches the abutment to the implant or the restoration and thus is not the result of peri-implant disease (Fig. 31-10).

        3. Severe mobility accompanied with discomfort also might indicate fracture of the implant itself.

4. Long-term mobility or misfit between the prosthetic components (e.g., screws between the crown and the implant) may lead to persistent inflammation, bone loss and the eventual complete failure of the implant.

  b. The technique for assessing mobility of a dental implant is similar to that used to assess a natural tooth. Two instrument handles are used to grasp the *implant restoration* and apply force back and forth in the facial and lingual direction. Remember that the implant *restoration* can be mobile, while the implant itself is healthy and not mobile. The use of two instruments with plastic handles is recommended if the implant itself must be touched.

  c. Radiographic evaluation is recommended when any mobility is noted. Loose internal screws or components will often be seen as a gap between the implant components on a radiograph.

 B. Radiographic Signs of a Failing Implant

   1. Radiographic signs of peri-implantitis include vertical destruction of the crestal bone around the implant—which assumes the shape of a saucer—while the bottom portion of the implant remains osseointegrated (42).

   2. Another radiographic indicator of peri-implantitis are wedge-shaped defects along the implant (42).

   3. A peri-implant radiolucency usually indicates advanced bone loss adjacent to the implant (Fig. 31-11).

4. Treatment Modalities for Failing Implants

 A. There are various methods available for the treatment of peri-implantitis including nonsurgical periodontal instrumentation, the use of antiseptics, local and/or systemic antibiotics, and access flap surgery (42).

   1. All these treatment modalities have been used with varying degrees of success, but at this time, there is no standard protocol for the treatment of peri-implantitis (42).

   2. Surgical treatment in which the lost bone is reestablished through bone grafting shows promising results (42,43).

 B. Nonsurgical periodontal instrumentation of peri-implantitis lesions with adjunctive local delivery of microencapsulated minocycline, as well as periodontal instrumentation supplemented with chlorhexidine can be beneficial to patients with peri-implantitis (24,44–47).

 C. The available evidence suggests that subgingival glycine powder air polishing for biofilm removal may reduce clinical signs of peri-implant mucosal inflammation to a greater extent than periodontal instrumentation with plastic curets combined with adjunctive irrigation with chlorhexidine (48).

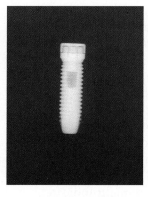

Figure 31-10. Loose Internal Screw. (Courtesy of Natalie A. Frost, DDS, MS, Omaha, NE.)

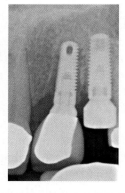

Figure 31-11. Peri-implant Radiolucency. A peri-implant radiolucency with advanced bone loss adjacent to the implant. (Courtesy of Natalie A. Frost, DDS, MS, Omaha, NE.)

Section 3
Clinical Monitoring of Peri-implant Disease

Routine monitoring of dental implants—as a part of a comprehensive periodontal examination and maintenance—is essential to the effective management of peri-implant disease.

1. **Probing**
   A. Initial probing of the implant should be done once the final restoration has been installed (22,49).
      1. In the past, routine periodontal probing of dental implants was not recommended by some authors. More recent literature, however, suggests that routine probing should be part of implant maintenance (22,49). Changes in probing depths can be used to detect changes in tissue/attachment health. Probing around osseointegrated implants does not appear to have detrimental effects on the soft tissue seal and, hence, does not seem to jeopardize the longevity of oral implants (50).
      2. Some implant surgeons recommend that probing should be avoided until postoperative healing is complete, approximately 3 months after abutment connection.
      3. A probing technique with light force (0.25 N, tip diameter 0.45) should be used since the biological seal is weakly adherent to the titanium surface (50). Heavy probing force will be invasive since the probe easily can penetrate through the biological seal and introduce bacteria into the peri-implant environment (9,51,52). The depth of penetration of the probe tip also is dependent on the health (or inflammatory stage of the peri-implant tissues) and thickness of the tissue around the abutment.
      4. Commercially available plastic probes have long been used when investigating the depth of the peri-implant sulcus (12). Recent literature recommends the use of conventional metal periodontal probes if probing pressures are kept light (53). Light lateral forces on the probe will protect against damaging titanium surfaces. However, plastic probes are more flexible and sometimes advantageous in probing excessive contours and angles found in implant restorations.
   B. Clinical attachment levels can be used to monitor peri-implant health.
      1. To interpret probe readings, the clinician must have baseline data recording previous probing levels of attachment, and a fixed reference point for repeatable probing comparisons.
         a. Initial probing of the implant should be done once the final restoration has been installed. Probing depth should be recorded and defined as the depth of probe penetration from the base of the implant sulcus to the crest of the mucosa. Similar to assessing natural teeth, the level of the crestal soft tissue can be measured using a fixed reference point on the restoration and should be noted as the clinical attachment level.
         b. ***Changes in probing attachment levels over time may be more important than the initial findings as implants may have deeper soft tissue probing depths.*** Due to variation in the depth of surgical placement, the tissue thickness at the site, as well as different lengths of the abutments and the connective tissue interface with the abutment, probing depths may be deeper than the 1- to 3-mm depths that are considered normal with natural teeth.
         c. A healthy peri-implant sulcus has been reported to range from 1.3 to 3.8 mm (54).
      2. The depth of penetration of the probe tip also is dependent on the health (or inflammatory stage of the peri-implant tissues) and thickness of the tissue around the abutment.

2. **Bleeding and Suppuration**
   A. Bleeding on probing is a good indicator of current tissue inflammation and should be recorded.
      1. *Lack of bleeding on gentle probing* is useful in predicting continuing tissue health around implants.
      2. Elimination of the bleeding on probing in peri-implant mucositis is important and should be accomplished with improved biofilm removal by the clinician and the patient.
      3. Increasing probing depth and bleeding are indicators for the need to perform an additional radiographic examination (15,55).
   B. Any suppuration should also be recorded at specific sites. Suppuration may be detected by probing, or by gently compressing the tissue over the implant with a gloved finger and observing for pus being expressed from the opening of the sulcus or pocket.
3. **Radiographs**
   A. Maintenance of bone levels around dental implants is an important criterion for determining treatment success. Radiographic evaluation of bone height and topography is necessary for the longitudinal monitoring of peri-implant stability (9,12,51,52).
      1. Vertical bone loss of less than 0.2 mm annually following the implant's first year of function is a criterion utilized to determine treatment success.
      2. Baseline radiographs should include the day of surgical implant placement, the day of final prosthesis insertion and periodically during implant maintenance (22). Bone remodeling during the first year after the final prosthesis insertion is expected, and then there should be less than 0.2 mm of bone loss annually thereafter.
      3. The shape and amount of bone remodeling following the final prosthesis insertion is different for different implant systems and configurations.
      4. If prior radiographs are not available, use 2 mm of bone loss from the expected bone level for the implant at that time point as the "decision point" for the diagnosis of peri-implantitis (53).
      5. Radiographs made on the day of the final prosthesis insertion (or re-cementation) should be reviewed for the presence of remaining excess cement. Cements that are visible radiographically should be used for implant restorations, especially if the margins and probable location of excess cements are subgingival.
      6. Radiographs also allow for the evaluation of the fit of the prosthesis and the integrity and adaptation of the different implant components.
   B. Dental implants should be evaluated radiographically at least once a year and should be checked more often in patients in whom periodontal breakdown around an implant was noted at a previous visit.

Section 4
Maintenance Therapy for Dental Implants

One of the most important factors in the long-term success of dental implants is the maintenance of the health of the peri-implant tissues. Successful maintenance requires the active participation of the patient and the dental team.

1. Considerations for Implant Maintenance
   A. Goals of Maintenance Therapy for Dental Implants
      1. Maintenance of Alveolar Bone Support
         a. Alveolar bone support is evaluated by use of good-quality radiographs taken with a long-cone paralleling technique at specific time intervals.
         b. The bone height and density around the implants is compared with previous radiographs of the site.
      2. Control of Inflammation
         a. Patient and professional biofilm control is important for proper gingival health.
         b. Patient self-care must be reevaluated and, if necessary, reinforced each time the patient is seen for maintenance. The better the patient self-care, the better the possibilities of maintaining stable results.
      3. Maintenance of a Healthy and Functional Implant
         a. Implant components should be checked for prosthesis integrity (such as mobility, loose screws, cement washout, material wear), implant, screw, or abutment fracture; unseating of attachments and proper adaptation of all components.
         b. *Any mobility of an implant or its restorative components requires immediate consultation with a dentist or specialist.*
   B. Patient Provided Information. Before beginning an examination, it is very important to obtain information from the patient related to implant-supported restorations or prostheses. The patient can often identify problems for clinicians that are otherwise difficult to find. Implant patients should be encouraged to share their perceptions of any changes in the fit, tightness, or feel of the implant restoration including the occlusion. Helpful questions to ask the patient include the following:
      1. Questions About Daily Self-care of Implant-supported Restorations/Prosthesis
         a. Are you able to clean around the neck portions of your implants easily?
         b. Do you still have enough cleaning aids to perform daily oral self-care?
      2. Questions Concerning Patient Satisfaction. General questions regarding the patient's satisfaction with the implant-supported restorations/prosthesis are part of a quality management concept for maintenance.
         a. Are you satisfied with the way your implants function?
         b. Are you satisfied with the appearance of your implants?
      3. Questions Regarding Patient-perceived Changes Since Last Appointment
         a. Do you think any part of the implant is loose?
         b. Do the gums around your implants bleed?
         c. Do you notice a bad taste coming from your implants?
         d. Have you noticed any changes in your implants?
   C. The Dental Implant Maintenance Visit
      1. Modern dental implants may be difficult to recognize intraorally since their restorations often have the same appearance as the crowns and fixed bridges used to restore natural teeth (Fig. 31-12). *For this reason, dental implants should be clearly noted in the chart, so that all dental team members are*

alerted to the fact that this is a dental implant patient. Also, the patient's radiographs should be reviewed before the start of periodontal instrumentation.

2. The following may be included in a maintenance visit; however, each maintenance visit should be individualized based on previous examinations, history, and judgment of the clinician: evaluation of peri-implant tissue health, examination of prosthesis/abutment components, evaluation of implant stability, occlusal examination, assessment of patient's self-care, radiographic examination, and treatment (e.g., periodontal instrumentation).

D. Maintenance Frequency

1. Maintenance intervals should be determined on an individual basis because there is a lack of data detailing precise intervals (4).

   a. A 3-month maintenance interval is usually appropriate for the first year following restoration of the implant (12). The clinician, however, must determine the best interval for each specific case.

   b. After the initial 12-month period, a 3- to 6-month maintenance interval may be used (56). Periodontal maintenance appointments should be scheduled as frequently as necessary to keep the periodontium and peri-implant tissues healthy.

   c. The risk factors identified for each patient are essential in the estimation of the prognosis for the implants and these factors should be included in the determination of the appropriate maintenance interval.

2. The following are indications for more frequent maintenance intervals.

   a. Reduced Bone Support Around Implants. Reduced bone support indicates that close monitoring of bone support is needed or the dental implant might be lost.

   b. Inflammation. A patient who has signs of inflammation around implants, even in the presence of good plaque control, needs more frequent maintenance visits.

   c. Host Response. Systemic conditions or diseases, such as diabetes, may affect the host-bacterial interaction. A shorter maintenance interval is needed for these patients.

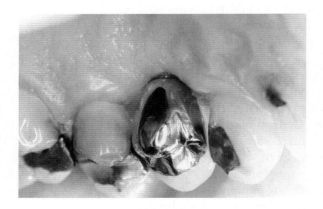

Figure 31-12. Fixed Prosthetic Crown. The first premolar in this photo is a prosthetic crown supported by a dental implant. During an intraoral examination, it would be difficult to distinguish between a crown that is supported by a natural tooth and a crown supported by a dental implant.

2. Procedures for Professional Biofilm Removal

   A. Plastic Curets for Biofilm Removal. Traditionally, plastic curets have been used for professional biofilm removal from dental implants.

   B. A Recent Innovation in Biofilm Management: Subgingival Air Polishing

      1. Air polishing technology uses a combination of an abrasive powder with water and compressed air delivered to a tooth or implant surface through an air polishing nozzle. Recently an air polishing device—Hu-Friedy Manufacturing's

Air-Flow Perio—has been introduced in the United States and Canada that utilizes a specially designed subgingival nozzle and low-abrasive glycine-based powder for subgingival biofilm removal.

2. The Unique Technology for Subgingival Air Polishing
   a. Subgingival air polishing devices use a specially designed disposable nozzle to deliver a low-abrasive powder to the subgingival environment.
   b. Subgingival air polishing uses a glycine-based powder that is biocompatible and gentle on the soft tissues of the oral cavity and subgingival epithelium (57–59).
   c. ***Prior to using this new technology, clinicians require special training in the proper use of the subgingival air polishing device.*** Explaining the techniques for use of subgingival glycine powder air polishing is beyond the scope of this chapter, but clinicians should be aware of this emerging technology and seek formal training in its use.

3. Clinical Evidence for Subgingival Air Polishing with Glycine Air Polishing of Dental Implants
   a. Subgingival air polishing for the removal of biofilm from titanium surfaces is a relatively new technology with clinical research supporting its safety and efficacy for use in the treatment of peri-implant disease.
      1. Although subgingival air polishing is an emerging technology in the United States and Canada, this technology has been used and researched for several years in Europe.
      2. It is important to note, that subgingival air polishing will not remove calculus deposits.
      3. In June 2012, during the *Euro-Perio 7 Conference in Vienna* (59), a consensus conference on mechanical biofilm management took place to review the current evidence from the literature on the clinical relevance of subgingival use of air polishing and to make practical recommendations for the clinician.
   b. Box 31-1 summarizes these recommendations, as well as, additional current evidence from the literature on subgingival biofilm management.

Box 31-1. Summary of Current Evidence on Subgingival Air Polishing of Titanium Surfaces

- Glycine powder polishing is safe and effective on titanium surfaces of dental implants (60,61).
- Glycine powder air polishing is more effective and less invasive than plastic curets for maintenance of peri-implant soft tissues (62,63).
- Subgingival glycine powder air polishing may reduce clinical signs of peri-implantitis (periodontal destruction around a dental implant) to a greater extent relative to instrumentation using curets with adjunctive irrigation with chlorhexidine (48,64).
- Glycine powder air polishing has only a minute effect on the surface topography of dental implants (65).
- Clinical, microbiological, and histological studies have confirmed subgingival glycine powder air polishing is safe, efficient, and comfortable when used as recommended by a trained professional (57,59,66–68).

3. **Periodontal Instrumentation of Dental Implants**
   A. **Special Considerations in Instrumentation Selection**
      1. The use of traditional metal curets is contraindicated around titanium implant components (56,69–72). Implant components are made of titanium, a soft metal, or titanium alloy that can be permanently damaged (grooved, scratched) if treated with metal instruments (Fig. 31-13).
         a. There is an increased likelihood of plaque retention and peri-implantitis if the titanium is scratched.
         b. Metal instruments can also disturb the surface coating of the implant, reducing the biocompatibility with the peri-implant tissues.
         c. The use of ultrasonic or sonic devices with standard metal tips is also contraindicated on titanium surfaces. Several manufacturers, however, offer specialized ultrasonic tips for use on titanium surfaces.
      2. Instruments used for assessment and periodontal instrumentation of implants and other titanium surfaces should be made of a material that is softer than the implant. Plastic instruments are commonly used (Fig. 31-14).
         a. Plastic instruments are safe for use on all types of implants, abutments, and components and will not cause damage to the surface.
         b. Standard dental restorative materials; for example, gold and porcelain; can be cleaned with conventional periodontal instruments. Care must be taken, however, not to use these instruments apical to the margin of the prosthetic crown where titanium might be in contact.
         c. Usually calculus deposits are removed readily from smooth titanium surfaces because there is no interlocking or penetration of the deposit with the surface. Light lateral pressure with a plastic instrument is recommended. Some calculus deposits, however, are densely calcified and tenaciously attached to the titanium surface and require more vigorous removal attempts. In such cases, powered instrumentation with specially designed ultrasonic tips may be helpful.

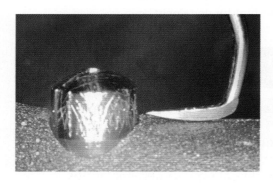

Figure 31-13. Surface Damage from Improper Instrumentation. Metal instruments can scratch the surface of the implant. (Courtesy of Drs. Mota and Baumhammers, University of Pittsburgh School of Dental Medicine, Pittsburg, PA.)

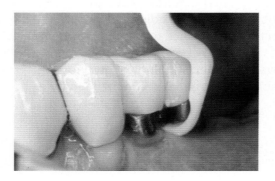

Figure 31-14. Plastic Curet. Plastic instruments are safe for use on dental implants.

3. Residual dental cement is a frequent finding when restorations have been cemented to abutments. These residual deposits are a definite contributor to peri-implant disease (36,37). Cement deposits are typically located subgingivally and are challenging to detect, especially if the cement is not visible radiographically. In addition, some of the advanced cement formulations used today are extremely strong and removal is very difficult. If removal efforts are not successful in a short time period, surgical access should be accomplished.

4. Some surfaces in implant systems are intended and manufactured to be rough. Rough surfaces are very common on portions or all of the implant body. These surfaces are usually intended to be adjacent to bone and not exposed to the oral environment. If an intentionally rough surface becomes exposed to the oral cavity, it will need to be cleaned and deplaqued as part of implant maintenance. Nonmetal instruments and air abrasives are the appropriate choices for instrumentation of such surfaces (71).

B. **Special Considerations for Polishing**
1. Implants, abutments, and components do not require routine polishing.
   a. When indicated, polishing of the implant restoration can be accomplished with rubber cups and nonabrasive polishing paste or by supragingival air polishing (12,56,71,73–78).
   b. Polishing has been shown to improve titanium surfaces *that have previously been roughened or scratched. However, if no surface alterations are noted, the titanium surfaces should not be polished.*
   c. A systematic review by Louropoulou of 34 papers indicates that *for rough implant surfaces,* air abrasives are the instruments of choice if surface integrity needs to be maintained (71). Air polishing with glycine powder may be considered as a better method to remove plaque biofilm from dental implants because glycine is less aggressive than sodium bicarbonate powder (74).

4. **Patient Self-care of Dental Implants**
A. **Considerations**
1. Meticulous self-care is of the utmost importance in preventing peri-implant disease. *An individualized self-care routine should be developed for each patient.*
2. Some patients undergoing implant therapy may have had a long history of dental neglect and/or poor plaque biofilm control.
3. The dental hygienist can assist the patient in maintaining dental implants by providing self-care education appropriate for implants and home care devices that are effective and simple to use.

B. **Care of Fixed Prosthetic Restorations**
1. A fixed prosthetic crown is an artificial tooth that fits over the abutment. These are made from a variety of routinely encountered restorative materials.
2. Self-care Challenges
   a. The single tooth prosthesis (crown) can present a challenge for biofilm control in that the patient may quickly begin to regard it to be just the same as a natural tooth.
      1. In fact, these restorations often have different designs and unusual contours that require focused self-care attention. The better the patient understands the design and contours, etc. that must be cleaned, the better the oral hygiene effectiveness will be.
      2. Self-care practices must be modified to include aids that can effectively clean the altered morphology of the peri-implant region.

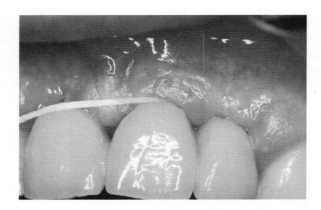

Figure 31-15. Implant Self-care. Dental floss is used to clean a single implant with a prosthetic crown. The "bulky" contours of the crown may contact the tissue and then "dip in" to meet the abutment at or below the gingival margin.

    b. The crown covering the implant abutment is larger in circumference than the abutment and will have contours added to it to make it look and function like a natural tooth.

       1. The "bulky" contours of the crown may contact the tissue and then "dip in" to meet the abutment at or below the gingival margin.

       2. Dental floss or tufted dental floss should be adapted along the margin of the crown and then pulled gently back and forth to direct it into the sulcus and around the abutment (Fig. 31-15).

    c. In some cases, the restoration may be similar to a fixed bridge (e.g., a pontic supported by two dental implants). Tufted dental floss, specially designed interdental brushes, and water flossers are effective cleaning devices for deplaquing the large embrasure spaces and into the sulci of these fixed bridge-type restorations.

    d. Restoration of multiple tooth replacement situations can involve complex, denture-like prostheses, which are attached to multiple implants and which are not removable by the patient.

       1. These prostheses are removable by the dentist or specialist at which time cleaning access is optimal.

       2. Daily care by the patient requires an individualized plan and a combination of devices to overcome the limited access often encountered.

  3. Techniques and Devices

    a. Standard multitufted, soft nylon bristle, manual toothbrushes can be used effectively by patients having sufficient dexterity and understanding of the task.

    b. Powered toothbrushes are safe for titanium surfaces and these devices are particularly helpful for implant patients in general.

    c. Interdental brushes can be effective in biofilm removal and may effectively clean the peri-implant sulcus (78).

       1. *Note that interdental brushes used to clean implants and components should have a soft protective coating on the twisted wire that secures the bristles.*

       2. The use a standard interdental brush (that does not have a plastic or nylon coating on the twisted wire) should be avoided since the exposed wire could scratch titanium.

d. Dental floss can be used with dental implants. Patients must be instructed as to the gentle use of dental floss in sometimes deep subgingival areas. Flosses with expanded spongy or fluffy sections along with a stiffer, floss threader section (tufted floss) are particularly helpful.

e. Oral irrigators may be safely used to deplaque dental implants.

    1. In a study, Magnuson et al. compared the efficacy of a manual toothbrush paired with either traditional dental floss or a water flosser. The study results demonstrate that the water flossing group had statistically significantly greater reduction in bleeding than the dental floss group. The authors conclude that water flossing may be a useful adjunct to implant maintenance (79).

    2. Patients should be instructed to use the lowest setting and direct the flow through the interdental contacts or perpendicular to the implants rather than directly into the implant sulcus (78).

f. Daily use of an antimicrobial mouth rinse is beneficial for many patients (80,81). The entire mouth can be rinsed twice daily after brushing. Or, if that is not acceptable to the patient, the mouth rinse can be applied topically to each implant area twice daily with a cotton-tipped applicator or with gauze.

C. Care of a Removable Prosthesis

    1. An implant supported removable prosthesis is similar to a traditional full denture except that in the case of implants, it is attached to the abutments by devices such as o-rings, magnets, or clips (Fig. 31-16).

      a. This type of prosthesis can also be designed as an implant and tissue supported prosthesis or as an overdenture.

      b. The patient can remove the prosthesis to clean it, the attachment devices, the abutments, and the remainder of the mouth.

    2. Techniques and Tools

      a. Selection of cleaning devices for the abutments that support a removable prosthesis should be based on the knowledge that implant components are made from titanium, which is a relatively soft metal.

      b. Cleaning devices must be selected for ease of use by each individual patient, and the recommendation of fewer, rather than more, devices is best. The cleaning aids that are recommended should be demonstrated for the patient and then evaluated by the hygienist to verify their effective use by the patient.

      c. In some cases, a metal bar connects the abutments and is used to attach the prosthetic denture in the mouth. Tufted dental floss or an unfolded 2 × 2 gauze square can be useful in cleaning underneath the metal bar and around the abutments (Fig. 31-17).

      d. Patients who have limited ability or poor success with mechanical plaque removal will benefit from the daily use of an antimicrobial mouth rinse (80,81). The entire mouth can be rinsed twice daily after brushing. Mouth rinses can be applied topically to the implant abutments or implants with cotton tipped applicators or other recommended cleaning devices if the patient cannot tolerate rinsing the entire mouth.

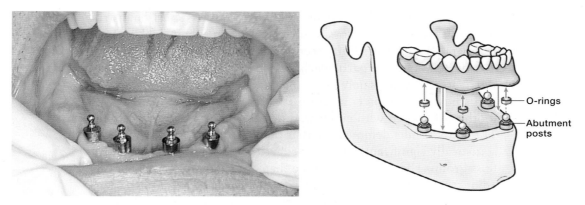

Figure 31-16. Implant Supported Removable Prosthesis. A: Abutment posts on the mandibular arch. **B:** An implant supported removable prosthesis is attached to the abutment posts by o-rings, magnets, or clips.

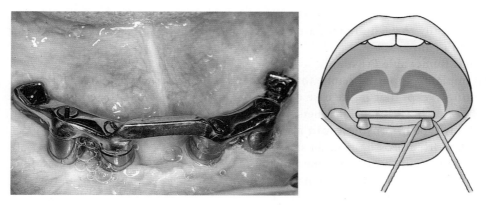

Figure 31-17. Abutments Joined by Metal Bar. Tufted dental floss is useful in cleaning the implant abutments and underneath the connecting metal bar.

Chapter Summary Statement

As dental implant therapy becomes more common, dental hygienists will care for increasing numbers of patients needing implant maintenance. A significantly higher incidence of peri-implantitis is found in patients with a history of periodontitis. The primary goals of treatment for peri-implantitis are to stop disease progression and maintain the implant in function with healthy peri-implant tissues.

Frequent professional maintenance is the most important step in the avoidance of peri-implantitis. An important role of the dental hygienist is the education of patients on the importance of meticulous self-care and frequent maintenance visits.

Implant restorations necessitate customized self-care instructions and devices. Implant maintenance appointments should include monitoring of plaque biofilm levels, examination of soft tissues, assessment of the restorative integrity, reinforcement of patient self-care measures, periodontal instrumentation of implant abutments and prostheses, and radiographic examination.

Section 5
Focus on Patients

Clinical Patient Care

CASE 1

While you are performing nonsurgical therapy on a chronic periodontitis patient, the patient tells you that he is thinking about having all of his teeth removed since they are not healthy anyway, and just having some implants placed. He tells you that this would be easier since he would not have to worry about the implants like he does his teeth. How should you respond?

CASE 2

You are scheduled to record the information needed to make a periodontal diagnosis for a patient new to your dental team. Radiographs have not yet been ordered for the patient. As you begin your probing, the patient informs you that she has two dental implants. Visual examination of the patient's dentition does not immediately reveal which teeth are replaced by the implants. How should you proceed?

CASE 3

At a maintenance visit for one of your team's patients you note obvious mobility of a crown supported by an implant. How should you (the dental hygienist) proceed?

References

1. Albrektsson T, Dahl E, Enbom L, et al. Osseointegrated oral implants. A Swedish multicenter study of 8139 consecutively inserted Nobelpharma implants. *J Periodontol*. 1988;59(5):287–296.
2. Cochran DL, Nummikoski PV, Schoolfield JD, et al. A prospective multicenter 5-year radiographic evaluation of crestal bone levels over time in 596 dental implants placed in 192 patients. *J Periodontol*. 2009;80(5):725–733.
3. Fugazzotto PA, Gulbransen HJ, Wheeler SL, et al. The use of IMZ osseointegrated implants in partially and completely edentulous patients: success and failure rates of 2,023 implant cylinders up to 60+ months in function. *Int J Oral Maxillofac Implants*. 1993;8(6):617–621.
4. Iacono VJ, Committee on Research, Science and Therapy, the American Academy of Periodontology. Dental implants in periodontal therapy. *J Periodontol*. 2000;71(12):1934–1942.
5. Patrick D, Zosky J, Lubar R, et al. Longitudinal clinical efficacy of Core-Vent dental implants: a five-year report. *J Oral Implantol*. 1989;15(2):95–103.
6. Sbordone L, Barone A, Ciaglia RN, et al. Longitudinal study of dental implants in a periodontally compromised population. *J Periodontol*. 1999;70(11):1322–1329.
7. Spiekermann H, Jansen VK, Richter EJ. A 10-year follow-up study of IMZ and TPS implants in the edentulous mandible using bar-retained overdentures. *Int J Oral Maxillofac Implants*. 1995;10(2):231–243.
8. Lang NP, Karring T, British Society of Periodontology. *Proceedings of the 1st European Workshop on Periodontology, Charter House at Ittingen, Thurgau, Switzerland, February 1–4, 1993*. London: Quintessence Publishing Co Inc.; 1994:478.
9. Bader H. Implant maintenance: a chairside test for real-time monitoring. *Dent Econ*. 1995;85(6):66–67.
10. Lang NP, Karring T, Lindhe J, European Federation of Periodontology, European Association of Osseointegration, Swiss Society of Periodontology. *Proceedings of the 3rd European Workshop on Periodontology: implant dentistry: Charter House at Ittingen, Thurgau, Switzerland, January 30–February 3, 1999*. Berlin: Quintessence Publishing Co Inc.; 1999:615.
11. Nevins M, Langer B. The successful use of osseointegrated implants for the treatment of the recalcitrant periodontal patient. *J Periodontol*. 1995;66(2):150–157.
12. Silverstein L, Garg A, Callan D, et al. The key to success: maintaining the long-term health of implants. *Dent Today*. 1998;17(2):104, 106, 108–111.
13. Albrektsson T, Zarb G, Worthington P, et al. The long-term efficacy of currently used dental implants: a review and proposed criteria of success. *Int J Oral Maxillofac Implants*. 1986;1(1):11–25.
14. Salvi GE, Aglietta M, Eick S, et al. Reversibility of experimental peri-implant mucositis compared with experimental gingivitis in humans. *Clin Oral Implants Res*. 2012;23(2):182–190.

15. Lang NP, Berglundh T, Working Group 4 of Seventh European Workshop on Periodontology. Periimplant diseases: where are we now?–Consensus of the Seventh European Workshop on Periodontology. *J Clin Periodontol.* 2011;38(suppl 11):178–181.

16. Mahesh L, Kurtzman GM, Shukla S. Microbiology of peri-implant infections. *Smile Dent J.* 2011;6:54–57.

17. Pye AD, Lockhart DE, Dawson MP, et al. A review of dental implants and infection. *J Hosp Infect.* 2009;72(2):104–110.

18. Atieh MA, Alsabeeha NH, Faggion CM Jr., et al. The frequency of peri-implant diseases: a systematic review and meta-analysis. *J Periodontol.* 2013;84(11):1586–1598.

19. Koldsland OC, Scheie AA, Aass AM. Prevalence of peri-implantitis related to severity of the disease with different degrees of bone loss. *J Periodontol.* 2010;81(2):231–238.

20. Marrone A, Lasserre J, Bercy P, et al. Prevalence and risk factors for peri-implant disease in Belgian adults. *Clin Oral Implants Res.* 2013;24(8):934–940.

21. Roos-Jansaker AM, Lindahl C, Renvert H, et al. Nine- to fourteen-year follow-up of implant treatment. Part II: presence of peri-implant lesions. *J Clin Periodontol.* 2006;33(4):290–295.

22. Rosen P, Clem D, Cochran D, et al. Peri-implant mucositis and peri-implantitis: a current understanding of their diagnoses and clinical implications. *J Periodontol.* 2013;84(4):436–443.

23. Heitz-Mayfield LJ, Lang NP. Comparative biology of chronic and aggressive periodontitis vs. peri-implantitis. *Periodontol 2000.* 2010;53:167–181.

24. Mombelli A, Lang NP. Antimicrobial treatment of peri-implant infections. *Clin Oral Implants Res.* 1992;3(4):162–168.

25. Quirynen M, De Soete M, van Steenberghe D. Infectious risks for oral implants: a review of the literature. *Clin Oral Implants Res.* 2002;13(1):1–19.

26. Renvert S, Roos-Jansaker AM, Lindahl C, et al. Infection at titanium implants with or without a clinical diagnosis of inflammation. *Clin Oral Implants Res.* 2007;18(4):509–516.

27. Shibli JA, Martins MC, Lotufo RF, et al. Microbiologic and radiographic analysis of ligature-induced peri-implantitis with different dental implant surfaces. *Int J Oral Maxillofac Implants.* 2003;18(3):383–390.

28. Shibli JA, Melo L, Ferrari DS, et al. Composition of supra- and subgingival biofilm of subjects with healthy and diseased implants. *Clin Oral Implants Res.* 2008;19(10):975–982.

29. Karoussis IK, Kotsovilis S, Fourmousis I. A comprehensive and critical review of dental implant prognosis in periodontally compromised partially edentulous patients. *Clin Oral Implants Res.* 2007;18(6):669–679.

30. Klokkevold PR, Han TJ. How do smoking, diabetes, and periodontitis affect outcomes of implant treatment? *Int J Oral Maxillofac Implants.* 2007;22(suppl):173–202.

31. Schou S, Holmstrup P, Worthington HV, et al. Outcome of implant therapy in patients with previous tooth loss due to periodontitis. *Clin Oral Implants Res.* 2006;17(suppl 2):104–123.

32. Van der Weijden GA, van Bemmel KM, Renvert S. Implant therapy in partially edentulous, periodontally compromised patients: a review. *J Clin Periodontol.* 2005;32(5):506–511.

33. Heitz-Mayfield LJ, Huynh-Ba G. History of treated periodontitis and smoking as risks for implant therapy. *Int J Oral Maxillofac Implants.* 2009;24(suppl):39–68.

34. Hinode D, Tanabe S, Yokoyama M, et al. Influence of smoking on osseointegrated implant failure: a meta-analysis. *Clin Oral Implants Res.* 2006;17(4):473–478.

35. Strietzel FP, Reichart PA, Kale A, et al. Smoking interferes with the prognosis of dental implant treatment: a systematic review and meta-analysis. *J Clin Periodontol.* 2007;34(6):523–544.

36. Linkevicius T, Puisys A, Vindasiute E, et al. Does residual cement around implant-supported restorations cause peri-implant disease? A retrospective case analysis. *Clin Oral Implants Res.* 2013;24(11):1179–1184. doi:10.1111/j.1600-0501.2012.02570.x.

37. Wilson TG Jr. The positive relationship between excess cement and peri-implant disease: a prospective clinical endoscopic study. *J Periodontol.* 2009;80(9):1388–1392.

38. Hudieb MI, Wakabayashi N, Kasugai S. Magnitude and direction of mechanical stress at the osseointegrated interface of the microthread implant. *J Periodontol.* 2011;82(7):1061–1070.

39. Rungsiyakull C, Rungsiyakull P, Li Q, et al. Effects of occlusal inclination and loading on mandibular bone remodeling: a finite element study. *Int J Oral Maxillofac Implants.* 2011;26(3):527–537.

40. Ericsson I, Lindhe J. Probing depth at implants and teeth. An experimental study in the dog. *J Clin Periodontol.* 1993;20(9):623–627.

41. Lang NP, Wetzel AC, Stich H, et al. Histologic probe penetration in healthy and inflamed peri-implant tissues. *Clin Oral Implants Res.* 1994;5(4):191–201.

42. Mahesh L, Kurtzman GM, Bali P, et al. Treatment of peri-implantitis. *Inside Dentistry.* 2013;9(3):84–90.

43. Kammerer PW, Lehmann KL, Karbach J, et al. Prevalence of peri-implant disease associated with a rough-surface dental implant system: 9 years after insertion. *Int J Oral Implantol Clin Res.* 2011;2(3):135–139.

44. Porras R, Anderson GB, Caffesse R, et al. Clinical response to 2 different therapeutic regimens to treat peri-implant mucositis. *J Periodontol.* 2002;73(10):1118–1125.

45. Renvert S, Lessem J, Lindahl C, et al. Treatment of incipient peri-implant infections using topical minocycline microspheres versus topical chlorhexidine gel as an adjunct to mechanical debridement. *J Int Acad Periodontol.* 2004;6(4 suppl):154–159.

46. Renvert S, Polyzois I, Persson GR. Treatment modalities for peri-implant mucositis and peri-implantitis. *Am J Dent.* 2013;26(6):313–318.

47. Schar D, Ramseier CA, Eick S, et al. Anti-infective therapy of peri-implantitis with adjunctive local drug delivery or photodynamic therapy: six-month outcomes of a prospective randomized clinical trial. *Clin Oral Implants Res.* 2013;24(1):104–110.

48. Muthukuru M, Zainvi A, Esplugues EO, et al. Non-surgical therapy for the management of peri-implantitis: a systematic review. *Clin Oral Implants Res.* 2012;23(suppl 6):77–83.

49. Heitz-Mayfield LJ, Needleman I, Salvi GE, et al. Consensus statements and clinical recommendations for prevention and management of biologic and technical implant complications. *Int J Oral Maxillofac Implants.* 2014;29(suppl):346–350.

50. Etter TH, Hakanson I, Lang NP, et al. Healing after standardized clinical probing of the periimplant soft tissue seal: a histomorphometric study in dogs. *Clin Oral Implants Res.* 2002;13(6):571–580.

51. Cochran D. Implant therapy I. *Ann Periodontol.* 1996;1(1):707–791.

52. Papaioannou W, Quirynen M, Nys M, et al. The effect of periodontal parameters on the subgingival microbiota around implants. *Clin Oral Implants Res.* 1995;6(4):197–204.

53. Sanz M, Chapple IL, Working Group 4 of the VIII European Workshop on Periodontology. Clinical research on peri-implant diseases: consensus report of Working Group 4. *J Clin Periodontol.* 2012;39(suppl 12):202–206.

54. van Steenberghe D, Klinge B, Linden U, et al. Periodontal indices around natural and titanium abutments: a longitudinal multicenter study. *J Periodontol.* 1993;64(6):538–541.

55. Lindhe J, Meyle J, Group D of European Workshop on Periodontology. Peri-implant diseases: consensus report of the sixth European workshop on periodontology. *J Clin Periodontol.* 2008;35(8 suppl):282–285.

56. Eskow RN, Smith VS. Preventive periimplant protocol. *Compend Contin Educ Dent.* 1999;20(2):137–142, 144, 146 passim; quiz 54.

57. Petersilka GJ, Tunkel J, Barakos K, et al. Subgingival plaque removal at interdental sites using a low-abrasive air polishing powder. *J Periodontol.* 2003;74(3):307–311.

58. Sahrmann P, Ronay V, Schmidlin PR, et al. Three-dimensional defect evaluation of air polishing on extracted human roots. *J Periodontol.* 2014;85(8):1107–1114.

59. Sculean A, Bastendorf KD, Becker C, et al. A paradigm shift in mechanical biofilm management? Subgingival air polishing: a new way to improve mechanical biofilm management in the dental practice. *Quintessence Int.* 2013;44(7):475–477.

60. Sahrmann P, Ronay V, Sener B, et al. Cleaning potential of glycine air-flow application in an in vitro peri-implantitis model. *Clin Oral Implants Res.* 2013;24(6):666–670.

61. Schwarz F, Ferrari D, Popovski K, et al. Influence of different air-abrasive powders on cell viability at biologically contaminated titanium dental implants surfaces. *J Biomed Mater Res B Appl Biomater.* 2009;88(1):83–91.

62. Mussano F, Rovasio S, Schierano G, et al. The effect of glycine-powder airflow and hand instrumentation on peri-implant soft tissues: a split-mouth pilot study. *Inter J Prosthodont.* 2013;26(1):42–44.

63. Schmage P, Kahili F, Nergiz I, et al. Cleaning effectiveness of implant prophylaxis instruments. *Int J Oral Maxillofac Implants.* 2014;29(2):331–337.

64. Sahm N, Becker J, Santel T, et al. Non-surgical treatment of peri-implantitis using an air-abrasive device or mechanical debridement and local application of chlorhexidine: a prospective, randomized, controlled clinical study. *J Clin Periodontol.* 2011;38(9):872–878.

65. Sahrmann P, Ronay V, Hofer D, et al. In vitro cleaning potential of three different implant debridement methods. *Clin Oral Implants Res.* 2013. doi:10.1111/clr.12322.

66. Graumann SJ, Sensat ML, Stoltenberg JL. Air polishing: a review of current literature. *J Dent Hyg.* 2013;87(4):173–180.

67. Petersilka GJ. Subgingival air-polishing in the treatment of periodontal biofilm infections. *Periodontol 2000.* 2011;55(1):124–142. doi:10.1111/j.1600-0757.2010.00342.x.

68. Petersilka GJ, Steinmann D, Haberlein I, et al. Subgingival plaque removal in buccal and lingual sites using a novel low abrasive air-polishing powder. *J Clin Periodontol.* 2003;30(4):328–333.

69. Guidelines for periodontal therapy. The American Academy of Periodontology. *J Periodontol.* 1998;69(3):405–408.

70. Supportive periodontal therapy (SPT). *J Periodontol.* 1998;69(4):502–506.

71. Louropoulou A, Slot DE, Van der Weijden FA. Titanium surface alterations following the use of different mechanical instruments: a systematic review. *Clin Oral Implants Res.* 2012;23(6):643–658.

72. Speelman JA, Collaert B, Klinge B. Evaluation of different methods to clean titanium abutments. A scanning electron microscopic study. *Clin Oral Implants Res.* 1992;3(3):120–127.

73. Chairay JP, Boulekbache H, Jean A, et al. Scanning electron microscopic evaluation of the effects of an air-abrasive system on dental implants: a comparative in vitro study between machined and plasma-sprayed titanium surfaces. *J Periodontol.* 1997;68(12):1215–1222.

74. Cochis A, Fini M, Carrassi A, et al. Effect of air polishing with glycine powder on titanium abutment surfaces. *Clin Oral Implants Res.* 2013;24(8):904–909.

75. Huband ML. Problems associated with implant maintenance. *Va Dent J.* 1996;73(2):8–11.

76. Jovanovic SA. Peri-implant tissue response to pathological insults. *Adv Dent Res.* 1999;13:82–86.

77. Matarasso S, Quaremba G, Coraggio F, et al. Maintenance of implants: an in vitro study of titanium implant surface modifications subsequent to the application of different prophylaxis procedures. *Clin Oral Implants Res.* 1996;7(1):64–72.

78. Mengel R, Buns CE, Mengel C, et al. An in vitro study of the treatment of implant surfaces with different instruments. *Int J Oral Maxillofac Implants.* 1998;13(1):91–96.

79. Magnuson B, Harsono M, Stark PC, et al. Comparison of the effect of two interdental cleaning devices around implants on the reduction of bleeding: a 30-day randomized clinical trial. *Compend Contin Educ Dent.* 2013;34(Spec No 8):2–7.

80. Balshi TJ. Hygiene maintenance procedures for patients treated with the tissue integrated prosthesis (osseointegration). *Quintessence Int.* 1986;17(2):95–102.

81. Ciancio SG, Lauciello F, Shibly O, et al. The effect of an antiseptic mouthrinse on implant maintenance: plaque and peri-implant gingival tissues. *J Periodontol.* 1995;66(11):962–965.

 STUDENT ANCILLARY RESOURCES

A wide variety of resources to enhance your learning and understanding of this chapter are available on thePoint®.

- Visit thePoint to access:
  - Audio Glossary
  - Animations
  - Suggested Readings
  - Answers to Review Questions
  - Case Studies

Periodontal—Systemic Associations

Clinical Application. This chapter reviews current literature findings concerning periodontitis as a potential contributing factor to the severity of certain systemic diseases. The possibility of an association between periodontal disease and systemic disease suggests that periodontal therapy may play a role in decreasing the incidence and severity of certain systemic diseases. Interprofessional relationships between dental team members and other healthcare providers should be established early to provide the highest standard of care for patients with systemic disease.

Learning Objectives

- Contrast the terms "association" and "cause" between a given factor (A) and a systemic disease (B).

- Educate patients at risk for cardiovascular diseases about the possible impact of periodontal infection on cardiovascular health and encourage oral disease prevention and treatment services.

- Educate pregnant women and those planning pregnancy regarding the possible impact of periodontal infection on pregnancy outcomes and encourage preventive oral care and treatment services.

- Educate patients with diabetes about the probable bidirectional association between periodontal disease and diabetes; encourage oral disease prevention and treatment services.

- Educate family members and caregivers about the association between periodontal disease and pneumonia in health-compromised seniors in hospitals and long-term care.

- Establish collaborative relationships with other healthcare providers to insure the highest standard of care for periodontal patients with systemic diseases and conditions.

Key Terms

Atherosclerosis
Atheroma
C-reactive protein
Dyslipidemia
Lipoprotein

Low–birth-weight
  infants
Preeclampsia
Glycemic control
HbA1C

Community-acquired
  pneumonia
Hospital-acquired pneumonia
Ventilator-associated
  pneumonia

Section 1
Associations of Periodontitis with Systemic Disease

Current research suggests that there may be a bidirectional relationship between oral health and systemic health (1). On one hand, as discussed in Chapter 15, the presence of systemic disease may increase the likelihood of periodontal disease initiation or increase the severity of existing periodontitis. On the other hand, the presence of a chronic oral infection (periodontitis) may have an adverse effect on an individual's systemic health. Published evidence supports a modest association between periodontitis and some systemic conditions. Dental professionals should be aware that currently there is limited evidence to support or refute an association between periodontitis and systemic disease (2).

1. **Association versus Causality**
   A. **Association.** A large body of evidence documents an association of periodontitis with several systemic conditions including cardiovascular/cerebrovascular problems, diabetes mellitus, preterm labor, low–birth-weight delivery, and pneumonia (3). Current data indicates that the relationship between periodontitis and systemic diseases is a complex one.
   B. **Causation.** An association between a given factor (A) and a health effect (B) does not mean that the factor (A) caused the specific disease (B).
      1. For example, a cohort study finds that eating red meat is associated with a higher risk of heart disease.
         a. A reader of this study might incorrectly conclude that eating red meat causes heart disease.
         b. The study, however, showed that those who ate red meat actually had the lowest cholesterol levels (4). Instead this study demonstrates that a whole variety of unhealthy lifestyle factors (smoking, no exercise, alcohol consumption, diet) are all associated with a higher risk of heart disease. Therefore, the reader must be very cautious in leaping to the assumption that an *association* between factors A and B means that A *causes* B.
      2. ***Based on available research it is not possible to prove causality between periodontitis and systemic disease*** (2,3–5). It is possible that the association is the result of common risk factors and not causality.
2. **Possible Mechanisms for Impact on Systemic Disease.** Three mechanisms have been postulated as to how periodontitis may modify some aspect of certain systemic diseases to make those diseases more severe: (a) infection, (b) inflammation, and (c) immune response (6). All three of these mechanisms have the potential to impact the systemic inflammatory/immune response that in turn may mediate a range of systemic diseases.
   A. **Infection**
      1. A periodontal infection is not limited to the periodontium or even the oral cavity (7,8). The everyday acts of chewing and tooth brushing disseminate whole bacteria and their products to other nonadjacent organs or body parts (7).
      2. Oral bacteria from periodontal lesions and the DNA of periodontal pathogens can survive in the blood stream and adhere to nonoral body sites causing infections such as endocarditis, lung infections, abscesses of the brain or liver, and fatty deposits in the carotid arteries (9–11).

B. Inflammation
   1. Infection of the periodontal pocket can disseminate inflammatory mediators to the blood stream triggering significant systemic inflammation (12,13).
   2. Proinflammatory mediators—such as IL-1β, IL-6, TNF-α, and PGE$_2$—produced locally in the inflamed periodontal tissues disseminate into the blood stream and have a systemic impact (12,13).

C. Immune Response
   1. In chronic periodontitis, bacterial antigens are processed and presented to body's immune system and recognized by lymphocytes (T-lymphocytes and B-lymphocytes). In response to a microbial challenge, host immune cells secrete proinflammatory mediators. As discussed in Chapter 14, it is clear that the body's immune response plays a significant role in inflammation and tissue destruction.
   2. Systemic inflammation, defined by increased circulating TNF-α, is associated with obesity and periodontitis and has been proposed as a mechanism for the connection between these two conditions (14,15). Understanding of the mechanism in many inflammatory systemic conditions, such as obesity, diabetes, rheumatoid arthritis, and cardiovascular disease is incomplete.

Section 2
Linking Periodontitis to Systemic Disease

1. Periodontitis and Atherosclerotic Cardiovascular Diseases
   A. Atherosclerotic Cardiovascular Diseases
      1. Atherosclerotic cardiovascular disease (ACVD) is a group of heart or vascular diseases including angina, myocardial infarction, stroke, transient ischemic attack (TIA), and peripheral artery disease.
      2. Atherosclerosis, a major component of cardiovascular disease, is a process characterized by a thickening of artery walls. Complications that arise from atherosclerosis cause deaths from heart attack or stroke and have been reported to account for nearly three-fourths of all deaths from cardiovascular disease.
      3. An atheroma is a fatty deposit in the inner lining of an artery; also called arterial plaque.
   B. Summary of Research Studies
      1. A large body of evidence exists relevant to the association of periodontitis with cardiovascular disease (3). Severe periodontal disease has been linked to cardiovascular disease in cross-sectional and cohort studies (3,16–18).
      2. *It is important to note, however, insufficient evidence exists to show that the treatment of periodontal disease can reduce the risk for cardiovascular disease.* The impact of treatment for periodontitis on the cardiovascular disease is an area for ongoing research.
   C. Possible Biologic Explanations. How is Periodontitis Related to Cardiovascular Disease? Four biologic pathways have been proposed to explain the possible link between inflammation due to periodontitis and cardiovascular disease (19). These proposed biologic mechanisms are summarized in Figure 32-1.
      1. Inflammatory Mediators From Periodontal Lesions may Heighten Systemic Inflammation
         a. In this first proposed pathway, periodontal infections may contribute to atherosclerosis by repeatedly challenging the blood vessel walls and arterial walls with proinflammatory mediators.
         b. Subgingival plaque biofilm provides a large and persistent source of periodontal pathogens and proinflammatory mediators that can enter into the systemic blood stream. These bacteria activate the host inflammatory response by multiple mechanisms (20). The host immune response facilitates atheroma formation and exacerbation (19,21).
         c. Bacteria or proinflammatory mediators from periodontal lesions may stimulate inflammatory responses in tissues and organs distant from the oral cavity (22–24). Thus, the evidence suggests an association between periodontal infections and a heightened state of systemic inflammation (25).
            1. C-reactive protein (CRP) is a special type of plasma protein—produced by macrophages, endothelial cells, and smooth muscle—that is present during episodes of acute inflammation or infection (3,26). CRP is an important cardiovascular risk predictor (27–30). Elevations in serum CRP are well-accepted risk factors for cardiovascular disease (29,30).
            2. One hypothesis is that periodontitis is the source of the inflammation that triggers the production of CRP (30). Serum CRP levels are elevated

in individuals with periodontitis when compared to individuals without periodontitis (31–33).

   d. Evidence from clinical and epidemiological studies suggests that inflammation is important in atherosclerosis and cardiovascular disease. Bacteria or their products could promote inflammatory changes that contribute to the development of atheromatous lesions (fatty deposits in the inner lining of an artery) (25).

2. **Periodontitis may Initiate the Host Immune Response: Antibody Cross-Reactivity**

   a. In this second proposed biologic pathway, periodontal infections may contribute to atherosclerosis by inducing a local immune response. Patients with periodontitis have elevated systemic antibody responses to a variety of periodontal microorganisms and are able to induce antibody cross-reactivity (19).

   b. Cross-reactivity occurs when an antibody reacts with an antigen other than the one that induced its production. In this proposed pathway, the antibody reacts with the endothelial cells of the blood vessel walls instead of the periodontal pathogens (19).

   c. This pathway suggests that periodontal pathogens induce the body's immune response to mistakenly target cells in blood vessels leading to vascular inflammation and atherosclerosis.

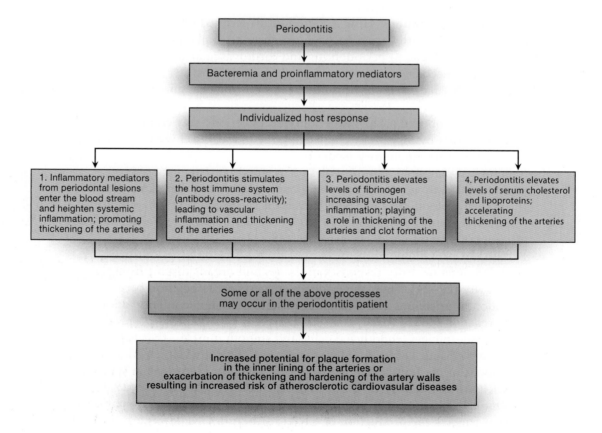

Figure 32-1. Proposed Biologic Pathways. A schematic representation showing the four biologic pathways that have been proposed to explain the possible link between inflammation due to periodontitis and cardiovascular disease.

3. **Periodontitis Elevates Levels of Fibrinogen: Increased Vascular Inflammation**
   a. In this third proposed biologic pathway periodontal infections may contribute to atherosclerosis by increasing circulating levels of fibrinogen in the blood stream and playing a role in vascular inflammation.
   b. Under normal circumstances, blood coagulation (blood clotting) is a protective process that slows and stops blood loss. For example, an individual cuts her finger and it starts to bleed. Immediately the platelets in the blood stream stimulate the production of thrombin. Thrombin, in turn, converts *fibrinogen* into fibrin, a protein substance that forms a network of threadlike structures and causes the blood plasma to gel. The blood cells and plasma enmesh in the network of fibrils to form a clot, stopping the flow of blood to the cut in the finger.
   c. A hypercoagulable state is a medical term for an abnormally increased tendency toward coagulation. In ACVD, blood coagulation can have an adverse effect when a blood clot forms in a coronary artery, obstructing blood flow to the heart.
   d. The coagulation and fibrinolytic systems play important roles in the thickening of the arteries and clot formation (34,35). *Elevated fibrinogen is a risk factor for atherosclerosis.*
   e. The association of periodontitis with blood clotting factors has been reported by a number of investigators.
      1. In an early study, Kweider reported that patients with periodontitis have higher plasma fibrinogen levels than age-matched control subjects (36).
      2. Recent studies note increased fibrinogen levels in patients with periodontitis (37–40) and an association between the number of periodontal pockets and fibrinogen levels (41).

4. **Periodontitis may Result in Dyslipidemia**
   a. In this forth proposed pathway, periodontal infections may contribute to atherosclerosis by elevating levels of serum cholesterol, as well as low-density lipoproteins (LDLs), triglycerides, and very low-density lipoproteins (vLDLs) (19).
   b. Dyslipidemia (dys·lip·id·e·mia) refers to abnormal amounts of lipids ("fats") and lipoproteins in the blood. A lipoprotein is a molecule that is a combination of lipid (fat) and protein. Lipoproteins are the form in which lipids are transported in the blood.
   c. Several studies indicate that blood serum concentrations of inflammatory lipids, including cholesterol, LDLs, triglycerides, and vLDLs are elevated in periodontitis patients. These inflammatory lipids may more easily enter the blood vessel wall and therefore are more likely to be incorporated into the atherosclerotic lesion (thickening of the vessel wall). This would accelerate development of the local lesions (42–46).

D. **Implications for Dental Hygiene Practice**
   1. Dental healthcare providers should be aware of the emerging evidence that periodontitis is a risk factor for developing ACVD. Dental hygienists should educate patients at risk for cardiovascular diseases about the possible impact of periodontal infection on cardiovascular health (47,48).
   2. There is evidence suggesting that periodontal therapy reduces systemic inflammation, but limited evidence on its effects on cardiovascular health in the long term (49). Well-designed research studies are needed to clarify associations of poor periodontal health on ACVD (50).

3. Comprehensive periodontal therapy should include patient education and advice on modifiable lifestyle risk factors such as smoking, diet, and exercise. Collaboration with appropriate specialists may facilitate the patient's efforts in making lifestyle modifications (47,48).
4. Periodontitis patients—with other risk factors for ACVD, such as smoking, hypertension, obesity, etc.—who have not been seen by a physician within the last year should be referred for a physical examination (47,48).
5. The American Journal of Cardiology and Journal of Periodontology published clinical recommendations for care of individuals with periodontitis (Table 32-1) (47).

TABLE 32-1. CLINICAL RECOMMENDATIONS: PATIENTS WITH PERIODONTITIS

Condition	CVD Risk Factors	Recommendations
Moderate to severe periodontitis	None	Inform patient that there may be an increased risk for CVD associated with periodontitis
Moderate to severe periodontitis	One known risk factor (smoking, family history of CVD, high cholesterol)	Recommend that patient seek a medical evaluation if he/she has not had one in the last 12 mo
Mild, moderate, or severe periodontitis	Two or more known risk factors	Refer patient for a medical evaluation if he/she has not had one in the last 12 mo

2. Periodontitis and Adverse Pregnancy Outcomes
   A. Introduction to Periodontitis and Adverse Pregnancy Outcomes
      1. Adverse pregnancy outcomes that have been associated with periodontitis include preterm birth, low–birth-weight, and preeclampsia. The strength of this association, however, is modest (51).
         a. Preterm delivery of low–birth-weight infants is a leading cause of neonatal death and of long-term neurodevelopmental disturbances and health problems in children.
         b. Preeclampsia is a serious complication of pregnancy characterized by an abrupt rise in blood pressure, large amounts of the protein albumin in the urine and swelling of the hands, feet, and face. Preeclampsia occurs in the third trimester (the last third) of pregnancy.
      2. Adverse pregnancy outcomes most likely involve additional shared risk factors with periodontitis, such as tobacco use, alcohol use, obesity, and diabetes.
   B. Two Possible Biologic Explanations. How is Periodontitis Related to Adverse Pregnancy Outcomes? Research demonstrates a modest association between periodontal disease and adverse pregnancy outcomes; however exact mechanisms remain unclear. Two major pathways have been proposed (52–54). Figure 32-2 shows these proposed biologic pathways.
      1. Pregnant women with severe periodontitis may develop bacteremia more frequently than those with healthy periodontium, exposing the fetus to aggressive periodontal pathogens.

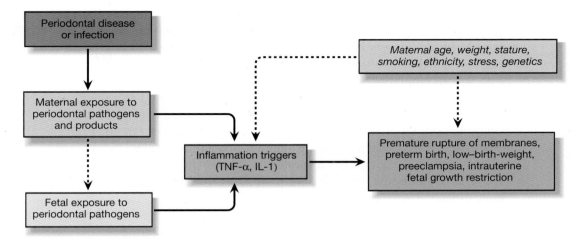

Figure 32-2. Proposed Biologic Pathway for Association Between Periodontal Disease and Adverse Pregnancy Outcomes. Reservoirs of gram-negative organisms, such as those found in periodontitis, may have a negative impact on pregnancy outcome.

2. Proinflammatory mediators produced within diseased periodontal tissues may enter the bloodstream and trigger systemic inflammation, thus leading to adverse pregnancy outcomes.

C. **Implications for Dental Hygiene Practice**

1. Several research studies show a significant association between chronic periodontitis and preterm delivery and low birth weight. Dental healthcare providers should be knowledgeable on the extent of these associations and their possible implications for health care.

2. The American Academy of Periodontology issued a statement in 2004, recommending, "Women who are pregnant or planning pregnancy undergo periodontal examinations. Appropriate preventive or therapeutic services, if indicated, should be provided. Preventive oral care services should be provided as early in pregnancy as possible. However, women should be encouraged to achieve a high level of oral hygiene before becoming pregnant and throughout their pregnancies." (55)

3. The European Federation of Periodontology and American Academy of Periodontology published clinical recommendations for care of females of childbearing age with periodontitis (51). A dental healthcare professional assessing a female patient of childbearing age should inquire whether she is currently pregnant or trying to become pregnant. If the patient responds affirmatively, the dental healthcare professional should always consider this pregnancy status in planning periodontal therapy.

a. Health promotion information should be provided including education about preventing and treating periodontal diseases for the oral health of the patient and future oral health of her children. Dental hygienists should educate patients about the association between adverse pregnancy outcomes and periodontal infection and provide early oral hygiene services for pregnant women and those considering pregnancy.

b. The patient should be educated about periodontal events usually occurring during pregnancy such as increased tissue response to biofilm, increase in vascularity, and possibility of increased bleeding or gingival enlargement.

c. The dental team should provide education on self-care for biofilm control; with special emphasis on interdental cleaning.

d. Periodontitis should be treated with nonsurgical periodontal therapy with the goal of reducing subgingival biofilm and the signs of periodontal inflammation. Emphasize that all preventive, diagnostic, and periodontal therapeutic procedures are safe throughout pregnancy. Elective procedures should be avoided in the first trimester.

e. The patient should be scheduled for periodontal maintenance at a later stage during pregnancy.

f. Interprofessional collaboration between the dental hygienist and other health professionals involved with pregnancy care are encouraged.

3. Periodontitis and Diabetes Mellitus

A. **Introduction to Periodontitis and Diabetes Complications.** To date, research studies suggest that there is a two-way relationship between diabetes and periodontal disease (3,56–59).

1. First, it is clear that diabetes increases the risk for and severity of periodontal diseases (58,60). The American Diabetes Association's Standard of Medical Care 2008 includes taking a history of past and current dental infections as part of the physician's examination (61,62).

2. Second, periodontal disease may exacerbate diabetes mellitus by significantly worsening glycemic control over time (62,63).

B. **Overview of Glycemic Control in Diabetes**

1. Overview of Glycemic Control

a. **Glycemic control** is a medical term referring to the typical blood glucose levels in those with diabetes mellitus.

1. Optimal management of diabetes involves patients measuring and recording their own blood glucose levels.

2. If left unchecked and untreated, prolonged and elevated levels of glucose in the blood will result in serious health complications, even death.

b. Blood glucose level is measured by means of a glucose meter, with the result either in mg/dL (milligrams per deciliter in the United States) or mmol/L (millimoles per liter in Canada and Europe) of blood.

1. The average person should have a blood glucose level of around 4.5 to 7.0 mmol/L (80 to 125 mg/dL).

2. In the patient with diabetes, a before-meal level of <6.1 mmol/L (<110 mg/dL) and a level 2 hours after the start of a meal of <7.8 mmol/L (<140 mg/dL) is acceptable.

c. Poor glycemic control refers to persistently elevated blood glucose and glycosylated hemoglobin levels, which may range from 200 to 500 mg/dL (11 to 28 mmol/L) and 9% to 15% or higher over months and years before severe complications occur.

d. **HbA1C** level is the average blood glucose level over the past 2 to 3 months (the lifespan of the red blood cell). The HbA1C test measures the amount of glycosylated hemoglobin in the blood. Glucose in the blood enters the red blood cell and attaches to the hemoglobin. The more glucose in the blood, the more will stick to the hemoglobin. A1C is reported as a percentage of total hemoglobin in the blood. For example, an A1C of 8 means that 8% of the hemoglobin has glucose attached. Normal HbA1C levels for nondiabetics are between 4 and 6.

C. **Proposed Biologic Pathway.** Periodontal diseases may serve as initiators of insulin resistance, thereby aggravating glycemic control. In this proposed pathway, systemic inflammation induced by periodontitis may increase insulin resistance, adversely affect glycemic control, and contribute to the development of complications in patients with diabetes mellitus. Figure 32-3 illustrates this potential biologic pathway.

    1. Evidence suggests that periodontitis raises the levels of proinflammatory mediators in blood serum (57,64–70).

    2. Several studies indicate that periodontal therapy may result in improved insulin sensitivity and eventually lead to improved glycemic control and overall outcomes of diabetes mellitus (71–73).

D. **Implications for Dental Hygiene Practice**

    1. Dental hygienists should educate patients with diabetes about the possible impact of periodontal infection on glycemic control and encourage oral disease prevention and treatment services.

    2. Patients with diabetes should be informed of other associated oral conditions, such as xerostomia, burning mouth syndrome, fungal infections, and slower wound healing.

    3. Collaboration with other healthcare professionals is encouraged to assist patients in managing diabetes. As our understanding of the relationship between diabetes mellitus and periodontitis deepens, collaboration among medical and dental professionals for the management of affected individuals becomes increasingly important (57).

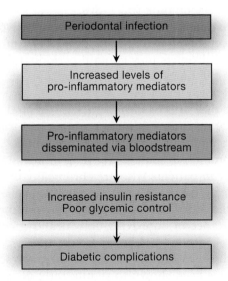

Figure 32-3. Proposed Biologic Pathway for the Association Between Periodontal Disease and Diabetes. Periodontal diseases may serve as initiators of insulin resistance, thereby aggravating glycemic control.

4. **Periodontitis and Pneumonia**
   A. **Introduction to Periodontitis and Pneumonia**
      1. Pneumonia is a serious inflammation of one or both lungs. It is caused by the inhalation of microorganisms and can range in seriousness from mild to life threatening. There are two types of pneumonia: community-acquired and hospital-acquired.
      2. **Community-acquired pneumonia** is pneumonia that is contracted outside of the hospital setting.
         a. Most cases of community-acquired bacterial pneumonia are caused by aspiration of oropharyngeal organisms such as *Streptococcus pneumoniae, Haemophilus influenzae,* and *Mycoplasma pneumoniae* (74).
         b. Community-acquired bacterial pneumonia generally responds well to treatment. There is no evidence that periodontal disease or oral hygiene alters the risk for community-acquired pneumonia.
      3. **Hospital-acquired pneumonia** is an infection of the lungs contracted during a stay in a hospital or long-term care facility.
         a. Hospital-acquired pneumonia usually results from organisms called *potential respiratory pathogens* (PRPs) that are generally found in the gastrointestinal tract but may colonize the mouth and oropharynx. Bacterial plaque biofilms can serve as reservoirs for PRPs, particularly during prolonged hospitalization (2,75,76).
         b. Oral colonization with PRPs increases during hospitalization, and the longer a patient is hospitalized the greater their prevalence.
      4. **Ventilator-associated pneumonia** is a type of hospital-acquired pneumonia developing after intubation for mechanical ventilation.
         a. In ventilator-associated pneumonia, placement of the endotracheal tube can transport oropharyngeal organisms into the lower airway.
         b. The oral cavity may serve as an important reservoir of infection for ventilator-associated pneumonia (2,77–80).
   B. **Proposed Biologic Explanations.** The proposed pathway between pneumonia and periodontitis involves the aspiration of fine droplets from the oral cavity and throat into the lungs. These droplets may contain periodontal pathogens that can breed and multiply within the lungs causing infection.
   C. **Implications for Dental Hygiene Practice**
      1. There is good evidence that improved patient self-care and frequent professional care reduce respiratory diseases among high-risk elderly patients living in nursing homes and those in intensive care units (2,75).
      2. Poor oral hygiene is common in patients residing in hospitals or long-term care facilities, especially in patients who are chronically ill. Oral healthcare providers should advocate for programs that enhance the access of dental care services to long-term care residents and collaborate with medical healthcare providers on the importance of improving daily oral hygiene care to this population.
      3. Application of 0.2% chlorhexidine gel to the teeth, gingiva, and other oral mucosal surfaces has been shown to significantly decrease the risk for pneumonia, especially in patients who are on ventilators (81). Clinicians should take these findings into account when providing oral care to intubated patients.

5. **Periodontitis and Chronic Obstructive Pulmonary Disease**
   A. Chronic obstructive pulmonary disease (COPD) is a group of lung diseases, mainly emphysema and chronic bronchitis, characterized by an obstruction of airflow during exhalation.
   B. Several investigators have hypothesized that periodontal infections may increase the risk of COPD. Reviews of the current evidence, however, indicate that at present there is no sufficient evidence for an association between periodontal disease and COPD (2,75,76).
6. **Periodontitis and Other Systemic Conditions**
   A. **Other Conditions**
      1. An association between periodontitis and various other systemic diseases has been postulated, including conditions such as cognitive impairment, obesity, cancer, rheumatoid arthritis, chronic kidney disease, and metabolic syndrome.
      2. Studies have shown modest associations between chronic periodontitis and various other systemic diseases. Very few of these studies meet stringent criteria to support or refute links between periodontitis and these systemic conditions (2).
   B. **Implications for Dental Hygiene Practice**
      1. Determining causation of a disease or condition is difficult. Diseases may be caused by a multitude of factors; causation often involves joint actions of complex mechanisms. There is still much to explore and understand concerning periodontitis, its negative impact on overall health, and the development of appropriate intervention protocols.
      2. Patients with periodontitis are increasingly aware of research into potential links between periodontitis and systemic diseases and conditions. Dental healthcare providers should know that there is currently limited evidence to support or refute such associations. Well-designed research studies are needed to clarify associations; clinicians should keep abreast of the emerging evidence.

Chapter Summary Statement

Periodontitis is a chronic oral infection that may be a risk factor for systemic disease. Research findings show weak associations between periodontitis and various systemic diseases and conditions. There is strong evidence that improved biofilm control by patient self-care and regular professional care has positive effects in the prevention of hospital-acquired pneumonia. Dental healthcare providers should be aware that other associations are weak and that, to date, there is no evidence that periodontal disease has a causative role in systemic disease. Education to encourage better periodontal health, patient self-care, and periodontal therapy may play roles in maintaining overall systemic health.

Section 3
Focus on Patients

Clinical Patient Care

A new patient in your dental office is 3 months pregnant with her first child. She is 38 years old and has chronic periodontitis. What counsel would you provide this patient about the association between adverse pregnancy outcomes and periodontitis?

Evidence In Action

You are a dental hygienist in a periodontal practice. Mr. O—a 45-year-old insurance executive—has been referred to the periodontal practice from his general dentist for treatment of chronic periodontitis. Today is his initial appointment with you.

Mr. O tells you that there is a history of heart attacks in his family and that he has been reading all about "how gum disease causes heart attacks." In addition, Mr. O states that he wants the periodontist to prescribe antibiotics for his gum disease, as he is quite convinced that the antibiotics will eliminate the gum disease and prevent him from having a heart attack when he gets older.

What education would you provide on the association between periodontitis and cardiovascular diseases? What information would you provide to Mr. O. on use of antibiotic therapy for the treatment of chronic periodontitis?

References

1. Kim J, Amar S. Periodontal disease and systemic conditions: a bidirectional relationship. *Odontology.* 2006;94(1):10–21.
2. Linden GJ, Lyons A, Scannapieco FA. Periodontal systemic associations: review of the evidence. *J Clin Periodontol.* 2013;40(14 suppl):S8–S19.
3. Van Dyke TE, van Winkelhoff AJ. Infection and inflammatory mechanisms. *J Clin Periodontol.* 2013;40(14 suppl):S1–S7.
4. Pan A, Sun Q, Bernstein AM, et al. Red meat consumption and mortality: results from 2 prospective cohort studies. *Arch Intern Med.* 2012;172(7):555–563.
5. Linden GJ, Herzberg MC, Working group 4 of the joint EFP/AAP workshop. Periodontitis and systemic diseases: a record of discussions of working group 4 of the Joint EFP/AAP Workshop on Periodontitis and Systemic Diseases. *J Periodontol.* 2013;84(4 suppl):S20–S23.
6. Thoden van Velzen SK, Abraham-Inpijn L, Moorer WR. Plaque and systemic disease: a reappraisal of the focal infection concept. *J Clin Periodontol.* 1984;11(4):209–220.
7. Chiang AC, Massague J. Molecular basis of metastasis. *N Engl J Med.* 2008;359(26):2814–2823.
8. Kinane DF, Riggio MP, Walker KF, et al. Bacteraemia following periodontal procedures. *J Clin Periodontol.* 2005;32(7):708–713.
9. Haraszthy VI, Zambon JJ, Trevisan M, et al. Identification of periodontal pathogens in atheromatous plaques. *J Periodontol.* 2000;71(10):1554–1560.
10. Raghavendran K, Mylotte JM, Scannapieco FA. Nursing home-associated pneumonia, hospital-acquired pneumonia and ventilator-associated pneumonia: the contribution of dental biofilms and periodontal inflammation. *Periodontol 2000.* 2007;44:164–177.
11. van Winkelhoff AJ, Slots J. Actinobacillus actinomycetemcomitans and Porphyromonas gingivalis in nonoral infections. *Periodontol 2000.* 1999;20:122–135.
12. Amar S, Gokce N, Morgan S, et al. Periodontal disease is associated with brachial artery endothelial dysfunction and systemic inflammation. *Arterioscler Thromb Vasc Biol.* 2003;23(7):1245–1249.
13. Elter JR, Hinderliter AL, Offenbacher S, et al. The effects of periodontal therapy on vascular endothelial function: a pilot trial. *Am Heart J.* 2006;151(1):47.
14. Al-Zahrani MS, Bissada NF, Borawskit EA. Obesity and periodontal disease in young, middle-aged, and older adults. *J Periodontol.* 2003;74(5):610–615.
15. Genco RJ, Grossi SG, Ho A, et al. A proposed model linking inflammation to obesity, diabetes, and periodontal infections. *J Periodontol.* 2005;76(11 suppl):2075–2084.

16. Janket SJ, Baird AE, Chuang SK, et al. Meta-analysis of periodontal disease and risk of coronary heart disease and stroke. *Oral Surg Oral Med Oral Pathol Oral Radiol Endod.* 2003;95(5):559–569.

17. Khader YS, Albashaireh ZS, Alomari MA. Periodontal diseases and the risk of coronary heart and cerebrovascular diseases: a meta-analysis. *J Periodontol.* 2004;75(8):1046–1053.

18. Pussinen PJ, Nyyssonen K, Alfthan G, et al. Serum antibody levels to Actinobacillus actinomycetemcomitans predict the risk for coronary heart disease. *Arterioscler Thromb Vasc Biol.* 2005;25(4):833–838.

19. Schenkein HA, Loos BG. Inflammatory mechanisms linking periodontal diseases to cardiovascular diseases. *J Periodontol.* 2013;84(4 suppl):S51–S69.

20. Preshaw PM, Taylor JJ. How has research into cytokine interactions and their role in driving immune responses impacted our understanding of periodontitis? *J Clin Periodontol.* 2011;38(11 suppl):60–84.

21. Reyes L, Herrera D, Kozarov E, et al. Periodontal bacterial invasion and infection: contribution to atherosclerotic pathology. *J Periodontol.* 2013;84(4 suppl):S30–S50.

22. Gibson FC, 3rd, Genco CA. Porphyromonas gingivalis mediated periodontal disease and atherosclerosis: disparate diseases with commonalities in pathogenesis through TLRs. *Curr Pharm Des.* 2007;13(36):3665–3675.

23. Gibson FC, 3rd, Yumoto H, Takahashi Y, et al. Innate immune signaling and Porphyromonas gingivalis-accelerated atherosclerosis. *J Dent Res.* 2006;85(2):106–121.

24. Hayashi C, Gudino CV, Gibson FC, 3rd, et al. Review: pathogen-induced inflammation at sites distant from oral infection: bacterial persistence and induction of cell-specific innate immune inflammatory pathways. *Mol Oral Microbiol.* 2010;25(5):305–316.

25. Teles R, Wang CY. Mechanisms involved in the association between periodontal diseases and cardiovascular disease. *Oral Dis.* 2011;17(5):450–461.

26. Van Dyke TE, Kornman KS. Inflammation and factors that may regulate inflammatory response. *J Periodontol.* 2008; 79(8 suppl):1503–1507.

27. Haverkate F, Thompson SG, Pyke SD, et al. Production of C-reactive protein and risk of coronary events in stable and unstable angina. European Concerted Action on Thrombosis and Disabilities Angina Pectoris Study Group. *Lancet.* 1997;349(9050):462–466.

28. Liuzzo G, Biasucci LM, Gallimore JR, et al. The prognostic value of C-reactive protein and serum amyloid a protein in severe unstable angina. *N Engl J Med.* 1994;331(7):417–424.

29. Ridker PM, Rifai N, Rose L, et al. Comparison of C-reactive protein and low-density lipoprotein cholesterol levels in the prediction of first cardiovascular events. *N Engl J Med.* 2002;347(20):1557–1565.

30. Ridker PM, Silvertown JD. Inflammation, C-reactive protein, and atherothrombosis. *J Periodontol.* 2008;79(8 suppl): 1544–1551.

31. Slade GD, Offenbacher S, Beck JD, et al. Acute-phase inflammatory response to periodontal disease in the US population. *J Dent Res.* 2000;79(1):49–57.

32. Wu T, Trevisan M, Genco RJ, et al. Periodontal disease and risk of cerebrovascular disease: the first national health and nutrition examination survey and its follow-up study. *Arch Intern Med.* 2000;160(18):2749–2755.

33. Wu T, Trevisan M, Genco RJ, et al. Examination of the relation between periodontal health status and cardiovascular risk factors: serum total and high density lipoprotein cholesterol, C-reactive protein, and plasma fibrinogen. *Am J Epidemiol.* 2000;151(3):273–282.

34. Davalos D, Akassoglou K. Fibrinogen as a key regulator of inflammation in disease. *Semin Immunopathol.* 2012;34(1): 43–62.

35. Popovic M, Smiljanic K, Dobutovic B, et al. Thrombin and vascular inflammation. *Mol Cell Biochem.* 2012;359(1–2): 301–313.

36. Kweider M, Lowe GD, Murray GD, et al. Dental disease, fibrinogen and white cell count; links with myocardial infarction? *Scott Med J.* 1993;38(3):73–74.

37. Amabile N, Susini G, Pettenati-Soubayroux I, et al. Severity of periodontal disease correlates to inflammatory systemic status and independently predicts the presence and angiographic extent of stable coronary artery disease. *J Intern Med.* 2008;263(6):644–652.

38. Buhlin K, Hultin M, Norderyd O, et al. Risk factors for atherosclerosis in cases with severe periodontitis. *J Clin Periodontol.* 2009;36(7):541–549.

39. Sahingur SE, Sharma A, Genco RJ, et al. Association of increased levels of fibrinogen and the –455G/A fibrinogen gene polymorphism with chronic periodontitis. *J Periodontol.* 2003;74(3):329–337.

40. Vidal F, Figueredo CM, Cordovil I, et al. Periodontal therapy reduces plasma levels of interleukin-6, C-reactive protein, and fibrinogen in patients with severe periodontitis and refractory arterial hypertension. *J Periodontol.* 2009;80(5):786–791.

41. Schwahn C, Volzke H, Robinson DM, et al. Periodontal disease, but not edentulism, is independently associated with increased plasma fibrinogen levels. Results from a population-based study. *Thromb Haemost.* 2004;92(2):244–252.

42. Katz J, Chaushu G, Sharabi Y. On the association between hypercholesterolemia, cardiovascular disease and severe periodontal disease. *J Clin Periodontol.* 2001;28(9):865–868.

43. Losche W, Karapetow F, Pohl A, et al. Plasma lipid and blood glucose levels in patients with destructive periodontal disease. *J Clin Periodontol.* 2000;27(8):537–541.

44. Losche W, Marshal GJ, Apatzidou DA, et al. Lipoprotein-associated phospholipase A2 and plasma lipids in patients with destructive periodontal disease. *J Clin Periodontol.* 2005;32(6):640–644.

45. Monteiro AM, Jardini MA, Alves S, et al. Cardiovascular disease parameters in periodontitis. *J Periodontol.* 2009;80(3): 378–388.

46. Pussinen PJ, Vilkuna-Rautiainen T, Alfthan G, et al. Severe periodontitis enhances macrophage activation via increased serum lipopolysaccharide. *Arterioscler Thromb Vasc Biol.* 2004;24(11):2174–2180.

47. Friedewald VE, Kornman KS, Beck JD, et al. The American Journal of Cardiology and Journal of Periodontology editors' consensus: periodontitis and atherosclerotic cardiovascular disease. *J Periodontol.* 2009;80(7):1021–1032.

48. Tonetti MS, Van Dyke TE, Working group 1 of the joint EFP/AAP workshop. Periodontitis and atherosclerotic cardiovascular disease: consensus report of the Joint EFP/AAP Workshop on Periodontitis and Systemic Diseases. *J Periodontol.* 2013; 84(4 suppl):S24–S29.

49. D'Aiuto F, Orlandi M, Gunsolley JC. Evidence that periodontal treatment improves biomarkers and CVD outcomes. *J Periodontol.* 2013;84(4 suppl):S85–S105.

50. Dietrich T, Sharma P, Walter C, et al. The epidemiological evidence behind the association between periodontitis and incident atherosclerotic cardiovascular disease. *J Periodontol.* 2013;84(4 suppl):S70–S84.

51. Sanz M, Kornman K, Working group 3 of the joint EFP/AAP workshop. Periodontitis and adverse pregnancy outcomes: consensus report of the Joint EFP/AAP Workshop on Periodontitis and Systemic Diseases. *J Periodontol.* 2013;84(4 suppl): S164–S169.

52. Ide M, Papapanou PN. Epidemiology of association between maternal periodontal disease and adverse pregnancy outcomes– systematic review. *J Periodontol.* 2013;84(4 suppl):S181–S194.

53. Madianos PN, Bobetsis YA, Offenbacher S. Adverse pregnancy outcomes (APOs) and periodontal disease: pathogenic mechanisms. *J Periodontol.* 2013;84(4 suppl):S170–S180.

54. Michalowicz BS, Gustafsson A, Thumbigere-Math V, et al. The effects of periodontal treatment on pregnancy outcomes. *J Periodontol.* 2013;84(4 suppl):S195–S208.

55. Task Force on Periodontal Treatment of Pregnant Women, American Academy of Periodontology. American Academy of Periodontology statement regarding periodontal management of the pregnant patient. *J Periodontol.* 2004;75(3):495.

56. Grossi SG, Genco RJ. Periodontal disease and diabetes mellitus: a two-way relationship. *Ann Periodontol.* 1998;3(1):51–61.

57. Lalla E, Papapanou PN. Diabetes mellitus and periodontitis: a tale of two common interrelated diseases. *Nat Rev Endocrinol.* 2011;7(12):738–748.

58. Mealey BL, Oates TW, American Academy of P. Diabetes mellitus and periodontal diseases. *J Periodontol.* 2006;77(8): 1289–1303.

59. Preshaw PM, Alba AL, Herrera D, et al. Periodontitis and diabetes: a two-way relationship. *Diabetologia.* 2012;55(1):21–31.

60. Papapanou PN. Periodontal diseases: epidemiology. *Ann Periodontol.* 1996;1(1):1–36.

61. American Diabetes Association. Standards of medical care in diabetes–2008. *Diabetes Care.* 2008;31(1 suppl):S12–S54.

62. Taylor GW, Burt BA, Becker MP, et al. Severe periodontitis and risk for poor glycemic control in patients with non-insulin-dependent diabetes mellitus. *J Periodontol.* 1996;67(10 suppl):1085–1093.

63. Taylor JJ, Preshaw PM, Lalla E. A review of the evidence for pathogenic mechanisms that may link periodontitis and diabetes. *J Periodontol.* 2013;84(4 suppl):S113–S134.

64. Chapple IL, Genco R, Working group 2 of the joint EFP/AAP workshop. Diabetes and periodontal diseases: consensus report of the Joint EFP/AAP Workshop on Periodontitis and Systemic Diseases. *J Periodontol.* 2013;84(4 suppl):S106–S112.

65. Engebretson S, Chertog R, Nichols A, et al. Plasma levels of tumour necrosis factor-alpha in patients with chronic periodontitis and type 2 diabetes. *J Clin Periodontol.* 2007;34(1):18–24.

66. Gupta A, Ten S, Anhalt H. Serum levels of soluble tumor necrosis factor-alpha receptor 2 are linked to insulin resistance and glucose intolerance in children. *J Pediatr endocrinol Metab.* 2005;18(1):75–82.

67. King GL. The role of inflammatory cytokines in diabetes and its complications. *J Periodontol.* 2008;79(8 suppl):1527–1534.

68. Loos BG. Systemic markers of inflammation in periodontitis. *J Periodontol.* 2005;76(11 suppl):2106–2115.

69. Pickup JC. Inflammation and activated innate immunity in the pathogenesis of type 2 diabetes. *Diabetes Care.* 2004;27(3): 813–823.

70. Shoelson SE, Lee J, Goldfine AB. Inflammation and insulin resistance. *J Clin Invest.* 2006;116(7):1793–1801.

71. Engebretson S, Kocher T. Evidence that periodontal treatment improves diabetes outcomes: a systematic review and meta-analysis. *J Periodontol.* 2013;84(4 suppl):S153–S169.

72. Simpson TC, Needleman I, Wild SH, et al. Treatment of periodontal disease for glycaemic control in people with diabetes. *Cochrane Database Syst Rev.* 2010(5):CD004714.

73. Teeuw WJ, Gerdes VE, Loos BG. Effect of periodontal treatment on glycemic control of diabetic patients: a systematic review and meta-analysis. *Diabetes Care.* 2010;33(2):421–427.

74. Ostergaard L, Andersen PL. Etiology of community-acquired pneumonia. Evaluation by transtracheal aspiration, blood culture, or serology. *Chest.* 1993;104(5):1400–1407.

75. Azarpazhooh A, Leake JL. Systematic review of the association between respiratory diseases and oral health. *J Periodontol.* 2006;77(9):1465–1482.

76. Scannapieco FA, Bush RB, Paju S. Associations between periodontal disease and risk for nosocomial bacterial pneumonia and chronic obstructive pulmonary disease. A systematic review. *Ann Periodontol.* 2003;8(1):54–69.

77. Craven DE. Preventing ventilator-associated pneumonia in adults: sowing seeds of change. *Chest.* 2006;130(1):251–260.

78. Craven DE, Duncan RA. Preventing ventilator-associated pneumonia: tiptoeing through a minefield. *Am J Respir Crit Care Med.* 2006;173(12):1297–1298.

79. Paju S, Scannapieco FA. Oral biofilms, periodontitis, and pulmonary infections. *Oral Dis.* 2007;13(6):508–512.

80. Scannapieco FA, Stewart EM, Mylotte JM. Colonization of dental plaque by respiratory pathogens in medical intensive care patients. *Crit Care Med.* 1992;20(6):740–745.

81. Labeau SO, Van de Vyver K, Brusselaers N, et al. Prevention of ventilator-associated pneumonia with oral antiseptics: a systematic review and meta-analysis. *Lancet Infect Dis.* 2011;11(11):845–854.

 STUDENT ANCILLARY RESOURCES

A wide variety of resources to enhance your learning and understanding of this chapter are available on thePoint®.

- Visit thePoint to access:
  - Audio Glossary
  - Animations
  - Suggested Readings
  - Answers to Review Questions
  - Case Studies

33

Oral Malodor and Xerostomia

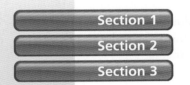

Clinical Patient Care. This chapter discusses two topics important to all dental healthcare providers: oral malodor and xerostomia. Though neither of the conditions is a disease of the periodontium, they both can be encountered in periodontal patients and can complicate the delivery of periodontal therapy and the maintenance of periodontal health. Dental hygienists need to be familiar with the basic issues involved with these conditions to allow them to participate in the comprehensive care of periodontal patients.

Learning Objectives

- Compare and contrast the terms oral malodor, breath malodor, and halitosis.
- Explain the significance of oral malodor.
- List chemical compounds that can cause oral malodor.
- Explain the association of oral malodor with other oral conditions.
- List some extraoral causes of breath malodor.
- Explain the diagnosis of oral malodor.
- Describe management of a patient with oral malodor.
- Define the term xerostomia.
- Explain the importance of saliva.
- Describe some causes of xerostomia.
- Explain the diagnosis of xerostomia in a dental setting.
- List some healthcare providers that might be involved in identifying an underlying systemic cause of xerostomia.
- Describe some principles of the dental management of patients with xerostomia.

Key Terms

Halitosis
Breath malodor
Oral malodor
Halitophobia

Volatile sulfur compounds
Tongue coating
Organoleptic evaluation
Xerostomia

Mouth breathing
Sjögren syndrome
Sialometry

Section 1
Oral Malodor

Perception of the odor of a patient's breath can be pleasant or unpleasant; if it is unpleasant, the terms **halitosis, breath malodor,** or simply bad breath have all been used to describe the perceived unpleasant odor. The term **oral malodor** is a bit more restrictive term, and this term has been applied to halitosis that has its origin within the oral cavity. Some breath malodors are not oral malodors, that is, they do not arise from the oral cavity. The focus of this part of the chapter is oral malodors (where the origin of the unpleasant odor is in the oral cavity), but members of the dental team must always be aware that some unpleasant breath odors indicate underlying systemic disease that must be managed by a physician. An oral malodor can indeed reflect some underlying oral pathology (such as caries or periodontal disease) in a patient, but this type of persistent odor should not be confused with the transient malodor caused by certain food intake, smoking, or breath odor encountered upon arising.

1. **Importance of Oral Malodor**
    A. **Halitosis.** Halitosis has been described as an important social problem in the United States; the magnitude of this problem is underscored by a reported consumer expenditure of between $1 billion and $3 billion each year in the United States on over-the-counter products purported to minimize bad breath (1). Breath malodor is a common complaint, with up to 50% of people worldwide assessing themselves as having frequent incidents of malodor (2). The American Dental Association Council on Scientific Affairs states that oral malodor is an identifiable condition that should be treated by the dental professional (3).
        1. It is safe to assume that the problem of halitosis will increase as the population of elderly adults in the United States increases. A Japanese study of more than 2,000 subjects reported that the volatile sulfur compounds (VSCs) (an accepted measure for halitosis) increases with age (4).
        2. No gender predominance seems to exist for halitosis, and the age of patients with halitosis includes all ages from childhood to the elderly.
    B. **Halitophobia.** It is important that members of the dental team be aware that in a small number of patients that complain of breath malodor the patients simply imagine that they have breath malodor in the absence of any clinical evidence of this condition.
        1. This illusionary breath malodor is called **halitophobia**.
        2. Management of a patient with this disorder is multidisciplinary and frequently involves the input of physicians including psychiatrists, ENT (ear, nose, and throat) specialists, and gastroenterologists as well as dentists.
    C. **Causes of Halitosis**
        1. In the majority of halitosis patients (approximately 90%) the underlying cause of the halitosis originates in the oral cavity (oral malodor), and malodor associated with gingivitis, periodontitis, low salivary flow, and tongue coating are the most common causative factors for this oral malodor (3).
            a. In most cases oral malodor is most evident upon awaking from sleep (5). For most individuals, the malodor is resolved with brushing, flossing, eating, and/or drinking water (5).
            b. Malodor of an intraoral etiology that is not resolved by simple self-care techniques usually involves periodontitis or dental caries, other factors such as gross dental neglect, smoking, or xerostomia (5).
        2. Even though the cause of halitosis is usually found within the oral cavity, in some patients the breath malodor results from extraoral sources such as an underlying systemic disease that can be difficult to identify. Approximately 10% of halitosis

cases are extraoral—originating from systemic conditions or a location other than the oral cavity (3,6). Dental professionals, therefore, should be diligent in completing a thorough medical history to understand all possible origins (3).

3. These extraoral causes are discussed briefly in this chapter and can include ear–nose–throat pathology, certain systemic diseases, hormonal problems, liver disease, kidney disease, bronchial carcinoma, or gastroenterological pathology (2).

D. **Chemical Origin of Oral Malodor**

1. Most oral malodors result from proteolytic degradation of peptides present in saliva, shed epithelial cells, food debris, and biofilm buildup on the teeth and tongue, gingival crevicular fluid, and blood.

2. The oral malodor is produced by microbial putrefaction of debris left in the mouth. The degradation of proteins that produces the unpleasant odor is the result of bacterial action. The most common bacteria involved are gram-negative anaerobic bacteria, such as Porphyromonas gingivalis, Prevotella intermedia, Fusobacterium nucleatum, Bacteroides forsythus, and Treponema denticola (2,5).

3. The oral malodor originates primarily from **volatile sulfur compounds** (usually referred to as VSCs) in the breath. These VSCs include hydrogen sulfide (H_2S), methyl mercaptan (CH_3SH), and dimethyl sulfide ($(CH_3)_2 S$) (2,3,5).

4. In addition to the VSCs, other chemicals may also contribute to an unpleasant breath odor; these chemicals include putrescine, cadaverine, indole, skatole, and butyric or propionic acid.

5. Box 33-1 shows some of the more important chemical compounds that can contribute to oral malodor.

2. **The Association between Oral Malodor and Other Oral Conditions.** Oral malodor is frequently associated with other oral conditions, some of which are actually quite common. Examples of some of these other conditions are discussed below. It is important for members of the dental team to identify these conditions and address them as part of the strategy for managing patients with oral malodor.

A. **Oral Malodor and Dental Caries**

1. In some patients oral malodor can be associated with existing dental caries.

2. Patients with deep carious lesions in teeth can exhibit oral malodor because of putrefaction of food that can lodge and remain in the tooth concavity created when carious lesions destroy tooth structure.

B. **Oral Malodor and Periodontal Disease**

1. Bacteria associated with periodontitis are almost all gram-negative, and many of these gram-negative bacteria are capable of producing VSCs.

2. In periodontitis patients the level of VSCs (and therefore the unpleasant breath odor) correlates with the depth of periodontal pockets (i.e., the deeper the periodontal pockets found in the patient, the more volatile compounds that are released).

Box 33-1. Chemical Compounds That can Contribute to Oral Malodor

- Hydrogen sulfide
- Methyl mercaptan
- Dimethylsulfide
- Putrescine
- Cadaverine
- Indole
- Skatole
- Butyric acid
- Propionic acid

3. In addition, in patients with periodontitis other molecules such as cadaverine and putrescine that result from decarboxylation of certain amino acids can also contribute to the oral malodor.

C. Oral Malodor and Dry Mouth

1. Dry mouth or xerostomia will be discussed later in this chapter, but it should be noted at this point that in patients with a dry mouth there can be an increased level of oral malodor because the VSCs are more likely to be released as gases when saliva is actually drying.

2. Thus these two conditions (oral malodor and dry mouth) can be related to some degree in selected patients.

D. Oral Malodor and Tongue Coatings

1. The dorsal (upper) tongue surface is so irregular that this surface provides a nearly ideal site for uninhibited bacterial growth within the contours of the irregularities in the surface (1).

2. In addition to the bacteria growing on the tongue surface, food remnants can be trapped in the irregular contours of the dorsum of the tongue, thus providing nutrients for bacteria already present.

3. In some patients there are anatomical variations of the tongue surface that result in even deeper fissures on dorsum of the tongue. These deep fissures can create even more sites for bacteria to grow and for food debris to lodge.

4. The dorsal surface of the tongue frequently accumulates a **tongue coating** that consists of bacteria, food debris, and desquamated epithelial cells (2,3,5).

    a. This tongue coating cannot be removed without special efforts during self-care because of the irregular contours of the surface. Craters, fissures, and peaks on the surface of the tongue are covered with a fine sticky substance that harbors the malodorous bacteria. Researchers report that a single epithelial cell in the oral cavity can harbor up to 25 bacteria, whereas one epithelial cell on the dorsum of the tongue can harbor up to 100 bacteria (7).

    b. High correlations have been reported in the literature between the presence of tongue coating and oral malodor.

E. Oral Malodor and Oral Infections. In patients with oral infections leading to purulent (pus) discharges into the mouth, there can be associated oral malodors because of the odor caused by the discharge of pus.

F. Oral Malodor and Acrylic Dental Appliances

1. Since the surface of an acrylic dental appliance is quite porous, the surface irregularities can also harbor bacteria.

2. Patients with certain oral appliances such as acrylic dentures can also display oral malodors.

3. Acrylic appliances are especially prone to oral malodor if the oral appliances are not cleaned thoroughly as a part of the patient's daily self-care regimen.

4. Box 33-2 shows examples of oral conditions associated with oral malodor.

Box 33-2. Examples of Oral Conditions Associated with Oral Malodor

- Dental caries
- Periodontal disease
- Dry mouth
- Tongue coatings
- Purulent infections
- Acrylic dental appliances

Box 33-3. Examples of Extraoral Causes for Breath Malodor

- Nose and throat conditions
- Diabetes
- Lung disease
- Gastrointestinal tract problems
- Liver disease
- Kidney disease
- Hormonal changes

---

3. **Extraoral Causes of Breath Malodor.** Even though in the majority of patients with breath malodor the unpleasant odor is due to an intraoral cause, bad breath can be a sign of a medical disorder in some patients (Box 33-3). Clinicians must have a high index of suspicion in any patient where breath malodor does not improve significantly following elimination of the more common intraoral causes of oral malodor.

   A. **Breath Malodor and Nose and Throat Conditions**
      1. Breath malodor can result from nose and throat conditions such as acute pharyngitis, sinusitis, and postnasal drip. Postnasal drip resulting in breath malodor can also be associated with the esophagitis resulting from damage to the nasopharynx following regurgitation of acidic stomach content.
      2. In patients with tonsillitis the deep crypts of the tonsils can accumulate food debris and bacteria that can also lead to breath malodor.

   B. **Breath Malodor and Diabetes**
      1. In uncontrolled diabetics there can be an accumulation of chemicals called ketones in the blood, and these chemicals can result in a typical breath malodor.
      2. Some clinicians have described the breath malodor associated with diabetes as being similar to the smell of rotten apples.

   C. **Breath Malodor and the Lung Disease.** Breath malodor has been associated with certain pulmonary (lung) causes including chronic bronchitis, bronchiectasis, and bronchial carcinoma.

   D. **Breath Malodor and the Gastrointestinal Tract**
      1. In a very small number of patients with breath malodor, the unpleasant odors can arise because of problems in the gastrointestinal tract.
      2. Among these gastrointestinal causes of breath malodor are herniated esophageal walls and gastric hernias.
      3. Also, a breath malodor can also result from intestinal gas production where some of the sulfide compounds can be transported to the lungs and exhaled in the breath.

   E. **Breath Malodor and Liver Disease.** In some patients with liver disease, such as seen in cirrhosis, ammonium can accumulate in the blood and later exhaled in the breath leading to a breath malodor.

   F. **Breath Malodor and Kidney Disease.** Kidney insufficiency can result in increased blood uric acid levels and can also result in breath malodor.

   G. **Breath Malodor and Hormonal Changes**
      1. In some women a breath malodor can develop when progesterone levels are increased as part of the normal menstrual cycle.
      2. VSC levels have also been reported to increase in the expired air near the time of ovulation.

   H. **Breath Malodor and Medications**
      1. Some medications have been reported to result in a breath malodor. For example, the antimicrobial drug metronidazole can cause breath malodor.
      2. The drug metronidazole can also be associated with patients' perceptions of a metallic taste in the mouth, which some patients may confuse with breath malodor.

4. Diagnosis of Oral Malodor
   A. The Medical History as a Foundation for Diagnosis
      1. The foundation for establishing a proper diagnosis of oral malodor is taking a thorough medical history.
      2. The medical history has been discussed in other chapters of this book, but when a patient complains of breath malodor, there are some directed questions that can help clarify the nature of the breath malodor problem.
      3. In patients with complaints of halitosis questions should be asked about the frequency of occurrence, the time of day the problem appears, whether others have noted the malodor, and whether the patient is aware of other symptoms such as dryness of the mouth.
   B. Techniques for Quantifying Halitosis
      1. There are several techniques that have been recommended for quantifying breath malodors (8–10). These techniques primarily include using organoleptic evaluation or the use of diagnostic machines.
      2. Organoleptic evaluation by a trained judge is the standard in the examination of breath malodor.
         a. Organoleptic evaluation is a sensory test that involves having a trained judge smell a patient's expired air to make an assessment whether or not the breath is unpleasant. This assessment depends upon the olfactory organs of the judge.
         b. Various scoring systems have been developed, however, most are based on a numerical scale of 1 to 5, with 1 being barely noticeable odor and 5 being extremely foul odor. An example of a rating scale is shown in Box 33-4.
         c. Since some adults have partial loss of smell acuity, testing of smell acuity is a part of the training for a judge.
         d. As part of a typical organoleptic evaluation, a trained judge would evaluate oral cavity odor, breath odor, tongue coating odor, and nasal breath odor.
      3. Diagnostic machines have also been used to detect volatile odor causing compounds, but it appears that many trained clinicians can be even more accurate in using their olfactory sense than these machines.
         a. Several diagnostic machines have been recommended for detection of breath malodor; examples of these machines are outlined below.
         b. A portable volatile sulfur monitor that is an electronic device has been used to detect hydrogen sulfide and methyl mercaptan (VSCs) in the breath (9). A major disadvantage of this instrument is that it does not detect unpleasant odors caused by compounds other than the VSCs such as dimethyl sulfide (6), putrescine, or cadaverine. Because of this limitation, the sulfur monitor may underestimate oral malodor (11).
         c. A portable gas chromatograph device has been developed for use in typical clinical settings to measure VSCs in the breath and can identify hydrogen sulfide, methyl mercaptan, and dimethyl sulfide (12). With these devices, the measurement of VSCs can be obtained and differentiated with samples from saliva, tongue coating, and breath. This assists in determining the origin of the malodor (9).
         d. The electronic nose is a handheld instrument that has the ability to "smell" and produce unique fingerprints for odors (13). This instrument has made odor analysis fast and simple. Although the electronic nose is used throughout the medical fields, few studies have been done to assess its effectiveness in clinically assessing oral malodor (13,14).

Box 33-4. Example of a Typical Rating Scale for an Organoleptic Evaluation

0 = no odor present
1 = barely noticeable odor
2 = slight but clearly noticeable odor
3 = moderate odor
4 = strong offensive odor
5 = extremely foul odor

---

   e. A saliva incubation test has been used to detect unpleasant odors in the air immediately above the incubated saliva. This test involves collection of a saliva sample in a glass tube and incubating the saliva in the tube over a 3-hour period. A gas chromatograph can be used to detect odor-producing compounds, but an organoleptic evaluation has also been recommended as part of this test.

5. **Management of Patients with Oral Malodor.** The strategies for management of patients with breath malodors can be complex, but since most breath malodors are oral malodors, the members of the dental team are ideally suited to manage most of these patients. The dental team should always have a high index of suspicion about any patient with breath malodor that does not respond to management strategies for oral malodors. Patients where the malodor persists should be referred to medical colleagues for further evaluation. It is helpful for members of the dental team to organize the therapeutic strategies employed for patients with oral malodor to include the steps outlined below.

   A. **Reduction of Contributing Oral Factors**
      1. Patients with dental caries should have carious lesions restored and the decay problem controlled.
      2. Patients with periodontal diseases should have the periodontal disease controlled through conventional periodontal therapy.

   B. **Patient Education for Malodor Control**
      1. Regardless of what may be the cause, mechanical removal of biofilm and microorganisms—meticulous daily self-care—is the first step in control of oral malodor (9,15). Self-care has already been discussed in other chapters of this book and would be employed to control both dental caries and periodontal disease, but it should be emphasized that self-care in the patient with oral malodor must include cleaning the dorsal surface of the tongue. It is estimated that approximately 60% of the VSCs originate on the surface of the tongue (9,10,16).
      2. Cleaning the dorsal surface of the tongue can be accomplished with a toothbrush, but using a tongue scraper is helpful if the tongue coating is well established.
         a. A Cochrane systematic review was conducted to determine reliable evidence concerning the effectiveness of tongue scraping or cleaning, compared with other interventions for controlling halitosis. The review included two trials involving a total of 40 participants. Based on the independent data from these two trials, the tongue cleaner or the tongue scraper demonstrated a statistically significant difference in reducing levels of VSCs when compared with the toothbrush (17).
            1. The technique for cleaning the tongue surface should include a gentle scraping with the brush or tongue scraper.
            2. The posterior part of the tongue collects the heaviest tongue coatings, and the gagging reflex can be a problem in some patients. Gagging seems

easier to control with tongue scrapers than with toothbrushes. In a clinical trial comparing tongue-cleaning methods conducted by Pedrazzi (18), patients reported that they preferred the tongue scraper to the toothbrush.

   3. Because patients often neglect tongue cleaning in their daily self-care routines as the result of lack of familiarity with the practice, dental hygienists should demonstrate the appropriate use of tongue scrapers.

   b. While mechanical tongue cleaning with or without chemical intervention can reduce bacterial load on the tongue, this effect is transient, and regular tongue cleaning is required to provide a long-lasting (overnight) reduction in bacterial numbers (19).

   c. In addition, for patients with acrylic oral appliances, the appliances should be removed at night and cleaned thoroughly before replacing them the next morning.

C. **Chemotherapeutic Reduction.** Chemical agents useful in plaque biofilm control have been discussed in other chapters of this book, but some of these agents have also been studied as aids to control oral malodor (20). A systematic review, published by Cochrane, concluded that mouth rinses containing antibacterial agents such as chlorhexidine and cetylpyridinium chloride may play an important role in reducing the levels of halitosis-producing bacteria on the tongue, and chlorine dioxide and zinc-containing mouth rinses can be effective in neutralization of odoriferous sulfur compounds. However, well-designed randomized controlled trials with a larger sample size, a longer intervention, and follow-up period are still needed (21).

D. **Alter Volatility of Sulfur Compounds**
   1. Certain metal ions can be used to trap some of the odor-producing sulfur-containing gases before they can be released (22–27).
   2. Zinc ions bind to sulfur radicals and thus can reduce the release of the VSCs.
      a. Because zinc is relatively nontoxic and does not accumulate in the body, zinc has been suggested for use in the control of oral malodor.
      b. Zinc chloride has been reported to reduce volatile sulfide compounds and zinc chloride is available is some over-the-counter products.
   3. Toothpastes containing baking soda have been shown to reduce VSCs, and there are many baking soda–containing toothpastes on the market today. The mechanisms for this reduction are not clear, but it appears that baking soda can change volatile sulfide compounds to a nonvolatile state.

E. **Increase Salivary Flow**
   1. Simply increasing the volume of saliva allows for more retention of larger volumes of sulfur compounds in the saliva, thus preventing their release.
   2. Strategies for increasing saliva are discussed in the next part of this chapter.
   3. As examples, these strategies include steps such as maintaining a proper liquid intake by the patient and using a sugarless chewing gum to stimulate saliva production.

F. **Mask the Oral Malodor.** Masking oral malodors with products containing volatiles with pleasant smells such as rinses, sprays, or lozenges does not have a lasting effect on oral malodor, but this strategy may be employed as part of a more comprehensive treatment plan to deal with the problem of oral malodor.

G. **Involve the Patient in Odor Management**
   1. Involving the patient in the assessment of control of oral malodor is helpful.
   2. This patient involvement can be critical in motivating the patient to perform the high level of self-care needed to control this condition.

3. Spitting some saliva into a cup, allowing it to dry a bit, and then smelling the result can be useful for a patient as self-examination for oral malodor. As the saliva dries, it releases volatile sulfide compounds if they are present.

4. It is sometimes helpful for a patient to scrape the back of the tongue gently with a metallic spoon and then smell the result as a mechanism for monitoring oral malodor; this is especially helpful if it appears that tongue coating is a major contributing factor to the unpleasant odor.

5. It should be noted that is not very helpful in making a meaningful assessment of breath malodor for a patient to breathe into cupped hands.

H. Reassess Malodor Control

1. Reassessment following dental treatment of a patient with a complaint of breath malodor is critical.

2. If breath malodor is not improved following the treatment strategies for oral malodor discussed above, then other sources of the odor should be investigated.

3. Other sources have already been discussed and patients with persistent breath malodor after thorough management for oral malodor has been implemented should be referred to their physician for a comprehensive physical exam.

Section 2
Xerostomia

1. Introduction to Xerostomia
   A. Xerostomia can be defined as dry mouth that results from a reduction in salivary flow.
      1. Dry mouth is a common patient complaint, and it affects about one in every four to five adults; the prevalence of xerostomia increases with age (28–33).
      2. Many medications include xerostomia as a potential side effect, and since there are more medications taken by older adults, it should not be surprising that dry mouth is a common complaint among this age group.
      3. Reduced salivary flow may be associated with decreased salivary gland function, but it may also be present in patients where the salivary glands are capable of producing an adequate flow of saliva under the right conditions.
   B. Importance of Saliva for Quality of Life
      1. Saliva has many functions in addition to moistening and lubrication of the mouth.
         a. Saliva is critical for its antimicrobial properties, in control of the pH of the oral cavity, for removal of food debris, in remineralization of teeth, and for maintaining the health of oral mucosa.
         b. In addition, saliva plays an important role in chewing, taste, swallowing, digestion, and speech.
      2. Reduced salivary flow decreases the oral pH and can significantly increase the development of dental caries; members of the dental team will manage many patients with dental caries resulting from a dry mouth.
      3. As discussed earlier in this chapter, xerostomia can also be associated with halitosis because drying saliva releases VSCs.
      4. Xerostomia can also be an indication of several systemic diseases and can promote oral infections such as candidiasis.
      5. Partially or fully edentulous patients with xerostomia are susceptible to pain from denture irritation, mucosal ulcerations, and fungal infections, in addition to loss of denture retention (33,34).
      6. Box 33-5 summarizes some of the important functions of saliva.

Box 33-5. Examples of Functions of Saliva

- Moistening and lubrication of the mouth
- Antimicrobial properties
- Maintaining pH of the oral cavity
- Removal of food debris
- Remineralization of teeth
- Maintaining the health of oral mucosa
- Aid in chewing
- Enhancing taste
- Aid in swallowing
- Aid in digestion

2. **Overview of Causes of Xerostomia**
   A. **Local Conditions Associated with Xerostomia.** A number of local and systemic causes may contribute to xerostomia. The American Dental Hygienists' Association (ADHA) has developed a useful screening tool for the recognition and management of hyposalivation and xerostomia. This screen tool is shown in Figure 33-1.
      1. As a general rule, decreased salivary flow resulting in dry mouth is due to systemic causes, not to intraoral problems. One exception to this general rule is mouth breathing.
      2. **Mouth breathing** can be defined as inhaling and exhaling through the mouth rather than through the nose.
         a. Patients normally breathe through the nose while either resting or performing light exercise, but they breathe through the nose and mouth only during more vigorous exercise.
         b. Continuous mouth breathing can cause a drying of oral tissues and lead to a patient complaint of dry mouth.
      3. Research suggests that the use of cannabis increases the risk of xerostomia and candidiasis (35). With the increasing prevalence of cannabis use, dental healthcare providers should be aware of cannabis-associated oral side effects.
   B. **Systemic Conditions Associated with Xerostomia**
      1. Xerostomia Associated with Sjögren Syndrome
         a. **Sjögren syndrome** (pronounced "show-grins") is the most common systemic condition associated with xerostomia (36–38).
         b. Sjögren syndrome is an inflammatory autoimmune disease that results in a general dryness caused by damage to the salivary and other similar glands such as tear glands.
            1. This syndrome occurs most frequently in postmenopausal women.
            2. One of the characteristics of the underlying pathology of this syndrome is infiltration of salivary as well as tear glands by lymphocytes.
            3. There are a variety of other patient complaints associated with Sjögren syndrome, and these can include symptoms such as blurred vision, oral soreness, smell alterations, taste alterations, fissures on the tongue and lips, fatigue, and dry nasal passages.
            4. There is no known cure for Sjögren syndrome, so therapy is directed at managing the symptoms of this disorder.
      2. Xerostomia as a Medication Side Effect
         a. More than 1,800 drugs have been reported to contribute to xerostomia; the majority of the most frequently prescribed medications in the United States can result in the feeling of dry mouth.
         b. For example, medications used to treat common ailments such as high blood pressure, anxiety, allergies, and weight loss can contribute to dry mouth.
         c. In addition, patients taking more than one medication have an increased chance of developing a dry mouth.
      3. Xerostomia Associated with Cancer Therapy
         a. Many cancer patients are treated with radiation therapy, and xerostomia is one of the most common side effects associated with radiation therapy to the head and neck.
         b. Radiation therapy can cause an inflammatory reaction in salivary glands and results in a condition referred to as acute xerostomia (39).

Name _____	/ /
HYPOSALIVATION with XEROSTOMIA SCREENING TOOL	**Points**

SOURCE BY DENTAL HYGIENE ASSESSMENT

CONTRIBUTORY HISTORY	☐None	☐Present (10 pts each); *indicate related history below*	
DIRECT RELATIONSHIP ☐Autoimmune Disorder: Sjögren's Syndrome or Other ☐Cancer Therapy: Recent Chemo and/or H&N Radiation ☐Diabetes (either type) ☐Dialysis ☐_____		☐Diet Disorder: Anorexia, Bulimia, and/or Dehydration ☐Infection: Hepatitis, HIV, Tuberculosis, or Other ☐Mental Condition or Dementia ☐Thyroid Disease: Hypo/Hyperthyroidism ☐_____ DIRECT RELATIONSHIP	

LONG-TERM DAILY INTAKE ☐None	☐One (5 pts); *check type below*	☐Two or more (10 pts total); *check type below*	
MORE THAN ONE MONTH ☐Alcohol (any form) ☐Antidepressant ☐Antidiarrheal ☐Antihistamine or Decongestant ☐_____	☐Antihypertensive ☐Antipsychotic ☐Bronchodilator ☐Caffeine (any form) ☐Diuretic	☐Garlic, Gingko, or Other ☐Non-Steroidal Antiinflammatory ☐Painkiller, Sedative, or Tranquilizer ☐Tobacco (any form) ☐_____ MORE THAN ONE MONTH	

SYMPTOM QUESTIONS BY DENTAL HYGIENE ASSESSMENT

Feeling Constantly Thirsty?	☐None	☐Slight (1 pt)	☐Moderate (2 pts)	☐Severe (3 pts)
Difficulty Chewing Food?	☐None	☐Slight (1 pt)	☐Moderate (2 pts)	☐Severe (3 pts)
Difficult Swallowing Food?	☐None	☐Slight (1 pt)	☐Moderate (2 pts)	☐Severe (3 pts)
Saliva Amount?	☐Regular	☐Low (1 pt)		☐Very Low (2 pts)
Dryness Amount?	☐Regular	☐High (1 pt)		☐Very High (2 pts)
Dryness Frequency?	☐None	☐Occasional (1 pt)		☐Constant (2 pts)
Dryness Duration?	☐None	☐Short-term (1 pt)		☐Long-term (2 pts)
Mouth Changes? *Select below*	☐None	☐One (1 pt)	☐Two (2 pts)	☐Three or More (3 pts)
ASK ☐Bad or Stale Breath? ☐Burning Mouth?	☐Denture Poor Hold? ☐Spicy Food Sensitivity?	☐Soreness in Mouth? ☐Stickiness of Tongue?	☐Taste Sensation Loss? ☐Tooth Sensitivity? ASK	
Additional Eye, Nose, Throat, Skin, Genital Dryness?			☐None	☐Yes (1 pt)

ORAL SIGNS BY DENTAL HYGIENE DIAGNOSIS

Tissue Changes? *If noted, circle specific signs* (1 pt each group)	☐None	☐Atrophy/ Redness	☐Cheilitis/ Fissured	☐Glossitis/ Stickiness	☐Ulcers/ Debris
Oral Diseases? (1 pt each)	☐None	☐Caries	☐Fungal	☐Halitosis	☐Periodontal
Saliva/Gland Changes? (1 pt each)	☐None	☐Enlarged	☐No Pooling	☐Stone(s)	☐Thick/White
Failure To Express? *Indicate gland(s)* (1 pt each)	☐None	☐Parotid	☐Sublingual/Submandibular		

RISK LEVEL BY DENTAL HYGIENE ASSESSMENT (tally points and circle level)		**TOTAL**
LOW RISK	**MODERATE RISK**	**HIGH RISK**
From 1 to 10 points	From 11 to 20 points	Greater than 20 points

DENTAL HYGIENE PLANNING AND IMPLEMENTATION

☐Document in patient record; ☐Correlate with other oral disease risk tools; ☐Recommend palliative management; ☐Monitor by evaluation over next 6-month period	☐Document in patient record; ☐Correlate with other oral disease risk tools; ☐Recommend palliative management; ☐Perform diagnostic salivary tests to evaluate for high risk 　☐If negative, monitor by evaluation over next 3-month period; 　☐If positive, consider high risk and proceed with planning	☐Document in patient record; ☐Correlate with other oral disease risk tools; ☐Recommend palliative management; ☐Perform diagnostic salivary tests for baseline ☐Refer to oral surgeon and/or physician for further testing if from unknown source or for prescribing medication(s), and follow-up evaluation/treatment

Copyright ADHA 2010 *ADHA Standards for Clinical Dental Hygiene*; Fox PC: Xerostomia: Recognition and Management, *Access Supplementary*, Feb. 2008.

Figure 33-1. Hyposalivation with Xerostomia Screening Tool.

c. As a result of radiation therapy there can also be an associated fibrosis of the salivary glands and this causes what is referred to as late xerostomia.

d. The degree of permanent xerostomia following radiation therapy depends upon the precise volume of salivary glands exposed to the radiation and depends upon the radiation dose used in the cancer treatment.

e. In addition to xerostomia associated with radiation therapy, some cancer chemotherapeutic agents can also decrease the salivary flow.

4. Xerostomia Associated with Aging

a. As patients age, there is a tendency to produce less saliva.

b. In general, this reduction in salivary output associated with aging is not dramatic enough to result in a complaint of oral dryness, but when combined with other factors such as the effects of medications, it can contribute to increased complaints related to xerostomia (40–42).

5. Xerostomia Associated with HIV Infection

a. In some young patients infected with HIV there can be an associated salivary gland disease that results in xerostomia.

b. This dry mouth usually follows enlargement of the parotid salivary glands and less frequently the submandibular glands.

6. Xerostomia Associated with Other Systemic Conditions

a. An array of other systemic conditions can cause xerostomia.

b. Systemic diseases that have been associated with dry mouth include sarcoidosis, rheumatoid arthritis, lupus erythematosus, nephritis, scleroderma, diabetes mellitus, hypertension, cystic fibrosis, and endocrine disorders.

c. In addition, other conditions associated with dry mouth include nutritional deficiencies, methamphetamine use, depression, anxiety, stress, and fear.

d. Dry mouth is often exacerbated by activities such as smoking or drinking alcohol.

3. **Diagnosis of Xerostomia in a Dental Setting.** It should be noted that confirming the presence of xerostomia can be much easier than identification of the fundamental underlying cause. The diagnosis of xerostomia in a dental office may be based on evidence obtained from the three primary clinical steps outlined below.

A. **First Diagnostic Step: Perform a thorough Patient History**

1. Patients with xerostomia usually complain of problems with eating, speaking, swallowing, or even wearing dentures.

2. A typical complaint would be that dry foods such as crackers are difficult to chew and swallow.

3. Box 33-6 outlines some typical patient complaints related to reduced salivary flow.

B. **Second Diagnostic Step: Perform a Comprehensive Examination of the Oral Cavity**

1. During examination of the oral cavity in a patient with xerostomia, the oral mucosa may appear dry and sticky; a wooden tongue depressor placed against the inner surface of the cheek may tend to stick to the mucosa.

2. Oral examination may reveal dental caries, parotid gland enlargement, inflammation and fissuring of the lips, inflammation or ulcers of the tongue or cheek mucosa, oral candidiasis, or halitosis.

3. There may be very little or no pooled saliva in the floor of the mouth.

4. The tongue may appear dry, and any saliva present may appear stringy or ropy.

Box 33-6.   Examples of Oral Complaints Associated with Reduced Salivary Flow Reported by Patients

- Difficulty in eating dry foods
- Problems with taste acuity
- Difficulty with swallowing
- Sensitivity of oral mucosa to foods
- Soreness of the tongue
- Increased tooth decay
- Difficulty in wearing dentures

Box 33-7.   Examples of Typical Salivary Flow Rates

Stimulated whole saliva   =   1–2 mL/min
Unstimulated whole saliva =   0.3–0.5 mL/min
Xerostomia   =   less than 0.1 mL/min

C. **Third Diagnostic Step: Measure the Salivary Flow Rate**
  1. Office tests can be utilized to determine the salivary flow rate; measuring the salivary flow rate is referred to as **sialometry**.
  2. Sialometry tests usually involve placing a collection device over the parotid gland duct orifice or the submandibular/sublingual gland duct orifices, and measuring saliva flow per minute with glands stimulated and with the glands unstimulated.
  3. A salivary flow rate of less than 0.1 mL/min is usually considered indicative of xerostomia.
  4. Examples of typical flow rates for saliva are outlined in Box 33-7.
D. **Identifying the Underlying Cause of Xerostomia: An Interdisciplinary Approach**
  1. Once the members of the dental team have determined that xerostomia exists, the actual diagnosis of the fundamental underlying cause of the dry mouth can require the input of a variety of healthcare providers in addition to dentists; the members of an advanced care team may include specialists in oral medicine, rheumatology, and ophthalmology.
  2. The type of information used by these healthcare providers to arrive at a definitive identification of the underlying cause is outlined below, but the details of this type of diagnosis are beyond the scope of this book.
     a. Complete history and clinical examination
     b. Salivary tests to measure both the flow rate of the saliva and the condition of the salivary glands themselves
     c. Tests on the eyes
     d. Special blood tests such as for antibodies associated with Sjögren syndrome, for rheumatoid factor, and for immunoglobulins
  3. Even prior to a definitive diagnosis of the cause of the xerostomia by an advanced care team, members of the dental team can implement strategies for management in patients with reduced salivary flow. Strategies for managing patients with xerostomia are outlined in the next section.

4. **Dental Management of Patients with Xerostomia**
   A. **Minimize the cause or symptoms of the xerostomia.** As already discussed, when possible the management of patients with xerostomia should include the identification of the underlying cause of the decreased salivary flow.
      1. In the event that steps can be taken to minimize the effect of the underlying cause, this should be done; frequently these steps will be in the hands of the patient's physician.
      2. For many patients, however, little can be done to alter the underlying cause of the dry mouth.
         a. For example, if the underlying cause is that the xerostomia is a side effect of medications taken to maintain the health of the patient, the patient must continue to take these medications even though this may mean that the xerostomia will persist.
         b. This means that in many patients with xerostomia the management should be focused on strategies to minimize the symptoms and to improve the quality of life for the patient.
      3. Strategies for dental management of patients with xerostomia are discussed below; the precise strategies that should be employed will depend upon the severity of the xerostomia in any individual patient (43,44).
   B. **Involve the patient in the management of the xerostomia.**
      1. Members of the dental team should make every effort to involve the patient in the active management of the dry mouth problem.
      2. This involvement should include participation in the identification of products and behaviors that are truly helpful for each individual patient.
      3. Patients should be encouraged to monitor the health of their oral cavities daily, and to report any suspicious findings to the dental team promptly.
      4. For example, patients should be instructed to watch for areas of redness or patches on the oral tissues that might indicate infection.
      5. Patients with xerostomia must be involved enough to practice vigorous preventive dentistry to minimize potential side effects such as dental caries. This involvement includes the motivation and skills for thorough daily brushing, flossing, and the use of fluorides.
   C. **Recommend helpful products.** Make the patient aware of over-the-counter products that can aid patients with xerostomia.
      1. Over-the-counter products are available to support patients with a dry mouth; these products include toothpastes, mouth rinses, sprays, gels, gums, and liquids (45).
         a. An example of these products are the Biotene brand of products; Box 33-8 lists some of these products.
         b. A quick search of the Internet will reveal a variety of over-the-counter products that can be helpful in some patients, and more products are available each year.
      2. Use of toothpastes and mouth rinses specially designed for individuals with xerostomia is recommended. Sodium lauryl sulfate—a foaming agent commonly found in toothpastes and mouth rinses—can further damage already fragile oral soft tissues. The use of sodium lauryl sulfate–containing products should be strongly discouraged for patients with xerostomia (46,47).
   D. **Instruct the patient in simple techniques for increasing existing salivary flow.**
      1. Some relatively simple techniques for increasing salivary flow (when there is some function of the salivary glands remaining) are outlined below.

2. Eating foods that require mastication can stimulate salivary flow; examples of these types of foods include carrots or celery.

3. Chewing sugarless gum can increase the flow of saliva.

4. In addition, some patients benefit from using acid-tasting sugarless candy (as recommended for diabetics).

5. For most individuals daytime dryness is easily managed; however, oral dryness is much more problematic at night while sleeping. One product, XyliMelts–a self-adhering, slowly dissolving disc that time-releases xylitol, a lubricant, and a humectant–is used to reduce oral dryness the occurs during sleep. In a 15-subject study, Burgess and Lee found that use of XyliMelts discs may be an effective strategy for managing oral dryness that occurs during sleep (48).

E. **Replace lost saliva with saliva substitutes.** Over-the-counter saliva substitutes specifically formulated for patients with xerostomia are available as solutions, spray, chewing gum, and gels (49,50).

1. Saliva substitutes can be used to replace some moisture in the oral cavity and to lubricate the mouth (51).

2. It should be noted that saliva substitutes are formulated to replace natural saliva, but they do not stimulate salivary production.

3. Examples of commercially available saliva substitutes containing carboxymethyl cellulose and hydroxyethyl cellulose that can be used in xerostomic patients are Salivart, Oralube, and Xerolube.

F. **Make the patient aware of simple behaviors to minimize the effects of dry mouth.** There are a variety of suggestions that can be made to patients to minimize the effects of dry mouth. Box 33-9 lists some suggestions for individuals with xerostomia.

G. **Consider the use of salivary stimulants.** There are several pharmacologic stimulants that can be prescribed to stimulate salivary flow.

1. Pilocarpine (Salagen)
   a. Pilocarpine is a prescription cholinergic parasympathomimetic agent that can stimulate functioning salivary glands.
   b. This drug has been used in some patients with xerostomia caused by Sjögren syndrome and in patients with xerostomia caused by radiation treatment for cancer (52,53).
   c. Research has shown that pilocarpine can significantly decrease dryness of the mouth and eyes in patients with Sjögren syndrome.
   d. Pilocarpine is available in an ophthalmic solution and gel as well as the oral tablet.
   e. This drug does have side effects, and the most common side effects are increased sweating and gastrointestinal intolerance.
   f. Hypotension, rhinitis, diarrhea, and visual disturbances have also been reported with the use of this drug.

2. Cevimeline (Evoxac)
   a. Cevimeline is a prescription cholinergic agonist that can lead to an increase in exocrine gland secretions including saliva.
   b. Cevimeline has been used for the treatment of symptoms of dry mouth in patients with Sjögren syndrome (54,55).

3. Chemical stimulants. There are several products containing citric acid; citric acid can stimulate salivary flow. "MouthKote" and "Optimoist" are examples of two such products.

H. Perform a comprehensive oral exam frequently
   1. Since dental caries can develop rapidly in patients with xerostomia and since these patients tend to develop infections that can affect the oral mucosa, they should be seen on relatively short recall intervals by members of the dental team.
   2. Of course, these recalls should include monitoring of the salivary flow rate, but they should also include both comprehensive oral examinations as well as dental radiographs.

Box 33-8. Examples of Biotene Brand of Products Formulated for Patients with Dry Mouth

- Biotene dry mouth toothpaste
- Biotene gentle mouthwash
- Biotene dry mouth gum
- Biotene dry mouth kit

Box 33-9. Useful Suggestions for Patients with Xerostomia

- Take frequent sips of water throughout the day or suck on ice chips.
- Use a humidifier in your bedroom at night.
- Chew your food slowly and thoroughly, and sip water with it before swallowing.
- Brush and floss your teeth thoroughly at least twice each day.
- Select and use a fluoride-containing toothpaste daily. (Your dentist may even prescribe a special fluoride-containing toothpaste.)
- Clean the surface of your tongue daily.
- Restrict your intake of sugar-containing foods and beverages.
- Use time-release xylitol lozenges (xylitol has properties that stimulate saliva). These products last for an hour or longer and some of these products can be used overnight.
- Chew gum that contains no sugar, but that does contain xylitol.
- Avoid your intake of spicy, salty, or very acidic foods.
- Limit your between-meal snacks.
- Do not smoke.
- Avoid intake of alcohol-containing products; many mouth rinses contain alcohol.
- Avoid intake of caffeine-containing drinks.
- Avoid products containing the chemical sodium lauryl sulfate.
- Do not wear dentures when sleeping.
- Visit your dentist at least three times a year.

Chapter Summary Statement

The focus of the first half of this chapter is oral malodors (where the origin of the unpleasant breath odor is within the oral cavity), but members of the dental team must always be aware that some unpleasant breath odors indicate underlying systemic disease that must be managed by a physician. An oral malodor usually reflects underlying oral pathology (such as caries or periodontal disease) that must be corrected as part of the management of patients with this condition. The chemical origin of oral malodor is primarily from VSCs, but there are other compounds that can contribute to the unpleasant odor. Therapy for this condition usually is directed toward eliminating both the bacteria and the nutrients that can lead to the unpleasant odors.

The focus of the second half of this chapter is xerostomia. Recognition of xerostomia in a dental setting is not difficult, but identification of the fundamental underlying cause of dry mouth can be difficult. In many patients the underlying cause of the xerostomia cannot be corrected, so management of many patients with xerostomia consists of controlling symptoms. There are many strategies that can be employed in the dental management of patients with xerostomia; the precise strategies employed for an individual patient should depend upon the severity of the xerostomia in the individual patient.

Section 3
Focus on Patients

Clinical Patient Care

CASE 1

A patient new to your dental team has a chief complaint of bad breath. Your dental team decides to treat this patient for oral malodor and reassess the results following treatment. What steps should be taken by the various members of your dental team to control the patient's oral malodor?

CASE 2

During a routine recall visit, an elderly patient taking several critical medications complains to you of dry mouth. Make a list of suggestions that you can give this patient to help minimize the effects of the patient's xerostomia.

Ethical Dilemma

Ava W. has been a patient in your practice for the last 15 years. She is a 48-year-old woman, who sees you every 6 months for periodontal maintenance.

When you escort her from the waiting room to your operatory, you notice that she is quite thin, appears weak and frail, and looks to be wearing a wig. As you review her medical history, she tells you that she was diagnosed with breast cancer right after her last appointment with you. She has been undergoing intensive chemotherapy and radiation, and in fact has been using medical marijuana to assist with the painful side effects.

During your intraoral examination, you notice that Ava has extremely bad halitosis and xerostomia. These conditions have not been noted in her chart in the past. You realize that she is unable to thoroughly clean her oral cavity due to her oral mouth sores, most likely from her cancer treatments.

You are aware of research that links the use of cannabis with increased risk of xerostomia. You, however, disagree with the use of marijuana for any purpose. As a result, you are unsure how to best educate Ava.

1. How would you discuss oral malodor/management with Ava?
2. What options could you discuss for management of xerostomia?
3. Are there ethical principles that are in conflict in this dilemma?

References

1. Lee SS, Zhang W, Li Y. Halitosis update: a review of causes, diagnoses, and treatments. *J Calif Dent Assoc.* 2007;35(4):258–260, 262, 264–268.
2. Porter SR, Scully C. Oral malodour (halitosis). *BMJ.* 2006;333(7569):632–635.
3. ADA Council on Scientific Affairs. Oral malodor. *J Am Dent Assoc.* 2003;134(2):209–214.
4. Youngnak-Piboonratanakit P, Vachirarojpisan T. Prevalence of self-perceived oral malodor in a group of Thai dental patients. *J Dent (Tehran).* 2010;7(4):196–204.
5. Scully C, Felix DH. Oral medicine–update for the dental practitioner: oral malodour. *Br Dent J.* 2005;199(8):498–500.
6. Tangerman A, Winkel EG. Intra- and extra-oral halitosis: finding of a new form of extra-oral blood-borne halitosis caused by dimethyl sulphide. *J Clin Periodontol.* 2007;34(9):748–755.
7. Haraszthy VI, Zambon JJ, Sreenivasan PK, et al. Identification of oral bacterial species associated with halitosis. *J Am Dent Assoc.* 2007;138(8):1113–1120.
8. Armstrong BL, Sensat ML, Stoltenberg JL. Halitosis: a review of current literature. *J Dent Hyg.* 2010;84(2):65–74.
9. van den Broek AM, Feenstra L, de Baat C. A review of the current literature on aetiology and measurement methods of halitosis. *J Dent.* 2007;35(9):627–635.
10. Yaegaki K, Coil JM, Kamemizu T, et al. Tongue brushing and mouth rinsing as basic treatment measures for halitosis. *Int Dent J.* 2002;52(suppl 3):192–196.
11. Klokkevold PR. Oral malodor: a periodontal perspective. *J Calif Dent Assoc.* 1997;25(2):153–159.
12. Tsai CC, Chou HH, Wu TL, et al. The levels of volatile sulfur compounds in mouth air from patients with chronic periodontitis. *J Periodontal Res.* 2008;43(2):186–193.
13. Nonaka A, Tanaka M, Anguri H, et al. Clinical assessment of oral malodor intensity expressed as absolute value using an electronic nose. *Oral Dis.* 2005;11(suppl 1):35–36.
14. Tanaka M, Anguri H, Nonaka A, et al. Clinical assessment of oral malodor by the electronic nose system. *J Dent Res.* 2004;83(4):317–321.
15. Hughes FJ, McNab R. Oral malodour–a review. *Arch Oral Biol.* 2008;53(suppl 1):S1–S7.
16. Allaker RP, Waite RD, Hickling J, et al. Topographic distribution of bacteria associated with oral malodour on the tongue. *Arch Oral Biol.* 2008;53(suppl 1):S8–S12.
17. Outhouse TL, Fedorowicz Z, Keenan JV, et al. A Cochrane systematic review finds tongue scrapers have short-term efficacy in controlling halitosis. *Gen Dent.* 2006;54(5):352–359, 360, 367–368.
18. Pedrazzi V, Sato S, de Mattos Mda G, et al. Tongue-cleaning methods: a comparative clinical trial employing a toothbrush and a tongue scraper. *J Periodontol.* 2004;75(7):1009–1012.
19. Bordas A, McNab R, Staples AM, et al. Impact of different tongue cleaning methods on the bacterial load of the tongue dorsum. *Arch Oral Biol.* 2008;53(suppl 1):S13–S18.
20. Blom T, Slot DE, Quirynen M, et al. The effect of mouthrinses on oral malodor: a systematic review. *Int J Dent Hyg.* 2012;10(3):209–222.
21. Fedorowicz Z, Aljufairi H, Nasser M, et al. Mouthrinses for the treatment of halitosis. *Cochrane Database Syst Rev.* 2008;(4):CD006701.
22. Jonski G, Young A, Waler SM, et al. Insoluble zinc, cupric and tin pyrophosphates inhibit the formation of volatile sulphur compounds. *Eur J Oral Sci.* 2004;112(5):429–432.
23. Thrane PS, Young A, Jonski G, et al. A new mouthrinse combining zinc and chlorhexidine in low concentrations provides superior efficacy against halitosis compared to existing formulations: a double-blind clinical study. *J Clin Dent.* 2007;18(3):82–86.

24. Young A, Jonski G, Rolla G. A study of triclosan and its solubilizers as inhibitors of oral malodour. *J Clin Periodontol.* 2002;29(12):1078–1081.

25. Young A, Jonski G, Rolla G. Inhibition of orally produced volatile sulfur compounds by zinc, chlorhexidine or cetylpyridinium chloride–effect of concentration. *Eur J Oral Sci.* 2003;111(5):400–404.

26. Young A, Jonski G, Rolla G. Combined effect of zinc ions and cationic antibacterial agents on intraoral volatile sulphur compounds (VSC). *Int Dent J.* 2003;53(4):237–242.

27. Young A, Jonski G, Rolla G, et al. Effects of metal salts on the oral production of volatile sulfur-containing compounds (VSC). *J Clin Periodontol.* 2001;28(8):776–781.

28. Lee E, Lee YH, Kim W, et al. Self-reported prevalence and severity of xerostomia and its related conditions in individuals attending hospital for general health examinations. *Int J Oral Maxillofac Surg.* 2014;43(4):498–505.

29. Malicka B, Kaczmarek U, Skoskiewicz-Malinowska K. Prevalence of xerostomia and the salivary flow rate in diabetic patients. *Adv Clin Exp Med.* 2014;23(2):225–233.

30. Minicucci EM, Pires RB, Vieira RA, et al. Assessing the impact of menopause on salivary flow and xerostomia. *Aust Dent J.* 2013;58(2):230–234.

31. van Eijk J, van Campen JP, van der Jagt H, et al. Prevalence of xerostomia and its relationship with underlying diseases, medication, and nutrition: a descriptive observational study. *J Am Geriatr Soc.* 2013;61(10):1836–1837.

32. Villa A, Polimeni A, Strohmenger L, et al. Dental patients' self-reports of xerostomia and associated risk factors. *J Am Dentl Assoc.* 2011;142(7):811–816.

33. Diaz-Arnold AM, Marek CA. The impact of saliva on patient care: a literature review. *J Prosthet Dent.* 2002;88(3):337–343.

34. Turner M, Jahangiri L, Ship JA. Hyposalivation, xerostomia and the complete denture: a systematic review. *J Am Dent Assoc.* 2008;139(2):146–150.

35. Versteeg PA, Slot DE, van der Velden U, et al. Effect of cannabis usage on the oral environment: a review. *Int J Dent Hyg.* 2008;6(4):315–320.

36. Carr AJ, Ng WF, Figueiredo F, et al. Sjogren's syndrome-an update for dental practitioners. *Br Dent J.* 2012;213(7):353–357.

37. Jensen SB, Vissink A. Salivary gland dysfunction and xerostomia in Sjogren's syndrome. *Oral Maxillofac Surg Clin North Am.* 2014;26(1):35–53.

38. Pinto A. Management of xerostomia and other complications of Sjogren's syndrome. *Oral Maxillofac Surg Clin North Am.* 2014;26(1):63–73.

39. Kaluzny J, Wierzbicka M, Nogala H, et al. Radiotherapy induced xerostomia: mechanisms, diagnostics, prevention and treatment–evidence based up to 2013. *Otolaryngol Pol.* 2014;68(1):1–14.

40. Desoutter A, Soudain-Pineau M, Munsch F, et al. Xerostomia and medication: a cross-sectional study in long-term geriatric wards. *J Nutr Health Aging.* 2012;16(6):575–579.

41. Enoki K, Matsuda KI, Ikebe K, et al. Influence of xerostomia on oral health-related quality of life in the elderly: a 5-year longitudinal study. *Oral Surg Oral Med Oral Pathol Oral Radiol.* 2014;117(6):716–721.

42. Liu B, Dion MR, Jurasic MM, et al. Xerostomia and salivary hypofunction in vulnerable elders: prevalence and etiology. *Oral Surg Oral Med Oral Pathol Oral Radiol.* 2012;114(1):52–60.

43. Rayman S, Dincer E, Almas K. Xerostomia: diagnosis and management in dental practice. *Today's FDA.* 2011;23(6):56–61.

44. Singh M, Tonk RS. Xerostomia: etiology, diagnosis, and management. *Dent Today.* 2012;31(10):80, 82–83; quiz 4–5.

45. Lopez-Jornet MP, Garcia-Teresa G, Vinas M, et al. Clinical and antimicrobial evaluation of a mouthwash and toothpaste for xerostomia: a randomized, double-blind, crossover study. *J Dent.* 2011;39(11):757–763.

46. Daniels TE. Evaluation, differential diagnosis, and treatment of xerostomia. *J Rheumatol Suppl.* 2000;61:6–10.

47. Rantanen I, Jutila K, Nicander I, et al. The effects of two sodium lauryl sulphate-containing toothpastes with and without betaine on human oral mucosa in vivo. *Swed Dent J.* 2003;27(1):31–34.

48. Burgess J, Lee P. XyliMelts time-release adhering discs for night-time oral dryness. *Int J Dent Hyg.* 2012;10(2):118–121.

49. Gupta A, Epstein JB, Sroussi H. Hyposalivation in elderly patients. *J Can Dent Assoc.* 2006;72(9):841–846.

50. Rhodus NL, Bereuter J. Clinical evaluation of a commercially available oral moisturizer in relieving signs and symptoms of xerostomia in postirradiation head and neck cancer patients and patients with Sjogren's syndrome. *J Otolaryngol.* 2000;29(1):33–34.

51. Eisenrich T, Sullivan D. Salivary stimulants and saliva substitutes are equally effective in terms of patient-perceived comfort in patients with xerostomia (UT CAT #2188). *Tex Dent J.* 2012;129(6):586.

52. Abbasi F, Farhadi S, Esmaili M. Efficacy of pilocarpine and bromhexine in improving radiotherapy-induced xerostomia. *J Dent Res Dent Clin Dent Prospects.* 2013;7(2):86–90.

53. Kim JH, Ahn HJ, Choi JH, et al. Effect of 0.1% pilocarpine mouthwash on xerostomia: double-blind, randomised controlled trial. *J Oral Rehabil.* 2014;41(3):226–235.

54. Leung KC, McMillan AS, Wong MC, et al. The efficacy of cevimeline hydrochloride in the treatment of xerostomia in Sjogren's syndrome in southern Chinese patients: a randomised double-blind, placebo-controlled crossover study. *Clin Rheumatol.* 2008;27(4):429–436.

55. Takagi Y, Katayama I, Tashiro S, et al. Parotid irrigation and cevimeline gargle for treatment of xerostomia in Sjogren's syndrome. *J Rheumatol.* 2008;35(11):2289–2291.

 STUDENT ANCILLARY RESOURCES

A wide variety of resources to enhance your learning and understanding of this chapter are available on thePoint®.

- Visit thePoint to access:
  - Audio Glossary
  - Animations
  - Suggested Readings
  - Answers to Review Questions
  - Case Studies

CHAPTER

34 Documentation and Insurance Reporting of Periodontal Care

Clinical Application. Dental hygienists are responsible for making multiple entries in patients' records as a routine part of periodontal care. Legal ramifications related to the quality of the documentation in patients' records require hygienists to have a thorough understanding of how to document patient interactions accurately. In addition, this chapter provides guidance in the use of ADA-approved terminology for insurance reporting related to delivery of care for periodontal patients.

Learning Objectives

- Explain the foundations of tort law and how it applies to the profession of dentistry.
- Define the term liability as it applies to provision of periodontal care.
- Describe situations in the dental office that trigger liability for dental hygienists.
- Define the terms intentional torts and negligence and give examples of each.
- In the clinical setting, thoroughly document all periodontal treatment including treatment options, cancellations, patient noncompliance, refusal of treatment, and follow-up telephone calls.
- Define the terms insurance codes and insurance forms and explain their use in periodontal care.

Key Terms

Standard of care
Liability
Malpractice

Tort
Intentional torts
Negligence

Upcoding
Insurance codes
Insurance forms

Section 1
Legal Issues in the Provision and Documentation of Care

It is important for every dental hygienist to practice to the highest established standards of care, not only to insure the safety of the patient receiving treatment but also to avoid costly malpractice litigation (1). Potential liability is a reality for every healthcare provider. While patients can sue a dentist or dental hygienist for many reasons, the success of such a suit often depends on the quality of the chart notes. The dental hygienist has a moral and ethical obligation to deliver high quality care and maintain thorough chart notes for each patient visit to protect the practice against liability.

CONCEPTS OF MALPRACTICE AND TORT LAW

1. **Standard of Care.** The legal definition of standard of care varies in North America, in general terms dental healthcare providers are required to exercise the same degree of skill and care as could reasonably be expected of a prudent dental healthcare provider of the same experience and standing (1,2).
2. **Liability.** In the context of health care, liability is a healthcare provider's obligation or responsibility to provide services to another person (the patient). The healthcare provider's liability entails the possibility of being sued if the person receiving the services feels as if he has been treated improperly or negligently.
3. **Malpractice.** Malpractice is the improper or negligent treatment by a healthcare provider that results in injury or damage to the patient (3,4).
4. **Tort.** The legal basis for most lawsuits in dental and dental hygiene practice is founded on tort law. A tort is a civil wrong where a person has breached a duty to another. A tort is the law that permits an injured person to recover compensation from the person who caused the injury.
5. **Intentional Torts.** Intentional torts are actions designed to injure another person or that person's property. There are many specific types of intentional torts, including the following:
   A. Battery is the unlawful and unwanted touching or striking of one person by another, with the intention of bringing about a harmful or offensive contact. Forceful discipline of unruly children in the dental chair could be construed as battery.
   B. Assault is an unlawful threat or attempt to do bodily injury to another. A doctor who treats a minor patient without proper parental or guardian-informed consent could be charged with assault or battery.
   C. Infliction of emotional distress. An example is talking in a loud or harsh voice to an unruly child.
   D. Fraud is deception carried out for the purpose of achieving personal gain while causing injury to another party.
   E. Misrepresentation occurs when a healthcare provider deliberately deceives a patient about possible outcomes.
   F. Defamation is communication to third parties of false statements about a person that injure the reputation of or deter others from associating with that person. For example, a dental hygienist learns that another hygienist has been making disparaging comments about the quality of care that he provides. The hygienist being disparaged could sue for defamation.
   G. Trespass is to infringe on the privacy, time, or attention of another. An example is discussing a patient's personal information with someone without the patient's permission.

H. Defamation by computer. Email correspondence and other written documents are discoverable in court, so avoid disparaging remarks in email communications.

6. Negligence. **Negligence** is a failure to exercise reasonable care to avoid injuring others. It is the failure to do something that a reasonable person would do under the same circumstances, or the doing of something a reasonable person would not do. Negligence is characterized by carelessness, inattentiveness, and neglectfulness rather than by a positive intent to cause injury (2).

A. Negligence is different from an intentional tort in that negligence **does not require the intent** to commit a wrongful action; instead, the wrongful action itself is sufficient to constitute negligence.

B. Examples of negligence include accidentally spilling a chemical on a patient, not updating the patient's health history resulting in the patient's health being jeopardized, and incorrect treatment of periodontal disease. Professional liability insurance typically covers only unintentional torts or negligence.

7. Upcoding. **Upcoding** refers to reporting a higher level of service than was actually performed. A good example of upcoding would be recording a prophylaxis as periodontal instrumentation. The purpose of upcoding is to charge a higher fee. The fee for a quadrant of periodontal instrumentation is about three times the fee for a prophylaxis. Upcoding is unethical and dishonest. Dental boards have been known to levy serious disciplinary measures, including revocation of license, for clinicians that have been found guilty of upcoding.

AREAS OF POTENTIAL LIABILITY

In judging whether a professional has been negligent, the courts use a standard called the "*reasonable prudent person or professional.*" This means the court compares what a reasonably prudent person or professional would have done in a similar situation. For example, the standard of care for periodontal charting is that every adult patient will have a six-point periodontal charting with all numbers recorded at least once per year. Failure to include a service because the dental hygienist is unaware of the current standard of care will not hold up in court. The top ten areas of potential liability for dental hygienists are summarized below in Box 34-1.

Box 34-1. Top Ten Areas of Potential Liability for Dental Hygienists

1. Failure to ask and document whether the patient has taken his or her premedication.
2. Failure to detect and document oral cancer.
3. Failure to update the patient's medical history.
4. Failure to detect and thoroughly document the presence of periodontal disease.
5. Injuring a patient.
6. Failure to document treatment thoroughly in the patient chart or computerized record.
7. Failure to protect patient privacy or divulging confidential patient information.
8. Failure to inform the patient about treatment options and the consequences of nontreatment.
9. Practicing outside the legal scope of practice. All dental hygienists should be well informed about the state practice act and follow the rules and regulations explicitly.
10. Failure to provide care that meets the established standards of care.

Section 2
Documentation of Periodontal Care

The dental chart is a legal document. It is the first line of defense in a malpractice suit. *When a patient decides to file a lawsuit, the dental chart becomes the single most important piece of information relative to the suit. Faulty records can be the most important reason for the loss of a lawsuit* (5). All periodontal assessment, educational, and treatment services should be documented in the patient chart or computerized record. Recommendations for thorough documentation are summarized in Table 34-1 and Box 34-2.

PRINCIPLES FOR THOROUGH DOCUMENTATION

TABLE 34-1. DOCUMENTATION GUIDELINES	
Action	**Why It Is Recommended**
Format: • Write on the proper form or computer document. • Write or print legibly in blue or black ink. • Use correct grammar, spelling, and standard dental terminology. • Date each entry correctly.	• It is important to write or print legibly to avoid miscommunication. (Some lawyers infer sloppy care from sloppy entries or charting.) • The date that actions occurred or observations were made is an important element of the dental record, which is a legal account of care provided.

Content:
 • Only record care that you have given or observations that you have made. Do not make entries for another care provider.
 • Enter information in a complete, accurate, concise, and factual manner.
 • Entries may include the following:
   • Reason for today's appointment
   • Through documentation of medical and dental history
   • Patient's chief complaint
   • Symptoms reported by the patient
   • Findings from the clinical periodontal assessment
   • Treatment options and recommendations
   • Patient treatment choices
   • All assessment, educational, and treatment services
   • Items given to patient, such as educational materials or home care aids
   • Date or interval of next appointment
 • Remember that in a liability situation, care or recommendations not recorded were not provided.
	• By making an entry in a dental record, you accept legal responsibility for that entry.
	 • Use only commonly accepted dental terminology and standard abbreviations and symbols. Do not create your own abbreviations. Using correct terminology and abbreviations will prevent others from having to second-guess your meaning.
	 • Proper and conscientious recording protects the patient, your employer, and you.

(continued)

TABLE 34-1. DOCUMENTATION GUIDELINES *(Continued)*	
Action	**Why It Is Recommended**

Accountability:

- Check the patient's name on the dental record and on the form where you are recording.
- Always sign your first initial, last name, and title to each entry.
- All entries should be written on the lines. No entries should be made in the margins or below the last line on the page. No lines should be skipped.
- Do not use dittos, erasures, or correcting fluids. A single line should be drawn through an incorrect entry and words "mistaken entry" or "error in charting" should be printed above or beside the entry and signed. The entry should then be rewritten correctly.
- Identify each page of the record with the patient's name and chart identification number.
- Recognize that a patient record (chart) is permanent.

- By verifying the patient's identification information, you ensure that you are recording the person's information on the correct record.
- By signing your entry, you indicate that you are the person who needs to be consulted if further clarification of the information is needed. In addition, signing your entry indicates that you accept legal responsibility for what you have written.
- All lines should be used, so that there is no opportunity for anyone to add information after a lawsuit is initiated. Making entries in the margins or below the last line on a page can cause juries to wonder if the entry was made at a later date.
- Striking through an error is the only legal way to indicate a change in the dental record. Erasing or using correction fluid could be seen as an attempt to hide or change existing information.

Timing:

- Record information in a timely manner.
- Document care as closely as possible to the time of providing treatment.
- Do not record care as given before you have provided the care.

- If you wait until the end of the day to record, you may forget important information.
- Something may occur that prevents you from providing the anticipated care (the patient may become ill halfway through the appointment; the patient may refuse a fluoride treatment). If you record care as "provided" in the dental record but then do not actually complete this care, you will have committed fraud.

Confidentiality:

- Clinicians using patient records are bound professionally and ethically to keep in strict confidence all information they learn by reading patient records.

- Individuals have a moral and legal right to expect that the information contained in their patient dental record will be kept private.

Box 34-2. Determining How Much to Write—*The Amnesia Test*

Imagine that you have amnesia and cannot remember any of the treatment that you have performed for any of your patients since you started to work in a periodontal practice 5 years ago! Would you be able to read any one of your patient charts and be able to:

- *Know every assessment, educational, and treatment procedures that the patient has undergone and why this treatment was necessary?*
- *Know what additional treatment has been recommended and accepted by the patient and know why this treatment is recommended?*

Two criteria should dictate how much to write

1. Write sufficient information that would allow you or any other clinician to determine exactly which assessment, educational, and treatment procedures were performed at each appointment; why that treatment was necessary; and what treatment is next—based solely on your documentation.
2. Write sufficient information that meets all the record-keeping requirements of your state board.

---

1. **Recommendations for Thorough Documentation.** Jeffery J. Tonner, J.D. recommends several principles that every dental professional should follow when documenting periodontal treatment in the patient chart or computerized record (6).
   A. **General Guidelines for Chart Entries**
      1. All entries should be complete and accurate using accepted dental terminology and abbreviations. Chart Entry 34-1 is an example of a complete chart entry.
      2. It is helpful to organize the services documented in sequential order so that no information is omitted.
      3. If handwritten, entries should be legible and in *permanent* ink.
      4. The healthcare provider making the entry should sign the entry with his or her first initial, last name, and title. Since many different people write in the patient chart, it is important that each entry be signed. If there are multiple dentists in the practice, the dentist that examines the hygienist's patient should be identified also.
      5. Thorough chart entries provide valuable information for the next clinician that treats this patient.
      6. The patient should be thoroughly interviewed regarding his or her medical status at each visit. Patients do not usually volunteer information when they are taking a new medicine or if there has been a change in their medical history. The medical status should be thoroughly documented at each visit.
   B. **Treatment Options.** The healthcare provider should document all treatment options presented to the patient.
   C. **Appointment Schedule and Chart Entries**
      1. Chart entries should be consistent with the appointment schedule.
         a. With most dental software and computer scheduling, the patient's name must be on the schedule in order to make a chart entry.
         b. With manual appointment books, however, entries can be erased and changed.

2. In the event of a lawsuit, doubt may be cast on the reliability of the office's records if the treatment dates in the chart do not match the appointment book entries.

3. If the patient is being seen as an emergency patient this circumstance should be recorded in the chart.

D. **Cancellations and Missed Appointments.** All cancellations and missed appointments should be written in the patient chart. Infrequent periodontal maintenance appointments can lead to a recurrence and progression of periodontal disease. Chart Entries 34-2 and 34-3 provide examples of how to document missed and cancelled appointments.

E. **Patient Noncompliance and Refusal of Treatment**

1. Patient noncompliance with recommendations, such as (1) inadequate self-care, (2) continued smoking, (3) failure to regulate diabetes, or (4) failure to follow specific instructions, can lead to disease progression. Noncompliance should be noted in the chart (Chart Entry 34-4).

2. Instances when a patient opts not to have recommended treatment or declines a referral to a specialist should be documented. In such situations, it is recommended that patients sign a "Refusal of Treatment Recommendation" document. An example of a refusal of treatment form is shown in Figure 34-1. Further, when a patient is referred to a specialist, it is recommended that a copy of the referral letter be kept in the patient chart. Chart Entry 34-5 provides an example of documentation of inadequate self-care.

F. **Follow-up Telephone Calls.** Patients appreciate a follow-up telephone call from the dentist or hygienist following a long or difficult treatment procedure. For hygienists, a good rule of thumb is to call any patient who required anesthesia for periodontal instrumentation. Follow-up telephone calls should be documented (Chart Entry 34-6).

Date	Treatment Rendered
1/10/10	Reason for visit: 3-month periodontal maintenance. Medical history update: pat. now taking one aspirin a day per his physician's recommendation. Chief complaint: none. Oral cancer exam: normal. Periodontal probing: changes noted in charting. Plaque: light, calculus: light, bleeding areas noted on periodontal chart. Perio maintenance: perio instrumentation of all four quads; ultrasonic and hand instrumentation. Plaque removal by patient using toothbrush and interdental brush. Patient tolerated all procedures well. Patient education: reviewed use of tufted dental floss around distal surfaces of maxillary and mandibular molars. Tray fluoride application 1.23% APF gel for sensitivity. Four bitewing radiographs. Next maintenance visit in 3 months. *R. Zimmer, RDH*

Chart Entry 34-1. Complete Chart Entry. This chart entry is an example of a thorough chart entry that documents all the events of the patient's appointment.

Date	Treatment Rendered
1/10/10	Patient missed maintenance appointment because of illness. *R. Zimmer, RDH*

Chart Entry 34-2. Missed Appointment. This chart entry is an example of documentation of a missed appointment due to illness.

Date	Treatment Rendered
1/10/10	Telephoned patient to confirm her 3-month maintenance appt. Patient cancelled and said that she would call to reschedule later. I reminded her of the importance of regular maintenance. *R. Zimmer, RDH*

Chart Entry 34-3.   Cancelled Maintenance Appointment. This chart entry provides an example of the documentation for a cancelled periodontal maintenance appointment.

Date	Treatment Rendered
1/10/10	Discussed options for smoking cessation. Patient stated that "he is not interested in quitting smoking." *R. Zimmer, RDH*

Chart Entry 34-4.   Patient Noncompliance. This chart entry provides an example of the documentation for patient noncompliance with recommendations.

Date	Treatment Rendered
1/10/10	Patient reports brushing twice daily but "does not have time to use an interdental brush." Showed patient signs of periodontal inflammation in the interdental areas. Explained benefits of interdental plaque removal and several alternatives for interdental self-care. Patient decided that he was not interested and stated that "he only wants to brush." *R. Zimmer, RDH*

Chart Entry 34-5.   Inadequate Self-Care. This chart entry is an example of documentation of inadequate self-care by a patient.

Date	Treatment Rendered
1/10/10	Telephoned patient at home this evening to check on her. Patient reports that she "has no bleeding and rates her pain as a 2, on a scale of 1 to 10." Reminded her to use warm saltwater rinse before bedtime. *R. Zimmer, RDH*

Chart Entry 34-6.   Follow-up Telephone Call. This chart entry is an example of documentation of a follow-up telephone call after a long or difficult treatment procedure.

Date	Treatment Rendered
1/10/10	Px, Ex

Chart Entry 34-7.   Incomplete Chart Entry. Although this hygienist may have been quite thorough in delivering care, the chart does not reflect that.

Date	Treatment Rendered
1/10/10	Patient reports that his "gums no longer bleed during brushing." Tissue color, tone, and texture are much improved from 3 weeks ago. *R. Zimmer, RDH*

Chart Entry 34-8.   Patient Comments. This chart entry is an example of how to include a patient's comments at a periodontal maintenance visit.

Refusal of Treatment Recommendation

Patient Name _____ Date of Birth _____
  Last   First   M.I.

I am being provided with this information and refusal form so I may better understand the treatment recommended for me and the consequences of my refusal of the recommended treatment. I understand that I may ask any questions I wish regarding the recommended treatment.

It has been recommended that I have the following treatment: _____
_____

This recommendation is based on visual examination, on any X-rays, models, photos and other diagnostic tests taken, and on my doctor's knowledge of my medical and dental history. The treatment is necessary because of:

☐ Decay   ☐ Broken tooth/teeth   ☐ Infection   ☐ Periodontal disease   ☐ Pain   ☐ Other

Note: _____
_____

_____ I have had an opportunity to ask questions about the recommended treatment.
Patient's Initials

I understand that complications to my teeth, mouth, and/or general health may occur if I do not proceed with the recommended treatment. These complications include: _____
_____

Acknowledgment

Note: _____ , have received information about the proposed treatment. I have discussed my treatment with Dr. _____ and have been given an opportunity to ask questions and have them fully answered. I understand the nature of the recommended treatment and the risks of my refusal of the recommended treatment.

I personally assume the risks and consequences of my refusal. I have read this document in its entirety.

I do NOT wish to proceed with the recommended treatment.

Signed: _____ Date: _____
                    Patient or Guardian

Signed: _____ Date: _____
                    Treating Dentist

Signed: _____ Date: _____
                    Witness

Figure 34-1. Refusal of Treatment Form. Shown above is one example of a Refusal of Recommended Treatment form.

PITFALLS IN DOCUMENTATION

1. **Common Problems in Documentation.** Jeffery J. Tonner, J.D. outlines four common pitfalls in documentation (6).
   A. **Making Entries in Haste.** Chart Entry 34-7 is an example of an *inadequate* chart entry. For example, in her haste to stay on schedule, the dental hygienist simply forgets to record that she did a periodontal charting and evaluation. Later, if the patient develops periodontal disease, he may accuse the doctor of failure to diagnose. The dentist or hygienist may state to a jury that a periodontal evaluation is done on every patient. *In the eyes of a jury, however, if a procedure is not written in the chart, it was not done.*
   B. **Skipping Lines Between Entries or Writing in Margins**
      1. Keeping in the lines or skipping lines.
         a. Chart entries should be written with small enough strokes to be contained within the space provided.
         b. No lines should be skipped on a treatment record form. All lines should be used, so that there is no opportunity for anyone to add information *after* a lawsuit is initiated.
      2. Writing in margins or below the last line. All entries should be written on the lines, and no entries should be written in the margins or below the last line on the page. Doing so can cause juries to wonder if the entry was made at a later date.
   C. **Altering Chart Entries.** *The single most common cause of punitive damages in a dental malpractice suit is altering the chart.*
      1. Correction fluid should never be used to correct an entry. If an error is made, a single line should be drawn through the incorrect entry, so that it can still be read, the words *charting error or mistaken entry* written above it, and the correct entry made on the next available line. The revised entry should be signed.
      2. Additional information should never be added to an entry from a previous appointment. Juries perceive such added entries to be fraudulent and deceptive.
      3. Forensic ink dating analysis allows an expert to determine the date that ink was used on a particular document. Therefore, it is foolhardy to add things at a later date to a patient chart in an attempt to avoid or win a lawsuit.
   D. **Not Clearly Indicating Patient Comments.** Quotation marks should be used to indicate patient comments. This is especially important when making follow-up telephone calls after a difficult or invasive procedure. A sample chart entry is shown in Chart Entry 34-8.

Section 3
Computer-Based Patient Records

The development, implementation, and evaluation of computer-based dental records present both challenges and opportunities for the periodontal dental office (7,8).

ADVANTAGES OF COMPUTERIZED PATIENT RECORDS

1. Organization and Data Gathering
   A. *Standardization of* clinical *data* where all staff members use the same templates for gathering data and the same abbreviations.
   B. *Greater legibility.* Handwriting can often be illegible, which increases liability risk for the clinician.
   C. *Easier and faster access to information.* Information is only a few keystrokes away.
   D. *Enhanced use of clinical images and radiographs.*
   E. *Provision of new ways to analyze clinical information.* For example, digital radiography allows the clinician to view radiographs with digital tools designed to enhance the image and visualize bone levels around teeth.
   F. *Potential for greater security of patient data.* Paper records are vulnerable to fire, earthquake, and water damage from flooding. Computer-based patient records can be backed up offsite to preserve data. Note that computerized data is more secure only if it is continuously backed up to an offsite location separate from the dental office.
2. Processing of Information
   A. *Patient information is accessible across the network simultaneously.* For example, business assistants can read input from clinicians and be ready for patient checkout before the patient reaches the business office.
   B. *Facilitates submission of insurance claims.* Computerized information facilitates submission of dental insurance claim forms to insurance companies.
3. Communication
   A. *Faster and better multidisciplinary interaction with specialists.* Successful treatment of periodontitis requires a team approach involving the primary care (general) dental team, the periodontal dental team, and often, other dental specialists or physicians.
   B. Continuous communication among healthcare providers is critical to the success of diagnosis, treatment, and maintenance. Ongoing communication is needed because it is common for the patient to be treated in phases, going back and forth between the primary care dental practice and the periodontal practice. A computer-based patient record can greatly increase the effectiveness of communication among dental healthcare providers.

CAUTIONS REGARDING COMPUTERIZED RECORDS

Even with advancing technologies, practitioners and staff must realize that the transition to computer-based patient records is not seamless, totally safe, or problem free.
1. **Data Backup.** Anyone who has ever used a computer recognizes that computers crash, freeze-up, and frequently lose data. Computer-based patient records can be backed up offsite to preserve data. Data should be continuously backed up to a secure offsite location.
2. **State Regulations.** In some states, computerized records may not eliminate the need to keep paper records due to legal requirements in those states. In such cases, the dental office may need to maintain patient data on paper and in computerized versions.

Section 4
Insurance Codes for Periodontal Treatment

This section highlights the importance of understanding various numeric and alphanumeric codes for accurately billing dental-related services to private pay or third-party insurance carriers.

INSURANCE CODING OVERVIEW

In the United States, dental healthcare providers most commonly use **Common Dental Terminology (CDT) codes** to submit insurance claims (9). **Insurance codes** are numeric codes used by insurance companies and the government to classify different dental procedures (10). For example, periodontal maintenance procedures are designated by the insurance code D4910. The most important use of codes is for insurance billing purposes. Insurance codes are entered on **insurance forms**. Dental treatment is listed under the appropriate procedure number. These codes are very specific and should be reviewed carefully before specific dental treatment is coded (10). Claim submissions for care provided can be completed electronically or by means of paper forms. An example of a completed dental insurance claim form is shown in Figure 34-2.

DENTAL CLAIM FORM

Check One:
☐ Dentist's pre-treatment estimate
☐ Dentist's statement of actual services

If the cost of treatment is expected to exceed $300, a pre-treatment estimate should be completed. The physician or dentist must indicate: A list of every recommended dental procedure; and the charge for each procedure and provide supporting pre-treatment radiographs.

1. Patient name & address: Mr. Boyd Bogus, 22 S. Green St. Ardendale, NC 28759
2. Relationship to employee: ☒ Self ☐ Spouse ☐ Child
3. Sex: (M) / F
4. Patient birthdate: 05 / 14 / 50
5. Is dependent a full time Student? __ Yes __ No
6. Employee's name (Last, First, Middle Initial): UUP Benefit Trust Fund
7. Employee's SSN: 001-00-1-1000
7. Group number/Name: 3214192
9. Employee's mailing address: 22 S. Green Street
10. City, State, Zip: Ardendale, NC 28759
11. Other family members employed? If yes, member's name: Brenda Bogus — SSN#: 002-02-0000 — Spouse Birthdate: 09 / 05 / 53
12. Name and address of employer: 22 S. Green Street Ardendale, NC 28759
11. Is patient covered by another dental plan? __ Yes X No — Dental plan name — Group number
14. Name and address of employer

I have reviewed the following treatment plan, I authorize release of any information relating to this claim.
Signed (patient or parent if minor) ______ Date ______

I authorize direct **payment** of benefits to the dentist or supplier.
Signed (employee) ______ Date ______

14. Dentist's name: Harry M. Montigue
15. Dentist's address: 1212 Upward Avenue, Ardendale, NC 28759
16. Dentist's SSN or TIN
17. License#
18. Phone#
19. First visit date Current series
20. Place of treatment: ☐ Office ☐ Hospital ☐ ECF ☐ Other ______
21. Radiographs or models enclosed? __ Yes __ No How many? ____
22. Is treatment result of Occupational illness or injury? __ Yes X No — If **yes**, give brief description and dates
23. Is treatment result of Auto Accident? __ Yes X No — Other accident? __ Yes __ No
24. If **yes**, give brief description and dates
25. If Prosthesis, is this initial placement? __ Yes X No — If **no**, reason for placement
28. Date of placement
27. Is treatment for Orthodontics? __ Yes X No
28. If services already commenced: Date appliances applied: ______ Months of treatment remaining: ______

19. Identify missing teeth with "X"

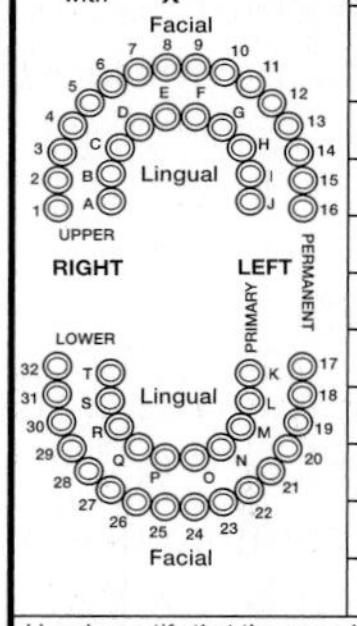

30. EXAMINATION & TREATMENT PLAN. LIST IN ORDER FROM TOOTH NO. 1 THROUGH TOOTH NO. 32 USE CHARTING SYSTEM SHOWN

TOOTH No. or Letter	SURFACE	DESCRIPTION OF SERVICE (Including X-rays, prophylaxis, materials used, etc.)	Date service performed Mo. Day Year	Procedure Code	FEE
		Complete intraoral radiographic series	3 / 28 / 10	D0210	
		Periodontal maintenance	3 / 28 / 10	D4910	
31	D	Localized delivery antimicrobial agent	3 / 28 / 10	D4381	
		Tropical fluoride treatment	3 / 28 / 10	D1204	
		Oral hygiene instructions	3 / 28 / 10	D1330	
			/ /		
			/ /		
			/ /		
			/ /		

I hereby certify that the procedures as indicated by Date ☐ Will be ☐ Have been completed
Signed ______ Date ______
REMARKS:

TOTAL FEE CHARGED	
MAXIMUM ALLOWABLE	
DEDUCTIBLE	
PLAN %	
PLAN PAYS	
PATIENT PAYS	

Figure 34-2. Insurance Claim Form. An example of a completed dental insurance claim form.

INSURANCE CODES FOR NONSURGICAL PERIODONTAL SERVICES

1. Evolution of Dental Terminology
   A. Members of the dental team should be aware that there is a continuous evolution of terminology used in dentistry and medicine.
      1. Changes in terminology occur as a natural result of scientific advances and improved understanding of disease pathogenesis.
      2. Terminology related to nonsurgical periodontal therapy is currently undergoing one such change.
   B. Traditionally in the dental literature, two terms have been used to describe the therapies employed to remove deposits from tooth surfaces. These terms are (1) *dental prophylaxis* and (2) *scaling and root planing.*
   C. Recently in the dental hygiene literature, increasing numbers of authors are using new terminology to describe periodontal instrumentation.
      1. The term "*periodontal instrumentation*" or "*periodontal debridement*" is suggested to replace the older terms dental prophylaxis and scaling and root planing.
      2. *In dental hygiene literature, periodontal instrumentation is defined as the removal or disruption of plaque biofilm, its by-products, and biofilm-retentive calculus deposits from coronal surfaces, root surfaces, and within the pocket space, as indicated, for periodontal healing and repair.*

2. Codes for Insurance Reporting. The ADA Current Dental Terminology continues to use the terms "prophylaxis" and "scaling and root planing" to describe periodontal instrumentation. *Dental team members will have to use the currently accepted insurance codes when filling out insurance forms and in communications with insurance companies or other third-party payers.*
   A. Examination Codes
      1. D0120—Periodic Oral Evaluation. An evaluation performed on a patient of record to determine any changes in the patient's dental and medical health status since a previous comprehensive or periodic evaluation. This includes periodontal screening and may require interpretation of information acquired through additional diagnostic procedures.
      2. D0180—Comprehensive Periodontal Evaluation—New or Established Patient. This code is used for patients showing signs or symptoms of periodontal disease and for patients with risk factors such as smoking or diabetes. This examination code may be used when the hygienist performs a comprehensive periodontal evaluation including full-mouth, six-point probing and recording, charting of recession, furcations, tooth mobility, or tissue abnormalities once per year.
   B. Currently Accepted Insurance Codes Pertaining to Periodontal Instrumentation
      1. D1110—Adult Prophylaxis (four quadrants). Removal of plaque, calculus, and stains from the tooth structures in the permanent and transitional dentition. It is intended to control local irritating factors. **This code usually is used for healthy patients and patients with gingivitis.** Scaling on this type of patient usually can be completed in a single appointment. This code may also be used to describe and report the cleaning of complete dentures in edentulous patients.
      2. D4341—Periodontal Scaling and Root Planing—Four or More Teeth Per Quadrant. This procedure involves instrumentation of the crown and root surfaces to remove plaque and calculus from these surfaces. *It is indicated for patients with periodontal disease and is therapeutic, not preventive in*

nature. This procedure may be used as a definitive treatment in some stages of periodontal disease and/or as a part of presurgical procedures in others.

3. D4342—Periodontal Scaling and Root Planing—One to Three Teeth Per Quadrant. This code is essentially the same as the D4341 code, the difference being the number of teeth present in a quadrant.

4. D4910—Periodontal Maintenance. *This procedure is instituted following periodontal therapy and continues at varying intervals for the life of the dentition or implant replacements.* It includes the removal of the bacterial plaque and calculus from supragingival and subgingival regions, site-specific scaling and root planing where indicated, and polishing of the teeth.

5. D4381—Localized Delivery of Antimicrobial Agents via a Controlled Release Vehicle. Synthetic fibers or other approved delivery devices containing controlled-release chemotherapeutic agents are inserted into a periodontal pocket.

6. D4355—Full-Mouth Debridement to Enable Comprehensive Evaluation and Diagnosis. **This code should not be confused with the term "periodontal debridement" as used in dental hygiene literature.** Full-mouth debridement is the gross removal of plaque and calculus that interfere with the ability of the dentist to perform a comprehensive oral evaluation. Full-mouth debridement refers to an *incomplete* removal of heavy calculus deposits only. This is a preliminary procedure and will necessitate the need for additional periodontal instrumentation.

7. D4921—Gingival Irrigation: Per Quadrant. Irrigation of gingival pockets with medicinal agent. Not to be used to report use of mouth rinses or noninvasive chemical debridement.

8. D5994—Periodontal Medicament Carrier with Peripheral Seal: Laboratory Processed. A custom fabricated laboratory-processed carrier that covers the teeth and alveolar mucosa. Used as a vehicle to deliver prescribed medicaments for sustained contact with the gingiva, alveolar mucosa, and into the periodontal sulcus or pocket.

C. **Codes for Radiographs.** The most common dental radiographs are
1. D0210—a complete intraoral radiographic series including bitewings.
2. D0220—an intraoral periapical (first film).
3. D0230—an intraoral periapical film (each additional film).
4. D0240—an intraoral occlusal film.
5. D0250—an extraoral first film, such as a cephalometric film.
6. D0260—an extraoral film (each additional film).
7. D0270—a single bitewing film.
8. D0272—two bitewing films.
9. D0274—four bitewing films.
10. D0330—a panoramic film.
11. D0277—vertical bitewings (7 to 8 films).
12. D0350—oral/facial images. The oral/facial image code includes traditional photographs or digital images obtained by intraoral cameras.

D. **Codes for Topical Fluoride**
1. D1206—topical application of fluoride varnish.
2. D1208—topical application of fluoride. This code is used to report prescription strength fluoride swishes, trays, isolates, or paint on fluorides, but not varnishes.

E. Codes for Patient Counseling
   1. D1310—nutritional counseling for control of dental disease. Counseling on food selection and dietary habits as a part of treatment and control of periodontal disease and caries.
   2. D1320—tobacco cessation counseling for control and prevention of oral disease.
   3. D1330—oral hygiene (self-care) instructions. Examples include toothbrushing technique, flossing, and the use of special oral hygiene aids.

Chapter Summary Statement

In judging whether a professional has been negligent, the courts use a standard called the *reasonable prudent person or professional*. Thus, providing and documenting periodontal care that meets or exceeds the standard of care is extremely important for dental health professionals.

The dental chart is a legal document. All periodontal assessment, educational, and treatment services should be documented in the patient chart or computerized record. When a patient decides to file a lawsuit, the dental chart becomes the single most important piece of information relative to the suit.

Insurance coding was developed to speed and simplify the reporting of dental treatments to third parties such as insurance companies and the government. These codes are very specific and should be reviewed carefully before specific dental treatment is coded.

Section 5
Focus on Patients

Clinical Patient Care

CASE 1

During a social gathering one evening, a dental hygienist tells her friend about an HIV-positive patient she had treated that day. As the news traveled down the grapevine and the patient learned that the hygienist had revealed his HIV status, he sued her. What specific charge could he bring against the hygienist? Would she be covered under the dentist/employer's malpractice coverage or her own personal malpractice coverage?

CASE 2

The dental hygienist performed an oral cancer screening on every patient, but she never wrote it in her progress notes. When a patient found out he had oral cancer, he sued his dentist and the dental hygienist. The patient had been seen for a prophylaxis and restorative care 6 months before his diagnosis of oral cancer, and the basis for his suit was that he felt the hygienist and dentist had been negligent in failing to detect the lesion. Why is it likely that the patient will win his suit against the dental practice?

CASE 3

During the informed consent process, the patient is informed of (1) his diagnosis; (2) purpose, description, benefits, and risks of the proposed treatment; (3) alternative treatment options; (4) prognosis of no treatment; and (5) costs. The patient asks questions and demonstrates that he understands all information presented during the discussion. Then the patient refuses any treatment. What, if anything, should the dental hygienist do?

Ethical Dilemma

Winnie RDH, has been working as a dental hygienist for Dr. Mooney for the last year. It is her first job after graduation. She is very happy with her working arrangements, enjoys her coworkers and patients, and has been given increased office responsibilities, as well as a pay increase.

Winnie RDH has been instructed to review all the patients' chart entries—for all the clinicians in the office—at the end of each business day for accuracy and make corrections as needed. Dr. Mooney has authorized Winnie RDH, to write and sign all of his patient notes, to maximize his time with patient treatments.

Dr. Mooney has also instructed each of the four other hygienists in his employ, as well as Winnie RDH, to bill each cleaning as "quadrant periodontal instrumentation" as opposed to a prophylaxis, so every patient will receive the ultimate dental hygiene experience. He also requires that all patients receive localized delivery of antimicrobial agents, and that the respective hygienists enter the proper insurance code for that service.

Dr. Mooney sent Winnie RDH, to a practice management seminar, to help improve the management of the office. At the course, Winnie RDH learned that many of the above office practices were unethical. Winnie RDH wants to continue working for Dr. Mooney but is concerned about her liability.

1. Discuss Winnie's potential liability with Dr. Mooney's current office practices and documentation of the care provided by the hygienists in the office?
2. Are there ethical principles in conflict in this dilemma?

References

1. Graskemper JP. *Professional Responsibility in Dentistry: A Practical Guide to Law and Ethics*. Chichester, West Sussex: Wiley-Blackwell; 2011:205.
2. Lai B, Lebuis A, Emami E, et al. New technologies in health care. Part 2: a legal and professional dilemma. *J Can Dent Assoc*. 2008;74(7):637–640.
3. Morse D. Dealing with dental malpractice, Part 2. Malpractice prevention. *Dent Today*. 2004;23(3):116–121.
4. Morse DR. Dealing with dental malpractice, Part 1. *Dent Today*. 2004;23(2):140–143.
5. Hapcook CP Sr. Dental malpractice claims: percentages and procedures. *J Am Dent Assoc*. 2006;137(10):1444–1445.
6. Tonner JJ. *Malpractice: What They Don't Teach You in Dental School*. Tulsa, OK: PennWell; 1996:218.
7. Schleyer T, Spallek H. Dental informatics. A cornerstone of dental practice. *J Am Dent Assoc*. 2001;132(5):605–613.
8. Schleyer TK, Thyvalikakath TP, Spallek H, et al. From information technology to informatics: the information revolution in dental education. *J Dent Educ*. 2012;76(1):142–153.
9. American Dental Association. *CDT 2014: Dental Procedure Codes*. 1st ed. Chicago, IL: American Dental Association; 2013:180.
10. Napier RH, Bruelheide LS, Demann ET, et al. Insurance billing and coding. *Dent Clin North Am*. 2008;52(3):507–527.

Suggested Readings

American Dental Association. *Dental Coding Made Simple: Resource Guide and Training Manual.* 1st ed. Chicago, IL: American Dental Association; 2013:300.

Gelbier S. 125 years of developments in dentistry, 1880–2005. Part 2: Law and the dental profession. *Br Dent J.* 2005;199(7):470–473.

Lopez-Nicolas M, Falcon M, Perez-Carceles MD, et al. Informed consent in dental malpractice claims. A retrospective study. *Int Dent J.* 2007;57(3):168–172.

Morse D. Dealing with dental malpractice, Part 2. Malpractice prevention. *Dent Today.* 2004;23(3):116–121.

Zinman E. Dental and legal considerations in periodontal therapy. *J West Soc Periodontol Periodontal Abstr.* 2006;54(1):3–12.

 STUDENT ANCILLARY RESOURCES

A wide variety of resources to enhance your learning and understanding of this chapter are available on thePoint®.

- Visit thePoint to access:
  - Audio Glossary
  - Animations
  - Suggested Readings
  - Answers to Review Questions
  - Case Studies

CHAPTER

35 Future Directions for Management of Periodontal Patients

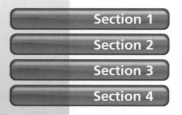
Clinical Application.
All dental healthcare providers should be excited about what the future holds for the management of patients with periodontal diseases. There are not many absolutes in periodontics, but there is undoubtedly one—the simple fact that strategies for the management of patients with periodontal diseases will continue to evolve and change over time. Dental hygienists must be prepared for changes in recommendations for the management of patients with periodontal diseases as research into these diseases continues. This chapter outlines a few ideas related to these directions for research.

Learning Objective

- Describe some strategies in the management of patients with periodontal diseases that are likely to evolve in the future.

Section 1
Diagnostic Technology for Periodontal Diseases

1. Probing Depths and Attachment Levels
   A. The diagnosis and monitoring of patients with periodontal diseases has been based on traditional clinical assessment methods for many years; one of these traditional clinical assessments is the use of manual periodontal probes to measure both probing depths and attachment levels.
   B. An experienced clinician can record probing depths fairly rapidly, and in many patients probing depths provide a reasonable assessment of periodontal health.
   C. On the other hand, attachment levels provide a more accurate assessment of the precise condition of the periodontium, but attachment levels are difficult to measure and record using manual periodontal probes.
   D. Computer-linked, controlled-force, electronic periodontal probes are already available to clinicians (1–3).
      1. These computer-linked probes can make it possible to measure both probing depths and attachment levels quickly, as well as provide automatic data entry features.
      2. This technology of computer-linked periodontal probes will continue to improve. As this technology improves, the use of these computer-linked probes in dental offices will undoubtedly become universal, making it much easier for clinicians to measure and record attachment levels while caring for patients with periodontal diseases.
2. Digital Radiographs
   A. Another traditional clinical periodontal assessment has been the evaluation of radiographic images, and advances in diagnostic technology also include advances in radiograph techniques (4–7).
   B. Digital (filmless) radiographic techniques have been developed to the stage where they are being used by most clinicians.
      1. Digital radiographic techniques allow members of the dental team to collect radiographic information using special sensors instead of printing the radiographic information on a film.
      2. These digital images are then stored on a computer and can be viewed on a computer screen or even printed when needed.
      3. Modern technology for viewing these images on computer screens has substantial advantages over the traditional use of radiographic film.
      4. Software for viewing these digitized images can eliminate distortion that is seen with traditional film, can allow for easy magnification of details, and can provide precise, anatomically correct measurements.
      5. The same software can also allow for enhancing aspects of a digitized image, providing members of the dental team with more details of the actual status of a tooth or of the periodontium.
      6. In addition, these digital images can be shared with other healthcare providers quite readily—as might be indicated during a patient referral or during consultation with a specialist.
3. Computed Tomographic Techniques
   A. Another interesting area of technology related to radiographic techniques is the use of computed tomographic techniques. Computed tomographic techniques provide clinicians with the ability to study minute details and precise dimensions of the jaws in a three-dimensional mode on a computer screen.
   B. These details can be so precise that they can include a three-dimensional radiographic image of a thin slice made through the jaws at any specific location.

C. Computed tomographic techniques are currently in use by many clinicians when planning for the placement of dental implants.

D. As these computed tomographic techniques become more accessible to the general dentist, treatment planning for many conditions, including periodontal diseases, will improve.

Section 2
Periodontal Disease/Systemic Disease Connections

Dental and medical researchers have been studying the connection between periodontitis and certain systemic diseases for some time. Research into this critical topic is ongoing and continues to offer insights into these connections (8–16). Review of the dental literature will reveal many studies about how systemic conditions may be linked to periodontal diseases, but all of these areas will require further scientific study.

1. **Systemic Diseases With a Link to Periodontal Disease**
   A. Some examples of systemic diseases or conditions that may have a connection to periodontitis are listed in Box 35-1.
   B. Discussion of these systemic conditions has been included in other chapters of this book, but it is of interest to review some of the relationships between one specific condition—diabetes mellitus—and periodontal disease.

2. **Diabetes Mellitus in Periodontal Patients**
   A. **Need for Additional Research.** It is clear that additional research into the connection between diabetes and periodontal disease will indeed impact the practice of dental hygiene.
      1. As discussed in other chapters of this book, research has demonstrated that patients with poorly controlled diabetes have an increased risk for periodontitis (17–22).
      2. Since periodontitis is a type of infection, and since diabetes can lower the body's resistance to infections in general, it is not surprising that there is a connection between poorly controlled diabetes and periodontitis in some patients.
      3. In addition, research suggests that periodontal infection and the elimination of the periodontal infection through proper periodontal therapy have the potential for altering the body's control of blood sugar levels.
      4. It has even been suggested that thorough treatment of periodontitis in a diabetic patient may make it easier for a patient's physician to control the diabetes (23).

Box 35-1. Examples of Systemic Diseases or Conditions that may have a Connection to Periodontitis

- Bacterial endocarditis
- Cardiovascular disease
- Diabetes mellitus
- Adverse pregnancy outcomes
- Pulmonary disease
- Osteoporosis
- Smoking
- Rheumatoid arthritis

B. **Research Questions.** There are many research questions that need to be answered related to the periodontitis/diabetes connection, but a few of those questions that can have a direct impact on the practice of dental hygiene are outlined below.
  1. Are the measures used to prevent or control periodontitis in the patient without diabetes mellitus adequate for the patient with diabetes mellitus?
  2. Since wound healing appears altered in patients with diabetes, are there adjustments clinicians need to make when delivering dental hygiene therapy to maximize the potential for healing in these patients?
  3. What precise periodontal maintenance protocols are the most effective for patients with diabetes?
  4. When a dental hygienist treats a patient with diabetes, what communication protocols can be most effective in insuring that the patient's physician is aware of the patient's periodontal status, so that adjustments in the therapy for diabetes can be made where needed?

C. **Use of Intensive Therapies for Diabetes Mellitus.** In examining the periodontitis/diabetes connection there is another line of inquiry that will also affect dental hygiene practice—the type of medical therapy used in diabetic patients (24).
  1. In medicine there have been dramatic improvements in the treatment regimens for patients with diabetes, and these regimens now frequently include intensive treatment with oral agents and with insulin.
  2. Unfortunately, some of these medical treatments have increased the risk for medical emergencies (such as hypoglycemia) during dental office treatment of a patient with diabetes.
  3. This medical trend in intensive therapies for patients with diabetes will continue.
  4. As physicians use more intensive therapies to manage patients with diabetes, the dental hygienist of the future will need to have more knowledge about these therapies, about how to manage these patients in a dental setting, and about how to respond when a medical emergency arises.

Section 3
Protocols for Maintaining Dental Implants

1. **State of Dental Implantology.** In modern dentistry dental implants are a viable option as one alternative for replacing most missing teeth. It should be noted that dental implants available today have a remarkable success rate. Even though dental implantology has been intensively studied for several decades, there are still many unanswered questions related to this field, and research will continue.
2. **Research Questions Related to Maintenance of Dental Implants.** Much additional investigation is needed in the area of dental implantology, and some examples of questions related to dental hygiene that are in need of further study are listed below. Answering these types of questions with appropriate scientific investigation is quite likely to have a substantial impact on clinical care delivered by the dental hygienist.
  A. What self-care measures can best prevent peri-implant infections?
  B. What are the most effective protocols for effective maintenance of implants?
  C. Should clinicians recommend the same techniques for minimizing the bacterial challenge to an implant that apply to a natural tooth?
  D. When treating dental implants patients what types of instruments provide the greatest chance of maintaining periodontal health?

Section 4
Treatment Modalities in Periodontal Care

Treatment modalities for patients with periodontal diseases are constantly evolving. This section suggestions some of these modalities that can be expected to enhance more effective periodontal therapy as they evolve further.

1. Lasers in Periodontal Care
   A. Lasers have been widely used in many fields of medicine since the early 1960s. Lasers produce a narrow beam of light with a single wavelength that can produce intense energy at precise locations.
      1. In dentistry these intense light beams can be passed down narrow optical tubing and can be focused on a small area of tissue within the mouth and within the periodontium.
      2. Some laser beams are so intense that they can actually be used to remove oral soft tissue or to cut tissues in the mouth.
      3. There are different types of lasers that have been studied for use in dentistry, and each type has a somewhat different effect on soft tissue, enamel, dentin, pulp, and bone.
   B. Lasers have been suggested for use in dentistry for a variety of dental applications. Some of these devices even have Food and Drug Administration (FDA) safety clearance for some intraoral soft tissue procedures.
      1. More study is needed, however, to clarify how these devices can be used appropriately in subgingival applications in patients with periodontal diseases and some of these studies are in progress (25,26).
      2. Some investigations have suggested a possible use for these devices as part of periodontal therapies such as instrumentation of root surfaces.
      3. Additional research will clarify appropriate uses for these devices in patients with periodontal diseases and may impact some of the therapy provided by dental hygienists for patients with periodontitis.
      4. If further study of these devices confirms that patients with periodontal diseases do benefit from their use, they may one day be a routine part of the care of patients with periodontitis and perhaps even a part of the practice of dental hygiene.
   C. *An American Academy of Periodontology statement on the efficiency of lasers in the nonsurgical treatment of inflammatory periodontal disease (27) states that there is minimal evidence to support use of a laser for the purpose of subgingival periodontal instrumentation, either as a monotherapy or adjunctive to SRP.*
2. Genetic Technology in Periodontal Care
   A. Clinicians have known for a long time that there are many factors that can increase the risk of developing periodontitis.
      1. One factor that is known to increase the risk of developing periodontitis is failure to control bacterial plaque growth on the teeth, thereby increasing the bacterial challenge to the periodontium.
      2. Scientific studies also indicate that certain genetic factors determine how an individual patient's host defenses actually react to an increased bacterial challenge.
      3. Based upon the current research literature available, it now appears that a key factor in determining whether a patient develops periodontitis in response to the bacterial challenge is how the body reacts to that bacterial challenge.
      4. One major determinant of how the body reacts to the bacterial challenge is genetics (or inherited characteristics).

B. Much more study into the genetic factors that increase the risk for periodontitis is needed, but it is already possible to use some types of genetic information to guide clinical decision-making in a small group of selected patients.

   1. Genetic testing can identify patients carrying gene mutations for several rare syndromes that are often accompanied by a form of periodontal disease.

   2. In addition to identifying patients with rare syndromes, there is already a commercially available genetic susceptibility test for severe chronic periodontitis.

   3. In this test specific gene polymorphisms (forms) that have been associated with the development of periodontitis can be detected.

   4. Ongoing scientific investigations will undoubtedly clarify how such genetic testing can be used in periodontitis patient management.

C. As more and more scientific information about identifying genetic control of host defenses becomes available, it is quite likely that this information will impact how we manage patients with periodontal diseases and will impact the practice of dental hygiene.

3. **Local Delivery Mechanisms in Periodontal Care**

A. As already discussed in other chapters of this book, research has demonstrated that using local delivery mechanisms for antimicrobial chemicals in patients with periodontitis has a small but measurable impact upon clinical parameters such as attachment levels (28). Reported analyses of the long-term effects of chemotherapeutic agents usually do not extend beyond a few months to a year. Nonsurgical periodontal instrumentation remains the gold standard for the treatment of inflammatory periodontitis (26).

B. There are several areas of research investigation that are needed related to these local delivery mechanisms, and some examples of research questions about this topic that need to be answered are listed below.

   1. Can local delivery mechanisms be designed that have a greater clinical impact than those currently available for clinical use?

   2. What specific local delivery treatment protocols should be followed to produce the most benefit for individual patients?

   3. Are there additional antimicrobial agents that can be delivered safely using the local delivery concept?

   4. Can other therapy provided by the dental hygienist be enhanced by using some of these local delivery mechanisms?

C. Research into the modification of polymers, manufacturing technologies, and carrier systems will undoubtedly lead to vastly improved drug delivery systems that may have an impact on periodontal therapy strategies.

D. Research into the use of local delivery mechanisms for antimicrobial agents continues. It is probable that as this modality improves in clinical effectiveness, using local delivery mechanisms may become more and more useful in the care of the periodontal patient by the dental hygienist.

4. **Host Modulation Therapies in Periodontal Care**

A. As already discussed, research has demonstrated that host defenses can play a significant role in the actual development of attachment loss and alveolar bone loss in patients with periodontitis.

   1. A variety of host modulation therapies have been investigated that could be used as adjunctive (supplemental) treatment in patients with periodontitis (29–31).

   2. Host modulation therapies usually involve using medications that can alter biochemical pathways in a manner that will (1) slow attachment loss, (2) slow alveolar bone loss, or (3) decrease inflammation.

B. Investigations into possible host modulation therapies have already resulted in one commercially available medication (low-dose doxycycline hyclate) that can be used as adjunctive treatment in patients with chronic periodontitis.

1. This medication can be used to lower levels of collagenase, an enzyme involved in the destruction of collagen.

2. Collagen is one of the components of many of the structures that make up the periodontium, and lowering the levels of collagenase can slow the progress of periodontitis.

3. Investigations are ongoing into a number of other possible host modulation therapies that include studies into (1) modulation of cytokines (chemicals involved in periodontitis that can result in increased periodontal disease progression), (2) reduction of prostaglandins (chemicals that enhance inflammation in the gingiva and in the periodontium), and (3) slowing alveolar bone loss with chemical agents.

C. In addition, an interesting future direction for research will include local delivery systems that can deliver varied concentrations of chemicals. Variable concentrations could be used to achieve the maximum therapeutic effects when planning individualized nonsurgical treatment for patients with periodontal disease.

D. As further scientific investigations improve our understanding of host modulation therapies in the management of patients with periodontitis there are likely to be a variety of new therapeutic options for members of the dental team to use in patient management.

5. **Disease Risk Assessment in Periodontal Care**

A. Recently there has been increased interest in identifying clinical tools that can be used to quantify a patient's risk for developing periodontitis (32–34).

1. Traditionally clinicians have assessed the risk of developing periodontitis subjectively, but studies have shown that subjective risk assessment is surprisingly variable even among clinicians who are experts (34).

2. Objective periodontal disease risk assessment tools would be quite useful to members of the dental team if they provided a method of risk assessment that could accurately predict which patients are most likely to develop periodontitis.

3. Examples of risk factors that have been suggested to be predictive of periodontal disease activity are listed in Box 35-2.

4. Using risk assessment tools to identify the patients with the highest risk for developing periodontitis would allow members of the dental team to provide more aggressive treatment for those patients.

5. In addition, these tools might identify which patients with periodontal diseases should be referred to a specialist early in their treatment and which patients can best be managed in a general dental setting.

Box 35-2. Examples of Factors that may Help Predict Periodontal Disease Activity

- Smoking
- Poorly controlled diabetes
- Poor patient self-care
- Severity of alveolar bone loss
- Positive family history
- Presence of pocket depths >6 mm
- Age
- Gender
- Gingival bleeding
- Number of missing teeth
- Presence of periodontal pathogens

B. Studies have already been published that document that some of these risk assessment tools are predictors of alveolar bone loss and loss of periodontally affected teeth.

1. It is likely that some of these tools for quantifying a patient's risk will soon be in widespread use in dental offices.

2. Guidelines from the American Academy of Periodontology indicate that periodontal disease risk assessment should be part of every comprehensive dental and periodontal evaluation.

3. The American Academy of Periodontology has even developed a simplified form of risk assessment for use by patients. This web-based patient self-assessment can be viewed at www.perio.org.

4. These risk assessment tools would be useful to the dental hygienist and the dentist in planning therapy and in identifying patients in need of immediate referral.

6. Advances in Stem Cell Biology

A. Stem cell biology is an emerging field of medical research that can have a profound effect on medical therapy available for certain systemic diseases and that may have utility in regeneration of periodontal tissues in the future (35–40).

B. Human stem cells have already been isolated from the periodontal ligament, dental pulp tissue, exfoliated deciduous teeth, dental papillae, and dental follicles.

C. Dental stem cells apparently can differentiate into specific components of the periodontium (such as periodontal ligament and cementum).

D. As understanding of the biology of these stem cells develops, their use in periodontal regeneration has the potential to influence periodontal treatment strategies.

Chapter Summary Statement

Dental hygienists should expect many changes to take place in recommendations for the management of patients with periodontal diseases as study of these diseases continues. This chapter presented a brief overview of a few of the possibilities for future directions in the management of patients with periodontal diseases by dental hygienists.

References

1. Mullally BH, Linden GJ. Comparative reproducibility of proximal probing depth using electronic pressure-controlled and hand probing. *J Clin Periodontol*. 1994;21(4):284–288.
2. Tupta-Veselicky L, Famili P, Ceravolo FJ, et al. A clinical study of an electronic constant force periodontal probe. *J Periodontol*. 1994;65(6):616–622.
3. Wang SF, Leknes KN, Zimmerman GJ, et al. Reproducibility of periodontal probing using a conventional manual and an automated force-controlled electronic probe. *J Periodontol*. 1995;66(1):38–46.
4. Armitage GC; Research, Science Therapy Committee of the American Academy of Periodontology. Diagnosis of periodontal diseases. *J Periodontol*. 2003;74(8):1237–1247.
5. Eickholz P, Kim TS, Benn DK, et al. Validity of radiographic measurement of interproximal bone loss. *Oral Surg Oral Med Oral Pathol Oral Radiol Endod*. 1998;85(1):99–106.
6. Jeffcoat MK, Reddy MS. Digital subtraction radiography for longitudinal assessment of peri-implant bone change: method and validation. *Adv Dent Res*. 1993;7(2):196–201.
7. Jeffcoat MK, Wang IC, Reddy MS. Radiographic diagnosis in periodontics. *Periodontol 2000*. 1995;7:54–68.
8. Parameter on systemic conditions affected by periodontal diseases. American Academy of Periodontology. *J Periodontol*. 2000;71(5 suppl):880–883.
9. El-Shinnawi U, Soory M. Associations between periodontitis and systemic inflammatory diseases: response to treatment. *Recent Pat Endocr Metab Immune Drug Discov*. 2013;7(3):169–188.
10. Gulati M, Anand V, Jain N, et al. Essentials of periodontal medicine in preventive medicine. *Int J Prev Med*. 2013;4(9):988–994.
11. Gurav AN. The association of periodontitis and metabolic syndrome. *Den Res J*. 2014;11(1):1–10.
12. Huck O, Tenenbaum H, Davideau JL. Relationship between periodontal diseases and preterm birth: recent epidemiological and biological data. *J Pregnancy*. 2011;2011:164654.
13. Jeffcoat MK. Osteoporosis: a possible modifying factor in oral bone loss. *Ann Periodontol*. 1998;3(1):312–321.
14. Otomo-Corgel J, Pucher JJ, Rethman MP, et al. State of the science: chronic periodontitis and systemic health. *J Evid Based Dent Pract*. 2012;12(3 suppl):20–28.
15. Shangase SL, Mohangi GU, Hassam-Essa S, et al. The association between periodontitis and systemic health: an overview. *SADJ*. 2013;68(1):8, 10–12.

16. Zhu M, Nikolajczyk BS. Immune cells link obesity-associated type 2 diabetes and periodontitis. *J Dent Res.* 2014;93(4): 346–352.
17. Gurav AN. Advanced glycation end products: a link between periodontitis and diabetes mellitus? *Curr Diabetes Rev.* 2013;9(5):355–361.
18. Leite RS, Marlow NM, Fernandes JK. Oral health and type 2 diabetes. *Am J Med Sci.* 2013;345(4):271–273.
19. Löe H. Periodontal disease. The sixth complication of diabetes mellitus. *Diabetes Care.* 1993;16(1):329–334.
20. Mealey BL, Oates TW; American Academy of Periodontology. Diabetes mellitus and periodontal diseases. *J Periodontol.* 2006;77(8):1289–1303.
21. Pradhan S, Goel K. Interrelationship between diabetes and periodontitis: a review. *JNMA.* 2011;51(183):144–153.
22. Taylor GW. Bidirectional interrelationships between diabetes and periodontal diseases: an epidemiologic perspective. *Ann Periodontol.* 2001;6(1):99–112.
23. Bascones-Martinez A, Matesanz-Perez P, Escribano-Bermejo M, et al. Periodontal disease and diabetes-Review of the Literature. *Med Oral Patol Oral Cir Bucal.* 2011;16(6):e722–e729.
24. Mealey BL. Periodontal implications: medically compromised patients. *Ann Periodontol.* 1996;1(1):256–321.
25. Cobb CM. Lasers in periodontics: a review of the literature. *J Periodontol.* 2006;77(4):545–564.
26. Drisko CL. Periodontal debridement: still the treatment of choice. *J Evid Based Dent Pract.* 2014;(14 suppl):33–41 e1.
27. American Academy of Periodontology statement on the efficacy of lasers in the non-surgical treatment of inflammatory periodontal disease. *J Periodontol.* 2011;82(4):513–514.
28. Gottumukkala SN, Sudarshan S, Mantena SR. Comparative evaluation of the efficacy of two controlled release devices: chlorhexidine chips and indigenous curcumin based collagen as local drug delivery systems. *Contemp Clin Dent.* 2014;5(2):175–181.
29. Bhatavadekar NB, Williams RC. New directions in host modulation for the management of periodontal disease. *J Clin Periodontol.* 2009;36(2):124–126.
30. Gokhale SR, Padhye AM. Future prospects of systemic host modulatory agents in periodontal therapy. *Br Dent J.* 2013;214(9):467–471.
31. Oringer RJ, Research Science Therapy Committee of the American Academy of Periodontology. Modulation of the host response in periodontal therapy. *J Periodontol.* 2002;73(4):460–470.
32. American Academy of P. American Academy of Periodontology statement on risk assessment. *J Periodontol.* 2008;79(2):202.
33. Page RC, Martin J, Krall EA, et al. Longitudinal validation of a risk calculator for periodontal disease. *J Clin Periodontol.* 2003;30(9):819–827.
34. Persson GR, Mancl LA, Martin J, et al. Assessing periodontal disease risk: a comparison of clinicians' assessment versus a computerized tool. *J Am Dent Assoc.* 2003;134(5):575–582.
35. Fawzy El-Sayed KM, Dorfer C, Fandrich F, et al. Adult mesenchymal stem cells explored in the dental field. *Adv Biochem Eng Biotechnol.* 2013;130:89–103.
36. Feng R, Lengner C. Application of stem cell technology in dental regenerative medicine. *Adv Wound Care.* 2013;2(6):296–305.
37. Han J, Menicanin D, Gronthos S, et al. Stem cells, tissue engineering and periodontal regeneration. *Aust Dent J.* 2014;59(suppl 1):117–130.
38. Hynes K, Menicanin D, Gronthos S, et al. Clinical utility of stem cells for periodontal regeneration. *Periodontol 2000.* 2012;59(1):203–227.
39. Research Science Therapy Committee of American Academy of P. Informational paper: implications of genetic technology for the management of periodontal diseases. *J Periodontol.* 2005;76(5):850–857.
40. Ulmer FL, Winkel A, Kohorst P, et al. Stem cells–prospects in dentistry. *Schweiz Monatsschr Zahnmed.* 2010;120(10):860–883.

 ## STUDENT ANCILLARY RESOURCES

A wide variety of resources to enhance your learning and understanding of this chapter are available on thePoint®.

- Visit thePoint to access:
  - Audio Glossary
  - Animations
  - Suggested Readings
  - Answers to Review Questions
  - Case Studies

36

Comprehensive Patient Cases

Learning Objective

- Apply the content from the chapters in this book to the decision-making questions for Fictitious Patient Cases 1, 2, 3, 4, and 5.

Section 1
Fictitious Patient Case 1: Mr. Karn

PATIENT PROFILE

Mr. Karn is a 47-year-old high school administrator who has recently moved to your city. He came to the dental office because he would like to know if it is possible to replace his missing upper right first molar tooth with a dental implant.

During Mr. Karn's first office visit, he informs you that he has been too busy lately to get a dental checkup and that he has not seen a dentist for quite a few years. Mr. Karn states that he brushes his teeth twice daily when he has time and that he does not floss regularly even though he knows that he should. He also uses an over-the-counter mouth rinse occasionally.

PATIENT HEALTH HISTORY

- On the day of his first visit to your dental office Mr. Karn's blood pressure is 130/80 mm Hg and his pulse is 62 beats per minute.
- A review of Mr. Karn's health history reveals that he takes two medications: Zocor and Nifedipine.
- Mr. Karn also states that he smokes between one-half and one pack of cigarettes each day.

CLINICAL PHOTOGRAPHS FOR MR. KARN

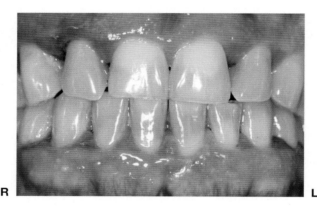

R   L

Figure 36-1. Anterior Teeth, Facial View.

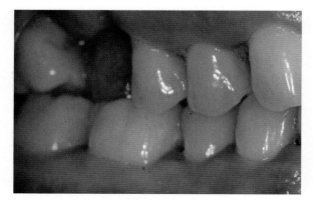

Figure 36-2. Right Side, Facial View.

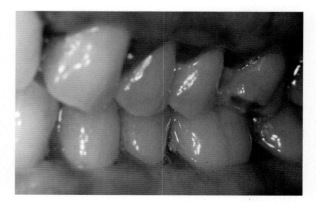

Figure 36-3. Left Side, Facial View.

CLINICAL PHOTOGRAPHS FOR MR. KARN

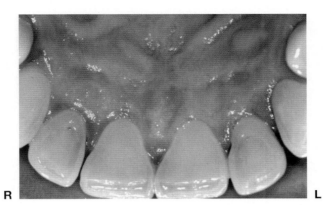

Figure 36-4. Maxillary Anterior, Lingual View.

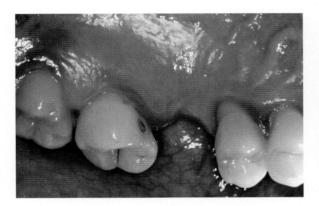

Figure 36-5. Maxillary Right, Lingual View.

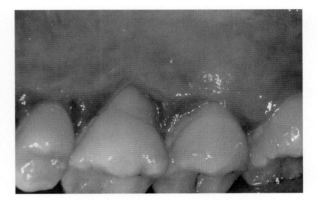

Figure 36-6. Maxillary Left, Lingual View.

CLINICAL PHOTOGRAPHS FOR MR. KARN

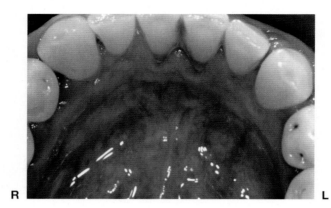

R   L

Figure 36-7. Mandibular Anterior, Lingual View.

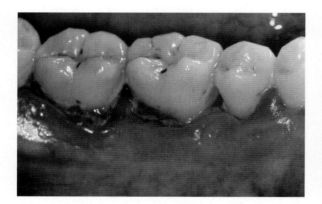

Figure 36-8. Mandibular Right, Lingual View.

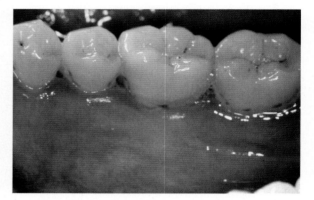

Figure 36-9. Mandibular Left, Lingual View.

CASE #1

Maxilla

1	2	3	4	5	6	7	8	9	10	11	12	13	14	15	16	
					I	I						I			I	Mobility (I, II, III)
+	+		+	+	+	+			+	+	+	+	+	+	+	Bleeding/Purulence (+)
646	647		535	536	415	322	322	334	425	435	536	626	638	846	746	Attachment Level (CEJ to BP)
646	635		325	536	525	435	433	334	425	435	536	626	638	846	746	Probing Depth (FGM to BP)

Facial

Palatal

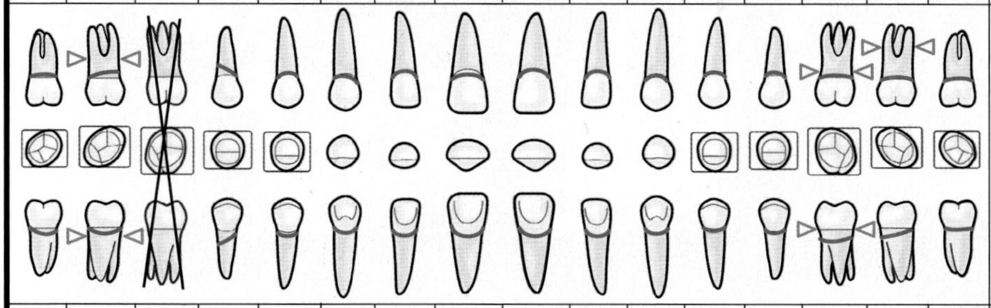

1	2	3	4	5	6	7	8	9	10	11	12	13	14	15	16	
+	+		+	+	+	+	+	+	+	+	+	+	+	+	+	Bleeding/Purulence (+)
646	646		546	526	536	425	443	324	424	525	535	626	859	937	736	Attachment Level (CEJ to BP)
636	525		335	526	536	425	443	324	424	525	535	626	627	827	736	Probing Depth (FGM to BP)
																ᶠ/ₚPlaque
	✓		✓	✓				✓	✓				✓	✓	✓	Supragingival Calculus
✓	✓		✓	✓	✓	✓	✓	✓	✓	✓	✓	✓	✓	✓	✓	Subgingival Calculus

PSR Code		
4	3	4

Right   *Left*

Mandible

32	31	30	29	28	27	26	25	24	23	22	21	20	19	18	17	
		I				I	I									Mobility (I, II, III)
+		+	+	+	+	+		+		+	+	+		+	+	Bleeding/Purulence (+)
546	746	736	635	435	534	324	534	434	324	324	434	435	536	746	635	Attachment Level (CEJ to BP)
546	736	626	635	535	534	324	423	323	324	324	434	435	536	746	635	Probing Depth (FGM to BP)

Lingual

Facial

32	31	30	29	28	27	26	25	24	23	22	21	20	19	18	17	
+	+	+	+	+		+	+	+		+		+		+	+	Bleeding/Purulence (+)
546	736	625	535	635	534	324	423	323	324	324	434	435	526	736	625	Attachment Level (CEJ to BP)
546	736	625	535	635	534	324	423	323	324	324	434	435	526	736	625	Probing Depth (FGM to BP)
																ᴸ/ꜰPlaque
					✓	✓	✓	✓	✓			✓	✓			Supragingival Calculus
✓	✓	✓	✓	✓	✓	✓	✓	✓	✓	✓	✓	✓	✓	✓	✓	Subgingival Calculus

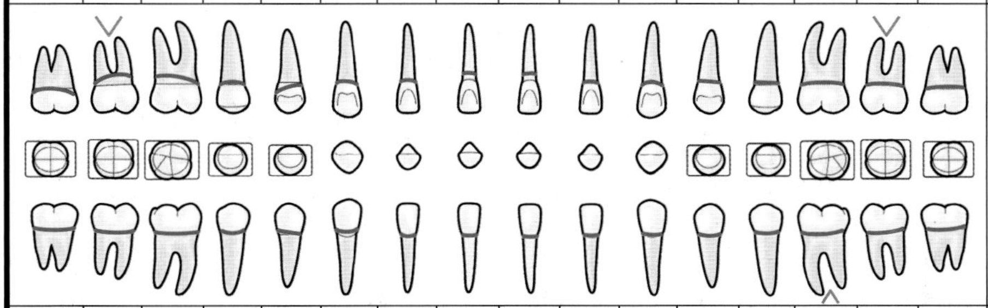

PSR Code		
4	3	4

Figure 36-10. Mr. Karn's Periodontal Chart.

RADIOGRAPHIC SERIES FOR MR. KARN

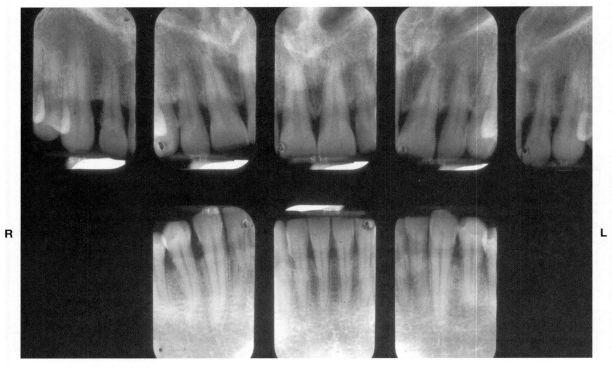

Figure 36-11A: Radiographs: Anterior Teeth.

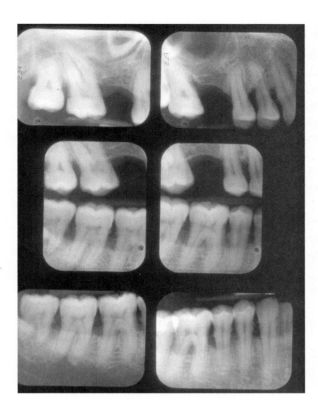

Figure 36-11B: Radiographs: Right Posterior Teeth.

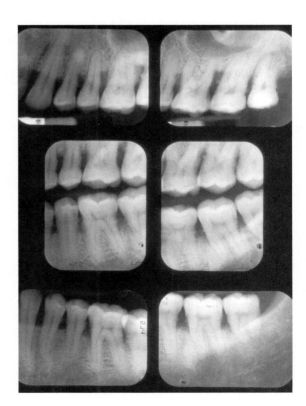

Figure 36-11C: Radiographs: Left Posterior Teeth.

DECISION-MAKING QUESTIONS FOR CASE 1: MR. KARN

1. What should Mr. Karn be told about the possibility of replacing his maxillary right first molar tooth with a dental implant? Note that this question was what prompted Mr. Karn to make an appointment in your dental office.
2. What factors in Mr. Karn's profile indicate that achieving an acceptable level of patient self-care may be a problem for the dental team?
3. What factors revealed in Mr. Karn's health history will be critical for the dental team to consider during treatment?
4. What signs of gingival inflammation are evident in Mr. Karn's clinical photographs?
5. What etiologic risk factors for gingival and periodontal diseases are evident in Mr. Karn's clinical photographs?
6. How might the presence of the furcation involvements found during Mr. Karn's periodontal evaluation affect his periodontal treatment?
7. Does Mr. Karn's periodontal evaluation indicate that he has attachment loss present on some teeth?
8. What etiologic factors for gingival and periodontal diseases are evident in Mr. Karn's dental radiographs?
9. On Mr. Karn's radiographs what specific findings indicate that he has alveolar bone loss present?
10. How would you characterize Mr. Karn's periodontal condition? Do you think that he has gingivitis, periodontitis, neither, or both? What clinical or radiographic findings did you use to reach your conclusion?
11. Develop a suggested step-by-step plan for nonsurgical periodontal therapy for Mr. Karn.
12. What information should your team give Mr. Karn about his periodontal condition?
13. What should Mr. Karn be told about the possible need for periodontal surgery later in the treatment?
14. What should Mr. Karn be told about the need for continuing treatment such as periodontal maintenance?

Section 2
Fictitious Patient Case 2: Mr. Wilton

PATIENT PROFILE

Mr. Wilton is a 52-year-old manager of a local gardening store who has come to your dental office for an initial visit. During his patient interview, Mr. Wilton informs you that he made this appointment at his wife's insistence. He states that his wife wants to know if there is anything that can be done about his bad breath. Mr. Wilton informs you that he cannot seem to get his bad breath under control using mouth rinses.

PATIENT HEALTH HISTORY

- At the time of his initial visit, Mr. Wilton's blood pressure is 164/100 mm Hg and his pulse rate is 74 beats per minute.
- Mr. Wilton informs you that he is taking Amoxicillin prescribed by his physician for an ear infection.
- Mr. Wilton tells you that he had high blood pressure once and that he did take a prescribed medication a few years ago for that condition. He tells you that he was feeling just fine, so he stopped taking the prescribed blood pressure medication.

CLINICAL PHOTOGRAPHS FOR MR. WILTON

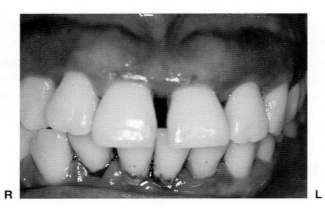

Figure 36-12. Anterior Teeth, Facial View.

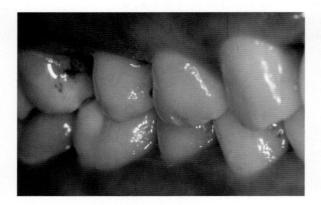

Figure 36-13. Right Side, Facial View.

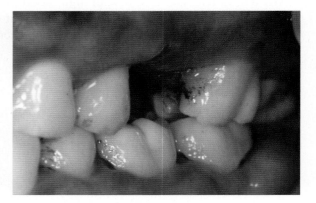

Figure 36-14. Left Side, Facial View.

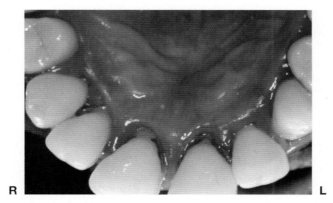

Figure 36-15. Maxillary Anteriors, Lingual View.

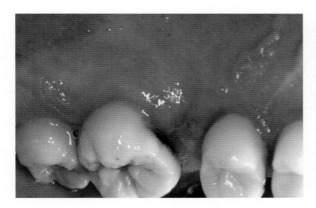

Figure 36-16. Maxillary Right, Lingual View.

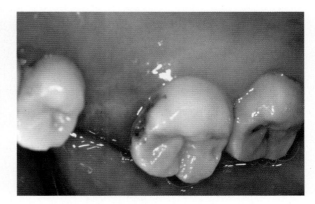

Figure 36-17. Maxillary Left, Lingual View.

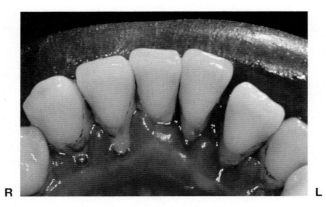

Figure 36-18. Mandibular Anteriors, Lingual View.

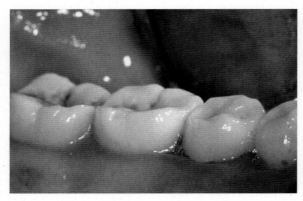

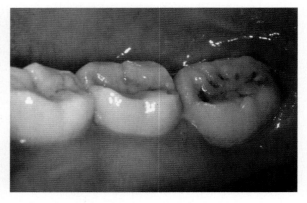

AU2

Figure 36-19. Mandibular Right, Lingual View.

Figure 36-20. Mandibular Left, Lingual View.

CASE #2

Maxilla

	1	2	3	4	5	6	7	8	9	10	11	12	13	14	15	16	
Mobility (I, II, III)				I			I	I	II	I		I					
Bleeding/Purulence (+)	+	+			+		+	+	+		+	+	+		+	+	
Attachment Level (CEJ to BP)	635	634		338	535	537	626	736	537	625	536	725	524		435	535	
Probing Depth (FGM to BP)	635	634		338	535	537	626	625	537	625	536	725	524		435	535	

Facial / Palatal tooth diagrams

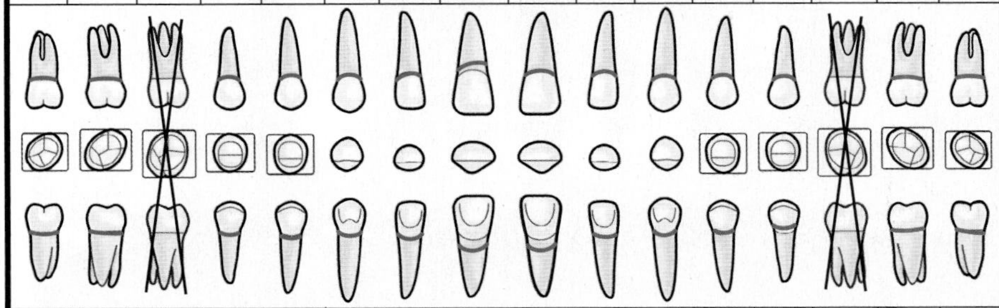

	1	2	3	4	5	6	7	8	9	10	11	12	13	14	15	16	
Bleeding/Purulence (+)	+	+		+	+	+		+	+		+	+	+		+		
Attachment Level (CEJ to BP)	535	634		438	534	636	536	646	746	535	536	726	423		426	535	
Probing Depth (FGM to BP)	535	634		438	534	636	536	535	635	535	536	726	534		426	535	
Plaque (F/P)																	
Supragingival Calculus				✓	✓	✓	✓	✓	✓		✓		✓	✓			
Subgingival Calculus	✓	✓		✓	✓	✓	✓	✓	✓	✓	✓	✓	✓		✓	✓	
PSR Code			4					4						4			

Right   Left

Mandible

	32	31	30	29	28	27	26	25	24	23	22	21	20	19	18	17	
Mobility (I, II, III)				I			II	II	II	II							
Bleeding/Purulence (+)		+	+	+		+	+	+	+	+	+	+	+	+		+	
Attachment Level (CEJ to BP)		435	536	545	524	535	746	656	647	748	635	524	535	535	636	645	
Probing Depth (FGM to BP)		535	536	545	524	535	635	545	536	637	635	524	535	635	636	635	

Lingual / Facial tooth diagrams

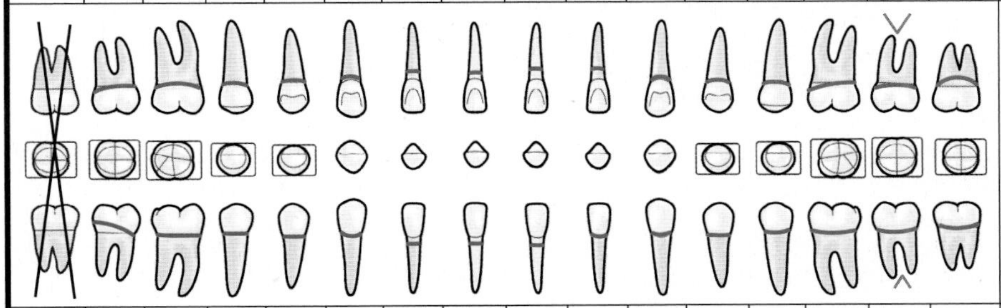

	32	31	30	29	28	27	26	25	24	23	22	21	20	19	18	17	
Bleeding/Purulence (+)		+	+		+	+	+	+	+	+	+	+		+	+	+	
Attachment Level (CEJ to BP)		435	526	535	424	535	735	646	636	536	524	525	425	525	526	625	
Probing Depth (FGM to BP)		535	526	535	424	535	624	535	525	536	524	525	425	525	526	625	
Plaque (L/F)																	
Supragingival Calculus						✓	✓	✓	✓	✓	✓					✓	
Subgingival Calculus		✓	✓	✓	✓	✓	✓	✓	✓	✓	✓	✓	✓	✓	✓	✓	
PSR Code			4					4						4			

Figure 36-21. Mr. Wilton's Periodontal Chart.

RADIOGRAPHIC SERIES FOR MR. WILTON

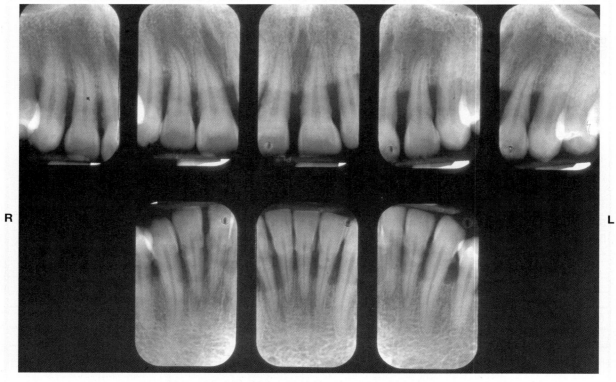

R   L

Figure 36-22A: Radiographs: Anterior Teeth.

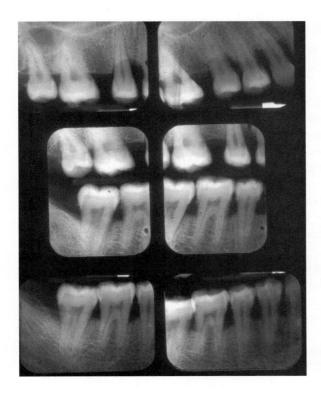

Figure 36-22B: Radiographs: Right Posterior Teeth.

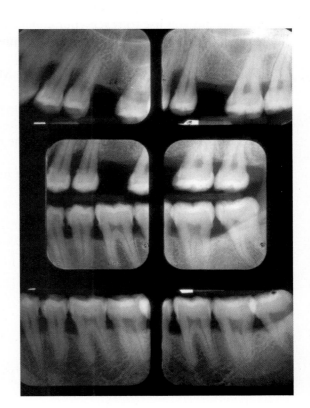

Figure 36-22C: Radiographs: Left Posterior Teeth.

DECISION-MAKING QUESTIONS FOR CASE 2: MR. WILTON

1. What information should your team give Mr. Wilton regarding his wife's concern about his bad breath? Note that this was the complaint that prompted Mr. Wilton to make an appointment in your office.
2. What factors in Mr. Wilton's profile indicate that achieving an acceptable level of patient self-care may be a problem for the dental team?
3. What factors revealed in Mr. Wilton's health history will be critical for the dental team to consider during periodontal evaluation or treatment?
4. What signs of gingival inflammation are evident in Mr. Wilton's clinical photographs?
5. What etiologic risk factors for gingival and periodontal diseases are evident in Mr. Wilton's clinical photographs?
6. Does Mr. Wilton's periodontal evaluation indicate that he has attachment loss present on some teeth?
7. In response to your questions, Mr. Wilton informs you that the spaces between his front teeth were not there a few years ago. What do you think may be causing these spaces between his teeth to appear?
8. What etiologic factors for gingival and periodontal diseases are evident in Mr. Wilton's dental radiographs?
9. On Mr. Wilton's radiographs, what specific findings indicate that he has alveolar bone loss present?
10. How would you characterize Mr. Wilton's periodontal condition? Do you think that he has gingivitis, periodontitis, neither, or both? What clinical or radiographic findings did you use to reach your conclusion?
11. Write a suggested step-by-step plan for nonsurgical periodontal therapy for Mr. Wilton.
12. What information should your team give Mr. Wilton about his periodontal condition?
13. What should Mr. Wilton be told about the possible need for periodontal surgery later in the treatment?
14. What should Mr. Wilton be told about the need for continuing treatment such as periodontal maintenance?
15. What should your team tell Mr. Wilton if he refuses your team's recommendations for periodontal therapy?

Section 3
Fictitious Patient Case 3: Mrs. Sandsky

PATIENT PROFILE

Mrs. Sandsky is a 42-year-old department store manager who has come to your dental office to get her dental condition in order. She states that she has neglected her dental care because she has been taking care of the dental needs of her children for many years, but now she is ready to take care of herself.

She informs your dental team that some years ago she was told that she had a gum disease, but elected not to receive any care for that condition at the time. She states that she brushes and flosses daily now in hopes that these actions can help her keep her teeth.

PATIENT HEALTH HISTORY

- At the time of Mrs. Sandsky's initial dental visit her blood pressure measures 130/83 mm Hg and her pulse is 75 beats per minute.
- She explains that she has problems with gastroesophageal reflux disease and elevated cholesterol level.
- She reports that currently she is taking Omeprazole and Simvastatin prescribed by her physician and that she is also taking multivitamin tablets because she thinks she needs them.
- Mrs. Sandsky informs you that she smoked one pack of cigarettes daily for about 8 years when she was younger, but that she quit smoking 10 years ago and has not smoked since that time.

CLINICAL PHOTOGRAPHS FOR MRS. SANDSKY

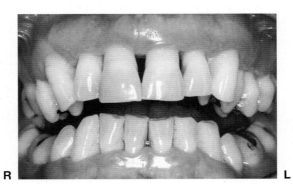

R   L

Figure 36-23. Anterior Teeth, Facial View.

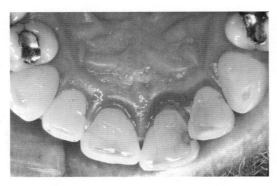

Figure 36-24. Maxillary Anterior Teeth, Lingual View.

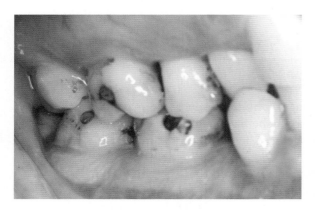

Figure 36-25. Right Side, Facial View.

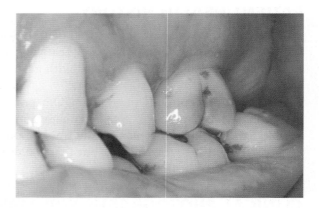

Figure 36-26. Left Side, Facial View.

CASE #3

1	2	3	4	5	6	7	8	9	10	11	12	13	14	15	16	Maxilla
							I	I			I					Mobility (I, II, III)
	+	+	+	+		+	+	+		+	+		+			Bleeding/Purulence (+)
	646	544	535	545	646	656	656	656	756	655	646		545			Attachment Level (CEJ to BP)
	646	545	535	545	535	545	545	545	645	545	635		545			Probing Depth (FGM to BP)

Facial / Palatal

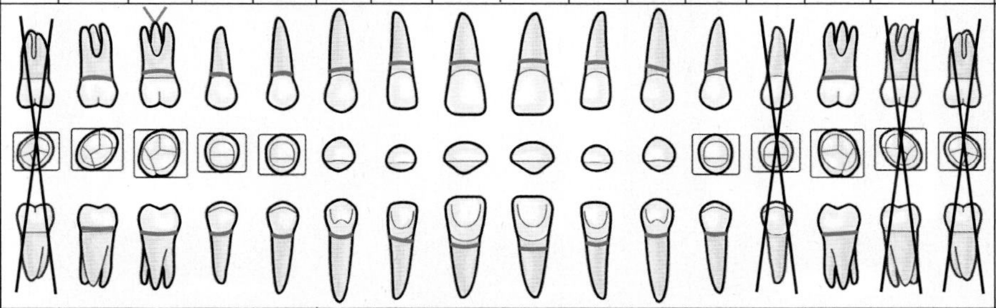

1	2	3	4	5	6	7	8	9	10	11	12	13	14	15	16	
	+	+	+	+	+	+	+	+	+	+	+		+			Bleeding/Purulence (+)
	645	545	543	545	545	645	656	656	666	545	535		545			Attachment Level (CEJ to BP)
	645	545	545	545	545	645	545	545	555	545	535		545			Probing Depth (FGM to BP)
																^F_P Plaque
	✓	✓	✓	✓		✓			✓	✓			✓			Supragingival Calculus
	✓	✓	✓	✓	✓	✓	✓	✓		✓	✓		✓			Subgingival Calculus
																PSR Code

Right   Left

32	31	30	29	28	27	26	25	24	23	22	21	20	19	18	17	Mandible
																Mobility (I, II, III)
	+	+	+	+	+	+	+	+	+	+	+	+	+	+		Bleeding/Purulence (+)
	455	545		545	545	544	444	544	545	543	543	434	545	545		Attachment Level (CEJ to BP)
	455	545		545	545	544	444	544	545	545	434	434	545	545		Probing Depth (FGM to BP)

Lingual / Facial

32	31	30	29	28	27	26	25	24	23	22	21	20	19	18	17	
											I						Bleeding/Purulence (+)
	355	545		545	544	444	444	445	545	545	535	525	545	545		Attachment Level (CEJ to BP)
	455	545		544	544	444	444	445	545	545	535	646	545	545		Probing Depth (FGM to BP)
																^L_F Plaque
	✓	✓		✓	✓	✓	✓	✓	✓	✓	✓	✓	✓	✓		Supragingival Calculus
	✓	✓		✓	✓	✓	✓	✓	✓	✓	✓	✓	✓	✓		Subgingival Calculus
																PSR Code

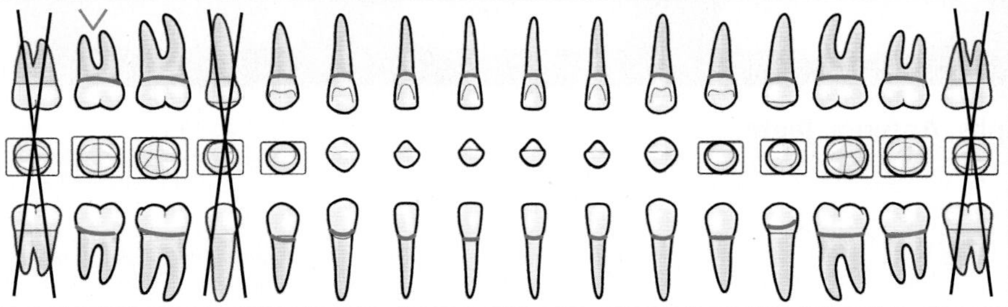

Figure 36-27. Mrs. Sandsky's Periodontal Chart.

RADIOGRAPHIC SERIES FOR MRS. SANDSKY

R

L

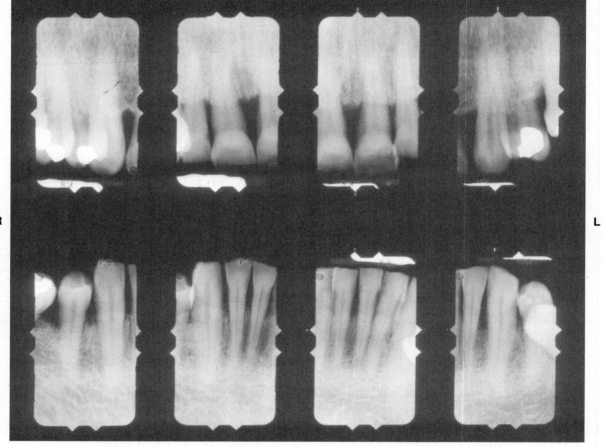

Figure 36-28A: Radiographs: Anterior Teeth.

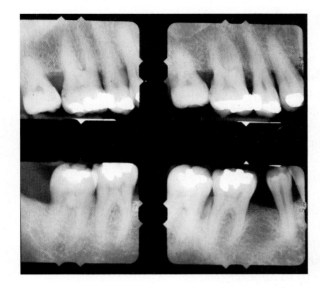

Figure 36-28B: Radiographs: Right Posterior Teeth.

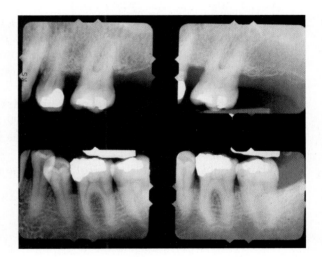

Figure 36-28C: Radiographs: Left Posterior Teeth.

DECISION-MAKING QUESTIONS FOR CASE 3: MRS. SANDSKY

1. What factors in Mrs. Sandsky's profile indicate that achieving an acceptable level of patient self-care may *not* be as difficult for her as it is for many patients?
2. Will the medications being taken by Mrs. Sandsky require any special precautions during treatment by the members of the dental team?
3. How might the history of smoking relate to Mrs. Sandsky's past and current risk for periodontal disease?
4. What signs of gingival inflammation are evident in Mrs. Sandsky's clinical photographs?
5. What etiologic risk factors for gingival and periodontal diseases are evident in Mrs. Sandsky's clinical photographs?
6. Does Mrs. Sandsky's periodontal evaluation indicate that she has attachment loss present on some teeth?
7. In response to your questions, Mrs. Sandsky informs you that the open triangular space between her upper front teeth was not there a few years ago. What do you think may be causing this space between her teeth to appear?
8. What etiologic factors for gingival and periodontal diseases are evident in Mrs. Sandsky's dental radiographs?
9. How would you characterize Mrs. Sandsky's periodontal condition? Do you think that she has gingivitis, periodontitis, neither, or both? What clinical or radiographic findings did you use to reach your conclusion?
10. Develop a suggested step-by-step plan for nonsurgical periodontal therapy for Mrs. Sandsky.
11. What information should your team give Mrs. Sandsky about her periodontal condition?
12. What should Mrs. Sandsky be told about the possible need for periodontal surgery later in the treatment?
13. What should Mrs. Sandsky be told about the need for continuing treatment such as periodontal maintenance?

Section 4
Fictitious Patient Case 4: Mr. Verosky

PATIENT PROFILE

Mr. Verosky is a 62-year-old recently elected to a local city council. He has become very interested in getting his oral health up to par following his election.

   During his initial visit, Mr. Verosky explains that he has always had spaces between his front teeth and is not really worried about that. He tells you that his major concern is that he has been told he has periodontal disease, and he doesn't want to lose his teeth.

PATIENT HEALTH HISTORY

- On the day of his first visit to your dental office Mr. Verosky's blood pressure is 142/90 mm Hg and his pulse is 66 beats per minute.
- Review of Mr. Verosky's health history reveals that he is supposed to be taking two medications: losartan/Hctz tablets and low-dose aspirin, but he readily admits that he frequently "forgets" to take his medications.
- Mr. Verosky also states that he smoked cigarettes prior to the age 40, but that he quit smoking during his early 40s.

CLINICAL PHOTOGRAPHS FOR MR. VEROSKY

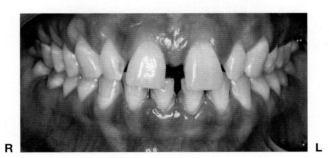

Figure 36-29. **Anterior Teeth, Facial View.**

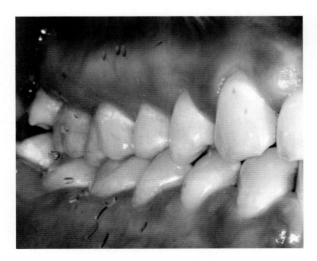

Figure 36-30. **Right Side, Facial View.**

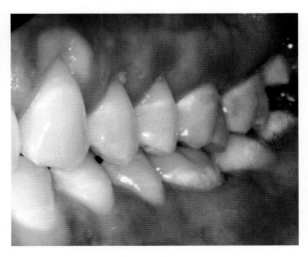

Figure 36-31. **Left Side, Facial View.**

CLINICAL PHOTOGRAPHS FOR MR. VEROSKY

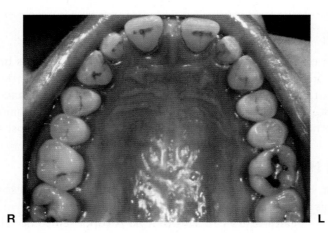

R   L

Figure 36-32. Maxillary Arch, Lingual View.

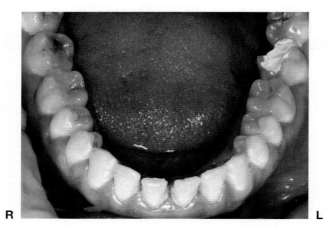

R   L

Figure 36-33. Mandibular Arch.

1	2	3	4	5	6	7	8	9	10	11	12	13	14	15	16	**Maxilla**
		I											I			Mobility (I, II, III)
+	+	+	+	+	+	+	+	+	+	+	+	+	+	+	+	Bleeding/Purulence (+)
336	867	646	241	342	151	242	111	111	233	232	234	313	425	447	544	Attachment Level (CEJ to BP)
558	756	535	322	423	222	323	313	313	324	323	325	424	425	446	655	Probing Depth (FGM to BP)

Facial

Palatal

1	2	3	4	5	6	7	8	9	10	11	12	13	14	15	16	
+	+	+	+	+	+	+	+	+	+	+	+	+	+	+	+	Bleeding/Purulence (+)
233	665	676	212	222	444	222	223	323	222	222	223	312	555	558	410	Attachment Level (CEJ to BP)
555	654	545	323	333	555	333	334	434	333	333	334	423	424	437	633	Probing Depth (FGM to BP)
✕	✕	✕	✕	✕	✕	✕	✕	✕	✕	✕	✕	✕	✕	✕	✕	ᶠ/ₚPlaque
✓	✓	✓											✓	✓	✓	Supragingival Calculus
✓	✓	✓	✓	✓					✓		✓	✓	✓	✓	✓	Subgingival Calculus
			4				3						4			PSR Code

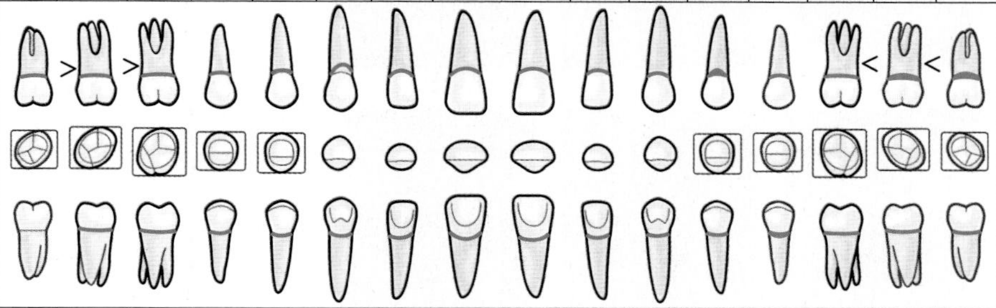

Right   Left

32	31	30	29	28	27	26	25	24	23	22	21	20	19	18	17	**Mandible**
I															I	Mobility (I, II, III)
+	+	+	+	+	+	+	+	+	+	+	+	+	+	+	+	Bleeding/Purulence (+)
336	444	433	333	222	222	222	221	122	331	121	232	244	443	534	434	Attachment Level (CEJ to BP)
547	555	544	434	323	323	323	322	223	422	222	333	345	544	545	655	Probing Depth (FGM to BP)

Lingual

Facial

32	31	30	29	28	27	26	25	24	23	22	21	20	19	18	17	
+	+	+	+	+	+	+	+	+	+	+	+	+	+	+	+	Bleeding/Purulence (+)
344	444	432	222	222	222	232	222	232	222	222	232	232	233	435	423	Attachment Level (CEJ to BP)
555	525	523	323	323	323	333	323	333	323	323	323	323	324	526	533	Probing Depth (FGM to BP)
✕	✕	✕	✕	✕	✕	✕	✕	✕	✕	✕	✕	✕	✕	✕	✕	ᴸ/ꜰPlaque
					✓	✓	✓	✓	✓	✓						Supragingival Calculus
✓	✓	✓	✓		✓	✓	✓	✓	✓	✓	✓		✓	✓	✓	Subgingival Calculus
		3					3						4			PSR Code

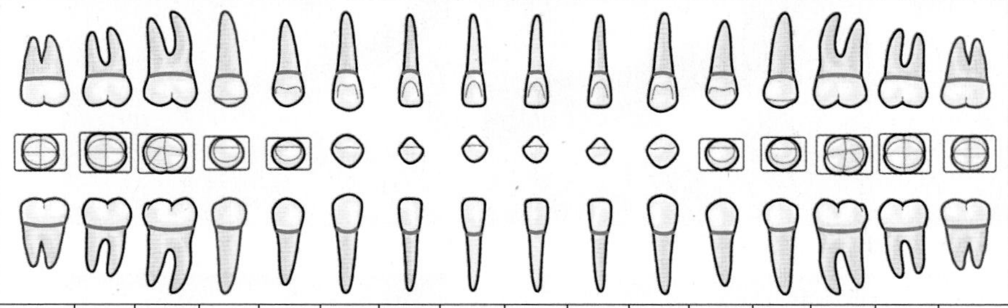

Figure 36-34. **Mr. Verosky's Periodontal Chart.**

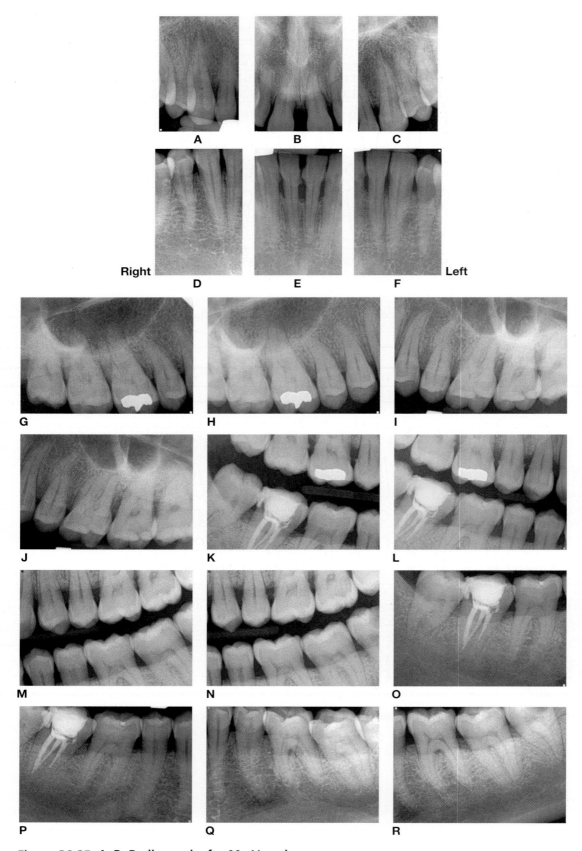

Figure 36-35. A–R: Radiographs for Mr. Verosky.

DECISION-MAKING QUESTIONS FOR CASE 4: MR. VEROSKY

1. What should Mr. Verosky be told about the spaces between his anterior teeth?
2. What factors in Mr. Verosky's health history will be critical for the dental team to consider during treatment?
3. What signs of inflammation are evident in Mr. Verosky's clinical photographs?
4. What etiologic risk factors for gingival and periodontal diseases are evident in Mr. Verosky's clinical evaluation?
5. Does Mr. Verosky's periodontal evaluation indicate that he has attachment loss on some of his teeth? How did you arrive at your conclusion?
6. What etiologic risk factors for gingival and periodontal diseases are evident in Mr. Verosky's radiographs?
7. On Mr. Verosky's radiographs what specific findings indicate that the alveolar bone level is normal or abnormal?
8. How should you characterize Mr. Verosky's periodontal condition? Do you think that he has gingivitis, periodontitis, neither, or both? What clinical or radiographic findings did you use to reach your conclusion?
9. Develop a step-by-step plan for nonsurgical periodontal therapy for Mr. Verosky.
10. What information should your team give Mr. Verosky about his periodontal condition?
11. What should Mr. Verosky be told about the possible need for periodontal surgery later in his treatment?
12. What should Mr. Verosky be told about the need for continuing treatment such as periodontal maintenance?
13. Mr. Verosky has a temporary restoration in a lower molar tooth. What should he be told about this restoration?

Section 5
Fictitious Patient Case 5: Mr. Tomlinson

PATIENT PROFILE

Mr. Tomlinson is a 48-year-old patient who is new to your dental office. He works as a computer technician in a large local firm. This is his first job following an extended tour of military duty.

   During his initial visit, Mr. Tomlinson explains that he has no dental problems, but he decided to make an appointment for a "cleaning" since he has a new dental insurance plan. He tells you that everyone in his family has always had pretty good teeth, so he is certain that you won't find anything wrong with his teeth or with his old fillings.

PATIENT HEALTH HISTORY

- On the day of his first visit to your dental office Mr. Tomlinson's blood pressure is 132/82 mm Hg and his pulse is 64 beats per minute.
- Review of Mr. Tomlinson's health history reveals that he is taking two medications: atorvastatin tablets and fluticasone propionate nasal spray.
- He states that he is currently under treatment for posttraumatic stress disorder (PTSD) that has resulted from his multiple military deployments.

CLINICAL PHOTOGRAPHS FOR MR. TOMLINSON

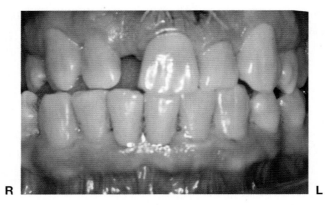

R   L

Figure 36-36. Anterior Teeth, Facial View.

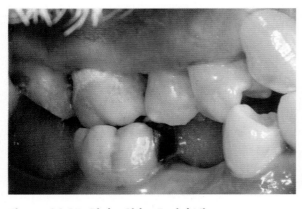

Figure 36-37. Right Side, Facial View.

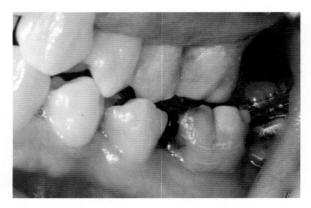

Figure 36-38. Left Side, Facial View.

CLINICAL PHOTOGRAPHS FOR MR. TOMLINSON

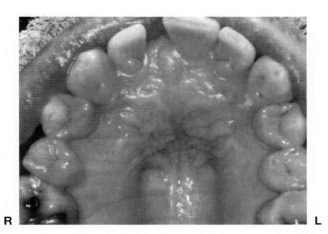

R   L

Figure 36-39. Maxillary Arch, Lingual View.

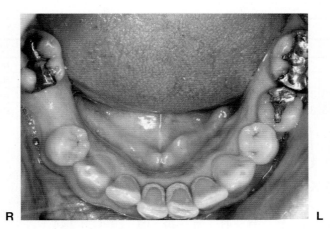

R   L

Figure 36-40. Mandibular Arch.

1	2	3	4	5	6	7	8	9	10	11	12	13	14	15	16	**Maxilla**
													I			Mobility (I, II, III)
	+	+	+	+	+	+				+	+	+	+			Bleeding/Purulence (+)
	546	745	323	312	312	311		112	213	213	424	447	747			Attachment Level (CEJ to BP)
	324	523	323	312	312	311		112	213	213	424	447	747			Probing Depth (FGM to BP)
																Facial
																Palatal
	+		+	+	+	+			+	+	+	+	+			Bleeding/Purulence (+)
	766	654	223	321	113	112		312	122	322	222	222	334			Attachment Level (CEJ to BP)
	513	423	223	321	113	112		312	122	322	222	222	223			Probing Depth (FGM to BP)
																^F_PPlaque
	✓	✓	✓	✓	✓	✓							✓			Supragingival Calculus
	✓	✓	✓	✓	✓	✓				✓	✓	✓	✓			Subgingival Calculus
	4				2					4						PSR Code

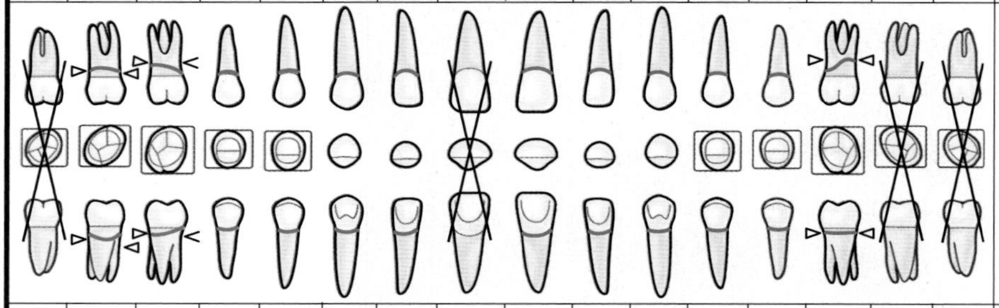

Right   *Left*

32	31	30	29	28	27	26	25	24	23	22	21	20	19	18	17	**Mandible**
																Mobility (I, II, III)
		+		+	+	+	+	+	+	+	+	+	+		+	Bleeding/Purulence (+)
		645		323	323	323	222	223	323	444	323	323	536		556	Attachment Level (CEJ to BP)
		423		323	323	323	222	223	323	333	323	323	424		334	Probing Depth (FGM to BP)
																Lingual
																Facial
		+		+	+	+		+	+	+	+	+	+		+	Bleeding/Purulence (+)
		545		434	423	334	424	224	223	223	212	124	755		334	Attachment Level (CEJ to BP)
		323		324	423	334	424	224	223	223	212	113	533		223	Probing Depth (FGM to BP)
																^L_FPlaque
				✓		✓	✓	✓	✓				✓		✓	Supragingival Calculus
		✓		✓	✓	✓	✓	✓	✓	✓	✓	✓	✓		✓	Subgingival Calculus
		4				3					4					PSR Code

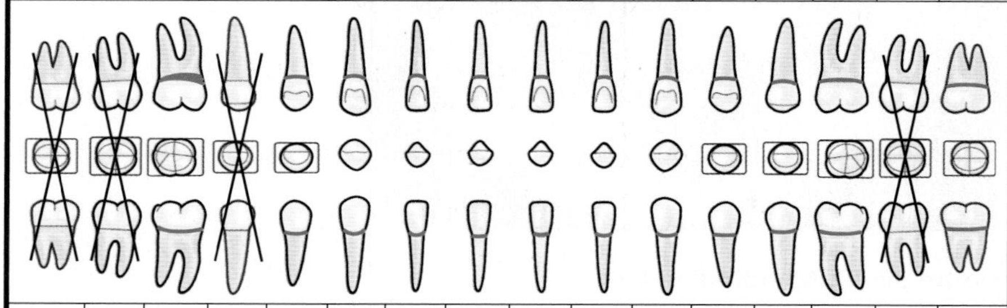

Figure 36-41. Mr. Tomlinson's Periodontal Chart.

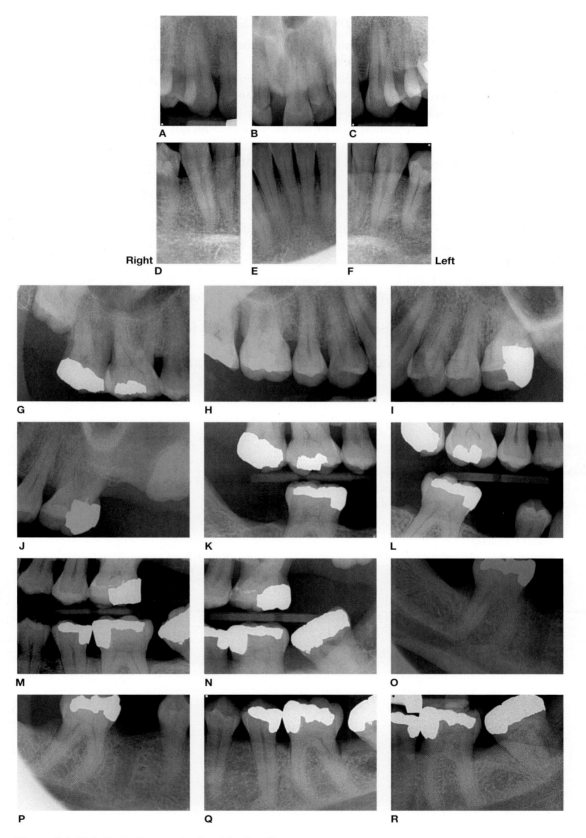

Figure 36-42A–R: Radiographs for Mr. Tomlinson.

DECISION-MAKING QUESTIONS FOR CASE 5: MR. TOMLINSON

1. What factors in Mr. Tomlinson's health history will be critical for the dental team to consider during treatment?
2. What signs of inflammation are evident in Mr. Tomlinson's clinical photographs?
3. What etiologic risk factors for gingival and periodontal diseases are evident in Mr. Tomlinson's clinical evaluation?
4. Does Mr. Tomlinson's periodontal evaluation indicate that he has attachment loss on some of his teeth? How did you arrive at your conclusion?
5. What etiologic risk factors for gingival and periodontal diseases are evident in Mr. Tomlinson's radiographs?
6. On Mr. Tomlinson's radiographs what specific findings indicate that the alveolar bone level is normal or abnormal?
7. How should you characterize Mr. Tomlinson's periodontal condition? Do you think that he has gingivitis, periodontitis, neither, or both? What clinical or radiographic findings did you use to reach your conclusion?
8. Develop a step-by-step plan for nonsurgical periodontal therapy for Mr. Tomlinson.
9. What information should your team give Mr. Tomlinson about his periodontal condition?
10. What should Mr. Tomlinson be told about the possible need for periodontal surgery later in his treatment?
11. What should Mr. Tomlinson be told about the need for continuing treatment such as periodontal maintenance?

 STUDENT ANCILLARY RESOURCES

A wide variety of resources to enhance your learning and understanding of this chapter are available on thePoint®.

- Visit thePoint to access:
  - Audio Glossary
  - Animations
  - Suggested Readings
  - Answers to Review Questions
  - Case Studies

Index

Note: Page numbers in *italics* denote figures; those followed by "t" denote tables and b box respectively.